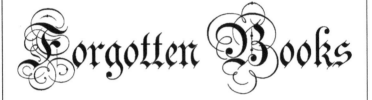

ISBN 978-0-282-86653-2
PIBN 10870548

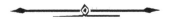

English
Français
Deutsche
Italiano
Español
Português

www.forgottenbooks.com

Mythology Photography **Fiction**
Fishing Christianity **Art** Cooking
Essays Buddhism Freemasonry
Medicine **Biology** Music **Ancient
Egypt** Evolution Carpentry Physics
Dance Geology **Mathematics** Fitness
Shakespeare **Folklore** Yoga Marketing
Confidence Immortality Biographies
Poetry **Psychology** Witchcraft
Electronics Chemistry History **Law**
Accounting **Philosophy** Anthropology
Alchemy Drama Quantum Mechanics
Atheism Sexual Health **Ancient History**
Entrepreneurship Languages Sport
Paleontology Needlework Islam
Metaphysics Investment Archaeology
Parenting Statistics Criminology
Motivational

MANUAL

OF

HOMŒOPATHIC PRACTICE,

FOR THE USE OF

FAMILIES AND PRIVATE INDIVIDUALS.

BY

A. E. SMALL, A. M., M. D.,

Professor of Physiology and Medical Jurisprudence in the Homœopathic Medical College
of Pennsylvania, and late one of the Consulting Physicians of the
Homœopathic Hospital in Philadelphia.

PHILADELPHIA:
PUBLISHED BY RADEMACHER & SHEEK, 239 ARCH STREET.
NEW YORK: WM RADDE.—BOSTON : OTIS CLAPP.
PITTSBURGH : J. G BACKOFEN.—CHICAGO: D. S. SMITH, M. D
NEW ORLEANS: D. R. LUYTIES, M. D.—MANCHESTER, ENG.: H TURNER
1854

KING & BAIRD, PRINTERS, SANSOM STREET, PHILA.

CONTENTS.

1   5

CHAPTER II.

CHAPTER III.

CHAPTER IV.

CHAPTER V.

CHAPTER VII.

1*

CHAPTER XIII.

CASUALTIES.

CHAPTER XV.

DISEASES OF NEW BORN INFANTS AND YOUNG CHILDREN.

CONTENTS.

XV

CHAPTER XVI.

RANGE OF USE OF THE MORE PROMINENT REMEDIES USED IN THIS WORK·

PREFACE.

IN offering to the public the following Manual of Homœopathic Practice, the author is by no means unmindful of the responsibility he has incurred. For more than half a century the science of Homœopathia has been gaining access to the more intelligent and reflecting classes of the community—and did not his convictions assure him of its entire truth and its perfect and satisfactory reliability, he would shudder at the thought of offering such a work as this to a patronizing people; and, moreover, he would lament that others of a like character had preceded this. But, without a shadow of doubt of the truthfulness of Homœopathy, and its adaptation to the wants of mankind, he hesitates not to add something to the stock of popular knowledge upon the subject. The Manual of Homœopathic Practice is herewith offered. It must pass for what it merits. It has been the endeavor of the author to point out, in a systematic way, a useful code of hygienic rules, and an explicit treatment for most of the diseases incident to the human family.

It will be perceived that extensive dietetic rules are laid down for general consideration, while at the conclusion of the given treatment for each malady, the specific diet for the case is noted. It is quite likely errors may be found, in this diet arrangement, when an application is made in particular cases; under such circumstances, any particular idiosyncrasies of the patient must be taken into account, as, for instance: some persons have a particular relish for *cabbage*, while a cracker or other kinds of bread would not be relished at all. When such a patient is sick, the *cabbage* may not be denied, if still craved, as in health. Numerous cases of this kind may be found, all of which will require an extempore prescription of diet to suit the individual, as well as the case.

It will be perceived also that the dose of each remedy is explicitly stated when prescribed. In most cases the medicines are prescribed both in dilutions and globules, and in order to avoid all confusion with regard to the matter, it may be stated that the globules are generally the most convenient and useful form. They are for the most part prescribed to be dissolved in water; but it is proper to remark, that this is the most preferable way, but it is not always necessary, nor always to be commended. For convenience sake, powders are often required; when such is the case, about two grains of sugar of milk and three globules may serve to make a powder, and a dose of this kind may be given dry upon the tongue under all circumstances, where any medicine is otherwise prescribed, if preferred in this way--Never-the less in acute cases a solution of the medicine in water is considered to be the best.

It is better to make no rapid changes from one medicine to another; for this is not generally attended with good results. Those who have an implicit faith in Homœopathy cannot fail of regarding it the providential means of affording them relief from suffering, and when a remedy is taken, it is with a confident reliance, that induces the patient to wait a sufficient length of time to obtain its legitimate effects; and to those who have less faith in the practice, we would caution to exercise patience and make a fair and critical trial of the remedies as prescribed.

Many of the diseases described, and the mode of treatment given, have been the result of the author's experience; others have been taken from reliable sources, and put into form, so as to obviate confusion where ever the manual is used; and it is believed that the work will give positive satisfaction where ever it is put to a practical test.

The object having been to impart information in popular language a glossary of medical terms has been deemed unnecessary and is therefore omitted. For the sake of plainness, the most common names of the various diseases have been given, as well as those pertaining to the same in nosological works.

The work has been divided into chapters, so as to

preserve a distinctness of classification favourable to the
design of the book. Constant reference has been had
in the preparation of this Manual to what is of the most
positively practical value.

With the hope that the book will fulfil its design and
answer the requirements of the lay-practitioner as well as
the novitiate members of the profession, if not, the more
experienced practitioners, and, also, that it may tend to
disseminate the true idea of disease and its treatment,
and prove a source of benefit to the human race, the
work is commended for careful perusal. It is the sincere
desire of the author that it may prove acceptable and
useful.

INTRODUCTION.

THE modern achievements of science, are fast ridding the world of that exclusiveness which has so long been upheld and practised in the medical profession; and light begins to break in from all directions, enlightening society in general upon such matters, as really pertain to the solid comforts of life.

It is obvious that medicine has not kept pace with other improvements since the revival of learning; and the reason is, the medical profession has labored to impress its patrons with the idea, that no one should study medicine except those who intend to follow it as a calling. For a long time it was thought that the honor and dignity of the profession required this course; that it would prove ruinous to its interests, and the interests of mankind, to make medical learning so plain and accessible that all classes of society might study it; and the consequence has been, the stifling of medicine itself, because kept in worse than Mahomedan seclusion.— There has not been that free strife for advancement, that usually characterizes those who lead the van of the intelligent classes in the community—there has been indolence, bigotry and intolerance hoarded up among the few, under the idea that the ignorance of the community did not render it necessary for them to strive for new attainments;—but that time has passed away; and the patrons as well as the profession of medicine itself seem disposed to inform themselves about the matter,

2   (1)

and the result is, new life is being instilled into the profession, and every effort consistent with reason and common sense is being made to promote its correspond-ing advancement; for is it not evident that it only requires that the patrons of medicine should be kept in ignorance, in order that its condition should remain stationary? But let the people become intelligent about the matter—yea, as intelligent as books can make them, and then the profession must start; they must advance or sink into insignificance. A school master cares about knowing but little when his pupils are ignorant,—place him over a class of intelligent pupils, and he wakes up; he strives for advancement. Therefore it may be said to the public, if a good intelligent class of physicians is desired, the people must inform themselves as correctly as possible concerning the very matters they are to preside over, and then they will be upon the lookout to keep themselves a little ahead of their customers; this is the only apology for offering another domestic work on the Homœopathic Practice of Medicine. It matters not how fast works of the kind multiply, provided they are well calculated to impart proper instruction to those who read them.

Frequent objections are urged against Domestic Manuals because they interfere so much with the legiti-mate uses of the profession; but men willing to rest on real worth will hardly offer this complaint, and those who have too much indolence to keep in advance of their patrons in the knowledge and requirements of their own profession, deserve all the obstacles that the intelligence of their patrons can throw in their way.

When we look back upon the past to see the mistaken zeal that has been manifest for the honor of medicine, and the disguise and concealment of an art so much needed among men; we have not wondered that authors wrote in a foreign tongue and tried to conceal the nature of their prescriptions. Their strife was not to gain additional knowledge, but to keep away from their patrons what they had. Therefore they wrote their medical disquisitions in an unknown tongue except to themselves; studied them in the same tongue, carefully prohibiting the promulgation of any of those secrets thus locked up from the common people: was there ever a scheme better calculated to intercept all progress in medicine?

It may be laid down as a settled rule, that intelligence among the masses, will tend to enoble and dignify the learned professions; and the better common people understand medicine the stronger will be the impetus for the profession to improve, and the same is eminently true of theology and law.

There was a time when every branch of human learning was regarded the privilege of a chosen few, but now nearly every branch of science is universally studied and open to all, and we see no reason why the science of anatomy or physiology or any of the collateral branches of medicine, may not be as accessible to all, as any branch of science that tends to ameliorate the condition of the human race.

In the present work every effort will be made to avoid all ambiguous terms, and to present a Manual of the Practice of Homœopathy in plain English: and instead of being governed by the fear, that remedies will be tampered with, an effort will be made to be so explicit, that any one who attentively reads, may be led to adopt a correct course.

A brief exposition of disease and its mode of treatment may be regarded as a piece of useful information for every man, woman or child in the community, and in order to facilitate the study, the work will be divided into chap- ters, with the headings rendered palpable and distinct, and moreover every paragraph will be duly marked so as to avoid confusion.

In concluding our Introduction we are free to express our regret that so many entertain views adverse to medicine as a popular science. There is certainly no valid reason why valuable knowledge should be confined to a few, while all the rest are taught to wholly neglect it, if not to despise it; and it is a matter of regret, that such futile objections have been raised as the following : " That people who dip into medical knowledge become fanciful and believe themselves afflicted with every disease of which they read." This is certainly a mistake with regard to sensible people, who seldom attempt a mode of procedure until duly informed. To render the most acceptable service to mankind, is to impart to them that kind of knowledge that will aid them in well meant endeavours to eradicate dangerous and hurtful practices; that will tend to extinguish unwarrantable prejudices, and afford security against quacks and impostors, and, lastly, to show what measures are at hand to preserve health, to prevent or cure disease, and to promote in the best manner the humane and benevolent operations of society.

CHAPTER I.

OBSERVATIONS ON DIET, AIR AND EXERCISE, ABLUTIONS, &c.

1.—Observations on Diet.

IT is manifest from observation that health in a great measure depends upon a judicious and well selected diet, that must be regularly supplied, and taken into the system with great care.

To prevent disease or promote health is certainly as desirable as to restore it when lost. One of the efficient means of preserving health is a well regulated diet. This can only be brought about by attending to a few simple rules, such as the following :

1. The first consideration that should influence every one is, that he "*eats to live*," and that he merely requires such aliments as will best promote the general health and strength of the body; he should always consult the real wants of the system, instead of the temporary gratification of the appetite.

2. In the selection of food, such articles as may be included among the common aliments, may always be regarded the best, because experience has sanctioned their use.

3. The manner in which food should be cooked in order to preserve its nourishing properties should be attentively studied.

2* (5)

4. The mode of seasoning food should be such as to avoid any unnatural stimulation of the stomach, or such as will tend by any irritating or corroding property to impair its tone. Strong acids, peppers, mustard, and articles of kindred properties, afford no nourishment, and a craving for them only argues some morbid derangement of the appetite, which, if it does not fore-warn the approach of more serious disease, ought to be resisted. The use of such articles ought to be tolerated only in great moderation, and never unless the stomach can receive them without the remotest inconvenience or derangement.

5. The proper times for eating should be established, and regularly observed. It is usual in this country to subsist upon three meals a day, and this from experience has been found amply sufficient to sustain the vigor and tone of the bodily health. It is not merely *the taking* of three meals a day that is required, but the taking of them in a proper way, and at proper hours, allowing sufficient length of time to elapse between each meal.

6. The exercise of eating should be performed in accordance with the indications of nature. The teeth are the proper organs of mastication, and every particle of food that requires mastication should be subjected to this operation; not a particle, susceptible of being further reduced by the teeth should be taken into the stomach, for it is evident that the economy of the system requires that the teeth should perform faithfully their proper office, without leaving any of their appropriate work to be done in the stomach. It is true that a vigor-ous, healthy stomach will for a time perform a service that in reality should have been performed by the teeth, but it is hazarding considerable to tax this useful organ

in this way; for when it becomes thus burthened by labor not properly its own, it may refuse to perform any labor at all, and the consequence is a disordered condition of the stomach and bowels.

7. There is no practice more to be deplored on the account of the injury which it inflicts than rapid eating ; it is therefore requisite that food should be taken into the system no faster than it can be thoroughly comminuated by the teeth, and even then it would be better if a short interval were to elapse between the times of supplying the masticatory organs.

To the foregoing rules we may append a few practical remarks. It is not best to be confined to any one kind of food a great length of time, for no creature is capable of subsisting on so great a variety of food as man. He inhabits all climates, and is capable of subsisting upon the productions of them all ; and if they do not suit the particular tastes which by habit he has acquired, the art of cooking is called into requisition to divest them of disagreeable qualities. The art of cooking is especially designed to prepare food, so that what is crude and hurtful may be rendered wholesome and salutary.

As much that serves for food is derived from the animal kingdom, and much from the vegetable, it may be regarded unsafe in the present state of the world to be confined to either. Man's habits are such that he requires a mixture, duly adjusted, with regard to the proportion of each. To be confined exclusively to a diet of animal food would fever the system, and sometimes render putrescent the contents of the stomach and bowels; and bring on violent colics, dysenteries, and diarrhœas. On the other hand, to be confined exclusively to a vegetable diet would deteriorate the powers of the whole system, unless the habit of being restricted to this kind of diet had been formed from childhood.

It is difficult to give any definite directions with regard to the proportion of the two kinds of aliments necessary. It cannot have escaped observation that the laboring man requires more animal food than the sedentary man, and one that labors in the open air than one in confined apartments. Therefore, we may lay it down as a rule, that a hard laboring man requires animal food at every meal he eats, and the sedentary not so often; not exceeding perhaps once or twice in twenty-four hours. Animal food is a great deal more stimulating than vegetable, and on this account it is prone to give rise to diseased conditions, such as scurvy. We have no better proof of the baneful effects of an exclusively animal diet, or perhaps a diet confined to bread and meat, than what is furnished by scorbutic affections, and it is well known that we have no means of curing the malady, unless the patient is allowed the free use of vegetables.

Perhaps it might be regarded a safe rule to observe, not to eat animal food except with potatoes or other vegetables; there is nothing at all necessary, to fix, with regard to proportion, for this may vary according to circumstances, climate, and weather; less animal food being required in warm weather and warm climates, than in cold weather and cold climates.

Certain descriptions of animal food are less to be commended than others, and the same remark may be made about certain kinds of vegetable food. Some are more nutritious—some are easier of digestion—some are too stimulating, while others excite unhealthy activities in the system.

It therefore becomes necessary to classify the aliments in such a way as to facilitate the selecting of those the best adapted for common use, either in sickness or in health. Most of the nutritious aliments taken when in the enjoyment of sound health, may be used as articles of diet when under homœopathic treatment, provided they are served up without condiments, and are found not to disagree.

But in preparing any article of diet for the sick, it should be a settled rule to make no use of any of the condiments except salt, and also, all flavors that savor in the least of a medicinal character should be avoided and let the cooking be of that character, the best calculated to adapt the food for the capacity and wants of the body.

2.—Articles of Diet that may be allowed under Homœopathic Treatment.

Gruel, made of oatmeal, wheat flour, corn starch, farina, powdered crackers, rice, corn meal, sago, tapioca, pearl barley.

Soup or broth, made of the lean of fat mutton, beef, or chicken, to which may be added rice, vermicelli, maccaroni, young peas, pearl barley, or any other farinaceous material, but it must have no seasoning except a moderate quantity of salt.

Cooked meats. Broiled beef or mutton steaks, roasted tender loin of beef, roast mutton; roasted or broiled chickens, pigeons, larks, rabbits, venison, reed birds, and quail, may be partaken of in moderation.

Cooked fish. Boiled rock fish, trout, smelts, perch, and flounders, may be partaken of in great moderation, provided none of them are found to disagree with the patient. The same kinds of fish fried are not so easy of digestion, nor so well suited for invalids; yet, in some instances where the preference for the fried is very great, it may be partaken of if found to relish and agree with the stomach.

Shell fish. Oysters, roasted in the shell, or stewed in a little water, boiled with their liquor and a few crumbs of bread for a few minutes only, are not only nutritious, but easy of digestion.

Vegetables. Irish potatoes, sweet potatoes, green peas, French beans, tomatoes, cauliflower, spinach, rice, hominy, carrots, and every kind of bean raised in gardens, when young and tender; all kinds of vegetables must be well cooked; potatoes, if boiled, should not remain in the water after being sufficiently cooked, and, if baked, care should be exercised to remove them from the oven when they are *done.* French beans and peas may be cooked and served up in the gravy of meats, or with butter, or milk instead of butter.

Puddings. Made of water crackers, (powdered) and of tapioca, sago, arrow root, corn starch, rice, farina, bread, and even with eggs and milk, merely sweetened with sugar.

Bread and cakes. Made of wheat flour, not recently baked, and bread made of the unbolted wheat flour, simple cakes, (composed of flour or meal, eggs, sugar, and *good new butter*,) sponge cakes and fritters.

Eggs. Served up in several ways, by being lightly boiled, poached, or made into custards. Sometimes, when the stomach has been known to reject almost every form of food, a gruel made of the flour of the yolks of hard boiled eggs has not only proved palatable, but so nutritive as to impart much vigor and strength.

Fruit. Roasted apples, or apples made into sauce, or

preserved or baked pears, raspberries, strawberries, grapes, plumbs, or any wholesome fruit not of an acid quality fully ripe, prepared in any of the usual forms of serving up fruits.

Beverages. Water, milk, cocoa, unspiced chocolate, rice water, toast water, (provided the toast is not *charred*) sugar and water, and any other non-medicinal beverage.

Any thing mentioned in the above list that is known to disagree, must not be used. So differently constituted are individuals, that oftentimes, what is one's meat is another's poison, and besides, some people have certain peculiarities that give them an antipathy to some one or more of the most wholesome aliments. Some aliments will in some persons induce a state of disease, owing to certain congenital peculiarities. Any article known to have this effect should be avoided. Any article not relished by a patient on account of some disagreeable sensation it imparts, ought not to be forced upon him. It is impossible to form a regimen free from all exceptions; variations will have to be made to suit particular cases, with due reference to the circumstances that surround them.

3.—Articles of Diet that may sometimes be allowed under Homœopathic Treatment.

Meats. Ham, veal, tripe, the dark meat of the turkey, and other poultry, (either roasted or boiled.)

Fruits. Watermelons, cantelopes, muskmelons, gooseberries, currants, whortleberries, oranges and lemons.

Beverages. Tea, coffee, and bromer.

It sometimes happens, that individuals have been so long accustomed to a single course of diet, that a deprivation of it, even when under homœopathic treatment, proves more injurious than useful. Those who have formed the habit of drinking tea at breakfast and supper, and have never found it to disagree with them, may still be allowed it, when under treatment. Others who have always been accustomed to *drink coffee* in the morning and have never found it to disagree or produce any departure from sound health, may still be allowed it in moderation, provided they suffer for the want of it. And so with regard to meats, some persons accustomed to eat ham, and always find it to agree with them, need not be deprived of it, unless it is found to derange the stomach. And the same remark is true of veal, tripe, and poultry. As none of the meats can be regarded injurious, only because they are more difficult of digestion, they have no property that interferes with the action of remedies, except the tax they lay upon the organs of digestion, for a little more force. Thus it will appear evident, if the stomach receives them with impunity, and suffers no inconvenience or derangement, they may be allowed; *Watermelons, Cantelopes, and Muskmelons* have often been allowed in certain febrile diseases with no inconvenience or injury to the patient, and some are led to believe that nature has furnished these watery materials for this purpose. Facts elicited by observation go very far to prove that ripe melons very rarely if ever prove a source of injury or disease when persons are so situated as to enjoy them; the same remark may be made in relation to all ripe fruits. They may be enjoyed with impunity in the season of *them;* they neither induce disease nor prove an obstacle to a return to health, provided the patient has no ailment that would render them incompatible. As *fruits and ice cream* are so nearly allied, it may be mentioned here, that the latter may very generally be allowed in fevers, provided it is not flavored with anything of a medicinal property. That flavored with the orange or strawberry is regarded the best, but those base imitations and colorings resorted to for gain, are always to be avoided as pernicious.

4.—Articles of diet that cannot be allowed under Homœopathic Treatment.

Meats. Fat pork, ducks, geese, calves' head, sausages, kidney, and every kind of salted, or fat meat.

Soups. Every description of seasoned soups, such as turtle, pepper-pot, and mock-turtle.

Fish. Salt codfish, pickled salmon, salt shad and mackerel, eels, smoked herring, and all smoked or fermented fish whatever.

Shell fish. Crabs, lobsters, clams.

Vegetables. Cucumbers, onions, celery, asparagus, greens, cabbage, radishes, parsley, horse-radish, leeks, garlic, and every description of pickles, salads and raw vegetables of every description.

Pastry of every description, whether boiled, baked, or fried.

All artificial Sauces, such as catsup, pickles, condiments mustard and vinegar; spices, aromatics, *distilled and fermented liquors.*

Rancid cheese and butter.

All kinds of nuts, such as chestnuts, filberts, walnuts, almonds, peanuts, cocoa nuts, and all others of a kindred character.

5. Sometimes invalids may be allowed chestnuts, roasted or boiled, but under certain restrictions. There may be some articles in the prohibited list that under certain circumstances may be permitted—and perhaps the regulations of diet as given may be subjected to

other modifications. The design of the tables being to point out in a general way the most reasonable course to be pursued, in the absence of direct experience. For the sake of imparting further practical knowledge concerning diet we will now insert what has been ascertained by experiment, with regard to the time required for the digestion of many of the prominent aliments.

These results were obtained by experiments made by Doctor Beaumont on St. Martin, who had an opportunity of observing the process through a fistulous opening into the stomach, under such circumstances as enabled him to note very accurately the time required for digesting the aliments noted in the list.

		h. m.
Apples—sweet, raw,	digested in	1 50
sour, hard, raw,	" "	2 50
Barley—boiled,	" "	2
Broiled rock fish,	" "	3
Beans boiled in pod,	" "	2 30
Beans and green corn boiled, (suckertash,)	" "	3 45
Beef, roasted or boiled,	" "	3
Beef, dried or salted, boiled,	" "	4 15
Beets, boiled,	" "	3 45
Bread made of wheat,	" "	3 30
Bread made of corn,	" "	3 15
Butter, melted,	" "	3 30
Cabbage, raw,	" "	2 50
Cabbage in vinegar,	" "	2
Cabbage, boiled,	" "	4 30
Cheese, old and strong,	" "	3 30
Chicken, stewed,	" "	2 45
Cod fish, dry, boiled,	" "	2

		h.	m,
Duck, roasted,	digested in 4		
Eggs, hard boiled,	"	" 3	30
" soft "	..	" 3	
" raw,	"	" 2	
Goose, wild, roasted,	"	" 2	30
Lamb, broiled,	"	" 2	30
Liver, beef's, broiled,	"	" 2	
Meat and vegetables, hashed,	"	" 2	30
Milk,	"	" 2	
Mutton,	"	" 3	
Oysters, raw,	"	" 2	55
Oysters, stewed,	"	" 3	30
Pork, roasted,	"	" 5	15
Pork, stewed,		" 3	
Potatoes, Irish, boiled,	"	" 3	30
Potatoes, roasted, baked,	"	" 2	30
Rice, boiled,		" 1	
Sago,	"	" 1	15
Salmon, salted,	"	" 4	
Tapioca, boiled,	"	" 2	
Tripe, "	"	" 1	
Trout, "	"	" 1	30
Turkey, "	"	" 3	55
Turnips, "	"	" 2	30
Veal, broiled,	"	" 4	
Venison steak,	"	" 1	35

Although we have in this table the comparative time required for the digestion of the aliments named, yet we are not to be governed by this consideration, but by the nature and quantity of nutritive material which each contains, as well as its adaptation to the wants of the body. A table which affords explicit information as to the time required for the digestion of the various kinds of food, is in some respects valuable as a reference in select- ing a diet for a given case. Nevertheless, an appeal to experience with regard to the particular aliments known to relish the best, and agree the best with the individual, is the criterion, the most to be commended.

The relative proportion of nutritious properties of the several kinds of aliment may be interesting to observe; the following table will show the relative amount of nitrogen contained in the aliments named, taken from Carpenter's Physiology. In the table *human milk is taken as the standard of comparison.*=100.

In regard to the nutritious properties of different articles of food, they are to be estimated by the propor- tion of nitrogen they contain. The food of man consists in general of two distinct kinds.

1. That which contributes to the formation of *animal heat*,—compound of oxygen, hydrogen, and carbon; the aliments containing these properties in abundance, are termed *non-nitrongenized.*

2. That which serves for *nutrition*, is composed mainly of nitrogen, and termed *Nitrogenized* or azotized.

Nearly all kinds of food may be regarded a mixture of that which *produces animal heat*, and that which *serves for nutrition.*

6.—Nutrition Table.

Vegetable.

Rice,	81	Barley,	125	Brown bread,	166
Potatoes,	84	Oats,	138	Peas,	239
Turnips,	106	Wheat bread,	142	Lentils,	276
Rye,	106	Wheat,	119, 144	Mushroom,	289
Maize,	100–125	Carrots,	150	Beans,	320

Animal.

Human milk,	100	Skate, boiled,	956
Cow's milk,	237	Herring, raw,	910
Oysters,	305	—— boiled,	808
Yolk of eggs,	305	—— milt of,	924
Cheese,	331, 447	Haddock, raw,	920
Eel, raw,	434	—— boiled,	816
—— boiled,	428	Flounder, raw,	898
Mussel, raw,	570	—— boiled,	954
—— boiled,	663	Pigeon, raw,	756
Ox liver, raw,	570	—— boiled,	827
Pork, ham, raw,	570	Lamb, raw,	833
—— boiled,	809	Mutton, raw,	773
Salmon, raw,	776	—— boiled,	852
—— boiled,	610	Veal, raw,	873
Portable soup,	764	—— boiled,	911
White of egg,	845	Beef, raw,	880
Crab, boiled,	859	—— boiled,	941
Skate, raw,	859	Ox lung,	931

7.—Observations on Air and Exercise.

It is well known from observation that an ample supply of good food, without the benefit of a pure atmosphere and exercise, avails but little in the way of promoting health. An atmosphere, contaminated with noxious vapors, may frequently prove the source of disease in despite of all the resistance that the best of food and exercise can offer.

We respire nearly twenty thousand times in twenty-four hours, and at each inspiration we imbibe a fresh portion of the air, and if this vast quantity possesses in the least degree any deleterious property, is it not evident that the delicate and sensitive tissues of the lungs

3*

which it permeates, may become impaired, so as to pour the seeds of disease into the circulation, and thus throughout the whole body?

It is by the aid of the atmosphere, that venous blood, which is, in the main, formed from the food taken into the stomach, becomes changed into arterial, and fitted to perform its use in the body. · The atmosphere is composed of one part of oxygen and four parts of nitrogen, and a small quantity of carbonic acid. That part, the most essential to life is the oxygen, and if this becomes diminished in quantity, the consequences are fatal, because the proportion of the three elements entering into the composition of the atmosphere cannot be altered in the least, without rendering it totally unfit for respiration.

It is therefore of the utmost importance to preserve the air, as nearly as possible, in that condition which promotes healthy respiration. It is at once evident, that this cannot be accomplished except by a thorough system of ventilation. When several persons are together in a closed room, the air after a while becomes vitiated; by ventilating the room the vitiated air passes out, and permits fresh air to take its place. The apartments of the sick are not to be regarded as exceptions to this rule, for no influence is more needed to facilitate restoration to health than that of fresh air. But every precaution should be exercised to prevent a draught from passing over the patient, or coming in contact with the head or any part of the body.

So important is it, that a well digested system of ventilation should be observed in all departments of life, that the study of works upon the subject may be commended. A very ingenious apparatus for ventilating confined apartments has been invented by Prof. Espy, which has proved of immense service in ventilating our naval ships, as well as public halls, churches, and other resorts, where the people are accustomed to come together in masses.

Ventilation should always be had from the top of a room if possible. It is true that it can be had by opening a window from the side, but this is liable to an objection on the account of its being difficult to avoid at all times the influence which a draught might occasion by being admitted from the side. This is particularly the case in rooms for public gatherings; and many are the instances where persons, heated and perspiring, in public assemblages, have suddenly had a window opened upon them, admitting a draught of cold air that has made them uncomfortable at the time, and subjected them to serious disease afterwards as the consequence.

The tendency of heated air in a room is to rise to the top, while that which is colder sinks to the bottom; therefore it will be seen that ventilation from the top of a room appears to be the most natural way of disposing of a heated and rarified air in the apartments of the sick.

Whether in the house, or out of doors, it is incumbent on every one to seek pure air; whether in sickness or in health, he must inevitably suffer without it.

Every thing that has a tendency to vitiate or corrupt the atmosphere, ought to be studiously avoided as far as possible, at all times, under all circumstances, and in all places. A few simple rules might aid in securing the blessing of a pure air, when otherwise it might be overlooked or heedlessly disregarded.

1. In sleeping apartments, or in apartments occupied during the day, let everything that has a tendency to deteriorate the air be removed; let them be kept clean and free from filth of every description.

2. In the apartments of the sick, avoid perfumery of every description, such as cologne, otto of roses, musk, camphor, scent bags, and everything that modifies in the least degree, the pure, clean, fresh, and invigorating effects of the atmosphere.

3. Always avoid attempting to extinguish one unpleasant odor by producing another. Some burn linen rags, some pour vinegar upon a hot shovel, others burn aromatic substances, hoping thereby to get rid of some unpleasant odor, but all these practices are pernicious. It is far better to provide for a due supply of fresh air, and if this does not prove sufficient, some disinfecting agent, as a solution of chloride of soda or lime, may have a decided preference.

4. It should always be observed as a rule, not to allow bouquets or flowers in a sick room, for it is manifest, that they soon begin to change after being plucked, and the perfume they then impart has a tendency to so corrupt the air as to exert a depressing, and sickening influence upon the patient.

The atmosphere is often made the vehicle of conveying deleterious matters from bogs, swamps, or marshes, that so diffuse themselves around, as to be the occasion of much disease; therefore, it is well to avoid an atmosphere tainted with such miasms as these locations may engender. Damp cellars may corrupt the air of all the apartments of a house. Animal or vegetable decomposition will do the same for a whole neighborhood, or region of country, and prove the frequent source of disease and death.

Without particularizing further, it may be remarked in general terms, that everything must be avoided that renders the air moist, and damp, or prevents its free circulation all about us; the more pure the air, the better. In childhood, it is instinctively craved, because it promotes a healthy development of the system. Infants ever delight to be tossed about where they can breathe the invigorating atmosphere.

It will be seen from the foregoing that *exercise promotes health*, and particularly when it is indulged in at the same time we are in the enjoyment of pure air. Gentle exercise, and a pure atmosphere, go hand in hand, in preserving man from evil; and, besides, exercise may be regarded the chief condition of animal life. It is exercise that causes the muscle to increase in size, strength, and power, the joints to become flexible and easy of motion; that invigorates the nerves, and imparts to the blood a vigorous movement. It creates a stimulus of demand for food, and brings life and activity to every part of the system. As an example, look at the muscles of the feet of opera dancers, and the muscles of the blacksmith's arm, and behold how strong, healthy and firm they appear. Bodily exercise is required of all, whether high or low, rich or poor, in order to promote health and strength.

But notwithstanding so great importance is attached to exercise, and particularly that in the open air, it may be indulged in to excess, and at improper seasons, when such conditions are present as will render it a positive evil. It therefore seems requisite to regard exercise useful only within certain bounds, and these may be set by a few appropriate rules.

1. Violent exercise should never take place either immediately before or after eating; for in the former case the system becomes too violently agitated to receive food into the stomach with impunity, and in the latter

instance the power that goes to sustain the upper and lower extremities during violent exercise, is in a measure abstracted from the power of digestion.

2. Exercise in the open air should take place at an interval of one hour after eating, provided it is practicable.

3. Exercise in any violent way should not be indulged in after the system has been reduced to a state of fatigue, for under such circumstances it induces fever, prostration, and rheumatic difficulties.

4. When the health is infirm, and the physical energies are prostrated by disease, it is highly detrimental to force an indulgence in exercise; by so doing, more injury can be done in one half hour, than can be repaired in weeks. When the system is laboring under the influence of fever, rest is better than exercise.

5. It should always be a rule to avoid that kind of exercise that aggravates any local irritation, such as prolapsus uteri, or falling of the womb, or any other local difficulty.

6. For persons of feeble constitution and feeble digestion, gentle walking is an exercise sufficiently vigorous, but those of strong constitution and feeble digestion may indulge in more active exercise.

7. Always exercise at regular intervals, if acustomed to sedentary employment, for this will regularly tend to keep the system in order.

8. It is better to exercise moderately in the morning before eating and if possible in the open air. It is not good to exercise immediately after dinner, especially after dining upon roast beef, mutton, turkey or other solid aliments : at least one hour should elapse before any considerable amount of exercise should be permitted.

9. During childhood and youth, running, romping, dancing, and other exercises of a vivacious character are not only requisite, but absolutely indispensable.

10. But in more advanced life, when the mind has to be exercised more intensely and with greater precision in the cares of life, these vivacious exercises may be supplanted by those of a more grave character, yet serving to promote the same or similar purposes. The sedentary student should regularly seek gymnastic exercises. The accountant should do the same. The operator bound up to a single kind of exercise, and one that requires sameness of position, should seek counter-acting exercises for relaxation. Violent exercises, throwing the whole system into an intense heat, and perspiration, are of but little service under any circum-stances, and should be avoided; because they too frequently become the source of rheumatic difficulties, and the occasion of exposures, fraught with serious, consequences.

11. There is an appropriate time of day for exercise, it is in the morning, before noon, because in the afternoon, towards evening, the air is damper and not so healthy, as at an earlier hour of the day.

12. Finally, it may be said that exercise must be so regulated as to accord exactly with the condition and capacity of the subject, and so must the temperature of the atmosphere; a cold air, ever so fresh, will not suit every one, neither will a hot one. A dense invigorating atmosphere may be the very thing for nervous weaknesses and debility after acute affections, but it is not beneficial for consumptives; it is too bracing and too likely to produce cough; neither is exercise always good for all descriptions of chronic ailments; some will derive

benefit and some will not; a very little exertion, beyond the capacity of the system to endure, is certainly worse than no exercise at all. Gymnastic exercises are reduced to a system; and every kind of subject may find such an one, as will suit his capacity and strength. The commencement should always be with light and moderate feats, gradually preparing the way, for becoming accustomed to those, which are more difficult and laborious.

8.—Ablutions and Bathing.

None of the elements of hygiene are superfluous or of inferior consideration. Water was not only designed as a beverage, but for ablutions, and its use in this respect is as indispensable as in the other; "cleanliness promotes health" is as true as any proverb recorded in *the book*, and this is the chief use of water as an external agent.—While considering the various modes of employing water to promote cleanliness of the body, we by no means shall render ourselves obnoxious to those who style themselves hydropathists; for although we do not prize water so highly as some do, as a therapeutic agent, yet we are willing to recommend its use, either cold, tepid, or warm, wherever it can perform a use,—but in one or the other of these forms it is requisite, under every possible circumstance in which a person can be placed, whether sick or well.

The common practice of washing the face and hands after a season of repose, is so natural that it may almost be considered an instinctive act; but even in the performance of this common ablution a few suggestions may not be inappropriate. During the warm weather the water coming from the hydrants or house-wells, without undergoing any change of temperature, other than what the atmosphere may occasion, is all that is required for the performance of this ablution; soap may be used to soften the water, provided there are no tetters or eruptions upon the skin; otherwise it is better that it should be dispensed with.

In cold weather, when the atmosphere is cold and bracing, and the water from the hydrants is cold also, there are many persons who cannot stand washing even the face and hands in it, on rising in the morning, without becoming chilled and thrown into paroxysms of fever; under such circumstances, common sense dictates that the water should be warmed, so as to be of a tepid temperature. The same rule with reference to the use of soaps, may be observed, as above.

Bathing has begun to be looked upon in the light which it merits; *baths* are now regarded indispensable in homœopathy, because they aid materially in preparing patients for the more certain and salutary action of remedies. There are only two of the modern appliances called *baths*, that can safely be recommended as being consonant with homœopathic treatment: viz. The FRESH WATER BATH and the SALT WATER BATH. The former may be either *cold* or *tepid*, and the latter, only to be indulged in during the heat of summer, may be of the *temperature of the salt water of the ocean*. The use of these baths may form a subject of study,—how often, when to be avoided, when to be cold, and when to be warm, are severally to be determined by proper rules.

1. A cold bath should never be taken during the presence of an eruption or rash. The sponge filled with water and gently pressed, may be passed quickly over the body in such a condition, but nothing approximating nearer to a bath can be recommended.

4

2. Cold baths should be avoided if they produce headache, or any other constitutional disturbance; if they are followed by chilliness instead of a glow, or if the body is in a perspiration, or suffering from any inflammatory disease. They should be avoided when the temperature of the atmosphere is declining, as in the evening; and when the water feels warm and the air cold, and in cold and chilling weather.

3. Cold bathing is beneficial when it is followed by a glow, in affections of a nervous character, in nearly all affections arising from indigestion, or from debility of the stomach.

4. The appropriate time for the cold bath is in the early part of the day, because the air becomes warmer than the water. In-door bathing may be kept up during the year, provided it is done in a moderately warm room. Persons that can swim may indulge in this exercise during warm weather.

5. In going into the water to swim, immerse the whole body at first, and not the lower extremities merely. It is better to lay down in the water, than to plunge, because this latter method of immersing the body, may induce headache or temporary deafness, by the shock which it occasions.

6. Do not remain in the water without exercising the limbs; do not stand still or remain too long in the water. About six minutes is allowed for a bath, and this is quite long enough to secure all the benefits to be derived. It defeats the object to remain so long as to become chilled.

7. If cramps ensue when bathing, leave the water at once, and apply a rough coarse towel, as briskly as possible over the body until it becomes perfectly dry, and

then, dress immediately. Gentle exercise, after bathing, is commendable.

8. Sea-bathing is found beneficial for those who have led a sedentary life, and are somewhat inclined to dyspepsia; but if it produces anything like nausea, or derangement of the stomach, it had better be avoided. Whenever any one finds himself invariably afflicted with some constitutional disturbance when indulging in *seabathing*, it is an indication for him to refrain altogether.

9. Warm baths are generally debilitating, and should seldom be indulged in. In cold weather, they are very apt to enervate the frame, and predispose the system to colds. Under some circumstances, however, a tepid bath may be preferable to a cold one, provided it be resorted to in warm weather or in a warm room.

10. Persons should not avail themselves of the bath oftener than once a day, and then in the early part of the day.

11. It is a safe rule to observe, not to bathe when the habit produces, invariably, some constitutional disturbance, or gives rise to a debilitated feeling not easily overcome.

12. The cold bath for very young children should never be countenanced; generally the temperature of the water should be such as to communicate a slight sensation of warmth to the hand; for older children a bath more nearly approaching the temperature of *the cold* may be used with impunity, provided great caution is used to wipe them thoroughly dry, and to supply them with warm clothing immediately after. It is very probable that experience may suggest many modifications with regard to the use of the baths not hinted at in the above rules.

So far as ablutions are necessary to promote thorough cleanliness of the body, they are always to be com- mended. The wet sponge or towel may be used very generally for this purpose, provided care is always taken to dry the body with dry towels immediately, and then resume the clothing; with regard to partial bathing, the same or similar rules are to be observed. *The shower bath* is so frequently attended with bad consequences that but little can be said in its favor. *Vapor baths* are still more objectionable, as being enervating and liable to be followed by bad results. *Medicated baths* may be looked upon with distrust by the patrons of homœo- pathy; they are strictly prohibited as belonging to that kind of practice which deserves only, to be classed among the merest quackeries of the day.

9.—Clothing.

Under the head of clothing there is considerable worthy of particular remark. That which is designed for the protection of the body should be of such a character as to answer the purpose; and in despite of fashion, which is too frequently regardless of the pro- tection which clothing should afford, we may lay down a few simple rules.

1. The body should be warmly clad during cold weather, and thinly clad during warm weather; this rule is imperative for the promotion of health.

2. The fashion of clothing the feet with thin soled boots or shoes in cold, damp weather, should be dis- countenanced as being destructive to health, and a fell destroyer of human life.

3. Linen or cotton fabrics may be regarded the most suitable clothing for warm and dry weather, and woolen

for cold weather; the same that is worn next to the skin in warm weather, may be continued in cold weather, provided a thicker and warmer suit of woolen clothing is worn as an external covering.

4. Persons exposed to the extremes of temperature should wear woolen flannel next to the skin, because this fabric is known to possess the power of stimulating the skin to greater action, and at the same time absorbs the perspiration; and besides, wool is a bad conductor of caloric, and on this account is better calculated to retain the natural warmth of the body in cold weather.

5. In regulating the quantity of clothing to correspond with the seasons, great care should be exercised not to make a change in advance of the coming season, but only after the season has fully made its appearance. It is by no means safe to dispense with the under-clothing until the warm weather has fully set in. The summer clothing may be worn, until the fall weather fully justifies a change.

6. Clothing should be so constructed as to allow the greatest freedom of movement, and so as not to incommode the body, whether in motion or otherwise. This is particularly required for the comfort of the feet; tight boots or shoes, by hampering the feet, may cause them to smart and ache with pain, while corns, and other excrescences, may make their appearance, inflicting a severe chastisement, as well as a good and wholesome admonition to refrain from wearing them. Tight lacing is another foul practice indulged in by some ladies, for the purpose of enhancing the symmetry of the form; but this practice embitters their enjoyment, and too frequently engenders consumption or other lung difficulties.

7. The feet should be kept warm, and when wet

4*

from exposure, the sooner a change is made the better. The same may be remarked of the other clothing; a neglect on this score may be the cause of lingering disease or even death.

8. Young ladies, as they approach the period of puberty cannot be too careful in protecting the feet, and the body in general, from exposure to damp and cold.

9. Clothing should never be removed suddenly after violent exercise; neither should any attempt be made to cool off, except in the most gradual way, keeping the body duly covered as the temperature diminishes.

10.—Observations on Sleep.

When the voluntary activity of the body has been kept up a given time, it requires an interval of repose, or otherwise the organs would soon become worn out or disabled by disease. It is therefore provided in the economy of life, that a certain proportion of every twenty-four hours should constitute a season of repose. The legitimate design of sleep is to afford an opportunity for the bodily powers to become renovated and strengthened; on this account the poet has styled the phenomenon,

"'Tired nature's sweet restorer."

When in the performance of manual labor the bodily powers gradually waste; but during sleep they become repaired, as no counteracting waste prevents. The hours of life, whether we are in wakefulness or sleep, whether feasting, in motion, or at rest, should be carefully disposed of with due regularity and order.

1. Labor of body and mind is requisite for every individual when in the enjoyment of health.

2. Eating is required to furnish materials for nutrition; and the chief meal should be taken in the after part of the day.

3. *Sleep should follow eating* at a given period, so as to afford an opportunity for the blood, which contains all the essential elements, to be incorporated into the different organs of the body. Doctor Franklin recommended that the season of sleep should be between the hours of 8 P. M. and 4 A. M., but no definite rule can be laid down of this character.

4. With regard to the number of hours required for repose, they vary according to age and habits of life. It may be laid down, however, that the normal condition of certain classes requires as follows,—

1. Infants require eighteen hours of repose in every twenty-four, until they are three months old; from three to six months, about fifteen; from six months to a year, about fourteen; and for the first seven years of life, children require about thirteen hours of sleep in every twenty-four; and from seven to fourteen years of age, they require about twelve.

2. After the age of puberty, males require less sleep as a general rule than females. The former require, between the ages of fourteen and twenty-one, about nine hours in every twenty four, and the latter about ten.

3. Those that have attained adult age will require an amount of sleep corresponding to constitution, temperature, and employment. Sedentary men and women do not require so many hours for sleep, as those who are subject to constant and severe exercise of body and mind; because the nervous energy becomes more exhausted in these, and of course the system requires longer intervals of repose, to repair the waste. In fleshy and lymphatic

persons there is not so great a demand for sleep, although in the opinion of some there is more.

4. Nervous, sanguine, or muscular constitutions may require from six to eight hours of sleep, from nine or ten o'clock in the evening, till four, five or six o'clock in the morning. Females perhaps may require an additional hour. For persons of bilious and sympathetic constitutions, six hours, or at most seven, of sound repose, are all that are required; but it should be the effort of every one to ascertain for himself what number of hours in every twenty-four is required for repose.

5. The time for sleep is evidently a matter worthy of consideration; the best period for lying in bed is during the middle portion of the night, from nine or ten o'clock in the evening to four or five in the morning. Early rising has so many advantages that it is hardly worth while to recount them; it contributes to health and happiness, and, in a certain sense, adds much to life that otherwise would be lost.

6. Sleeping rooms should not be upon the lower floor of a house, if it can be avoided, because the confined air during the night, in such apartments, is not so suitable for respiration.

7. Sleeping rooms should be large and well ventilated; during the day, their windows should be open, and the bed-clothing must be well aired.

8. Cots or beds should be, if possible, made of hair, because the hair-mattrass affords the best surface to sleep upon, and combines all the necessary qualities for the purpose. During sleep the covering ought to be sufficient, and so constructed as to be easy of regulation.

9. The best position for sleep is lying upon the side. This is the most healthy and natural posture; either side

will suffice, though many believe the right side the best; —with the head slightly elevated by one pillow. It is impossible to lay down explicit rules in relation to sleep, without remarking as many exceptions as rules. While too little sleep does not promote the due support of the organs, too much deteriorates them ; it is therefore enjoined upon every one to ascertain if possible the measure of sleep his system requires.

11.—Observations on Occupations and Professions.

The particular employment or occupation of a man may have a greater or less effect on his health, mentally as well as bodily. Statistical tables have shown that the comparative longevity of persons of some occupations or professions is greater than others. We present a table of statistics made at Berlin, 1834, which we find also inserted in a work entitled, " Sources of Health," by Dr. Tarbell.

Of 100 Clergymen,........only 42 attained the age of 70 yrs. and upwards.
"   Farmers, ..."...40........."........."........."........."...........
"   Commercial men,.."...35........."........."........."........."...........
"   Military men,........"...33 ...."........."........."........."...........
"   Lawyers, ..."...29........."......,.. "........."........."...........
"   Artists,.............."...28........."........."........."........."...........
"   Teachers,............"...27........."........."........."........."...........
"   Physicians, ..."...24........."........."........."........."...........

We would infer from the above, that the quiet pursuits of life, such as contribute to an evenness of temper, and a constancy of a moderate degree of mental and bodily activity, are most conducive to longevity. It will be seen that the average age attained by the clergy is the greatest of all, and the reason is, the labors of a minister of the gospel, though constant and unremitting, are by no means attended with so many irregularities and excitements as those of the physician, which, it will be perceived, stands lowest on the list. The table is interesting as showing the tendency of anxieties and ambitious enterprises to abridge the duration of life. A sterner adherence to duty, and less unchecked passion and ambition may often prove efficient in prolonging life.

CHAPTER II.

A GENERAL VIEW OF THE BODILY ORGANS.

1.—Digestive Organs.

As the derangement of the digestive organs is a fruitful source of many of our physical sufferings, a concise account of them is manifestly proper.

The succession of distinct changes that occur after food is taken into the mouth, before it is suitable for the nourishment of the various parts of the body, is worthy of being well understood.

1. The food is masticated, or chewed; by this pro. cess, it becomes broken up, and finely comminated. *The teeth* are furnished for the consummation of this work.

2. During mastication, the food becomes intimately mixed with the saliva or spittle of the mouth, and this fluid is furnished by six glands, situated about the mouth, viz.: the *parotid*, one under each ear; the *sub-maxillary*, one under each side of the under jaw, and the *sub-lingual*, two small glands under the tongue. Each

of these glands has small ducts, that empty themselves into the mouth; the motion of the jaws, and the stimulus of the food, during mastication, excites these glands to pour forth the saliva or spittle into the mouth, to mingle with the food.

3. The *mastication and insalivation* of the food, by the aid of the tongue, forms it into a ball, and then, by the act of swallowing, it passes into the œsophagus, or gullet, which is the passage, or tube, through which the food passes from the mouth into the stomach.

4. The stomach receives the food in the form of balls from the mouth; every mouthful of food taken at a meal forms one of these balls. As soon as received, the stomach begins to perform the work of *digestion;* it assumes a churning motion, that keeps the balls moving about, so as to come in contact with the walls of the stomach.

In the lining coats of the stomach are numerous little glands, called the *gastric follicles*, because they furnish the *gastric fluid* in the stomach, that dissolves the food. The motion of the balls, coming in contact with these little glands, excites them to pour this fluid into the stomach, and it acts upon the food as a solvent, and reduces the balls to a pulp, or homogenious mass of chyme, of a thick, pappy appearance. By this process, the different kinds of food and materials taken into the stomach at a single meal, become mingled together, so as to scarcely admit of recognition.

5. The stomach is a membranous bag, containing two openings; one for the ingress of the food from the mouth, the other for its egress into the intestines. The former is termed the cardiac orifice, because it is near the heart, and the latter is called the pylorus or pyloric orifice,

because it closes the entrance into the intestinal canal. After a meal, both of these orifices become closed; the former to prevent the return of the food into the gullet, and the latter, to prevent its entrance into the intestinal canal, until the stomach has reduced it to *chyme*. After this is accomplished, the pyloric orifice opens, and the food passes into the upper portion of the intestinal canal; this portion is called the *duodenum*, or second stomach.

6. In the *duodenum* the chyme received from the stomach, is acted upon by the bile and fluid secretion of the *pancreas*, (a gland that furnishes a fluid secretion resembling saliva, and on this account has been styled the salivary gland of the stomach.) The chyme is also acted upon by the secretions of several small glands embedded in the lining membrane of the intestines.

7. The change that takes place in the chyme in consequence of the action of the bile and the other secretions, is that of separation into the nutritious and non-nutritious portions. The former resembles milk, and is taken up by the absorbent vessels and conveyed into the veins, while the latter mingled with the bile, is carried off or ejected in fæces.

This process is always taking place when the body is in health, and with so much ease as to produce no sensation that would lead to its detection, but if anything interrupts the progress of the work, the digestive system is thrown into derangement, and pain and suffering is the result.

The great variety of diseases that assail the digestive system, renders it inexpedient to give a catalogue of them in this place. Numerous are the affections arising from over-eating and drinking — of eating improper food — of eating at improper times, &c., while many others arise from the careless use of cathartics, and others from stimulants, and others from other sources of disease, coming in contact with the body.

As the process of digestion merely prepares the food for being imbibed into the system, or rather into the blood, it has to undergo other changes through the agency of other organs before it is fully prepared to become flesh and bone. One of the most important of these, is effected by respiration, the organs of which we will now consider.

2.—Respiratory Organs.

1. We accomplish the act of breathing through the aid of the lungs. The whole cavity walled in by the ribs and breast-bone, is filled with the lungs and heart. Every time we draw in a breath, the ribs rise and expand the chest, just in proportion to the quantity of air inhaled. The air is received through the nose and mouth, and passes through the wind-pipe into the lungs.

2. The atmosphere taken into the lungs, parts with its oxygen, in exchange for carbonic acid, and this being heavier than common air, falls every time the breath is exhaled. This prevents its return into the lungs at the next breath, so it will be seen that oxygen is supplied from the air at every breath, which is exchanged for carbonic acid given off in the lungs.

3. The benefit that is done to the system by this process, is this: the food, that by the process of digestion, became changed so as to enter into the veins, is conveyed first to a chamber in the heart, called the right auricle, and from this, to another chamber called the right ventricle, and from this chamber it is forced through a large artery into the lungs; this artery

5

divides and subdivides continually—spreading like a tree, until branches of it permeate every part of the lungs. The blood that is sent through this artery, is unsuited to the wants of the body, it contains too many impurities—it contains carbonic acid, which, if suffered to accumulate, will so burthen the system, as to cause disease and death. Now it will be seen that respiration is the act by which these impurities are abstracted from the blood. The quantity of air taken into the lungs, and the quantity of carbonic acid thrown off, at every breath, keeps up a perpetual renovation of the blood, and fashions it into pure blood, such as can be made to lay open its bosom and furnish material for the nourishment of every part of our frames. After the blood is thus prepared in the lungs, it is returned through other channels to a chamber upon the left side of the heart, called the left auricle, and from this it is forced into another, called the left ventricle, and from the left ventricle it is forced into the main artery of the body, which furnishes a channel for the ascent and descent of the blood throughout every part of the body. The great artery after it leaves the heart, divides into ascending and descending branches, and these branches divide and subdivide continually until millions of little branches may be counted supplying every organ; penetrating every structure; supplying a portion of the blood to bone; a portion to muscle; a portion to nerve; a portion to skin, &c., &c.

4. The blood thus prepared in the lungs, and returned to the heart, to be sent forth through arteries to replenish the body, is not all converted into the solid parts during its first round. A portion of it, after parting with what assimilates with the different tissues, is returned again

through the veins, which receive and mingle with it fresh supplies of the nutritive portion of the food from the intestinal canal, reconveying it to the heart, and thence to the lungs, to be sent on the same round as before. This is what is termed the *circulation* of the blood, holding an intermediate relation between digestion, respiration and nutrition.

3.—Circulatory Organs.

The heart is the centre of the circulatory system in man. It has a double structure; one portion may be considered as the starting point of the circulation through the lungs, called pulmonic circulation; the other is the starting point of the circulation throughout the whole system, called systemic circulation. The blood is conveyed from the heart through arteries, and conveyed to the heart through veins. The heart, the arteries, and the veins, are considered the circulatory organs.

When digestion, respiration and circulation are severally going on in an orderly manner, there is complete harmony in their operations; when the organs of digestion are impaired, the supply of nutritive materials becomes obstructed; when the respiratory organs are impaired, the blood does not become duly renovated and vitalized; and when the circulatory organs are the seat of disease, the body fails of receiving throughout the equible distribution of the blood. The various diseases incident to these organs will be described, and the mode of treating them will be pointed out in the following chapters of this work.

4.—Urinary Organs.

The urinary organs are the kidneys, bladder and appendages; they hold an important relation to the other organs. The kidneys secrete the urine from the blood, and by this process the blood is relieved of many impurities, that if not abstracted by this defecatory process, would prove a source of disease in the system. The secretion of the kidneys is passed into the bladder, through little ducts, called the *ureters*, and when the bladder is filled, the urine is passed off through the urinary canal. When nature dictates, that the act of urinating should be performed, it is dangerous to disobey. An effort to retain, throws back upon the system, what it has attempted to reject as worthless, and derangement and disease may be the consequence.

5.—Biliary Organs.

The *liver*, and the *gall bladder*, the largest gland of the body, located in the right hypochondrium, or right side of the abdomen beneath the right lung; the office of this gland is to secrete the bile;—it is a purificatory organ, it separates impurities from the nutritious part of the food received from the stomach and intestines.

1. It also separates impurities from the venous blood. It acts in concert with so many organs, in its work of defecation, that it will be impossible to impart more than a general idea of its office.

2. The gall bladder is the reservoir into which the dirty, black, and acrid materials, separated from the blood by the liver, are collected; this reservoir empties itself into the duodenum, where, by a peculiar affinity, it unites with the innutritious part of the chyme, and both

together, are ejected from the system, through the intestinal canal.

3. If the functions of the liver or gall bladder are in anywise interrupted, it is manifest that impurities will remain in the blood, productive of the most serious consequences.

4. The most inveterate diseases known to humanity, result from an interruption of the defacatory process of the liver. When such interruption occurs, it is shown in the color of the skin, under the eyes, sometimes occasioning a dark sallow, and sunken expression of the countenance.

5. Biliary diseases often prove the most prostrating and violent, because the system being so burthened, is aroused to the most violent struggle to compensate for the interruption. A more particular account will be given in succeeding chapters.

6. The liver, pancreas and spleen, appear to be a class of organs associated together in the work of purifying the blood, and when the office of either is interrupted, it is reasonable to suppose that disease will be the inevitable result.

The proper performance of the office of any of the organs that have been named, depends upon another class of organs which we have yet to consider.

6.—The Nervous System.

This system being the central source of all the vital movements of the body, is worthy of a concise description.

1. The nervous system in man, includes the great nervous centres, and all the nerves that proceed from them. *The brain* and spinal cord, are the great centres

5*

where the nervous force is generated, that communicates through nerves, the vital endowment of all the organs.

2. The ganglionic or sympathetic system, which is dependant on the two great centres named in the preceding paragraph, presides over the functions of digestion, respiration and defecation. This system is sometimes called the pneumogastric or lung and stomach nerve, hence,

3. The brain is divided into the *cerebrum* or large brain, the cerebellum or small brain, and the *medulla oblongata*, by which is understood the nervous system of the senses and actions. The large brain includes all the top of the head, the small brain lies at the bottom below the point even with the top of the ears, and the medulla oblongata is the commencement of the spinal cord in the cranium.

4. There are twelve pairs of nerves that issue from the brain. One pair is the olfactory that goes to the nose and contributes to form the sense of smell; another pair supplies the eyes with power of being impressed with light; another supplies the ears; another the face; another the tongue, &c.; thus showing that the nervous system is the source from whence the special organs derive their vigor and life.

5. The spine is but a continuation of the brain all down the back, and from this centre all the nerves that supply the muscles with life and animation are derived; and the power of locomotion is promoted by this apparatus, and the power of standing, walking, or running, is also promoted by it.

6. The skin also is endowed from the nerves with the sense of touch. Therefore it is plain that the nervous system is the source from whence we derive the senses of sight, hearing, smell, taste and touch; that it is the

power that makes the muscles act, and sets the limbs in motion; that enables us to walk, work with the hands, &c.; that causes the digestive organs to digest our food, or that causes the lungs to breathe, the heart to beat, the liver to secrete the bile and purify the blood, that causes the kidneys to perform their office. The nervous system is so perfectly present in the whole body, that if all the rest of the material of which the body is composed were abstracted, still the human shape would not be destroyed.

It must be perceived from this account of the nerves, that any violence done to them, will derange the system very much. Any disease in the nervous system cuts off the supply of healthy nervous force from the body. If the optic nerve is diseased, the sense of sight is impaired; if the olfactory, the sense of smell; if the nerves that supply the stomach,—as a matter of course, the stomach is diseased; and so with every organ and function of the body.

An insight into diseases of the nervous system, will constitute a valuable piece of information, and a chapter will be devoted to the special consideration of them.

There are other organs and apparatus that might be remarked upon concisely, but it is not in accordance with the plan of this work to give anything more than a mere outline of the organs and their functions, that the range of diseases might be better comprehended. Those who would like a farther insight into these matters, will find themselves amply repaid by perusing Esreys' Anatomy and Physiology, for sale by Rademacher & Sheek.

7.—Temperaments.

As occasionally certain temperaments will be referred to in detailing the treatment of disease, it is proper to define what is meant by temperament.

1. By temperament is meant the modification or influence that any one of the class of organs or humors may exert, when it predominates in the system. Thus, when the blood-vessels are of large capacity, and the quantity of blood so great in the system as to show its modifying influence upon all the other parts of the body, it is called the *sanguine temperament.* When the biliary organs predominate, the subject is of the *bilious temperament.* When the nervous system predominates, it is termed the *nervous temperament.* When the lymphatic system predominates, it is termed the *lymphatic temperament.* We will proceed to explain each as follows :—

1. *Sanguine temperament.*—This may be known by the great activity of the circulation, with rather a full habit, florid complexion, blue eyes, red, auburn, or yellowish red hair, great activity of mind and body, somewhat restless and fond of change.

2. *Bilious temperament.*—This may be known by great firmness of the flesh, black hair, dark eyes, dark skin, sometimes of a yellow appearance, moderately full habit; a determined expression of the countenance, indicating firmness and energy of character, violent and lasting ill-will, when crossed ; strong pulse, of moderate frequency; not easily turned aside from any undertaking.

Nervous temperament.—This is indicated by the predominant activity of the brain and entire nervous system ; fine hair, thin skin, small muscular frame, rapid speech and walk, quick of decision, and somewhat changeable; head rather large, in proportion to the rest of the frame; hasty movements, and of quick perception and judgment.

Lymphátic temperament is indicated by softness of the muscular system, inactive brain, slow movement, an abundance of fatty substance throughout the entire body, fair hair, pale skin, sluggish expression of the countenance, dull and inanimate expression of the eyes, quiet, and prone to lazy habits, and the circulation is correspondingly of a sluggish character.

Besides these *temperaments*, others have been noted, which do not appear to be pure, but of a mixed character, as

Melancholic temperament.—We see persons having all the characteristics of the bilious; black hair, dark eyes and complexion. Though less active in body and mind, of a very grave disposition, suspicious, wearing what is commonly called a *long face*, and very meditative. These persons may be said to be of the melancholic temperament, and they are perpetually subject to derangement of the biliary system, prone to constipation of the bowels, feeble pulse, of a wiry slow beat, and a dry skin.

Other forms of mixed temperaments are very frequently found, indeed, it may be said that temperaments are oftener found of a mixed character than pure.

There is the *nervous-sanguine*, which partakes of the character of the two, as expressed in the term.

The *lymphatic-sanguine*, characterised by a robust constitution, sometimes termed *nutritive*, because the subjects are fond of good living, and care but little about anything aside from the gratification of the appetite. Such persons, appear to be characterised by selfishness, conceit, are sanguine that they can perform a great deal, but have so little perseverance, that frequently nothing is accomplished.

The *nervous lymphatic* is indicated by large brain, and at the same time an abundance of the fatty material; somewhat active, easily fatigued, and prone to seek long intervals of rest.

The *nervous-bilious* is indicated by large brain, active nervous system, with all the other indications of the pure bilious.

There are other mixtures of the temperaments; we have only named the more frequent and prominent, but, in a practical point of view, other terms, distinguishing the variety of habits or constitutions, are preferable, as follows :—

Debilitated constitution, is one characterised by feebleness of frame, capable of but little physical endurance.

Plethoric constitution, is indicated by corpulence, full, hale and hearty appearance.

Lean habit as the term implies, denotes the reverse of the plethoric.

In the same manner, we make use of terms to express the predominant moral characteristics, as

Melancholly disposition, *mild disposition*, sensitive, &c., as indicating that, which is prominent in the character.

The practical utility of becoming familiar with the classification of temperaments, habits and dispositions, is with reference to the adaptation of remedies in cases of sickness. Remedies adapted to the sanguine temperament are not always adapted to the bilious, &c.

And remedies well suited to persons of a *mild* disposition, are often found less serviceable to those more *passionate and irritable.*

Medicines that act speedily upon persons of a full habit, are often found inactive upon those of spare and lean habit, even if the indications for their use in both cases are otherwise the same. The following chapter upon medicines, will contain an account of the remedies best adapted to *the different* temperaments, habits and dispositions, so arranged as to facilitate reference.

CHAPTER III.

1.—List of remedies ; principle of applying them, &c.

THE following list, comprises all the medicines used in this work. It is remarked that every medicine has a certain range of action in the body. Some will act upon one kind of organs in a peculiar way, and some on others;—or some medicines will always direct their energies to one locality, and others to another, therefore, it must first be ascertained, how a remedy will effect the healthy system, and this will determine the locality of its action, or in other words, it will manifest the symptoms of its effect; it is a record of these symptoms that gives us an idea of the range of a medicine.

In the following list, we shall only place such medicines as have been thus tried, and their range of use ascertained. In the concluding chapter of this work, will be found a concise statement of the range of use of each medicine.

List of remedies.

1. Aconitum napellus,	27. Digitalis purpurea,	53. Petroleum,
2. Alumina,	28. Drosera rotundifolia.	54. Phosphorus,
3. Ammonium carb.,	29. Dulcamara,	55. Phosphoric acid,
4. Antimonium crud.,	30. Eupatorium,	56. Platina,
5. Apis melifica,	31. Euphrasia off.	57. Pulsatilla,
6. Arnica montana,	32. Ferrum metallicum,	58. Rheum,
7. Arsenicum album,	33. Graphites,	59. Rhus toxicodendron,
8. Aurum metallicum,	34. Helleborus,	60. Ruta graveolens,
9. Belladonna,	35. Hepar sulph. calc.,	61. Sabina,
10. Bromine,	36. Hyoscyamus niger,	62. Sambucus nigra
11. Bryonia alba,	37. Hamamelis,	63. Sanguinaria.
12. Calcarea carb.	38. Ignatia amara,	64. Secale cornutum,
13. Cannabis sativa,	39. Iodine,	65. Senega,
14. Cantharis,	40. Ipecacuanha,	66. Sepia succus,
15. Carbo vegetabilis,	41. Kali carbonicum,	67. Silicea,
16. Causticum,	42. Kali bichromicum,	68. Spigelia anthelmin.,
17. Chamomilla,	43. Lachesis,	69. Spongia marina tosta,
18. China officinalis,	44. Lycopodium,	70. Stannum,
19. Cina,	45. Mercurius subl. corr.,	71. Staphysagria,
20. Cocculus,	46. Mercurius vivus,	72. Stramonium,
21. Coffea cruda,	47. Mezereum,	73. Sulphur.
22. Colchicum,	48. Moschus,	74. Sulphuric acid,
23. Colocynthis,	49. Natrum muriaticum,	75. Tartarus emeticus,
24. Conium maculatum,	50. Nitric acid,	76. Uva ursi,
25. Crocus sativus,	51. Nux vomica,	77. Veratrum album,
26. Cuprum metallicum,	52. Opium,	78. Zincum metallicum.

Tinctures for External Use.

79. Arnica,	82. Causticum,	85. Staphysagria,
80. Calendula,	83. Hypericum,	86. Urtica urens,
81. Cantharis,	84. Ruta graveolens,	

2.—Medicines the best adapted to the different temperaments, habits, &c.

1. *For the sanguine temperament.*—Acon., Arn., Bell., Bry., Calc., Hep., Merc., Cham., Nux v., Phos., &c.

2. *Bilious temperament.*—Bry., Nux v., Ars., Sulph., Merc., Cocculus, &c.

3. *Nervous temperament.*—Sepia, Coff., Platina, Ignatia, Puls., Nux v., Cham., &c.

4. *Lymphatic temperament.*—Ant., Arn., Ars., Nit acid., Calc., Puls., Sulph., Con., Clematis.

5. *Melancholic temperament.*—Aurum, Ars., Nux v., Verat., Ipec., Chin., &c.

6. *For plethoric habit.*—Acon., Bell., Calc., Puls., Merc., Sep., &c.

7. *Debilitated habit.*—Ars., Chin., Bry., Lachesis, Arn.

8. *Lean habit.*—Sil., Lach., Graph.

9. *Melancholy disposition.*—Ars., Verat., Aurum., Puls., Acon., Bry.

10. *Mild disposition.*—Puls., Sep., Calc., Ignat.

11. *Sensitive disposition.*—Calc., Ignat., Plat., Bell., Bry., Graphites.

NOTE.—The above affords only a partial view of the distribution of remedies according to temperaments, habits, &c.; reference will be had more fully to the subject, in detailing the treatment of specific diseases, in the following chapters.

CHAPTER IV.

OBSERVATIONS ON THE METHOD OF NOTING DISEASES.

IN order to determine upon the appropriate administration of remedies, it is necessary to ascertain correctly, the condition of the patient and the nature of his malady. It is, therefore, requisite to observe certain regulations that will tend to consummate the object.

1. In learning the character of disease, the first thing requisite is, to know the general condition of the patient—the constitution and temperament—and if practicable, it would be well to ascertain the hereditary constitutional character.

6

2. After noting the sex, age, and whatever is individually peculiar to the patient, inquire into the relative state of the secretions, and into the circumstances by which they become modified; and then for the part *most* affected,—whether of long standing, or of recent date;—and also inquire into the general habits, occupation, mode of living, diet, and other influences to which the patient has been exposed.

1.—Examination of Patients.

1. If a patient possess a full habit of body—an active circulation, great animation and energy when in health, florid complexion, full frame, and general appearance of being warm, ardent and active, we recognise a *plethoric or sanguine constitution*, and one peculiarly subject to inflammatory influences, and predisposed to local inflammatory difficulties. Proceeding then, from this consideration, an inquiry for the affected parts, will next be in order, and wherever an extreme local suffering is manifest, an inflammation or congestion may be apprehended, and the treatment may be directed accordingly.

2. If on the other hand, a patient possesses a *feeble constitution*, unable to bear exertion; if the breath is easily exhausted by rapid motion, or there appears to be deficiency of warmth and animation in the system; it is not difficult to infer a retarded performance of the bodily functions, and such a patient would be liable to diseases of a torpid character. The digestion might be difficult, the circulation feeble, the liver inactive, or there might be alternations of condition in the secretory organs, varying from excess to deficiency. In making further inquiry into any specific ailment, it is of course necessary to bear the tendency of the constitution in mind.

3. When the liver is the most susceptible of any organ of the body, the skin will often wear a yellow tinge, and almost any exposure will contribute to biliary derangement, with numerous concomitant symptoms. Persons of this habit, generally have dark skin, and are subject to dark colored urine and stools, and a wiry pulse ; costiveness and piles, or else diarrhœa and prostration, affect the *bilious constitution* more readily, perhaps, than other difficulties.

4. When a person of short neck, high shoulders, thick set, or full frame, subject to flushes of blood to the brain, comes under our notice, we cannot avoid recognising *an apoplectic subject.*

5. And also we recognise a *nervous constitution*, when we come in contact with a person whose body and mind are prone to be excitable ;—whose ideas, habits, or inclinations, are extremely variable ; with such, the pulse is also variable, and purely nervous difficulties may assume every variety of form; the slightest touch may prove sufficient to aggravate suffering, almost beyond endurance, and spasmodic affections and fits may occur, which cannot be referred to any definite cause.

6. Were a patient of firm, wiry muscles and tendons, swarthy complexion, sharp set features, searching glance, persistent expression of the countenance, to be presented for treatment, there would be no difficulty in recognising a *fibrous constitution*, and the distinct, wiry pulse, the deficiency of flesh, the want of perspiration, the scanty urine and hard stools, that under other circumstances, might indicate disease, are viewed only, as the characteristics of this kind of constitution. But a patient of this description is prone to inflammatory affections, more particularly of the intestines. Yet also, any other disease

may befal this constitution, as a consequence of super-abundant activity.

7. On the other hand, we find opposed to the fibrous constitution, a *lax* or *lymphatic constitution*, characterised by a fleshy, flabby appearance. Not lean, but fat; not active, but dull; fair skin, rounded frame, the whole appearance lazy, as if all the muscles and tendons were relaxed or unstrung. Such an individual is subject to chilly sensations, because sensitive to cold. Such a normal condition, is sufficient to impart to every disease a sluggish character: hence, in such, we are more apt to find *chronic difficulties*, as persistent in their features, as the constitution is slow of action.

8. It is always well, to know something of a patient's *hereditary constitution*. This can only be ascertained by reference to the antecedents of the family. If he is of scrofulous or consumptive parents, whatever afflicts him may strongly tend in this direction,—and even a gouty or psoric diathesis may be inherited from parents. Therefore, in the treatment of such maladies as may afflict a patient of the kind, reference must be had to the restraining or counteracting of the hereditary tendency.

9. The investigation of disease in a *psoric constitution*, would lead us to perceive that almost every form would be strongly attracted to the skin,—and every acute malady would be preceded or followed by general foulness of the skin, ulcerative sores, &c.

10. *Persons of a consumptive habit*, which is easily determined by the clear transparent skin, bright flush spot on the cheeks, especially on the left cheek, flatness of the chest, &c., are especially subject to complications affecting the lungs, from every inflammatory or irritative process. The treatment of this class of patients must

also be with reference to restraining or subduing the consumptive diathesis.

11. By reference to what is remarked on the temperaments at the conclusion of Chapter II., it will be seen that patients are subject to an infinity of peculiarities, usually associated with the peculiar habits and constitution of the body, which must be taken into account, in forming a correct estimate of disease. Whatever the natural condition is, must be regarded the standard by which to measure the extent of any departure caused by disease.

12. In prescribing for the sick, it is requisite to note the obvious peculiarities of each sex. The male, in general, is not so sensitive as the female,—he possesses more strength, vigor and energy, and disease, of course, may be viewed in comparison with what is regarded the natural characteristics. It is obviously impossible for a weaker frame to endure so much as a stronger.

13. Human life has been divided into five distinct periods, viz: 1st. Infancy. 2d. Infancy. 3d. Adolescence. 4th. Virility. 5th. Old-age. Each of these periods is marked by peculiar characteristics, that exert a modifying influence upon disease. The first period extending from birth to the age of seven years, is marked by great tenderness and excitability, consequently alive to any irritation produced by teething or other slight causes.— The second period, is from seven to fourteen years, and may also be regarded a period of life, somewhat subject to disease, in consequence of second dentition and other natural changes taking place in the system. Until the completion of the second period, but very little can be predicated of the difference between the sexes; both require nearly the same physical or medical treatment,

6*

because both are subject to similar natural influences. But on the approach of the *third period*, those natural developments appear, that mark the wide difference between the physical character of the two sexes. This period is a growing period,—the functions become more fully established, and the whole frame acquires vigor, in proportion as the constitution is good. It may be remarked of this period, which may terminate at about the age of twenty-one years, that constitutional peculiarities will begin to show themselves; latent hereditary difficulties will very likely begin to be disclosed, and this would indicate the particular care that should be exercised, in striving to modify or overcome any constitutional defects; for it may safely be remarked, that these defects must be overcome during this period, if controlled at all. The *fourth period*, may be regarded as one of vigorous maturity of both sexes, if the constitution be good, when all the functions are well established. The *fifth*, is the period of *old age*, when, according to the course of nature, some of the functions cease, and the whole frame begins to decline. This period usually begins at an earlier period of life with the female than with the male. There are diseases incident to each of these periods of life, and many are the ailments common to the approach of old age, that require peculiar hygienic and medical treatment.

14. The importance of taking into consideration the natural constitution, age, sex and temperament of the patient, cannot fail of being recognised, when an effort is made to investigate the nature and character of disease. Having premised this, we will proceed to the second consideration in the examination of patients.

2.—The Special Examination of Disease.

For the purpose of adapting homœopathic treatment, it is necessary to become acquainted with the character-istics of disease, and we can only acquire this knowledge, by strict attention to the following rules:

1. Make particular inquiries in relation to the general, specific, or local causes of any disease.

2. Observe the general character of the disease, whether it be febrile or otherwise.

3. Note carefully the symptoms of the disease.—Observe the condition of the PULSE,—its varities and indications.

4. Note the discharges generally.

5. Examine the condition of the mouth and tongue and the digestive system.

6. Observe the character of the respiration.

7. Note the condition of the brain, and the nervous system in general.

By observing the above rules, there will be no difficulty in forming a tolerably correct idea of the nature and extent of disease, provided there is a correct interpretation of facts. That a more definite idea may be had, an illustration will be given of what is meant by "a correct interpretation of facts."

1. If in the examination of a patient, we elicit the fact that he is afflicted with a constitutional infirmity, inherited from the antecedents of his family, it is safe to suppose, that this alone may be the cause of seasons of acute suffering,

2. If the fact be elicited that a patient has become sick about the same time that many others in the same region of country have become so, it is perfectly safe to regard the malady as *endemic ;*—that some evil influence

in the atmosphere is operating to impress disease upon all who are in an impressible condition.

3. If facts are elicited of patients becoming afflicted from over exercise, or exposure to cold, or damp weather, we must interpret them, so as to form a definite idea, of the difficulty to be overcome.

4. It is by reference to the PULSE in connection with the various manifestations of disease, that we are able to judge correctly of its character. When the nerves are the seat of pain, the pulse is not much accelerated; but when the muscles are in pain, the pulse *is* accelerated, often, in a very marked degree. It will be seen, then, that pain is not the criterion to be governed by, but the pulse in connection with the pain.

5. *Of the urine.* This secretion is regarded indicative of health, when it is clear and of the color of amber, or of a pale, or brightest yellow; and if it precipitates no sediment after standing; and is devoid of all loathsome odor. The best time to examine urine, is about six hours after a meal.

6. The urine in fevers changes its character, at each stage of the disease; at first it is clear, but after the fever has passed its crisis, it is commonly cloudy, and forms a cloud which appears to float in the *chamber*.

7. At the crisis of a fever, the urine precipitates a sediment, which is, for the most part, a favorable indication.

8. If the *urine* be of a very dark color, it indicates a putrid condition; if it be yellow, or red, it is the usual characteristic of an intermittent type of disease, or something of inflammatory rheumatism; if white and gritty, it indicates some concrete substance in the canal; if irregular or disturbed, of a purple color, and muddy, it is an indication of bad health.

9. If the urine be red, when the pulse is accelerated, there is unmistakable signs of inflammatory action. If of a deep yellow hue, accompanied with fever and yellowness of the skin, it indicates jaundice; if the urine be black, or nearly so, with much sediment, it indicates the presence of gangrene, or a near approach to it in the system.

10. If the urine is bloody, turbid, and thick, with much sediment, a dropsical condition of the system may be inferred, because there is evident signs of the decomposition of the blood. If milky, as is sometimes the case, in children, it indicates worms; if it be thick, but pale, and often changeable during a fever, we have reason to decide upon the character of the fever, as being nervous; if clear, transparent, and watery, and a continual urging to pass it, the nature of the affection is spasmodic; if it be bloody or slimy, we may infer inflammation of the kidneys, or catarrh of the bladder.

11. If the discharge of urine be involuntary, it indicates a local paralysis, and is a serious manifestation in fevers; if the reverse condition, or difficult, painful, or impeded discharge, the indication represents some local inflammatory, or spasmodic difficulty.

12. A copious perspiration will diminish the quantity of urine, and so will a watery diarrhœa.

13. *Of the Stools.*—Constipation of the bowels, or deficient stools, indicate a febrile condition of the system, or torpidity of the bowels; very dark stools indicate a profuse quantity of bile; very light colored stools indicate a deficiency of bile, and a torpid condition of the liver.

14. Copious and relaxed stools indicate nervous irritability of the intestines, or an inflammatory condition of them. If greenish, they indicate griping or acidity, as in the case of infants.

15. The stools are sometimes *urgent* and *spontaneous* when the contents of the bowels are liquid; when they are purely involuntary, they indicate paralysis of the intestines, and usually occur in the last stage of postrating typhoid fevers.

16. Dysenteric stools are accompanied with straining or tenesmus, and are usually mixed with bloody mucus, and sometimes of pure blood.

17. *Of Flatulency.*—Wind may accumulate in the stomach, from various causes; sometimes it results from bad digestion; sometimes it indicates worms in children, when the belly is distended; and in some fevers it imparts a drum-like distension of the bowels, which is painful to the touch.

18. *Indications of nausea and vomiting.*—Habitual nausea and vomiting indicate an organic derangement of the stomach. If food and drink are vomited up as soon as swallowed, it indicates inflammation of the organ. If vomiting is preceded by pain in the stomach, it indicates indigestion, especially if the stomach is relieved by the act. If vomiting is preceded by intense pain in the head, it may be sympathetic; if by severe pain in the right side, accompanied by cramps, it may indicate inflammation of the liver. Cramp, and habitual vomiting in the morning, may indicate *gravel.*

19. Vomiting may result from sympathy with the brain, or with diseased conditions of the womb, or with inflammation of the kidneys, or intestines, in which event there is a continuance, and obstinate constipation of the bowels.

20. *The appetite.*—In acute febrile diseases, the appetite is usually suspended; weakness of the power of digestion or any organic derangement of the stomach,

may occasion loss of appetite. Over-charging 'the stomach with food and drink, may so derange and injure the organ as to create entire loss of appetite. Sudden emotions of joy or grief may take away the appetite for a time.

Certain morbid conditions of the system may give rise to a ravenous appetite, and then the patient may crave food, not because ·the system requires it, but because some morbid difficulty stimulates his appetite.

The old domestic saying, that a patient must or ought to be allowed what the appetite craves, in sickness, is entirely false; for the appetite when in a morbid state may crave the most deleterious kinds of food, not because it is adapted to the nourishment of the system, but because it accords with the morbid fancy and appetite of the individual.

The state of the appetite is not always indicative of the health; for there are some severe maladies which do not impair the appetite at all. In *rheumatic fever* it may not be impaired. Neither is it in *hectic fever;* yet it may be variable in both of these diseases, on the account of other qualifying circumstances.

21. In most all cases of fever, the subjects complain of *thirst.* It is, therefore, probable, that a continual thirst indicates some febrile or inflammatory difficulty. But as dryness of the mouth and throat may result from other influence than fevers, it is necessary to exercise care in discriminating between that, indicating a want of the system when in health, and that which indicates a diseased constitution.

22. The *kind of thirst* which merely indicates a healthy demand for some diluent drink, is but the provision of nature, suggestive of what the body needs

to compensate for the natural absorption of fluids constantly going on in the body, or for the loss of fluids
constantly thrown off from the body by perspiration and
the urinary secretion.

23. The *kind of thirst* which takes place without
reference to compensation for natural losses, accompanied with increased heat and dryness of the skin,
furred tongue and accelerated pulse, may be regarded an
indication of FEVER. If very *intense* and *insatiable*, with
frequent and tense pulse, the FEVER is of an inflammatory character, and the thirst results from the deficiency
of the watery constituents of the blood.

24. An acid condition of the stomach may give rise
to *thirst*, and under such circumstances it will be accompanied by acrid risings, &c.

25. Certain spasmodic difficulties may give rise to
thirst even though no fever is manifest, but rather a
coldness.

26. Next in importance are the *indications* of disease
which the TONGUE affords. Many are the conditions in
which the tongue is found.

When thickly furred with dirty or brownish white,
and moist, with no other indication of derangement, it
may be inferred to be recent and principally confined to
the lining membrane of the mouth, and easily removed.

When coated with slimy matter, leaving the tip and
edges of the tongue red, it still indicates an affection of the
lining membrane, but less favorable and more enduring
in its character.

A yellow coat upon the tongue indicates derangement
of the biliary organs; a naturally moist and clean red
tongue, with an unnatural prominence of the pappillæ,
indicates a recent derangement of the stomach, affecting

its nerves; but if the tongue be swollen and slightly furred with white, it indicates a nervous derangement of the digestive organs and a sympathetic action upon the brain. *A dry, red and glassy tongue*, indicates somewhat of a chronic derangement affecting the nerves of the stomach.

When the tongue is swollen, furrowed or cracked, it indicates a *severe* derangement of the nerves of the stomach.

When the tongue is coated with a bright white, with the edges and tip red and swollen withal, it indicates a diseased condition of the mucus coat and nerves of the stomach, of an obstinate character, and long standing. A condition that reacts upon the brain, and often attended with great despondency and depression of spirits.

A *dark colored coating* upon the tongue, with dry streak in the middle, and tremulous, or paralytic, indicates a severe form of low fever, either a putrid abdominal, or typhus.

The appearance which the tongue presents is always to be associated with other symptoms in determining what it indicates.

27. VARIOUS KINDS OF COUGH.—Coughs, in general, indicate some irritation of the lining membrane of the respiratory organs. This irritation may be of two kinds : it may have its seat in the respiratory organs themselves, or these organs may become sympathetically affected from the irritation of other organs.

If produced from indigestion and derangement of the liver, it can only be removed by overcoming these difficulties.

A short dry cough and sneezing are frequently the precursor of measles and other eruptive diseases.

An exceedingly painful hacking cough, accompanied with acute febrile symptoms, indicates some degree of inflammation of the lungs. A cough with profuse expectoration, indicates a bronchial disease, confined principally to the mucus membrane. When the cough is hard, whistling or crowing, it indicates incipient croup. When the cough appears to be *spasmodic* and comes on *in paroxysms*, without leaving any distinct marks of prostration, it indicates the *whooping cough*. When *deep* and *hollow*, attended with *emaciation and expectoration of purulent matter*, it indicates deep seated tubercular disease of the lungs.

Many persons have a predisposition to cough, from almost any exciting cause, and this condition indicates great feebleness of the pulmonary organs, and admonishes such patients to avoid as much as possible all kinds of exposure, beyond their power of endurance.

A cough with wheezing or whistling respiration, and difficulty of breathing, indicates the ASTHMA.

28. PERSPIRATION, AND THE SKIN.—In a state of health the skin is neither *moist or dry*, but of a moderate warmth, and agreeable to the touch, that is, if at rest, in a temperate climate. But *exercise* may induce perspiration which is of a healthy character; and *disease* may induce perspiration, which indicates morbid derangement of some of the organs. It may be the termination of some slight febrile disease that has first produced *dryness* of the skin. In this event it is but a favorable sequence, and only requires that it should be followed by great care to guard against exposure, &c., that no return of the disease may take place. *Sweating*, also, under certain circumstances, may take place without affording relief, indicating merely the progress of disease.

The *former takes* place at the crisis of a disease, and is followed by convalescence; but the latter occurs before the *crisis*, and always leaves the patient more prostrated and weighed down by the influence of the disease upon him. Of this latter kind may be mentioned,

Night or morming sweats, accompanying *hectic fever.*

, Offensive sweats, in typhus and typhoid fevers.

Sour sweats, accompanying miliary fever.

Sweating stage of the paroxysms of intermittent fevers.

Cold sweats, attending vital prostration.

Local sweats, indicating congestion to the part, as of the chest or head.

Debilitating sweats, such as occur from extreme debility of the system.

Wherever sweating occurs without affording relief, it is to be regarded merely as a symptom, associated with other indications of the presence of disease. The former kind of sweat which marks the crisis of disease, and is followed by convalescence, may be distinguished from the other by the general relief which it affords the system, and the subsidence of the irregularities of the pulse, and by its being warm, and leaving the skin when it subsides in a normal state of warmth, as in health. FEVERS frequently run from nine to fourteen days, and terminate favorably in this way.

29. THE COUNTENANCE.—A well-directed observation may often detect certain diseased conditions by the appearance of the countenance alone. The physiognomy of disease is in many respects worthy of attentive study, for not a few of the morbid derangements may be detected through this channel, as for instance,

An habitually *blue and livid countenance,* indicates organic disease of the heart.

A *sallow countenance,* usually indicates intestinal derangement.

A *yellow countenance,* and yellowness about the eyes, denotes jaundice.

A ˉred, *flushed countenance*, denotes rush of blood to the head.

Redness, or red spots upon the cheeks of a flushed appearance, denotes a hectic predisposition.

A sunken pallid countenance in children, denotes worm difficulties.

A white and cold appearance of the countenance, indicates green sickness in young females.

A *pale countenance, and livid spots* in persons advanced in life, may indicate an apoplectic predisposition.

In estimating any disease from the appearance of the countenance, reference must be had to the attendant symptoms and condition of the system in general.

29. OF THE PULSE, *and its indications.*—The usual rate of the pulse in healthy individuals, is somewhat variable according to temperament, habits, &c., as for instance:

The PULSE in children one year old, will beat from 110 to 120 per minute.
"   five years "   "   "   100 to 120   "
"   from ten to fourteen,   "   100 to 110   "
A youth   "   fourteen to twenty, "   95 to 105   "
The pulse of a healthy male adult in the prime of life, is from   70 to 80   "
"   of a healthy female adult in the prime life, is from   80 to 90   "

In advanced life, the pulse usually declines a little in frequency in both sexes;—and in all periods of life, the pulse of the female beats from 10 to 15 times more in a minute, than that of the male.

The healthy pulse may vary in the frequency of its beats, to correspond with the alternations of labor or exercise, and repose.

The healthy pulse, is regular, moderately full, of a soft and yielding beat.

An intermittent pulse, indicates great debility or disease of the heart.

A full, tense, jerking beat of the pulse, indicates aneurism near the heart.

A very rapid and violent pulse, indicates fever, (when the skin is warm.)

A rapid, weak pulse, indicates irritability from pulmonary disease.

A wiry pulse, indicates inflammation of some of the internal organs.

A slow and scarcely perceptible pulse, indicates a sluggish circulation.

A full, tense, and hard pulse, not much accelerated, may indicate the inflammatory stage of typhus fever.

A rapid, fluttering pulse, accompanied with vomiting, often indicates the approach of severe eruptive disease, such as *scarlet fever.*

Without associating the condition of the pulse with other conditions or symptoms, it cannot be relied upon, in determining the character of disease.

3.—Rules for the Administration and Repetition of Remedies.

1. In acute diseases, a remedy, if well chosen, may be repeated at intervals of one or two hours, until some amelioration or aggravation of the malady becomes manifest; in either case, it would be well to discontinue the remedy for awhile, to await the result.

2. If the aggravation is persistent without reaction, there is reason for change of remedy, and another should be chosen, according to indications.

3. If convalescence follow the administration of a remedy, it need not be repeated unless the patient ceases to improve before he is quite recovered ; and the same rule will apply, in cases of amelioration, after an aggravation of symptoms.

7*

4. When the improvement in a patient becomes inter-rupted, without a change of symptoms, recourse may be had to the same remedy as at first ; but if such arrest is accompanied by a development of other symptoms, a more appropriate remedy must be sought for.

5. In obstinate cases, a change of remedy is admissable, when the continuance of one, has been so long as to ren-der its action doubtful.

6. In chronic cases, a well-chosen remedy need not be repeated oftener than once in one, two, or three days.

7. In the selection of a remedy, great care should be exercised, that no symptoms of the disease should be uncovered by the characteristic symptoms of the remedy.

4.—The Form of Medicines Designed for Domestic Use.

The only forms, in which homœopathic medicines are prepared, may be comprised under the head of tinctures, triturations, dilutions, and globules. The two last, are the only forms requisite for general use, the two former being only the primary or preparatory stages of the two latter. Therefore, either the *dilutions*, or *globules* saturated with them, are the only forms of medicines accompany-ing this work.

When either of the forms is administered in water, contained in a tumbler or other open vessel, it should be well covered between the periods of administration, and kept in a dark place, away from any corrupting odor ;— and all other medicines, teas or odors, are strictly pro-hibited during its administration. External applica-tions of anything in the form of poultices, washes, lotions, such as camphor, liniments, cologne, mustard-plasters, medicated poultices, onions, burdocks, or anything con-taining any medicinal property whatever, must be strictly avoided when taking the medicine.

5.—Of Preserving the Purity of Medicines.

1. The medicines should be kept in a chest constructed for the purpose.

2. The chest should be kept closed, and in a cool place, or if in a warm climate, as much so as possible.

3. In uncorking a vial, be careful to replace the identical cork, or a new one, if the first should get broken or unfit for use.

4. Do not change the corks of different remedies, nor put medicine of one kind, into a phial that has contained another kind.

5. It is better to destroy empty phials, than to put any medicine in them, other than that which they originally contained.

6. Every medicine should be carefully labelled or numbered.

7. Do not prepare a solution without first being assured that the glass and spoon are perfectly clean; and if it be necessary to prepare two at a time, use separate spoons for each, and be careful to keep them apart.

6.—Antidotes, and Changing Medicines.

When any medicine produces aggravation of suffering, that cannot well be endured by the patient, the administration of one drop of camphor in a spoonful of water, will generally antidote its effect. And when it is thought requisite to change a remedy, avoid doing it suddenly. A period from two, to four or six hours should elapse, before a remedy should follow one that has been given; a teaspoonful of coffee, or a few drops of wine, may also be employed as antidotes to an unfavorable medicinal action.

7.—External Applications.

When it is desired to hasten suppuration, a piece of lint *saturated with cold water*, and kept constantly moist, with a dry bandage on the outside, so as to exclude the air, will be found one of the simplest and best applica-tions that can be used.

It is doubtful whether cold applications to local irritations or tension of parts, are of any use; warm applications, either of warm water or non-medicinal fomentations are better, as they may palliate suffering during the administration of internal remedies. Cold applications to the head, to counteract heat in that region, more frequently prove injurious than beneficial. Mode-rately hot water, applied by means of saturating a flannel, is by far the most preferable.

The same remedies, prescribed internally for local affections, may be applied externally as a lotion, by dis-solving them in water, and applying them to the affected part.

8.—Remedies suitable to follow others.

8. In the treatment of diseases, it has been observed that some remedies act very beneficially, after others have been employed, and the following list may be referred to as a partial guide;—only, let it be understood, that the remedy must be selected, homœopathic to the case.

ACONITUM NAPELLUS, may be often followed by Calc., Petr., Puls., Sulph.

ALUMINA, by Bryonia if indicated.

ANTIMONIUM CRUD., by Puls. and Merc., if either appear to be indicated.

ARNICA MONT., by Acon., Ipec., Rhus., Sulph., &c., if either be indicated.

ARSENICUM ALBUM, by Chin., Ipec., Nux vom., Sulph., Verat., if specifi-cally indicated.

BELLADONNA, by Chin., Ipec., Hep., Rhus. and Seneg.,—either if indicated.

BRYONIA, by Alum. and Rhus,—according to indication.

CALC. CARB., by Lyc., Sil., Phos., and Nit. ac., provided any one of them
    is indicated.
CARBO. VEG., by Ars. and Merc., according to indication.
CHINA OFF., by Ars., Verat., and Puls., if suitable.
CUPRUM MET., by Calc. and Verat.,   "
HEP. SULPH., by Bell., Merc., and Spong. "
IPEC., by Am., Ars., Chin., and Nux.,   "
LACHESIS, by Alum., Ars., Bell, Con., and Nux vom., if suitable.
LYCOPODIUM, by Graph., Phos., and Sil.,   "
MERCURIUS, by Bell., Dulc., Puls., and Sil.   "
NUX VOM., by Bry., Puls., and Sulph.,
OPIUM, by Calc., Petr., and Puls.,
PHOSPHOR., by Petr., Rhus., and Sulph.,
PULSATILLA, by Asa., Bryon., and Sep.,
RHUS TOX., by Ars., Bry., Calc., Con.,
SEPIA SUC., by Carbo v., and Sulph.,
SILICEA, by Hep., Lach., Lyc. and Sep.,
SPONGIA, by Hep. Sulph.,
SULPHUR, by Acon., Bell., Calc., and Puls.,
TART. EMETIC, Ipec., Puls. and Sep.,   "
VERATRUM ALBUM, by Ars., Am., Chin., Cuprum, and Ipec., if suitable.

CHAPTER V.

DISEASES INVOLVING THE VARIOUS ORGANS AND THEIR TREATMENT

1.—Fevers.—(*Febres.*)

FEVERS in general, are characterised by chilliness and
heat, functional disturbance, acceleration of the pulse,
thirst, restlessness, and prostration; there are a variety of
disturbances produced by fever, as many organs are
involved;—sometimes, there is intense action of the
blood-vessels,—sometimes, serious disturbance of the
nerves,—sometimes, bilious derangement,—and some-

times, severe prostration of all the powers. The different kinds of fevers, are owing to differences of character in the tissues of the organs involved. Thus, a simple inflammatory fever is characterised by intense heat, rapid pulse, &c., because the *arterial excitement* is great, and the nerves are only implicated in a secondary degree. But a nervous fever may be characterised by great prostration, dulness of the senses, and stupefaction, without much alteration in the pulse, because the *nerves* are the most implicated, and the blood *vessels* or *arteries*, only in a secondary degree. Sometimes the inflammatory, after exhausting the system, may merge into the nervous or typhus.

A simple fever by being neglected, or by improper treatment, may assume the inflammatory form, and this again may assume some other form, thus one attack may ssume a variety of forms.

A simple fever may come on and run a fortunate course to its height, and then decline as it came on.

Nearly all fevers are preceded by what is termed a cold stage, succeeded by a hot stage, which increases to a crisis, then decreases, and convalescence follows, if they terminate favorably. Thus, there are five stages: the *commencement, increase, crisis, decrease, convalescence.* When the result is fatal, some important part becomes the seat of disorganisation during the progress of the fever, or the vital energy of the patient becomes exhausted by its intensity.

The value of homœopathic treatment in fevers, consists in the power the remedies can exert over the disease, to shorten the duration of the several stages, and to ameliorate the sufferings of the patient, and in hastening ✝he crisis.

Sometimes the crisis is manifested by perspiration sometimes by diarrhœa, sometimes by alteration of the secretions, either in quantity or quality, sometimes by the appearance of an eruption, and sometimes by hemorrhage from the bowels; after which, if the crisis brings about a reaction in favor of convalescence, the skin becomes moist, and the pulse becomes natural, as in health.

Although the treatment of all varieties of fever must be in accordance with the peculiar symptoms manifest in each individual case, yet to avoid confusion, it is proper to adopt a general classification.

1. Fevers that arise without any obvious local cause in the system.

2. Fevers that are dependant upon local irritation.

The first class we shall arrange for consideration as follows :—

1. Simple fever,   4. Bilious or gastric fevers,
2. Inflammatory fever,   5. Intermittent fevers,
3. Typh'd and typh's fevers, 6. Eruptive fevers.

This arrangement is for the sake of convenience merely, as no fever can be treated by its name. Every attack of fever presents peculiar features, and is to be looked at as it presents itself—an individual affection, having no necessary connection with any generalisation, and to be treated according to the nature of its symptoms.

2.—Conditions of treatment in fevers.

1. A patient suffering from fever must be at rest in body and mind.

2. The apartment of the patient should be well ventilated, and of a medium temperature.

3. The patient's bed should be a hair, or other kind of mattrass, when practicable, and the bed clothes should be only sufficient.

4. The drink should be water.

5. Abstinence from all kinds of food when the fever runs high, is a condition proclaimed by the voice of nature herself.

6. When the fever is somewhat abated, toast-water, weak barley or rice water, flavored with raspberry syrup or orange, may be allowed in great moderation, but even the use of these must be with great care, not to provoke a relapse. The wholesome fruits enumerated in the diet table, are very generally allowable in fevers unattended with diarrhœa.

7. Drinks ought to be given frequently and in small quantities.

1.—Simple Fever.

This is usually an ephemeral disease, but as it often is the precursor of more serious disorders, it requires attention.

SYMPTOMS.—Shivering succeeded by heat, thirst, general uneasiness, accelerated pulse and some degree of prostration, terminating in profuse perspiration.

TREATMENT.*—When it cannot be traced to any particular cause, and particularly when the skin is hot and dry, *Aconitum* should be prescribed, and if it should be simple fever, this remedy will speedily dissipate the symptoms; but if it be the precursor of eruptive diseases, or typhus, the Aconite will still be the remedy as indi-

* In the administration of a remedy it is not necessary that all the symptoms that call for its use should be present; it is sufficient if some of the more prominent and unmistakable ones only are present.

cated by the symptoms; and it will tend very materially to modify the malignity of the succeeding disease.

DOSE.—Dissolve a drop or four globules in half a tumbler of water, and give a teaspoonful every two hours, until the skin becomes moist, and the pulse begins to diminish in frequency, which result will take place in a few hours.

2.—Inflammatory Fever.

SYMPTOMS.—This fever commences with a chill of some duration followed by burning heat, strong, hard and accelerated pulse, dry skin, and dryness of the mouth, lips, and tongue, white coating upon the tongue, or of a bright red appearance, intense thirst, urine red and scanty, constipation, hurried breathing. As the pulse assumes a more regular condition many of the symptoms disappear. It runs its course in about fourteen days, progressing rapidly to a crisis, which may show itself by bleeding at the nose, or diarrhœa, or by profuse perspiration. Under homœopathic treatment, the natural duration of the disease is abridged, and the perfect crisis takes place at a much earlier period. This disease easily merges into the typhoid or typhus, from improper or careless treatment, or it may fall upon some important organ.

CAUSE.—Sudden check of perspiration, exposure to damp, wet, or piercing winds; intense mental emotions, high living, local inflammation, or mismanaged febrile attacks.

Those of a sanguine temperament or plethoric habit, are particularly subject to this fever, previous to the age of thirty-five years.

It has been regarded a kind of fever that requires the most vigorous treatment, and the allopathic physicians have hitherto resorted to bleeding and saline purgatives

8

at a very early stage. But this course has often rendered the system less able to bear the disease than before, and as a consequence the result has been unfavorable. Inflammatory continued fever not unfrequently becomes complicated with cerebral disturbances, and the reducing treatment, so far from being a barrier against this, often paves the way for, and renders such a complication more certain.

TREATMENT.—It is at once evident that the most successful treatment of this disease would be that which will most successfully allay the arterial excitement. Aconitum is the remedy, the most likely to produce the desired effect, if the group of symptoms resemble those detailed, as marking the character of the disease.

DOSE.—Dissolve two drops or six globules in six tablespoonfuls of water, and give a spoonful every three hours, until a change for the better is noted in the pulse and skin, and then at intervals of six hours, until amelioration or convalescence becomes established.

This disease is frequently attended with delirium, chiefly at night, and unless there is a threatening of inflammation of the brain, Aconite will prove the only remedy needed. But if inflammation of the brain becomes apparent, or in any degree threatened, *Belladonna* must be called into requisition. This remedy is especially useful after the previous use of *Aconite.*

Belladonna may be prescribed in an early stage of the disease when there is a strong tendency to the head, which is manifested by violent pain in the forehead, redness of the face, violent throbbing and distension of the arteries in the temples, sleeplessness at night, with furious delirium; red shining and fiery appearance of the eyes; and general heat throughout the body, with intense thirst.

DOSE.—Dissolve two drops or six globules in four table-spoonfuls of water, and give a teaspoonful every four hours, until amelioration takes place. If medicinal aggravation be apparent, the suspension of administration is recommended until the reaction has taken place. In the event of distinct improvement, the interval should be extended to six, and even to eight or twelve hours.

Bryonia is indicated when the disease is concentrated in the internal of the chest, or there is a *bilious* complication; and the fever inclines to become continued, or of a typhoid character, and also when in addition to the usual symptoms of inflammatory fever already given, there is a *heavy* stupefying headache, and a feeling as if the head would burst at the temples, aggravated by movement; *vertigo and giddiness on rising up or moving; burning heat of the head and face*, with redness and swelling of the face. *Oppression at the pit of the stomach*, excessive thirst, and sometimes sickness at the stomach. Shooting pains in the limbs, hacking cough, oppressed and laborious breathing.

DOSE.—One drop or six globules may be dissolved in four table-spoonfuls of water, and a teaspoonful may be given every four hours until the violence of the disease has been subdued, and the patient continues to improve, then the administration may be suspended.

Cantharis is indicated when the fever is very intense during the night, accompanied by burning heat of the skin, redness of the surface, dry mouth, violent thirst, and rapid pulse. It is also indicated when the patient complains of pains in the right side, attended with intense anxiety and raving.

Chammomilla is especially useful when the fever is mainly irritative, with burning heat and redness of the cheeks, tremulous, anxious, palpitation of the heart; extremely irritable, acuteness of the senses; alternations of chilliness and heat; and also if the above symptoms have been excited by anger or vexation. When the derangement has been caused by this circumstance, a dose of *Aconite* may first be required.

DOSE.—Six globules or one drop of either of the above medicines, may be dissolved in four tablespoonfuls of water and given, a teaspoonful at a time, every three hours, until a favorable change takes place.

DIET.—Water is the best drink to rely upon in inflammatory continued fevers, and the draughts should be frequent and but little at a time.

When the fever is rising, nature has indicated that no food is required; but when the fever abates, rice or barley gruel, flavored with orange stripped of the peel, or strawberry syrup, may be allowed in great moderation.

When the fever disappears entirely, broth made of chicken may be allowed at first, with crums of stale bread, and as the appetite returns, the strength of the broth may be increased, and finally such articles of food and fruits may be allowed as will partially satiáte the appetite.

3.—Nervous Fever.—Febris Nervosa.—Typhoid or Typhus.

This fever sometimes is termed slow fever, and its general characteristics are a small, weak and unequal pulse; sometimes not much accelerated, but more frequently the reverse, great prostration of strength, and much cerebral disturbance. It varies in its duration from two to six weeks. It is either a continued or intermittent fever, and may manifest itself in either a mild or malignant form.

SYMPTOMS of the mild form, are slight shiverings at first, heavy stupefying headache, great oppression, anxious expression of the countenance, nausea, sighing, despondency, very drowsy, or a quiet delirium, slightly accelerated pulse, feeble and tremulous; the patient complains of no acute suffering, sometimes there is constipation, and at others a painless diarrhœa.

SYMPTOMS, of the malignant form, are alternations of rigors and heat, with very little if any perspiration; a tense hard pulse, sometimes quick but fluttering, at other times not much accelerated; pain over the forehead, and at the top of the head, sleeplessness and delirium, succeeded by stupor or low muttering delirium; putrid diarrhœa, bleeding from the nose, and discharges of dark bloody matter from the bowels, dark red or coppery spots upon the skin, and great tenderness of the abdomen.

Sometimes this fever has received the name of CONGESTIVE FEVER, because the balance or equilibrium of the circulation being destroyed, the blood determines to some of the internal organs, and the external surface of the body appears cold.

Death may take place from the complete exhaustion of the vital energies, or from local congestions, as of the brain or lungs, or in consequence of a change to the putrid form.

CAUSES.—A vitiated atmosphere arising from the decay of vegetable and animal matter, or from the crowding together of large numbers in restricted apartments on board of ships, or in work-houses where it is impossible to secure a good circulation of the air. A deleterious quantity of food, or a deficiency of wholesome nourishment, over exertion of body or mind, or excesses in eating, drinking and debauchery, and every circumstance tending to depress the vital energies, or to abridge the supply of the hygienic elements.

Inflammatory fevers are often made to assume the typhus form by the severely prostrating treatment they receive from the heroes of the lancet and drastic purges.

8*

Blood-letting or any other severe antiphlogistic treatment may as certainly be classed among the causes of typhus as any other deteriorating agencies.

TREATMENT.—The medicines employed are Acon., Ars., Arn., Bell., Bry., Chin., Cocc., Camph., Calc. c., Carbo. veg., Dig., Hyos., Helleb., Lyc., Lach., Nux v., Nit. ac., Nat. mur., Opium, Puls., Phosph., Phos. ac., Rhus., Stram., Sulph. and Verat.

ACONITE.—When inflammatory symptoms declare themselves at the commencement in epidemic typhus, such as full, tense rapid pulse, heat in the head, thirst, and other symptoms attendant upon *simple irritative fever.*

DOSE.—One drop or six globules in three tablespoonfuls of water, a teaspoonful every three hours until a change.

ARSENICUM.—Where there is extreme prostration of strength and falling of the lower jaw, open mouth, dull glassy eyes, bitter taste, inclination to vomit, dirty white coating upon the tongue, aching at the pit of the stomach, bursting headache, giddiness, low muttering delirium, or deep sleep, distension of the bowels, burning thirst, dry hot skin, tongue dry and cracked, watery, dark colored, acrid, diarrhœa, pulse extremely feeble and intermittent.

DOSE.—Of a solution of one drop or six globules in three table-spoonfuls of pure water, give a teaspoonful every half hour until a change or amelioration takes place, doubling or tripling the length of the intervals as soon as improvement becomes manifest.

ARNICA.—When the patient lies in an unconscious state, as if stunned, with half sleep, with eyes open, or delirium.

DOSE.—Of a solution of one drop or six globules to three tablespoon-fuls of pure water; give a desert spoonful every two hours.

BELLADONNA.—When there is a bloated appearance of the face, alternate heat and chills, or alternations of coldness and paleness, and burning heat and redness of the face, violent throbbing of the carotids or arteries of the neck, sparkling and protrusion of the eyes, dilitation of the pupils, extreme sensibility to light and strabismus or squinting, noises in the ears, wild expression of the countenance, violent shooting pains in the forehead, or dull heavy pain causing the patient to put his hand frequently to his head, furious delirium followed by loss of consciousness, parched lips and sores at the corners of the mouth, redness and dryness of the tongue, or foul and covered with a yellow coat, skin hot and dry, bitter taste in the mouth, intense thirst, unable to swallow liquids, nausea and pressure at the stomach, constipation or watery motions, scanty or red-colored urine, rapid breathing, pulse full, quick and wiry, inflammation of the parotid glands, and swollen.

DOSE.—The same as for Arnica.

BRYONIA.—When after a slight cold, the patient complains of pains in his limbs, and aching over the whole body, throbbing headache, aggravated by turning the eyes, or opening them, tenderness of the scalp, burning heat in the head, forehead frequently bathed in cold sweat, obliged to lie or sit from languor and heaviness of the limbs, and an aversion to cold air, disturbed at night, by congestion of blood, heat and anxiety; sighing and moaning during sleep; agonizing dreams, which often arouse the patient, and that continue to haunt him while awake; bitter taste, yellow furred or dry tongue; disgust of food; nausea, and inclination to vomit; pressure or weight, and pricking at the pit of the stomach; sensation of distension of lower ribs; costiveness.

DOSE.—Dissolve a drop or six globules in four tablespoonfuls of water, and give a desert-spoonful every three hours, until a change; if for the better, increase the intervals to six hours.

CHINA.—In the first stage, when there is paleness of the face; lancinating, rending, aching or pressing pains in the head; obscurity of vision; roaring in the` ears, 'and dulness of hearing; yellow or white coating on the tongue; dryness of mouth; insipid, clammy taste; inclination to vomit; sensibility and distension of the abdomen; thin, watery, and yellow stools; scanty, pale, or dark colored urine; oppression of the chest; shooting or dragging pains in the limbs; anxiety, sleeplessness, and general coldness and shivering.

DOSE.—The same as for *Bryonia.*

COCCULUS.—When the patient complains of giddiness and headache, or tendency to faint, or paralysis of the limbs; when there are symptoms of bilious or gastric derangement. Very suitable after Rhus or Camphor.

DOSE.—The same as for *Bryonia.*

CAMPHOR.—When there is heat of the head, with confusion of ideas, or violent delirium; giddiness; throbbing headache; burning heat in the forehead, cold *clammy skin;* continuous coldness of the hands and feet; debilitating and clammy sweat; tendency to diarrhœa; scanty, cloudy urine, which deposits a thick sediment; great weakness, and feeble pulse, scarcely perceptible; suitable after Rhus.

DOSE.—One drop of the tincture on a lump of sugar every half hour, until some change or amelioration takes place.

CALC. C.—When there is jerkings or twitching of the limbs, and for nose-bleed; after Phos. ac., Rhus, China. Some maintain that Calcarea is beneficial as an alternating remedy, with Bell., Arsenicum or Rhus, when the symptoms indicate, but there is a doubt, whether alternatives of the kind are at all useful.

DOSE.—Of the solution of six globules, or a drop in four tablespoonfuls of water, give a teaspoonful every six hours, until there is some indication to discontinue its use.

CARBO VEGETABILIS.—When in critical cases there is drowsiness, with rattling respiration, face pinched, sunken and death-like; pupils insensible to light, pulse scarcely perceptible, and the vital power rapidly sinking; cold perspiration on the face and limbs; involuntary evacuations of a very putrid odor, deep red urine, with a cloud floating over it, or rising towards the surface; burning in the abdomen, and at the pit of the stomach.

DOSE.—Of a solution of six globules, or one drop in three tablespoonfuls of water, give a teaspoonful every half hour until a change.

DIGITALIS.—When there is in the first stage a yellow jaundiced hue of the skin; violent bilious vomiting; spasmodic pains in the stomach; sensibility of the left side on pressure; frequent desire to urinate, particularly at night, with scanty, bilious urine; burning heat of the head and face, anxiety of mind, and dread of some imaginary impending misfortune; painful and difficult urination, or entirely suppressed.

HYOSCYAMUS.—When in addition to such symptoms as indicate the use of *Belladonna*, there are twitchings of the tendons; strong, full pulse; fulness of the veins; burning heat of the skin; sensation of pricking all over the body, and constant delirium, fancying wasps or other insects about the head; and frequent, but ineffectual desire to urinate.

HELLEBORUS NIG.—When the disease occurs as the sequel of other febrile affections: such as scarlet fever; measles; bilious fever; worm fever and cholera, with pain as from contusion, combined with tumefaction in the integuments of the head; disposition to sleep, with confusion of ideas and extreme restlessness; dark, cloudy urine; heaviness, or feeling of stiffness and powerlessness in the limbs; dulness of the faculties, and depression of spirits.

DOSE.—Of a solution of six globules, or one drop of either of.the three preceding remedies, give a desert-spoonful every three hours, until there is a change in the symptoms, that indicated the use of the remedy

LYCOPODIUM may be employed after *Calc. c.* in the second stage of typhus when miliary eruption is slowly and scantily developed and there is sopor with muttering delirium, confounding of words, stammering, picking of the bed clothes, twitching of the tendons, distension of the abdomen with constipation, affections of the bladder, or when there are shivering and heat alternately, circum-scribed redness of the cheeks, debilitating sweats, excessive debility, falling of the lower jaw, half closed eyes, slow respiration, or state of excitement without heat or congestion in the head or face, redness of the tongue, constipation, burning urine, tranquil and resigned state of the mind, or surliness .and malevolence, especially on waking.

DOSE. —Six globules, or one drop in four tablespoonfuls of water, may be administered, a teaspoonful at a time every four hours until a change may indicate a new remedy.

LACHESIS.—When there is vertigo on rising or sitting up, low muttering delirium, falling of the lower jaw, staring expression of the countenance, sunken features, bitter taste, yellowish tongue, red about the edges, cracked tongue, smooth, furred, or white slimy tongue, heaviness of the tongue, without the power of protruding it, and inarticulate speech, seeming paralysis of the eyelids, lethargic sleep, thirst with disinclination to drink, copi-ous urine of a brownish red color.

DOSE.—Three globules or half a drop may be given every three hours, dissolved in a teaspoonful of water.

NUX VOM.—When there are gastric or bilious symp-

toms, constipation with frequent inclination and ineffectual efforts to evacuate, spasms of the stomach and bowels,
painful and difficult emission of urine, painful pressure
and tension in the upper portion of the stomach and at
the sides under the ribs, general nervousness with restlessness at night, and slight delirium; weakness and
exacerbation of symptoms in the morning; sanguine
or bilious temperament; irritable and impatient disposition.

DOSE.—Three globules in a spoonful of water every four hours, or one
drop in the same way.

NITRIC ACID.—When there are hemorrhages and sen
sibility of the abdomen, with diarrhœa and slimy, acrid,
greenish-colored stools, tenesmus, sore mouth, ulcers in
the intestines, sorenes or pressure of certain parts of the
abdomen, shooting pains in the rectum, straining, and
greenish slimy diarrhœa, scalding urine, tendency to
collapse.

DOSE.—Of a solution, six globules, or one drop in three tablespoonfuls
of water, give a teaspoonful every three hours until a change. Phos. ac. is
useful after this remedy.

NATRUM MURIATICUM.—When there is great debility
and unquenchable thirst, dryness of the tongue, loss of
consciousness, and particularly when the fever is the
sequel of some previous debilitating disease.

DOSE.—The same as for Nitric Acid.

OPIUM.—When there is much stupor, drowsiness, or
sleep with the eyes half closed, labored breathing, with
low moaning noise, open mouth, fixed look, slight
delirium, or muttering, picking the bed clothes, difficult.
to arouse from sleep, dry offensive stools, which, together
with the urine, are passed involuntarily.

DOSE.—The same as for Nitric acid.

PULSATILLA.—When there are profuse bleedings from the nose in persons of a lymphatic temperament, or phlegmatic disposition.

DOSE.—Of a solution of six globules, or one drop in three table-spoonfuls of water, give a teaspoonful every hour until relieved, or change takes place.

PHOSPHORUS.—When there is great dryness of the tongue, heat of skin, small hard, quick pulse, painless diarrhœa, with rumbling in the bowels; or when there is congestion of the lungs, laborious breathing and anxiety, dulness in percussion, rattling of mucus, stitches during respiration, cough, with copious expectoration of mucus mixed with blood, or even offensive pus.

PHOSPHORIC ACID.—When at the very beginning of the disease there is great prostration, with wandering, when awake; or in almost hopeless cases, when the patient is found lying on the back in a drowsy state, exhibits a vacant stare when spoken to, but no reply; or else incoherent, constant talking or low muttering; picking the bed clothes; tries to escape from something alarming; black incrustations on the lips, dry hot skin, copious watery diarrhœa, involuntary; frequent and weak pulse, sometimes intermittent.

DOSE.—When either of the above remedies are indicated, six globules, or one drop of the dilution, may be dissolved in four tablespoonfuls of water, and a teaspoonful may be given every three. hours until a change takes place.

RHUS TOXICODENDRON.—When there is great debility and diarrhœa; congestion to the head and chest, and great prostration; stupefying headache, as if from a bruise; dirty yellowish coat upon the tongue; violent pain in the stomach when touched. This remedy is very nearly allied in many particulars, to Bryonia. The indications for its use in nervous fevers, are in many respects the same, and on this account, many practitioners use it in alternation with that remedy, still it is particularly indicated when there is hot, dark-colored urine, at first clear, but afterwards turbid; difficult swallowing, as if the throat had become too small; general trembling, debility and prostration, almost amounting to paralytic weakness of the limbs; shooting pains in various parts of the body, aggravated when at rest and at night,—relieved for a time by moving the part affected; small, quick pulse, or weak and slow; anxious, depressed, and inclined to weep.

DOSE.—One drop of the dilution or six globules, dissolved in four tablespoonfuls of water, and give a teaspoonful every three hours, until amelioration or change. Bryonia is a valuable remedy, either to precede or follow *Rhus*.

RHUS TOX.—When exposed to a thorough wetting, which brings on a diarrhœa, Rhus is also an invaluable remedy; or if the patient is seized with a violent diarrhœa from any other cause, accompanied by colic; chilliness, even when by the fire; aching pains in various parts of the body; stiffness of the nape of the neck and in the back.

DOSE.—The same as before.

STRAMONIUM may be administered after Belladonna, when there is twitching of the muscles of the face, and of the tendons, squinting, trembling of the extremities, tremulous motion of the tongue on protruding it from the mouth, burning heat of the body, stoppages of the urine, fantastic gesticulation, and a convulsive separation of the lips.

DOSE.—Of a solution of six globules or one drop in four tablespoonfuls of water, give a teaspoonful every three hours, until amelioration or or change.

SULPHUR, may follow Bryonia, Rhus, or Phos. ac.,

9

when there is pale collapsed countenance, burning itching eruptions on the lips, dryness of the mouth, foul, dry tongue, bitter taste, slimy or bilious vomiting, tenderness of the region of the stomach, and pain as from excoriation in the umbilical region, increased on pressure; rumbling in the bowels, frequent, watery, floculent, or yellow evacuations, cloudy urine, depositing a reddish sediment; purulent miliary eruption, bleeding at the nose, stitches in the chest, oppressed respiration, dry cough towards evening and at night; sleeplessness, whining during sleep, dry heat during the day, with moderately quiet pulse and profuse sweating at night.

DOSE.—One drop, or six globules, may be dissolved in a tablespoonful of water, and given every eight hours, until some amelioration or change.

VERATRUM.—When there is coldness of the inferior or lower extremities; it is useful to follow Arsenicum.

DOSE.—One drop, or six globules, may be dissolved in four tablespoonfuls of water, and a teaspoonful may be given every half hour.

DIET in *nervous fevers.*—During the inflammatory stage, abstinence. During the progress of the disease, the farinaceous gruels may be given from day to day—varying from one kind to another. After convalescence becomes established, and the appetite returns, the greatest care should be exercised in the supply of food. For, relapses often occur from over-eating, when the patient had, to all appearances, been out of danger. Therefore, as a rule, when a patient is recovering from typhus, toast and black tea, light bread puddings, mutton broth, and very little mutton steak, or surloin steak, or broiled chicken, may be allowed in great moderation, but never to the extent of the appetite.

When NERVOUS FEVER prevails as a pestilence, it is

sometimes termed the PUTRID TYPHUS, or MALIGNANT TYPHUS, or ABDOMINAL TYPHUS, but does not vary in its characteristics from that already treated of as indicating the use of *Arsenicum*, *Bryonia*, *Carbo vegetabilis*, *Rhus* and *Veratrum*.

4.—Bilious or Gastric Fever. Remittent Fever.

Bilious fever deranges the stomach, and digestive organs in general. It differs from the typhoid and typhus, (nervous fevers,) in being of a less torpid character, the nervous system not being so extensively involved. It differs also, in not being characterised by the extreme prostration, pain in the back of the head, and derangement of the ordinary senses.

These fevers, seemingly take place without any definite duration, they do not seem to have any fixedness of character, that is determined by any particular kind of crisis. They often occur in consequences of a derangement of the biliary organs, and terminate in vomiting from the stomach, a quantity of bile, or in bilious diarrhœa, and the patient being totally relieved, begins to recover. In other cases, only partial relief is gained by the vomiting and purging, and the fever continues until some other crisis marks its termination. This may be a general perspiration, or perhaps some 'change in the urine, or a dissipation of the febrile symptoms by the general recuperation of the system.

When a mere derangement of the stomach, attended with fever, occurs, it may terminate its course in a few days. When the liver is disturbed, and the mucus coat of the stomach and bowels are severally associated with the fever, its duration may be for several weeks, and in some instances, it may assume to a greater or less degree, an inflammatory character, and sometimes, it may degenerate into the purely *nervous*, especially, if improperly treated.

CAUSES.—It may be remarked of this disease, as of many other affections, that it originates by reason of malarius influences on the one hand, and of susceptible conditions of the system on the other ; or in other words, from the conjoint action of *predisposing* and *exciting* causes. Whenever one is disposed to great heat, the perspiration may be so rapid, as to create undue excite- ment of the biliary organs and stomach ; by reason ot their sympathy with the organs of perspiration ; exposure to the extremes of temperature in alternation, super- induces conditions of the stomach and bowels, easily impressed ; any irritable matters taken into the stomach, or that may be undigested therein, operate to develope febrile difficulties that may assume the gastric, bilious, or remittent character ; anger, emotion, grief, care, &c., acting upon impressible subjects, or on such as are already predisposed to biliary derangement, may be recorded among the exciting causes.

SYMPTOMS.—Bilious fevers are characterised in general by a sensation of weight or fulness in the region of the stomach, with nausea or inclination to vomit ; an offen- sive gulping of wind, and vomiting of acrid bile, or mucus mixed with bile from the stomach ; the tongue is thickly covered with a dirty-yellow coat; the bowels appear to be soft, though constipated. In a more advanced stage of the disease, the discharges from the bowels are often quite offensive, of a thin consistence, and mixed with portions of undigested food.

The HEAD is often afflicted with pain in the front part over the eyes. The *face* is pale, and the countenance distressed and sickly. The white of the *eyes* is more or less colored with yellow ; greater or less degree of chilliness, followed by heat and dryness of the skin. The *pulse* quick, not very tense, sometimes irregular or intermittent ; and the *urine*, dark-colored and cloudy, or of a thick, turbid appearance. The more the liver is implicated in the disease, the more aggravated will many of these symptoms appear. Sometimes the heat of the skin is very considerable, and the restlessness and thirst immoderate, and the coating of the tongue, which at first is of a pale yellow, often changes into that of a brown. There is an acrid, bitter taste in the mouth, and bitter risings in the throat, and the substance vomited from the stomach is of a greenish, bilious matter. When the bowels are not costive, the evacuations are either of a yellow, green, or brown color; sometimes there is burning in the region of the liver, and hardness and tension in the *right hypochondrium*.

Fevers are termed *remittent*, in consequence of a remission of the symptoms, which begins to take place after the disease becomes established; the remission is commonly preceded by a gentle perspiration, after which, the patient seems greatly relieved, but in a few hours the fever returns, and there may be a succession of these remissions, alternating with more prominent febrile symptoms, and the nearer these remissions approach to a complete intermission, the more favorable to the patient.

TREATMENT.—Inasmuch as it has been hinted that gastric and bilious fevers are mainly dependent upon the derangement of the abdominal organs—the stomach, the liver, and the intestines, it would appear evident, that the fever might accompany various groups of symptoms;

9*

and in every case, the name of the disease should be left out of the question for the purpose of acquiring a positive knowledge of the individual case. The actual symptoms in each case, must indicate the remedy.

The medicines to be employed in the treatment of gastric and bilious fevers are: Acon., Ars., Bell., Bry., Cham., Cocc., Coloc., China, Digitalis, Ipec., Mercurius viv., Nux vom., Puls., Rhus tox., Tart. emet.

ACONITE.—When there is bitterness in the mouth, so that every article of food tastes bitter; yellow coating upon the tongue; accelerated pulse; bitter risings in the throat; or when there is vomiting of greenish, bitter, or slimy matter; scanty stools, or constipation of the bowels; or else urging, with frequent small evacuations; swelling and tightness across the stomach; extreme tenderness in the region of the liver, and along the lower ribs; pulsating headache, aggravated by talking; sensation of heaviness and fulness in the forehead. When these symptoms are increased by exercise, standing or sitting, or speaking; or if they are mitigated by admitting the patient to a fresh atmosphere, this remedy is especially indicated.

DOSE.—One drop or six globules may be dissolved in four tablespoon-fuls of water, and a teaspoonful may be given every three hours, until some favorable change ensues, or the disease has taken another form.

ARSENICUM. When there is dryness of the tongue, accompanied with severe thirst and continual desire for drink, and unable to drink but a small quantity at a time, acrid bitterish, pungent eructations, saltish or bitter taste in the mouth, nausea, vomiting of greenish or dark-colored matter, great tenderness in the stomach, unable to bear any pressure, burning, cutting and cramp-like pains in the stomach and bowels, accompanied with anguish and chilliness; sensation as if a weight with burning at one point were in the stomach. The bowels either very torpid or continually relaxed, with violent urging, with greenish or brownish stools; *urine* burning and scalding as it passes from the bladder; movement provokes the discharges from the bowels, as does the drinking of any fluid; shivering, shuddering and anxiety; oppression of the chest, headache, labored respiration in the open air, especially *in the evening and after drinking;* hot, burning and stinging sensation communicated to the hand on feeling the skin. *Pulse* irregular, frequent, great prostration, and desire for recumbent posture.

DOSE.—One drop, or six globules, may be dissolved in four tablespoonfuls of water, and a teaspoonful may be given every two hours, until there is a change; if the symptoms are very violent, repeat the medicine every hour or every four hours, if only manifested in a moderate degree.

BELLADONNA.—When there is beating and throbbing of the arteries of the temples, and severe pain in the head, chiefly in the forehead above the eyebrows, with a feeling as if the head would burst, and as if the brain would fall out the forehead, and also reeling and giddiness; dryness of the mouth and throat, sometimes incessant nausea; *tongue* with a thick whitish or yellowish coating; sour taste; repugnance to food of every description, and usually to all kinds of drink; *vomiting of food,* or sour, slimy or bitter matters; full *pulse* and accelerated, evacuations of the bowels suspended, or otherwise loose with slimy evacuations; and especially if the symptoms about the head are aggravated by moving the eyes, or exercise of any kind, or by coming in contact with the fresh air.

DOSE.—One drop, or six globules, in a half pint tumbler of water, and give a teaspoonful every four hours, until change or mitigation of the head symptoms takes place.

BRYONIA, is particularly useful in the treatment of bilious fevers, when they occur in hot weather and the atmosphere is damp and sultry, if characterised by the following symptoms: taste insipid, clammy, foul and bitter, especially on waking; *mouth and throat* dry, and continual thirst; *tongue* coated with white or yellow fur, with a number of small blisters on its surface, morbid hankering after acid drinks and stimulants, but repugnance to solid food; offensive breath; *vomiting of bilious matters* after drinking; ineffectual retching and straining to vomit; sensation of fulness and tightness in the stomach after eating the smallest quantity; chilly feeling and shuddering; heat in the head, with redness of the face; oppressive headache, with sensation of extreme heat, fulness, aggravated by drinking and exercise, as in turning; sensation of dulness and confusion of the head, and constipation.

DOSE.—One drop or six globules, dissolved in a half pint tumbler of water, and give a teaspoonful every four hours until the dose is repeated three times, afterwards every six hours until a change.

CHAMOMILLA is useful in bilious fevers, when the *tongue* is red and fissured, or where it has a yellow coating, particularly if *Nux vomica* has failed of arresting the symptoms. Its use is particularly indicated when there is intense heat and redness of the face, particularly at night, restlessness and disturbed sleep, with much inquietude and tossing about; pressure and fulness of the head, and pain as if bruised; inflammatory redness and burning of the eyes; easily provoked to tears or anger; fretful, suspicious and quarrelsome, and at times great anguish of mind; *bitter* taste in the mouth, and every kind of food tastes bitter; loss of appetite; nausea and bitter eructations; vomiting of sour, greenish or bitter matters;

great anxiety and weight at the pit of the stomach, extending across the stomach and under the ribs; foul breath; ·looseness of the bowels; frothy evacuations; sour smelling slimy evacuations of the appearance of *muddled eggs;* greenish stools, or on the other hand, constipation and suspended evacuations. ·

DOSE.—One drop, or six globules, in a half-pint tumbler of water, and give a teaspoonful every two hours until a change of the symptoms or convalescence becomes manifest.

COCCULUS is applicable in bilious derangements and fevers, when the patient has been treated without success, with decoctions of chamomile under allopathic treatment. It is particularly indicated when there is absolute loathing for food, dryness of the mouth, with or without thirst; offensive eructations; nausea and inclination to vomit when eating, talking or riding in a carriage, or after sleeping; yellow coating upon the tongue; oppressed breathing, occasioned by fulness in the region of the stomach; loose and soft evacuations, and burning in the passage, or more frequently constipation; headache or pain above the eyebrows, attended with giddiness. The least physical exertion producing weakness and sweating.

DOSE.—Four globules may be given, and repeated every four hours until a change.

COLOCYNTH is particularly indicated when in connection with other symptoms of bilious derangement and fever, there is spasmodic colic and severe pain in the region of the navel, spasm of the stomach and vomiting, or loose discharges from the bowels after eating; cramps in the calves of the legs; shivering with general coldness, but with heat of the head, unattended with thirst, full and rapid pulse.

DOSE.—One drop, or six globules, in half a tumbler of water, a teaspoonful may be given every three hours, until amelioration or change.

CHINA is the appropriate remedy when there are frequent eructations, vomiting or regurgitation of food, loss of appetite, perfect satiation, as if one had eaten more than enough; offensive discharges of wind from the bowels, stools mingled with undigested food; painful sense of distension of the bowels, and weight in the region of the navel; sensation of chilliness and shuddering after *drinking;* diarrhœa, with watery slimy or bilious evacuations; hot skin; frequent and full *pulse,* sometimes headache, attended with delirium; burning sensation in the lips, red face, and dry mouth. This remedy is well adapted to those persons suffering from bilious febrile difficulties, who are naturally of debilitated constitutions.

DOSE.—One drop, or six globules, in four tablespoonfuls of water, give a teaspoonful every four hours, until amelioration or change.

DIGITALIS often proves of great service in fevers, accompanied by biliary derangement when the following symptoms are present, viz: looseness of the bowels, attended with great loss of strength; nausea, with bitter taste in the mouth after sleeping; thirst and vomiting of phlegm.

DOSE.—Give a teaspoonful every three hours of a solution of six globules, or one drop in half a tumbler of water.

IPECACUANHA is very serviceable when there is a disposition to vomit, with utter dislike to any kind of food, and especially to substances of a fatty or greasy nature; dryness of the mouth, the tongue either clean or else covered with a thick yellowish coating; bitter taste in the mouth; all food tastes bitter when taken into the mouth; offensive smell from the mouth and breath; violent gulping without raising any thing, attended with great straining; or copious vomiting of slimy matters; or vomiting food with a gush; looseness of the bowels, the evacuations of a very offensive or even putrid character; bilious colic, weight, and sense of fulness, with severe pain in the region of the stomach; yellowish pale hue of the skin; severe headache in the forepart of the head, and a sensation as if the head were crushed; chilliness and shuddering over the whole surface of the body; cold hands and feet.

DOSE.—Of a solution of one drop, or six globules, in a half-pint tumbler of water, give a teaspoonful every three hours, until a mitigation or change.

MERCURIUS VIV., is particularly useful in gastric and bilious fevers, when indicated by such symptoms as the following, viz., moist tongue, loaded with a *white* or yellowish *coating*; dry and burning lips, sickly, putrid or bitter taste, nausea with decided inclination to vomit, or actual vomiting of slimy or *bitter substances;* painful tenderness on each side between the ribs and the hips, and at the pit of the stomach, and also in the region of the naval, especially in the morning, with anguish and inquietude; desire to sleep by day and sleeplessness at night; peevishness, irritability, shiverings alternately with heat, burning thirst, and sometimes with aversion to drinks.

DOSE.—A teaspoonful of a solution of one drop, or six globules, in a half-pint tumbler of water, may be administered every three hours, until change, or amelioration of the symptoms.

NUX VOM.—This remedy is indicated when the following symptoms are present: Dry and white tongue, or yellowish towards the root; excessive thirst with burning in the throat; bitter or putrid taste; bitter eructations; continued nausea, especially in the open air, or vomiting of ingesta; pain in the stomach; pressure and painful tension in the whole abdomen, and in the sides under the ribs, or between the ribs and hips; spasmodic colic, with pinching and grumbling noise in the region of the navel; constipation, with frequent but ineffectual desire to evacuate, or, on the other hand, small, loose, slimy or watery stools; pressive pain in the forehead, with vertigo; fretful, peevish and melancholy; great weakness and fatigued feeling; red and hot or yellowish and earthy face; heat mixed with shivering and shuddering, sensation as if the limbs had been beaten; increase of the sufferings after midnight.

DOSE.—Dissolve six globules, or one drop, in four tablespoonfuls of water, and give a teaspoonful every three hours, until the disease mitigates, or there is some change.

PULSATILLA.—When there is attendant on the biliary or gastric derangement, the following symptoms, this remedy is especially indicated. Tongue loaded with whitish mucus, insipid, clammy or else bitter taste, especially after swallowing; risings, with taste of the food; aversion to food, especially to salt meat or to fat; hankering after acids and stimulants; food disposed to rise from the stomach into the mouth; disagreeable nausea, vomiting of slimy and whitish, bitter and greenish or acid substances; vomiting of partially digested food; pressure at the pit of the stomach and difficult respiration; constipation or evacuations, which are loose, white or slimy, bilious and greenish, or like eggs beaten up; headache on one side of the head; frequent shivering with flushes of heat, or dry heat with thirst; face at one time pale and at another red, or redness on one cheek and paleness on the other.

DOSE.—After being very particular to dissolve one drop, or six globules, in a half pint tumbler of water, give a teaspoonful every three hours. until there is some change in the symptoms or the disease.

RHUS TOX.—When there is a great weakness and prostration attending the ordinary bilious and gastric derangements, and slight delirium and offensive diarrhœa, somewhat of a putrid character, dryness of the mouth and tongue, intense thirst, strong tendency to nervous symptoms,—

DOSE.—If the liquid is used, one drop in four tablespoonfuls of water may be given, a teaspoonful at a time, and repeated every four hours. If globules, three may be given upon the tongue every three hours, until the condition of the patient may indicate the discontinuance of their use.

TART-EMET.—This remedy is particularly serviceable in such cases of bilious fever as are strongly marked with catarrhal symptoms, or loose cough, abundant secretion of mucus, and sinking respiration.

DOSE.—The same as for Rhus.

DIET.—In the early stage of this fever the appetite is usually suspended and there is no inclination to take food. This is a wise provision, and indicates that no food should be forced upon the patient. It is therefore improper to require the taking of any kind of solid food during the course of the fever. Wheat, barley, or rice gruel may be drank cold until convalescence has set in, when a little mutton or lamb soup, made very weak, may be given at first, and then as the fever entirely disappears a little broiled mutton or chicken may be allowed, but restricted to meagre limits; and during the whole period of convalescence the diet should be moderate in order to guard against a relapse; light custards, puddings made of rice, tapioca or sago, toast and black tea, and occasionally a little meat will be found sufficiently substantial to enable the patient to regain, in a safe and certain manner, his strength.

Intermittent Fevers.—(*Febris intermittens.*)

The peculiar characteristics of intermittent fevers may be stated in a few words. They consist of distinct periods in which the disease manifests itself; these periods are

10

called paroxysms, and between which there is a complete intermission of the disease in which no fever is present. There are several varieties of this disease—

1. There are those of which the paroxysms occur every 24 hours, called quotidian.

2. Those of which they occur every 48 hours, called tertian.

3. Those of which they occur every 72 hours, called quartan.

When the paroxysms occur at longer intervals, they are very apt to be irregular.

Each paroxysm of an intermittent is usually marked by three distinct stages, viz., the cold, the hot and the sweating stages.

CAUSES.—The *predisposing causes* are generally believed to be impurities in the atmosphere arising from low, boggy districts or marshes, from stagnant pools, when acted upon by the heat of summer, and from the fact that intermittents usually occur in the latter part of the warm season or early in the fall, when the temperature of the nights begins to diminish, it is very probable this is the case; living in a deteriorated atmosphere any great length of time evidently weakens or debilitates the sys- tem so that almost any *exciting cause* may develope the disease. After passing through the heat of a warm day, exposed to these influences, without very careful protec- tion against the change of temperature and dampness of the night, persons will be very liable to the disease.

SYMPTOMS OF THE COLD STAGE.—The first indication is usually a pain in the head, weariness of the limbs, pains in the loins and back, coldness of the hands and feet, stretching, yawning, and sometimes with sickness and vomiting; to which succeed shivering and oftentimes severe shaking.

SYMPTOMS OF THE HOT STAGE.—After the cold stage passes off, the body returns to a state of warmth, gradually increasing, though irregular at first, by transient flushes, soon becomes a steady dry or burning heat, much augmented above the natural temperature of the body. The skin, which was before pale or bluish, becomes now puffed up and red and often very sensitive to the touch. Pains in the head, flying pains all over the body; the pulse quick, strong and hard; the tongue white; intense thirst. The *urine* for the most part of a high color.

SYMPTOMS OF THE SWEATING STAGE.—Immediately succeeding the hot stage, a moisture will break out upon the face and neck, which soon becomes universal and uniform, and the heat falls to its natural standard. The pulse diminishes and becomes full and free. The urine changes its color. The bowels become laxed, respiration becomes full and free, and the functions generally resume their natural condition, and the intermission takes place.

During the intermission, the patient may feel quite well, until a given period passes away, and then a similar paroxysm of coldness, heat, and sweating occurs, and so on, until the disease is arrested.

Sometimes, the cold stage is not characterised by shivering and shaking; and sometimes, though rarely, the paroxysms pass off without the general sweat.

TREATMENT.—It is found by experience, that it is best to administer the treatment in this disease, between the recurrence of the paroxysms, but under some circumstances, the remedies may be given, either at the beginning or ending of the paroxysms. In the treatment, the type is to be regarded as of the utmost importance, as well as the other features of the disease.

The remedies found useful in curing this disease, are Arn., Ars., Bell., Bry., Carb. veg., Cham., China, Cocc., Ipec., Ign., Merc., Nux v., Nat. mur., Opium, Puls., Sep., Sulph., Rhus, Veratrum.

In the employment of any of these remedies, according to their specific indication, it must be borne in mind, that their use is *curative*, not to smother the disease, as has often been the case, in allopathic practice by the aid of *quinine*, to return again upon the slightest exposure. It is better that several paroxysms should occur during the process of a radical cure, rather than the creating of a mere suspension of them for a time, by overdoses of *quinine*. Therefore, when the remedy is properly selected, it is by far better to persevere with its use, until a change takes place, even though in the meantime, several paroxysms occur.

The mere stopping of the chills is by no means a cure, for we often see persons that have been drugged with *quinine* or *barks*, looking pale, sickly and debilitated, and in a more deplorable and-wretched state of health, from such treatment, though the chills were suspended for a time, than they would have been, had the ague been left undisturbed. It is, therefore, requisite to change the condition of the system by gentle and curative means; if a radical cure is to be expected, without such a sequel as the barks and quinine are prone to leave behind. In most cases, homœopathic treatment will not stop the paroxysms at once, it will, however, operate to bring about a healthy condition of the system, and the paroxysms gradually become less violent until they disappear altogether, and then the patient has less to fear from a return. Whenever any remedy is selected upon such grounds, as will warrant an anticipation of a favorable result, it is better not to change for several days, and not at all, if the paroxysms become lighter and later in the day.

ARNICA is indicated as a remedy for intermittent when the paroxysm comes on in the *evening*, marked by the following symptoms : pressing headache, as if caused by a blow; sore rheumatic pains in the joints; weariness or soreness as if from fatigue, succeeded by chilliness and a great deal of thirst, and also inclination to vomit; bitter taste in the mouth; stitches in the pit of the stomach, and bruised; sensation of drawing in the periosteum of all the bones, or pains in the limbs, as if bruised, succeeded by fever, but not so much thirst; bitter or putrid eructation, or vomiting of blood during the chill, or retention of the urine, with pressive sore pain in the bladder, or red or brown urine, with a brick-dust sediment.

DOSE.—One drop or six globules may be put in four tablespoonfuls of water, and a tablespoonful may be given immediately after the paroxysm, or at an early stage of the same, and repeated every six hours. Not to be given during the paroxysm. Treatment to be continued perseveringly until a change.

ARSENICUM is indicated, when shivering and heat appear at the same time, or when shivering and heat succeed each other in rapid alternations; as well as internal shivering, with external heat, or external shivering with internal heat; burning heat, as if boiling water were circulating in the veins; dry heat and absence of perspiration, or else appearing a long time after the heat, and principally at the commencement of sleep, or when heat and shivering are slightly developed; appearance of other affections with the shiverings, such as pains in the limbs; anxiety and restlessness; transient heat on speaking, or on the slightest movement; oppression of the

10*

chest; pulmonary spasms; headache, &c. During the *sweats*, humming in the ears; during the heat, restlessness, aching in the forehead; vertigo, and even delirium; great *debility*, vertigo, tenderness of the liver and spleen, after the fever, or during its course; nausea; violent pain in the stomach; sores in the corners of the mouth; bitter taste in the mouth; trembling; great anxiety; paralysis of the limbs, or *violent pains*; disposition to dropsical affections.

DOSE.—Of a solution of six globules in four tablespoonfuls of water, give a teaspoonful every three hours, between the paroxysms, if they occur daily ; or every four hours, if they occur every other day ; or one drop of the dilution in a half-pint tumbler of water, may be administered in the same manner, until a change.

BELLADONNA is of great value as a remedy in those intermittents of daily paroxysms, when they are characterised by violent headache, dizziness, violent shivering, followed by moderate heat; or when the shivering is ' slight, followed by intense heat, or partial shivering and shuddering, with heat in other parts; redness and heat of the face; violent pulsation in the carotids; complete absence of thirst, or the reverse; great susceptibility and tearfulness; *Tertian intermittents*, or those having the paroxysms every other day, characterised by the above symptoms, are also indicative of the use of this remedy. And also those called *double tertian*, as when the paroxysms of one become manifest every other day in the morning, and the paroxysms of the other occurring on the intermediate days, in the afternoon or evening, provided they are accompanied by similar symptoms.

DOSE.—Of a solution of six globules, or one drop, in four tablespoonfuls of water, give a tablespoonful every three hours during the interim between the paroxysms until a change takes place, or there is a perceptible mitigation of the violence of the disease.

BRYONIA is particularly indicated when there is a

predominance of cold and shivering, with redness of the cheeks, heat in the head and yawning, or predominance of heat followed by chilliness, or with stitches in the side; headache and vertigo during the heat; *thickly coated tongue*, bitter taste, aversion to food, nausea or vomiting, great thirst, constipation, or else the reverse. This remedy is also applicable to the different forms of the fever, when the symptoms indicate its use.

DOSE.—The same as that of Belladonna.

CARBO VEGETABILIS.—When the paroxysms come on *in the evening*, either every day, or every other day, or even every fourth day, *with thirst only during the shivering*, profuse perspiration followed by shivering; rheumatic pains in the teeth or limbs before or during the fever; vertigo; nausea; redness of the face during the hot stage.

DOSE.—Dissolve six globules in a half-pint tumbler of water, or one drop in the same way, and give a tablespoonful every four hours until some mitigation or change in the appearance of the paroxysms. This remedy should be administered in the interim.

CHAMOMILLA, for the quotidian or daily type, when there is pressure during the paroxysm at the pit of the stomach, *hot* perspiration on the forehead, exasperation and tossing, or bilious vomiting, diarrhœa and colic; *intense thirst;* predominance of heat and perspiration.

DOSE.—As soon as the paroxysm begins to subside, give four globules dissolved in a tablespoonful of water, and repeat every three hours until the period of the next paroxysm should it occur, or one drop in four tablespoonfuls of water may be given, a teaspoonful at a time every two hours until as before.

CHINA OFF.—In epidemic or endemic intermittents arising from the influence of marsh miasm, this remedy is indicated when the following peculiarities are present; when in the commencement, there is a sense of languor or general uneasiness of the heart, anxiety, headache, sneezing, great thirst, *bulimy* or voracious appetite, or when there is nausea and pain in the bowels. It is also indicated when there is at the commencement absence of thirst during the cold stage; but thirst during the hot and sweating stages, or between the cold and the hot stage; and further, when there is swelling of the veins, with heat in the head, natural warmth of the body, or determination of blood to the head, commonly with redness and heat in the face, frequently with chilliness of all other parts of the body, and even external coldness with only sensation of heat in the face, cold sweat on the forehead. This remedy in massive doses is fraught with evil consequences.

DOSE.—One drop in four spoonfuls of water may be given, a teaspoonful every two hours in the interim, or four globules may be given every two hours until amelioration or change, or one drop of the dilution, or four globules may be given immediately before the cold stage, and the same may be given immediately after the sweat.

COCCULUS is indicated when in addition to the usual symptoms of ague, there is in the interim between the paroxysms, spasms of the stomach and bowels, or cramps in the stomach, or constrictive pinching, tearing, burning, colicky pains in the bowels.   .

DOSE.—Precisely the same as directed for China, until the cramps disappear, then at intervels of four hours.

IPECACUANHA is indicated when there is much shivering, followed by moderate heat, or the reverse; or when external heat aggravates the shivering, or complete absence of thirst, or at least very little thirst during the chill, but violent thirst during the heat; or when the paroxysms are preceded by *vomiting* or other derangements of the stomach, with clean tongue, or moderately coated, and oppression of the chest; vomiting in the interim. This remedy if persevered in, will in most cases where it is indicated, produce a speedy cure; and if it fails of this, it usually produces a favorable change, and *Arnica, China* or *Nux vom.* may complete the cure.

DOSE.—Six globules may be dissolved in three tablespoonfuls of water, or one drop may be dissolved in the same, and a teaspoonful may be given every two hours during the interim

IGNATIA is applicable in ague, when there is thirst only during the cold stage, or when external heat tends to mitigate in some measure the cold, or when there is only external heat and internal shivering, or when there is nausea and vomiting, pale complexion, or when the exciting cause is grief or disappointment, and there is absence of thirst during the heat and headache, vertigo or delirium, alternate paleness and redness of the face, or redness of only one of the cheeks, pain in the head during the fever, *great fatigue and pain at the pit of the stomach*, drowsiness or profound sleep, with snoring; eruptions on the lips, and at the corners of the mouth; nettle-rash and itching during the fever.

DOSE.—Four globules may be given every two hours, on the tongue, or one drop in three tablespoonfuls of water may be given, a teaspoonful at a dose, every two hours, until a change. Nux vom. may be used to complete a cure, in the same way, if this remedy should only seem to palliate.

MERCURIUS may be employed, when there is in addition to the ordinary symptoms of ague, flushes of heat, commingling with the shivering, or heat with great anguish and thirst, or *profuse sour* perspiration, or perspiration of an offensive odor, with palpitation of the heart. It is also serviceable when there are flying pains in the region of the liver.

DOSE.—Of a solution of one drop of the dilution, or four pellets in two table-spoonfuls of water, give a teaspoonful every three hours during the interim, or until a change.

NUX VOM. is to be employed when the fever is pre ceded by great weakness and prostration, followed by shivering and commingling of heat, or heat before the shivering, or external heat with internal shivering, or internal heat with external shivering. The patient should be constantly covered during the heat and per-spiration, *during the shivering fit, coldness and blueness of the skin, hands and feet, face or nails,* or stitches in the side, and shootings in the abdomen, pains in the back and loins, or drawing pains in the abdomen, *headache,* and humming in the ears; *during the heat,* pains in the chest, heat in the head and face, with redness of the cheeks and thirst. Sometimes, craving for malt liquors during the chill and heat, derangements of the stomach, nausea, vomiting of bilious matter, vertigo, anguish, and constipation. This medicine is often suitable after *Ipec.,* when this remedy has had a palliative effect.

DOSE.—Two drops, or ten globules may be dissolved in a half-pint tumbler of water, and a teaspoonful may be given every three hours, until better or a change.

NATRUM MURIATICUM is particularly indicated where the cold stage is marked by *constant shivering, without any interruption,* heat and dizziness, cloudiness of the eyes, vertigo and redness of the face, violent headache, espe-cially during the heat; pains in the bones; yellowish complexion; great debility; ulceration in the corners of the mouth; violent thirst during the shivering, and especially during the hot stage; dryness of the pit of stomach to the touch; bitter taste in the mouth, and complete want of appetite.

DOSE.—Of a solution of one drop, or six globules, in four tablespoon-fuls of water; give a teaspoonful every four hours, until better or change.

OPIUM is particularly indicated where there is during the hot stage an inclination to sleep, or sometimes during the cold stage; snoring with the mouth open; convulsive twitches; hot perspiration; suppressed excretions; this medicine is better suited to aged persons or to children.

DOSE. Of a solution of one drop, or six globules, in a half-pint tumbler of water; give a teaspoonful every four hours.

PULSATILLA is a remedy well suited to intermittents, when in addition to ordinary symptoms, there is want of thirst throughout the entire period of the fever. *Aggravation in the afternoon or evening;* oppressive pain in the head; anxiety and oppression of the chest during shivering; redness and puffing of the face; perspiration on the face; shivering when uncovered, or redness only of the cheeks during the hot stage; *gastric or bilious affections;* bitter taste in the mouth; slimy, bilious or sour vomiting; diarrhœa; constipation; oppression of the chest; moist cough and headache during or between the paroxysms of fever. This remedy is particularly applicable when imprudent eating or indigestion has caused a relapse.

DOSE.—Dissolve six globules in four tablespoonfuls of water, and give a teaspoonful every three hours in the interim, or one drop may be dissolved in the same quantity of water, and given as before; it is suitable after *Nux vom.* or *Ignat.*

SEPIA is very useful when the usual symptoms of the ague are present, and in addition there is icy coldness of the hands and feet and numbness of the fingers.

DOSE.—The same as directed for Pulsatilla.

SULPHUR is particularly applicable where there is suppressed eruption of the skin, which is followed by paroxysm of fever, as that following repercussion of the itch, and when there are shiverings every evening, heat and perspiration at night, especially towards the morning, or when there is fever with palpitation of the heart and violent thirst, even before the cold stage.

DOSE.—Sulphur may be administered, a dose every morning, one drop in a spoonful of water, or six globules. This remedy is often useful in the treatment of those cases that have been severely treated with *quinine*, until the system has become weakened, without success, especially if the countenance is pale and haggard, and indications of dropsy are manifest.

RHUS TOX. is also extremely useful in the treatment of such cases as have the cold stage commingled with heat, and when the paroxysms come on at night or in the evening, and the perspiration comes on after midnight, or towards the morning, or when there is pains in the limbs during the shiverings; headache, toothache, vertigo, convulsive jerks, either during the paroxysms or between them, or when there is nettle-rash, colic, diarrhœa and other derangements of the stomach, or jaundice, sleeplessness with tossing, thirst at night, palpitation of the heart, with anxiety; pressure at the pit of the stomach.

DOSE.—Of a solution of six globules in three tablespoonfuls of water; a teaspoonful may be given every four hours; or one drop dissolved in three tablespoonfuls may be given in the same manner.

VERATRUM is applicable when during the paroxysm there is coldness all over, with cold, clammy sweat, especially on the forehead; shuddering and chilliness with desire for cold drink; or where there is severe chill, succeeded with little heat, slow pulse, prone to perspirations during the day, great anxiety, or when there is cutting colic, with violent painful diarrhœa.

DOSE.—Of a solution of six globules, or one drop of the dilution, in four tablespoonfuls of water; a teaspoonful may be given every three hours during the interim, or every two hours, if the paroxysms occur every day, until a mitigation or change.

With regard to the particular type, most of the above remedies are applicable to all types when the symptoms are present that indicate their use.

The quotidian or daily type, Arn., Ars., China.

The tertian, or every other day, Cham., Chin., Sulph., Nux vom.

Quartan, or that which occurs once in seventy-two hours, Carb. veg., Bry., Chin., Ars., Sulph. may be consulted, according to symptoms.

The symptoms, however, are the guide, and the remedies, under all circumstances, should be selected to accord with them. After a remedy has been well selected, a perseverance in its continuance is generally found best, and although the process of cure may seem slow, yet the gradual change wrought in the system will be effectual, while a resort to barks and quinine, may only smother the disease for a while, to break out again and again, thus consuming more time in the end, than if the genuine homœopathic remedy had been adhered to from the first.

DIET AND REGIMEN.—On the days which the paroxysms occur, nature generally indicates that but little food of any kind should be taken. The barley or rice gruel may be taken as a drink. In the interim, it is better not to tax the digestive organs with food of a solid character, for this alone may provoke a paroxysm. Great care should be taken, until the paroxysms disappear entirely, not to tax the digestive system. Therefore, we may regard it a rule, to take nothing, except farinaceous gruel, made of farina, flour, rice, arrow-root, or sago, on the days of the fever, or during the occurrence of a paroxysm; while in the interim, light puddings, made of bread, tapioca, arrow-root, or sago, may be indulged in; or sometimes delicate soups, made of mutton, chicken, or game, with rice boiled in them, may be allowed; as also, some delicate meats, taking the greatest care to masticate them well, may be taken.

As patients are often seemingly quite well, between the paroxysms, it is requisite to guard against out-door

11

exposures; patients should not venture into a chilly or damp atmosphere. They should not fatigue themselves with exercise, or stand, or sit, in any place where there is a draft of cold air, and the clothing should be ample and sufficient.

5.—Yellow Fever.

This very acute and dangerous febrile affection, is called yellow fever, because complicated in its second stage with jaundice, and at a later stage, accompanied by vomiting of black matter. Many writers on the subject, regard it as a variety of typhus; and others regard it simply a malignant bilious fever. Its regular occurrence is usually confined to tropical climates, but it has prevailed epidemically in the temperate regions. Some have also regarded the disease an inflammation of the mucus coat of the stomach and bowels, highly exasperated by atmospheric heat, so that it runs through its stages with much greater rapidity than in cooler climates. The yellow color of the skin is attributed to an obstruction of the gall-bladder, preventing the secretion of the liver from escaping, it is thus thrown back upon the system, and becomes universally present in the skin.

CAUSES.—There has been much speculation in relation to the cause of this malady; it is believed, however, to be the result of exposure in hot climates, to miasms arising from decaying vegetable matter on the one hand, and to a struggle in the system to become acclimated, on the other.

SYMPTOMS.—The premonitory symptoms of yellow fever, are giddiness; wandering pains in the back and limbs; slight chills; nausea, and frequent sensations of faintness. After these symptoms have continued awhile, a reaction occurs, the circulation becomes excited; the face flushed; the eyes red; there are violent pains in the head, back, loins, and extremities; distress of the stomach, and vomiting of acid, bilious matters; the surface becomes dry with intense thirst, and sometimes delirium.

The paroxysms continue about twenty-four hours, though sometimes they continue for a much longer period; after which there is a disappearance of the symptoms, except a distressed sensation in the stomach, with nausea and vomiting. Several hours. may pass away while the patient is in this state; after which, there is a return of the former symptoms in some degree of an aggravated form; the stomach now becomes extremely tender to the touch, and painful vomiting becomes incessant and violent; the matter vomited is darker in color; the skin and eyes acquire a yellow tinge, and the mind becomes confused and wandering. This stage lasts from twelve to forty-eight hours, with slight remission of the symptoms in some cases, towards the termination.

The third stage usually sets in immediately, and this is characterised by the complete *black vomit*. At this period, there is a rapid sinking of all the powers of the system. The pulse sinks, and perhaps, intermits; the tongue becomes dry, black, and shrivelled; the breath irregular and laborious; cramps seize the calves of the legs, and the bowels; the whole countenance loses its life-like expression; the extremities become cold; colliquative sweats; diarrhœa; hemorrhages, and loss of intellect; and finally, death ends the scene.

This is but a brief outline of some of the ordinary symptoms of this malady, given merely to furnish some idea of its course. The practitioner, however, will find this description only of general use, as each individual case will present its own peculiar character, when it comes up for treatment.

TREATMENT.—Wherever an opportunity has offered itself for the trial of homœopathic treatment in this fearful disease, it has signalised itself above every other mode of practice that has been brought to bear. Dr. Leon and others were eminently successful in combatting the late epidemic in New Orleans. The remedies found most successful are *Acon., Ars., Bell., Bry., Chin., Canth., Carbo veg., Ipecac., Lachesis, Mercurius, Nux vom., Rhus., Sulphur and Veratrum.*

ACONITE is suitable in the first and second stages when there are burning and dry skin, red cheeks, full and rapid pulse; red and sensitive eyes; tongue natural or covered with a whitish slimy coat; lips and mouth dry; vomiting of mucus and bile; urine dark red; violent febrile reaction; sensation of intense heat; great thirst; acute pains in the temples, forehead, or on the side of the head; vertigo on rising; the eyes weak and sensitive to light; pains and soreness in the back and limbs; nausea; general sense of debility; great heat and irritability of the stomach; short and anxious respiration. When the fever is on, great anguish, anxiety and restlessness, and for the most part delirium at night.

DOSE.—Dissolve two drops, or twelve globules, in four tablespoonfuls of water, and give a teaspoonful every hour or two hours until a change, or if another remedy is needed, Belladonna may often be used with advantage in alternation with this remedy in the first stage.

ARSENICUM is reported to have been used with signal success during the late siege of yellow fever at the South, and the following symptoms are believed to be indicative of its use: yellowish or bluish color of the face, eyes sunken and dull, with a mark under them; whites of the eyes yellow; nose pointed; general coldness of the body, with cold and clammy sweat; lips and tongue brown or black; colliquative sweats; pulse irregular or quick, weak, small and frequent, or suppressed and trembling sense of extreme debility; dull, throbbing, stunning or shooting pains in the head; burning or short darting pains in the region of the liver; frequent involuntary evacuations, or with tenesmus; oppression of the chest, with rapid and anxious breathing; cramps in the calves of the legs; violent vomiting, and great oppression at the stomach, especially after drinking; drawing and cramp-like pains in the abdomen; sensation as if a weight was pressing upon the bowels; great indifference; weakness of the memory; delirium, with great flow of ideas; loss of consciousness, and loss of sense.

DOSE.—Dissolve two drops, or twelve globules in four tablespoonfuls of water, and give a teaspoonful every half hour until some change is produced in the symptoms. In cases of less violent symptoms, the remedy may be repeated every hour or two hours, &c.

BELLADONNA may be given in the first stage when there is glowing redness and bloated appearance of the countenance, eyes red and sparkling, or fixed and glistening, or protruding; tongue loaded with foul, yellowish or brownish mucus; pulse variable, or when there is a dry burning heat upon the surface; sharp shooting pains in the head; violent throbbing of the arteries in the temples; cramp-like pains in the back and loins and legs, and also in the stomach, with pressure; violent vomitings, or inclination to vomit; great depression and melancholy during the remission, and when reaction comes on, with great agitation, continual tossing and anguish.   ·

DOSE.—Dissolve twelve globules in four tablespoonfuls of water, and give a teaspoonful every two hours, or two drops may be used instead of

11*

the globules. ⹁ This remedy may be advantageously used in alternation with Aconite at intervals of two hours.

BRYONIA is suitable for the first stage, when there are yellowness of the skin; redness of the eyes; dry tongue, loaded with white or yellow coating; rapid and full pulse, or else, weak and rapid; burning sensation in the stomach, with severe pain and vomiting, especially after drinking; burning thirst; pains in the back and limbs; pains in the head, aggravated by moving; eyes painful, on moving them; fulness and oppression in the stomach and bowels; great dread of the future, with much anxiety; loss of memory, and delirium.

DOSE.—Twelve globules may be dissolved in four tablespoonfuls of water, or two drops; and a teaspoonful may be given every hour, or every two hours, according to the severity of the symptoms, until a change, or some other remedy is required.

CHINA is of service in the first and second stages, when there is very apparent remissions; yellowness of the skin and eyes; tongue loaded with white coating, or of a brownish color; or when there is excessive weakness and prostration, after discharges of blood from the nose or from the bowels.

DOSE.—Dissolve twelve globules, or two drops, in four tablespoonfuls of water, and give a teaspoonful every two hours, until a change of the symptoms. This remedy is useful, after Sulphur, and may be alternated with *Bry.* or *Rhus.*

CANTHARIS is sometimes indicated in the third stage, when there is complete insensibility, cramps in the abdominal muscles and limbs; suppression of urine; discharges of blood from the bowels; and cold sweat on the hands and feet.

DOSE.—Dissolve twelve globules, or two drops, in four tablespoon-fuls of water, and a teaspoonful may be given every half hour, until there is a decided change, or a perceptible impression and modification of the symptoms.

CARBO VEG. is also one of the most useful remedies in

the third stage, and has sometimes proved curative. The symptoms that particularly indicate its use, are, putrid breath; dark colored coating, very thick, upon the tongue; vomitings of putrid, offensive matters; and the discharge of liquid, offensive, putrescent stools.

DOSE.—The same in all respects as Cantharis.

IPECACUANHA is one of the most important remedies in the earliest stage of the disease, when the first symptoms declare themselves as, dizziness; slight chills; pains in the back and limbs; uneasy sensations at the stomach, with nausea, vomiting, and fainting.

DOSE.—Dissolve twelve globules, or two drops, in four tablespoonfuls of water, and give a teaspoonful every two hours, until there is a decided change in the symptoms. If the disease is not arrested by this remedy in the first stage, it may be essentially modified, so that an alternation with some other remedy as indicated, may so mitigate the second and third stages, as to promote the recovery of the patient.

LACHESIS is particularly indicated for the third stage, when there is a sunken paleness of the countenance, with eyes sunken, and a black streak beneath them; or when there is continued burning in the stomach, with inclination to vomit; or vomiting of dirty, dark-colored matter; and burning discharges from the bowels, of a putrescent odor; great prostration, and loss of consciousness.

DOSE.—Twelve globules, or two drops, may be dissolved in four tablespoonfuls of water, and a teaspoonful may be given every half hour, until a change.

MERCURIUS VIV. is suitable in the first and second stages, when there is yellow color of the skin; redness of the whites of the eyes; paralysis of some of the limbs; thick, white, moist fur upon the tongue, or covered with white mucus stools, sometimes thin and watery; *pulse* irregular, strong and quick, intermittent, or weak and trembling; inclined to sleep, or restless from nervous irritation; sensation of fatigue and debility; rapid loss

of strength; dizziness, or pain in the head; violent convulsive vomiting of mucus and bilious matter; tenderness
of the stomach; constipation, or diarrhœa, with discharges
of slime, bile, or blood; coldness and cramps of the anus
and legs; great sensitiveness of all the organs; agitation;
loss of memory; forebodings;. depression of spirits;
sullen, or raving.

DOSE.—Dissolve twelve globules, or two drops, in four tablespoonfuls
of water, and give a teaspoonful every hour, until mitigation or change;
useful after Acon. and Bell.

NUX VOM. is often to be consulted for the first and
second stages, when indicated by yellow skin, pale
yellowish appearance of the face around the mouth and
nose; lower portions of the whites of the eyes, yellow;
eyes inflamed, with redness of the balls, or surrounded
with a dark circle and full of tears; *tongue* with a white
or yellow fur, or dry, cracked and brown, with red
edges; variable *pulse;* burning pains in the stomach
and pressing, cramp-like pains; vomiting of bilious,
acid or mucus matters; violent hiccough; sensitiveness
of the eyes to light; vertigo, or pains in the head;
tremors of the limbs; cramps in different parts; thirst
for beer and other stimulants; spasms in the bowels,
and contraction of the abdominal muscles; *stools* loose
and slimy, or bilious with blood; burning at the neck
of the bladder, with painful urination; cramps, coldness
and paralysis of the limbs and extremeties; great anxiety;
fear of death; muttering and moaning and loss of consciousness.

DOSE.—Twelve globules, or two drops, may be dissolved in a half-pint
tumbler half full of water, and a teaspoonful may be given every hour or
two hours; Veratrum is suitable after Nux vom.

RHUS TOX. is suitable when the surface is of a dirty
yellow color, eyes sunken and glassy; dry and black

tongue; brownish dry lips; pulse quick and small; delirium and disposition to talk; sleepy, with noisy breathing; constant moaning; pain and distressing burn; ing in the stomach; nausea and vomiting; paralysis of the lower extremities; spasms in the abdomen; want of power over the abdominal muscles; colic and diarrhœa - difficulty and pain in swallowing; dulness and cloudiness of the intellect; delirium and great inquietude.

DOSE.—Twelve globules, or two drops, in four tablespoonfuls of water, and give a teaspoonful every three hours; Bryonia is suitable for alternation with this remedy.

SULPHUR, in the first and second stages, is commended when the face is pale or yellowish; little sores in the mouth; dry, rough, reddish tongue, or coated with a brownish white; quick pulse and full; stools whitish, greenish, brownish or bloody; dizziness or sharp pains in the head; burning and itching pains in the eyes; roaring noises in the ears; nausea, with trembling and weakness; vomiting of bilious, acid, bloody or blackish matter; pressure and pain in the stomach; pains in the back and loins; melancholy, sad, timid, undecided, wandering.

DOSE.—Dissolve twelve globules in four tablespoonfuls of water, or two drops, and give a teaspoonful every four or six hours.

VERATRUM is adapted to the second and third stages, and should be resorted to when there is a yellowish or bluish color of the face; cold, and covered with cold perspiration; yellowish, watery, cloudy or dull eyes; dry tongue, brown and cracked; hiccough; coldness of the hands and feet; trembling and cramps of the feet, hands and legs; evacuations loose, blackish or yellowish; pulse slow, and almost extinct, or small, quick and intermittent; general prostration of strength; confusion of the head, or vertigo; deafness; difficult swallowing;

intense thirst; violent vomiting of green bile and mucus, or black bile and blood; burning in the stomach, abdomen and limbs; diarrhœa; timid, despondent, restless, loss of sense, coma, or violent delirium.

DOSE.—Of a solution of one drop, or six globules, in a wineglassful of water, ; give a teaspoonful every hour.

DIET AND REGIMEN.—During the course of this fever, in any of its forms, no solid food whatever can be allowed, and even thin gruels can only be allowed in small quantities at a time. 1. *Drinks.*—Water, toast water, barley tea, or tea made of groats. 2. *Food.*—Gruel, made thin, or rice flour, wheat flour and sago; all food and drink should be taken in exceeding small quantities at a time, and cold, and at regular intervals, say midway between the times of giving the medicine. In the first stage the patient must avoid exercise and keep quiet; he must be exposed, if possible, to only a moderate degree of heat, in well ventilated apartments. Great attention must be paid to proper ablutions with tepid water, and the air of the apartment should be changed as often as possible.

Eruptive Fevers.

By this term is understood those fevers, attended by some kind of eruption on the skin, varying in its character according to the nature of the disease; under this head are included, 1. Nettle rash. 2. Scarlet rash. 3. Scarlet fever. 4. Measles. 5. Erysipelas. 6. Chicken pox. 7. Varioloid, and 8. Small pox.

1. Nettle rash. Urticaria. Hives.

This affection is by no means regarded dangerous, although the burning, stinging and itching that attends it renders it exceedingly annoying.

SYMPTOMS.—The eruption is much like that produced

by the sting of the nettle, from which it takes its name; a pale, red or whitish eminence, surrounded by a purple color; on making its appearance it is attended with heat, burning, tingling and itching in the spots; the blotches are constantly changing from one position to another, or disappearing in a few hours on one part, and appearing on another; cold is more favorable to their appearance than warmth.

CAUSE.—Changes of the temperature; over-eating and drinking, by eating herring or shell-fish, or some kinds of fruit, as strawberries.

TREATMENT.—The remedies employed in the treatment of this affection, are Acon., Calcarea, Cham., Bryonia, Dulcamara, Ipec., Mercurius, Nux vom., Nit. acid, Pulsatilla, Rhus and Sulphur.

ACONITE.—When the eruption is attended with acceleration of the pulse.

BRYONIA.—When the rash is occasioned by damp weather, and attended with shivering, and also when the rash strikes in.

CALCAREA.—When the rash is of a chronic character.

DOSE.—Of the two former remedies, dissolve a drop, or six globules, in four tablespoonfuls of water, and give a spoonful every three hours until the rash disappears. Of the latter, the same solution, and give a teaspoonful morning and evening.

DULCAMARA.—When the rash is produced by a cold, preceded by stinging.

IPECAC.—When the rash is accompanied with nausea or a sick feeling at the stomach.

DOSE.—One drop, or six globules, of either of the above two remedies, may be dissolved in four tablespoonfuls of water, and a teaspoonful may be given every three hours.

MERCURIUS is useful when the rash is somewhat of a chronic character, attended with burning, itching and stinging sensation.

DOSE.—One drop, or six globules, in half a pint tumbler of water, a teaspoonful morning and evening.

NUX VOMICA is useful when the rash is occasioned by indigestion of ordinary food, or fruits, oysters, or other shell-fish.

DOSE.—One drop, or six globules, in half a tumbler of water, a teaspoonful every three hours until relieved. ꞏ

NITRIC ACID is useful when the rash is somewhat chronic, accompanied with sensation as if insects were biting, and itching and biting whenever the rash appears.

DOSE.—Similar to that of Nux vomica, to be given three times a day, at intervals of six hours.

PULSATILLA is particularly serviceable when the rash is produced by eating fat meats, or any greasy kind of food.

DOSE.—The same as directed for Nux vomica.

RHUS TOX. is suitable when the rash is of a red, shining appearance, accompanied with slight fever, occurring from cold or damp weather.

DOSE.—One drop, or six globules, dissolved in four tablespoonfuls of water, a teaspoonful every four hours until relieved.

SULPHUR is suitable in the more chronic cases, when the rash occasions scratching, which leaves an annoying itching and burning of the skin, and also when it accompanies any chronic derangement of the stomach.

DOSE.—One drop, or six globules, in a spoonful of water, may be taken morning and evening.

DIET AND REGIMEN.—Toast and black tea, or gruel thickened with wheat flour and milk, and other simple kinds of food, free from condiments or stimulants of any kind.

When the rash is without any complication with other diseases, it will generally disappear under the above treatment in a very short time, but should any accompanying disease be regarded the source of the rash, the treatment will be modified according to symptoms.

2.—Scarlet Rash.—(*Miliara purpura.*)

This affection consists of small granular elevations, easily felt by passing the hand over the surface; dark, red efflorescence, which leaves no white imprint from pressure of the finger. It is often mistaken for measles or scarlet fever.

SYMPTOMS.—Chilliness, alternating with heat; heaviness and fulness of the head; vertigo, and pain in the forehead at first, after which the eruption begins to appear on the covered parts and above the bend of the joints, sometimes soreness of the throat precedes the eruption, which subsides when it fully makes its appearance.

This affection is not regarded dangerous unless the eruption strikes in; in such an event, the throat usually becomes sore and inflamed, and may assume a dangerous form; great caution is requisite to keep the disease out, or otherwise it may affect some of the vital organs, producing derangement of the brain, &c. The disease is evidently of a contagious character, and it may appear in the same individual several times.

TREATMENT.—The remedies employed in the treatment of this affection are *Aconite, Belladonna, Bryonia, Coffea, Ipecac. and Opium.*

ACONITE is, for the most part, the only remedy required when the disease is uncomplicated, as it will affect a speedy cure.

DOSE.—One drop, or six globules, dissolved in a tumbler of water, give a spoonful every three hours, but under other circumstances,

BELLADONNA will be needed when there is fulness of the head, and the eyes seem red and suffused, and there is a proneness to start in opening and closing the eyes, and pain in the forehead.

12

DOSE.—One drop of the dilution, or six globules, may be dissolved in four tablespoonfuls of water, and a teaspoonful may be given every two hours until the symptoms disappear.

BRYONIA will be required when the eruption is slow in making its appearance, or when it suddenly disappears, and there is nausea or glairy vomitings.

DOSE.—The same as directed for Belladonna, until the particular symptoms disappear.

COFFEA will be indicated when there is a restless, whining mood, or pain in the head, back, and extremities.

DOSE.—The same as directed for Aconite, and it may be administered in alternation with this remedy, at intervals of three hours.

IPECAC. will be of service if there is nausea, and a retarded appearance of the eruption ; or if the eruption recedes, producing sickness at the stomach.

DOSE.—The same as that directed for Belladonna and Bryonia.

OPIUM is required when there is stupor, or fulness about the head, producing an inclination to sleep, without being restless.

DOSE.—One drop, or six globules, in four tablespoonfuls of water, a teaspoonful every three hours, until the particular symptoms disappear.

As this affection is often complicated with scarlet fever, and measles, the treatment required under such circumstances, may be the same as indicated in these diseases.

DIET AND REGIMEN.—Plain toast and black tea, or gruel made of wheat flour, arrow-root, or rice flour, or toast-water, or barley-gruel.

The greatest care should be exercised, not to take cold, for a serious relapse may be the consequence, attended with symptoms of a formidable character. Overloading the stomach, may also induce a relapse, that results in a dangerous sequel.

3.—Scarlet Fever. (*Scarlatina.*)

This disease, is generally believed to be of a contagious character, and is usually regarded as the most formidable of any of the eruptive fevers among children. There are three varieties of the disease, viz: the *simple*, anginose, and malignant.

THE SIMPLE SCARLET FEVER, is usually preceded by chilliness; weariness of the limbs; peevishness and fretfulness; pain in the head; nausea, or sickness at the stomach, and sometimes vomiting, after which, the eruption begins to appear in patches, covering the entire body with a bright, scarlet eruption; the breath appears foul; the tongue loaded with a white coating; inflammation of the tonsils, but without ulceration.

The ANGINOSE variety, makes its appearance with more violent symptoms; great acceleration of the pulse, and continual vomiting for hours, of green, bilious matter; when the vomiting subsides, there is an eruption of a paler appearance, that begins to manifest itself in patches; the tonsils become inflamed and swollen, and severely ulcerated; and the breath has an exceedingly offensive odor; and the tongue is loaded with a dirty, white coating, or appears red; and the papillæ swollen; there is great prostration, and swelling of the parotid glands, and also the glands of the under jaw; the fever is intense, and the chest seems afflicted with catarrhal difficulty; and not unfrequently, there is a constant discharge of hot, acrid mucus from the nose; the tongue is dry and swollen.

THE MALIGNANT FORM of the disease, manifests the most violent symptoms about the head, it is sudden in its appearance, and often terminates fatally, before the eruption has fully made its appearance; but when such is not the case, there is continual vomiting, violent pain in the head; stupor; eyes half closed; pale eruption in spots, of the color of brick-dust; and not unfrequently, thin, acrid, and burning discharges from the nose. These are the general characteristics of the three forms, but great variations in the symptoms, may be met with, that will call for corresponding treatment.

Scarlet fever rarely attacks persons of adult age; in general, it may be regarded a disease of childhood, though, in some cases, persons of mature age have been its subjects.

TREATMENT.—The remedies employed in the treatment of scarlet fever in its various forms, are, *Acon.,* *Arsenicum, Belladonna, Bryonia, Calc. carb., Chamomilla, Digitalis, Dulcamara, Helleborus nig., Hepar sulph., Kali carb., Lycopodium, Mercurius, Nitric acid, Nux vom., Opium, Phosphorus, Phosph. acid, Pulsatilla, Rhus tox., Sulphur, Silicea.*

ACONITE.—When the fever runs high in the first stage of simple scarlet fever, that has been preceded by chilliness, and there is throbbing of the temples, and vomiting of greenish matters.

DOSE.—Six globules, or one drop, in half a tumbler of water, a teaspoonful every hour, until the eruption is completely out, and then refer to Belladonna.

ARSENICUM is indicated when there is a heavy, fetid odor from the mouth, with continual inclination to vomit; great heat about the head, and strongly marked indications of cerebral disturbance; a discharge of hot, acrid water from the nose; fetid ulceration of the throat; great prostration, and loss of consciousness; pulse rapid, full and tense; stupor and delirium. This remedy is suited to the malignant form of the disease.

DOSE.—One drop, or six globules, in half a tumbler of water, a teaspoonful every two hours, until mitigation or change.

BELLADONNA is useful after Aconite, in simple inflammatory scarlet fever after the fever is somewhat subdued, and the throat appears to be seriously affected; tonsils swollen and red; the skin of a scarlet hue; the tongue coated, and red around the edges; the pulse quick and strong, and particularly, when the disease appears in its simple form, without any prominent febrile symptoms.

DOSE.—One drop of the dilution, or six globules, in four tablespoonfuls of water, a teaspoonful every three hours, until mitigation or change. It should be administered as soon as the throat and tongue become affected with dryness and burning, provided the other indications are present.

BRYONIA is indicated when there is vomiting of white glairy mucus, and the eruption is slow in making its appearance; it promotes the bringing out of the eruption after it has receded.

DOSE.—One drop of the dilution, or six globules, in four tablespoonfuls of water, a teaspoonful every three hours; this remedy may also be followed by Belladonna, the same as directed for the use of this remedy.

CALC. CARB. is particularly indicated in the more malignant form of the disease, when complicated with scrofula, or the subject has been known previously to be affected with herpetic eruptions, that have been sup-. pressed, and also by pale, sunken expression of the countenance; stupor; swelling of the parotid and submaxillary glands; red, glairy appearance of the tongue; disposition to sleep; pale color of the eruption and in patches.

DOSE.—One drop, or six globules, may be dissolved in four tablespoonfuls of water, and a tablespoonful may be given first, and Belladonna may be given if otherwise indicated three hours after; Calc. carb. should not be repeated oftener than once in two days; during the interval any remedy indicated by the acute symptoms may be given every three hours.

CHAMOMILLA is indicated when there is in the commencement great restlessness and inquietude, and also when there is pain in the stomach, preceding the appearance of the eruption; fretful, wheezing and moaning;

12*

the eruption red and distinct; slight indications of perspiration on some parts of the body, and particularly on
the face and forehead; tossing about or throwing about
the arms and legs, and also for rawness of the face.

DOSE.—This medicine may be given four globules at a time, every
three hours, either in water or dry upon the tongue, or one drop of the
dilution in four spoonfuls of water, a teaspoonful at a time, every three
hours, until amelioration or change.

DIGITALIS is particularly applicable in local affections
arising from scarlet fever, such as dropsy of the chest;
the symptoms which indicate its use are: small, quick,
soft *pulse;* labored breathing, as if the patient were
smothering; tumefaction of the countenance; pale, sickly
appearance of the face; great debility and want of
strength in the limbs; discharges of watery pus from
the ears.

DOSE.—One drop, or six globules, in four spoonfuls of water, a teaspoonful every four hours ; this remedy may be used in alternation with
Arsenicum, or Helleborus, or Calcarea carb.

DULCAMARA may be used to obviate deafness after an
attack of scarlet fever, attended with pains in the ears,
when there still remains heat and dryness of the skin,
or when the scarlet fever has appeared suddenly after a
cold.

DOSE.—The same in all respects as for Digitalis.

HELLEBORUS NIG. is particularly indicated when general
dropsy sets in, as an after effect of scarlet fever, and may
be associated with Arsenicum, Bryonia and Rhus.

DOSE.—Of either remedy, one drop, or six globules, may be dissolved
iu four spoonfuls of water, and one spoonful may be given three times a
day.

HEPAR SULPHUR is another remedy to be consulted in
obstinate dropsical difficulties, or discharges from the
ears, or stoppage in the nose, when they appear as the
after effects of scarlet fever.

DOSE.—Four globules, or one drop of the dilution may be given twice a day, or Hepar. may be given at night, and Puls. in the morning.

KALI CARBONICUM is indicated when there is continued inflammation of the parotid glands, and catarrhal difficulties implicating the chest, or sore throat, remaining after the fever has disappeared.

DOSE.—The same in all respects as for Hep. Sulph.

LYCOPODIUM is suitable for internal inflammation of the ears, discharge of pus, and for obstinate dropsical difficulties, after the use of Helleborus.

DOSE.—One drop, or four globules, twice a day.

MERCURIUS VIV. is a good remedy against soreness of the nose and face after the fever, with swelling of the sub-maxillary glands; it may be followed with Silicea or Sulphur.

DOSE.—One drop, or four globules, may be given twice a day; twenty-four hours should elapse in all cases after the use of this remedy, before either of the others are employed.

NITRIC ACID is a useful remedy in scarlet fever, when it assumes the typhoid form; when there is a kind of half sleep and stupor; severe and dangerous ulceration of the tonsils; snoring and difficult breathing; coldness of the lower limbs and feet.

DOSE.—One drop, or six globules, in four tablespoonfuls of water; a teaspoonful may be given every hour, until the vital energies appear to be aroused, or there is some amelioration or change.

NUX VOMICA is particularly indicated during the fever, when there is a large quantity of viscid mucus secreted from the inflamed surface of the throat, which adheres so closely that it is difficult to expel, and that sometimes threatens suffocation; it may be used in alternation with Pulsatilla.

DOSE. OF EITHER.—One drop, or four globules, two or three times a day, or in alternation every four or six hours.

OPIUM is a useful remedy to follow Belladonna when

there is burning heat of the skin; drowsiness; stupor; snoring respiration; open mouth; eyes half closed; restlessness, with vomiting and convulsions; furious delirium; restlessness, and continual movements of the hands in the commencement of the disease.

DOSE.—One drop, or six globules, may be dissolved in four tablespoonfuls of water, and a teaspoonful may be given every two hours, until the system becomes aroused, or there is some mitigation or change.

PULSATILLA is decidedly indicated when the face is pale, and bloated or red, and also when the stomach and digestive organs are deranged; when there is constipation of the bowels; or, on the other hand, looseness at night, and occasionally with pains in the bowels and shivering; disposition of a fretful, irritable, sensitive, melancholy character.

DOSE.—Of a solution of six globules, or one drop, in four tablespoonfuls of water, give a teaspoonful every two hours; when the patient is known to be of a scrofulous habit, one dose of four globules of *sulphur* may precede the use of pulsatilla.

PHOSPHORUS is an excellent remedy in the fever when there is dry and hard tongue, and lips covered with blackish scabs, loss of speech and hearing, difficulty of swallowing, inability to retain urine, excessive falling off of the hairs.

DOSE.—In all respects the same as directed for Pulsatilla.

PHOS. ACID is useful in the after-effects of the fever, when there are boils, clusters of red, fine rash pimples, gouty affection of the joints, stitching in the ears, difficulty of hearing, intolerance of music and noise, tough phlegm in the throat, swelling of the parotid glands, and discharge of thin pus from the ears.

DOSE.—Of a solution of six globules, or one drop, in four tablespoonfuls of water, give a tablespoonful morning and evening, until a change.

RHUS TOX. is particularly indicated if the eruption degenerates into a kind of vesicular erysipelas, with inclination to sleep; starting and agitation; stoppage of the urine, and violent thirst. It is also useful in the after-effects of the fever, when there is a tendency to general dropsy. It may be used alone or in alternation with Bryonia, Helleborus or Arsenicum, as the particular symptoms may indicate.

DOSE.—Rhus tox. may be given every three hours, four globules in a spoonful of water, or one drop may be dissolved in half a tumbler of water, and a teaspoonful may be given every three hours, or in alternation with either of the above named remedies every three hours.

SULPHUR may be employed in the commencement of an attack of scarlet fever, where there is any thing like a scrofulous habit, or where it is known that the patient has previously suffered from tetter or any herpetic eruption that has been suppressed, or where there is a head affection that will not yield to Belladonna, or lethargic sleep, starts, convulsions of the eyes or continued delirium; puffed and bright red face; obstruction of the nose; dry, cracked, red tongue, covered with brownish mucus; thirst and difficulty in swallowing, or in the after-affects when there is swelling of the glands; pains in the ears, and discharge of pus; or when there is loss of mind, or memory, or more positive indications of idiocy, it may be used in alternation with Phosphorus in this latter difficulty.

DOSE.—Sulphur when used in the commencement of the fever, may be repeated every six hours, one drop, or four globules ; but in the after-effects it is sufficient to repeat a dose of one drop, or six globules, every twenty-four hours.

SILICEA is particularly useful in the after-affects, when there is swelling of the glands, discharge of thick pus from the ears, or chronic stoppage of the nose, inflammation of the parotid glands.

DOSE.—One drop, or six globules, every twenty-four hours.

There are other remedies that may be employed in the treatment of scarlet fever, but the above group embraces the principal remedies.

Sometimes in severe cases attended with heat in the head, *cold water* has been applied, but this is seldom to be recommended; but more rarely hot or warm water applied to the head under such circumstances may be attended with favorable results; cloths dipped in very warm water may be applied to the head, while internal remedies are being administered, but they should be removed when there appears to be any mitigation of the symptoms.

DIET AND REGIMEN.—There is but little that can be taken of any kind of food during the raging of the fever; very thin rice gruel, or gruel made of arrowroot may be given in small quantities, when the mouth and throat are exceedingly dry or parched; a little warm milk and water may be given to moisten them; and also, when thick scales accumulate on the teeth and lips, or dry scabs, · warm milk and water may be employed to cleanse the mouth and to moisten the scabs; after the fever has abated, and there begins to be a craving for food, great care should be exercised to avoid taxing the digestive organs; a single portion of food unsuited to the condition of the stomach may provoke a relapse, attended with all the dangerous sequels of the disease; swabbing the mouth in the morning with warm water, or milk and water, even after convalescence becomes established, is recommended; a little plain or milk toast may be allowed at regular intervals after the fever has disappeared and the appetite returns; when it is found that digestion goes regularly on, a small quantity of digestible meat may be allowed, with bread once a day, until the normal strength is regained; beef or mutton, or chicken boiled, are best; the two latter may be made into a soup, with rice or barley; vegetables should be avoided for some weeks after convalescence from a serious attack of scarlet fever.

4.—Measles. (*Rubeola.*)

This disease for the most part, rages as an epidemic, and is generally confined to children, though adults, are by no means exempt from it. It is not regarded a dangerous disease, if properly treated, but sometimes, it is made formidable, by the injudicious treatment given it. In adults it has a more critical character than in children. It rarely attacks the second time. The disease is often followed by serious consequences, and the after effects may be regarded more painful and dangerous than the disease itself. .This is sometimes termed the *dreg* left behind, is simply the result of improper treatment, for instance: *It is manifestly improper to give a patient, when sickening with measles, any heating or stimulating teas, to bring out the eruption;* for the practice, in one case out of three, would be productive of severe cough and the incipient seeds of consumption. Cold drinks are preferable, and by far the most to be relied upon, as fulfilling the requirements of the system.

SYMPTOMS.—Measles, as well as other species of cruptive fevers, come on very much like a common cold, and it is not easy to discriminate the incipient stage of the disease, and that of many other maladies; when measles are prevailing epidemically, they are observed to come on with chilliness; short, dry cough; running from the eyes and nose; redness of the eyes; and fever, more or less intense, preceding the eruption from four to five days, which generally continues until the eruption is perfectly developed, and even throughout the disease, gradually diminishing as the eruption disappears.

The character of the eruption is that of small red spots upon the skin, often found in the shape of small, irregular arcs. They usually make their appearance on the face and neck, become confluent, and gradually extend down the body. About the sixth or seventh day after sickening, the eruption begins to turn pale on the parts, where it first made its appearance, and then on the remaining portions of the body, and generally about the ninth day, it entirely disappears, with a bran-like shedding of the outer skin; this is a distinguishing sign of this disease.

TREATMENT.—The apartments of the patient should be well-ventilated. The remedies employed, are *Aconite, Arsenicum, Arnica, Belladonna, Bryonia, Cham., Calc. c., Carbo veg., China, Conium, Drosea, Dulcamara, Hyosciamus, Hepar sulph., Ignatia, Ipecac., Lachesis, Mercurius, Nux vom., Phosphorus, Pulsatilla, Sepia, Sulphur.*

ACONITE may always be given in the first stage of measles, uncomplicated with any chronic difficulty when there is fever; full, tense, or bounding pulse; pain in the head, and back, and loins; dry heat of the skin; redness of the eyes; intolerance of light; general weakness or prostration, and when the fever is of an inflammatory type, this remedy may prove sufficient to effect a cure in a short time.

DOSE.—Of a solution of one drop, or six globules, in six tablespoonfuls of water, a tablespoonful may be given every three hours.

ARSENICUM is called into requisition in the treatment of measles, when there appears to be a great struggle for the eruption to come out; when there is burning at the pit of the stomach, and vomiting of acrid matters from the stomach, with severe and intense pain in the front part of the head, producing stupor and drowsiness; chilliness and heat simultaneously.

DOSE.—Of a solution of one drop, or six globules, in four tablespoonfuls of water, a teaspoonful may be given every three hours.

ARNICA is indicated when the febrile stage comes on with pains in the limbs, as if bruised; or soreness of the skin where the eruption makes its appearance; and also for swelling and inflammation of the parotid glands.

DOSE.—Of a solution of one drop, or eight globules, in six tablespoonfuls of water, give a teaspoonful every three hours, until amelioration or change.

BRYONIA is a useful and efficient remedy in bringing out the eruption, when there is a short, dry, spasmodic cough, and sometimes vomiting of glairy mucus; soreness and heat in the chest; snoring respiration, as if the air-passages of the lungs were filling up; nausea; tardy appearance of the eruption. It is mostly requisite after Aconite, when the fever is of an inflammatory type.

DOSE.—Of a solution of one drop, or six globules, in six tablespoonfuls of water, one tablespoonful may be given every four hours, until mitigation or change.

BELLADONNA is useful after Aconite has been given, in the inflammatory eruptive fever, when there are strongly marked congestive symptoms, either of the head or chest; or when there is intense pain in the top of the head; throbbing in the temples; hot, dry skin; thirst; sore throat; enlargement of the tonsils; drowsiness; snoring respiration; inflammation of the eyes; short, spasmodic cough, worse at night; great restlessness, and high nervous excitement, and delirium.

DOSE.—Dissolve one drop, or six globules, in four tablespoonfuls of water, and give a teaspoonful every three hours, until amelioration or change.

13

CHAMOMILLA is very useful, when there is great restlessness and anxiety, attending a short dry cough, and a disposition to be turning from side to side; slow appearance of the eruption, and pain in the stomach, or colic; better suited to very young children, than to persons of adult age.

DOSE.—Of a solution of one drop of the dilution, or six globules, in four tablespoonfuls of water, give a teaspoonful every three hours; or in alternation with Aconite every two hours.

CALC. CARB. is indicated when there is any indication of measles, being complicated with scrofula; or when it becomes known that a scrofulous habit exists in the family. One or two doses of this remedy may be given at first, and afterwards, Acon., Bell., or Bry., according to indication.

DOSE.—Of a solution of one drop, or six globules, in half a tumbler of water, give a tablespoonful, and repeat in twelve hours, afterwards use Acon., Bry., or Bell., &c., if indicated.

CARBO VEG. is better suited to some of the after-effects, when there is great debility and aching in the lumbar region; cold feet, and great difficulty in getting warm, with hard dry cough, or cough with fetid expectoration; ulceration of the throat; short respiration, and accelerated pulse.

DOSE.—One drop, or six globules, may be dissolved in six spoonfuls of water, and a spoonful may be given three times a day, until some benefit is derived, or change.

CHINA is very suitable for great debility after the disease, attended with diarrhœa, and particularly if there are neuralgic pains in the limbs, teeth or face.

DOSE.—Dissolve one drop, or six globules, in four tablespoonfuls of water, and give a tablespoonful three times a day, until better, or a change.

CONIUM is suited to the after effects, when from the inflammation of the eyes, there are spots left upon the cornea; spasmodic cough, with little expectoration of tough mucus; or when there is ulceration of the tonsils, or inflammation of the ears; accumulation of ear-wax, and purulent discharge from the nose.

DOSE.—One drop, or four globules, may be dissolved in a spoonful of water and given every twenty-four hours, at night.

DROSERA, in a majority of cases, when there is a cough remaining after an uncomplicated case of measles, will be specific; when the cough is violent or comes on in paroxysms, there can be but little doubt of its effecting a cure.

DOSE.—One drop, or six globules, in four tablespoonfuls of water, a teaspoonful every three hours.

DULCAMARA will often cure a cough that is left after measles, characterised by moisture, or hoarseness and much mucus expectoration, tightness of the chest, or indications of dropsy. (Hydrothorax.)

DOSE.—One drop, or six globules, dissolved in half a tumbler of water, may be given a teaspoonful at a time, every six hours.

HYOSCYAMUS, for a cough after measles, that resembles the whooping cough; or for a cough with expectoration of greenish mucus; or when there are paroxysms of deep hollow dry cough at night, affecting the head and eyes; or causing the appearance of dark spots before the eyes.

DOSE.—Dissolve a drop, or six globules, in four tablespoonfuls of water and give a teaspoonful every four hours, until better, or a change.

HEPAR SULPH., when there is a rough hoarse cough, without expectoration, dryness of the throat, and predisposed to croup.

DOSE.—One drop, or four globules, in a spoonful of water twice a day, or three times a day if the cough be of a croupy character.

IGNATIA is suitable for an after-cough, from constriction of the throat pit; or when there is soreness as if a plug were in the throat; or when there is swelling of the parotid glands; or sensitive disposition, and a dry cough with disposition to weep.

DOSE.—Of a solution of one drop, or six globules, in four tablespoonfuls of water, give a teaspoonful every four hours until better, or a change.

IPECACUANHA, when there are bilious vomitings or nausea previous to the appearance of the eruption; or when there is a cough with retching, either before the eruption comes out, or as an after effect of the disease; this remedy may follow the use of *aconite* when the indications for both remedies are present.

DOSE.—Dissolve six globules, or one drop, in four tablespoonfuls of water, and give a teaspoonful every two hours, if preceding the eruption, or every four hours, if after, or in alternation with *Bryonia*, every three hours.

LACHESIS is particularly indicated when there is an after cough with inflammation and gangrene of the tonsils; or when there is gnawing at the pit of the stomach, or dryness of the throat and mouth; or when there is diarrhœa with putrid discharges from the bowels after measles.

DOSE.—One drop, or four globules, two or three times a day.

MERCURIUS is indicated for the after effects of measles, when there is cough and derangement of the stomach; flow of watery saliva in the mouth; swelling of the parotid glands; dysenteric stools, or diarrhœa with bilious discharges from the bowels.

DOSE.—Dissolve one drop, or six globules, in four spoonfuls of water, and give a spoonful every three hours, until a disappearance of symptoms, or change.

NUX VOM. may be applicable after Aconite, when the disease is making its appearance. Its use is indicated by dry, hollow cough; pain in the head, back and limbs; nausea, chilliness and heat, or vertigo; redness of the eyes, and stoppage of the nose; tongue coated white and dry.

DOSE.—Of a solution of one drop, or six globules, in four tablespoonfuls of water; give a teaspoonful every three hours, or in alternation with Aconite every three hours.

PHOSPHORUS is indicated if there is dry, hollow cough; pain in the chest; stitchings from one side to the other; great inflammation of the eyes and dread of light; strong tendency of the disease towards the head; rapid pulse; eruption making its appearance irregularly, of a pale color, and also when cough and diarrhœa manifest themselves as an after effect, and tenderness of the skin.

DOSE.—Of a solution of one drop, or six globules, in four tablespoonfuls of water; give a teaspoonful every three hours, until better or change; Arnica and Phosphorus may be used in alternation at intervals of four hours.

PULSATILLA is one the most valuable remedies when there is derangement of the stomach, or cough, worse towards evening, or during the night, attended with rattling of mucus in the air passages, or much expectoration of thick, yellowish or white mucus, sometimes followed by vomiting, or symptoms approaching suffocation; also, when the discharge from the nose is of a thick, greenish or yellowish appearance.

DOSE.—Of a solution of one drop, or six globules, in four tablespoonfuls of water; give a teaspoonful every three hours. In scrofulous subjects, a dose of sulphur may be given once a day when administering the Pulsatilla, and in dark complexioned persons, of a bilious temperament, Nux vomica may be used in alternation every three hours.

SEPIA SUC. is a valuable remedy for an after cough in females, where there is considerable debility and fulness of the head, or sick headache.

DOSE.—Of a solution of one drop, or six globules, in four tablespoonfuls of water; give a teaspoonful every six hours.

SULPHUR is of great value when there is violent inflammation of the eyes, with slightly developed eruption, or violent pains in the ears, with purulent discharges; difficulty of hearing; tearing and throbbing in the head;

13*

pains in the limbs, and paralytic weakness; or if there be typhoid symptoms with loose cough and expectoration of mucus of a somewhat purulent form.

DOSE.—Dissolve one drop, or six globules, in half a tumbler of water, and give a tablespoonful morning and evening.

There are other remedies that may be called into requisition in the treatment of this disease, which must be selected according as they are indicated; all remedies, of course, must be selected in view of their applicability to corresponding symptoms. The treatment of the after effects of measles is generally of more difficult success than that of the disease itself.

As a precaution against an attack of measles when the epidemic is abroad, Pulsatilla and Aconite may be taken in alternation, morning and evening for about two weeks; and renewed after an elapse of a few days, if the epidemic has not disappeared.

DOSE.—One drop, or four globules of either may be taken in a spoonful of water.

DIET.—In the commencement give nothing but toast water, thin flour or rice gruel, barley water, black tea, not too hot; after the disease begins to abate, toast moistened with water and a very little sweet fresh butter may be allowed; and the allowance may be increased to a light tapioca or bread pudding, and even to a moderate quantity of venison, chicken, or beef steak, once a day, until the strength is fully regained, and the whole system appears to have recovered.

5.—Erysipelas.—(*St. Anthony's Fire.*)—Rose.

This disease is classed among the eruptive fevers, because inflammation of the skin appears to be a sequel of general fever. The inflammation is for the most part superficial, producing tension and swelling of the part; pain and heat more or less acute, and redness by no means circumscribed, disappearing when pressed upon by the finger, but returning as soon as the pressure is removed.

The disease presents two forms, one of which is termed *vesicular*, and the other *phlegmonous;* both are evidently dependent upon the same cause, and are in fact the same disease; the *former* presents the appearance of small vesicles on the inflamed part; the *latter* extends deeper into the sub-cutaneous tissue, and is in every respect dependent upon a more highly inflammatory fever than the former.

The termination of the *vesicular* is the drying up of the vesicles which fall off in the form of branny scales on the subsidence of the fever; the *phlegmonous* or that which extends deeper into the sub-cutaneous tissue, generally terminates by resolution, though in some instances it assumes an ulcerative or gangrenous form, which terminates in the same way as other suppurative processes.

CAUSES.—The disease may arise from derangement of the digestive functions, exposure to cold, or in consequence of powerful mental emotions, biliary derangements, menstrual difficulties, or from eating shell-fish, lobsters, &c.

TREATMENT.—The remedies employed in the treatment are *Aconite, Arsenicum, Belladonna, Bryonia, Lachesis, Rhus tox.,* and some others.

Aconite is required when there is high inflammatory fever, and hot dry skin in the commencement of the disease, and also during the continuance of the disease, until the vascular action abates.

DOSE.—Of a solution of six globules, or one drop, in four tablespoonfuls of water, give a teaspoonful every two hours, until the pulse becomes diminished in frequency, and the skin assumes its normal appearance or becomes moist; in mild cases no other remedy is necessary.

ARSENICUM is of great service when there is a blackish hue of the vesicles, with a tendency to degenerate into gangrene; great prostration of strength; burning in the stomach; acrid vomitings, with strong tendency towards the head; burning and stinging in the part affected.

DOSE.—Six globules, or one drop, may be dissolved in four spoonfuls of water, and a teaspoonful may be given every four hours until a change. Sulphur may be employed after Arsenicum to effect a cure.

BELLADONNA is indicated when there is violent pain in the head, and when the redness extends in rays, and an acute shooting pain with heat and tingling is experienced in the affected part, aggravated by motion; or when the erysipelas breaks out in the face, with burning heat, excessive swelling, so that the eyes are almost closed; hot dry skin; disturbed sleep or restlessness; delirium.

DOSE.—Of a solution of six globules, or one drop, in four tablespoonfuls of water, give a teaspoonful every three hours, until the peculiar symptoms disappear.

BRYONIA is indicated when the disease affects the joints, and particularly if the stomach is deranged, and there is great prostration, or pain in the joints, produced by motion.

DOSE.—Dissolve one drop, or six globules, in three tablespoonfuls of water, and give a teaspoonful every three hours, as long as required; should the gradual recuperation of the system not be apparent, the remedy may be changed to Rhus tox.

LACHESIS is a most important remedy, where *Belladonna* fails of completing a cure, and particularly, if the vesicles appear of a dark color, or the inflammation extends into the subcutaneous tissue, producing swelling of the parts.

DOSE.—Of a solution of six globules, or one drop, in four tablespoon-fuls water, give a teaspoonful every three hours; and if it should appear that this remedy only produces an alteration, instead of cure, resort may be had to Rhus tox. or Arsenicum, according to indication.

RHUS TOX.—This remedy is one of the principal ones, in the treatment of the disorder. When Aconite is indicated, and its use changes the, form of the disease, RHUS TOX. may follow to complete a cure; and also when *Belladonna has been previously given*, this remedy may succeed with marked benefit; or it may be used in alternation with *Belladonna*, or with *Lachesis*, or *Arsenicum.* It is particularly applicable after *Aconite in the vesicular form*, when the parts become very red, and swollen, and there is a strong tendency to the head, brain, or its membranes, and the symptoms indicate something like brain fever. This remedy is also useful when the disease is produced by eating certain kinds of shell-fish or lobster, or when any exciting cause operates upon constitutional peculiarities, which predisposes the patient `to such attacks.

DOSE.—If administered alone, six globules may be dissolved in four tablespoonfuls of water, and a teaspoonful may be given every two hours in severe cases. If after Aconite, a dose every six hours; if in alternation with Aconite, Belladonna, Arsenicum, or Lachesis, an interval of eight hours should elapse between the doses.

There are other remedies that may be called into requisition in the treatment of this disease, under pecu-liar circumstances, as *Caprum met.*, when inflammation of the brain appears to be threatened; or *Graphites*, in some forms of wandering or fugitive erysipelas; or *Nux vom.*, if the disease affect the knee, or foot, and the parts are red and swollen. It is also useful in spurious erysipelas of irritable subjects, females in particular, and even in gangrene of the subcutaneous tissue.

DOSE.—The dose of either of these remedies may be as follow: Of a solution of one drop, or six globules, of *Caprum Met.*, in half a tumbler of water, give a tablespoonful three times a day.   Of the same of Graphites, give a spoonful every twenty-four hours.   Of the same of Nux vom., give a teaspoonful every four hours, until a change.

DIET AND REGIMEN.—In acute attacks, rice-gruel, or gruel made of arrow-root, tapioca, *farina*, or corn-starch; during convalescence, weak soups, without any seasoning; toast and black tea, cocoa, broma, light puddings, made of bread, eggs, and milk.

The apartments should be well ventilated, and kept only of a moderate temperature.   In chronic cases, the diet must be plain, and free from condiments, stimulants, or anything of the kind.

6.—Chicken-pox.   (*Varicella*.)

This disease is characterised by vesicles or blisters scattered over the body, which are smooth and transparent, and of about the size of a pea; they appear in successive groups, are covered by a thin pellicle, and usually disappear about the third, fourth, or fifth day, by bursting at the tip, and concreting into small, puckered scabs, which rarely leave a pit in the skin. The disease is almost exclusively confined to childhood, and as it runs its course rapidly, it is attended with but little danger; although in some respects it resembles small-pox, yet, unlike this disease, it seldom attacks the face to any great extent, the eruption appearing more on the scalp, shoulders, neck, and breast.

There is always an ephemeral fever preceding the eruption, seldom continuing more than twenty-four hours.   The fever is sometimes attended with headache.

The eruption is distinguished from the small pox pustule, by having no dent on the top.

TREATMENT.   The remedies employed, are *Aconite*, *Belladonna*, *Coffea*, *Cantharides* and *Ignatia*.

ACONITE is required when there is considerable fever. BELLADONNA, when there is great pain in the head.

DOSE.—These remedies may be given alternately. Of a solution of six globules, or one drop, of each separately, in four tablespoonfuls of water, a teaspoonful of each may be given alternately every three hours, until better.

COFFEA is applicable when there is restlessness, and considerable nervous excitement; disturbed sleep, with dreams, and moaning.

DOSE.—Of a solution of one drop, or six globules, in three tablespoonfuls of water, give a teaspoonful every three hours until relieved.

CANTHARIDES is useful when there is strangury, or obstruction of the bladder.

DOSE.—The same as for Coffea.

IGNATIA is useful with Bell. in alternation, when there are spasms in teething children attending the disease.

DOSE·—The same as for Aconite and Belladonna in alternation.

PULSATILLA is well suited to mild cases, and abridges their duration.

DOSE.—One drop, or six globules, may be dissolved in half a tumbler of water, and a tablespoonful may be given every three hours, until better.

DIET AND REGIMEN.—As the disease almost uniformly occurs in young children, but little change from the ordinary diet is requisite. The clothing should be loose, and the apartments well ventilated.

7.—Varioloid. (*Modified Small Pox.*)

This disease is really small pox, modified by previous inoculation or vaccination, hence it is called *modified small pox*, and requires very nearly the same treatment as the unmodified form of the disease which is next described.

8.—Small Pox. (*Variola.*)

This is a contagious disease, and is marked by different stages, each of which requires different remedies.

1. *The febrile stage* usually commences in ten days or two weeks after exposure, and continues several days. It sets in with chilliness and fever, heat and dryness of the skin; hard and frequent pulse; derangement and pain in the stomach; pain in the head and back; nausea and vomiting; aching in the bones; soreness of the flesh; swimming of the head, and sometimes convulsions and delirium.

2. The *eruptive stage* begins on the third or fourth day, and the eruption makes its appearance on the face in the form of red points, which increase in extent and elevation, and at the same time on the arms, hands and whole body.

3. The *suppurative stage* is when the pustules complete their development, (usually the size of a pea,) and become filled with a yellowish fluid, which gradually changes its color, until it assumes a turbid appearance, and each pustule is surrounded by a red circle, and has on its top a dark indentation. The eruption becomes fully developed on some parts of the body, while it is only making its appearance on others. This stage generally continues three or four days, with considerable degree of fever, swelling, and flow of saliva.

The *fourth stage* is the drying up of the pustules; they present on the top a brown appearance, and some of them burst, forming scabs. The fever abates and the swelling gradually subsides. The scales peal off, leaving a cicatrice of the pustule of a deep red color. The patient is evidently better, and free from danger.

The disease is termed *distinct small pox* when the pustules are all isolated, and not running into each other. It is termed *confluent* when the pustules run into each other, forming an immense scab. This latter variety is regarded more severe, and is of longer duration than the former.

TREATMENT.—The remedies employed in the treatment of this disease are Aconite, Belladonna, Bryonia, Chamomilla, Coffee, Opium, Pulsatilla, Rhus tox., Stramonium, and Vaccinin.

ACONITE is applicable in the first or febrile stage of the disease, if there is severe pain in the head; full, bounding pulse; thirst; intolerance of light, and delirium.

BELLADONNA may follow Aconite when there is manifested a strong tendency to the head, characterised by a flushed countenance, intolerance of light, headache and delirium; great thirst; nausea and vomiting; or when there is redness of the tongue at the tip and margins; abdomen tumid and painful, particularly in the upper portion of the stomach, where it is tender to the touch; great prostration; loss of strength, and stupor.

DOSE.—If given separately, of a solution of one drop, or six globules, in three tablespoonfuls of water ; give a teaspoonful every three hours, or if in alternation, give a teaspoonful every two hours, until the eruptive stage fully sets in.

BRYONIA is of great use in the eruptive stage in aiding the natural course of the eruption. It is also indicated by derangement of the stomach; bitter taste in the mouth; foulness of the tongue; headache; rheumatic pains in the limbs, aggravated by motion; constipation, and irritability of disposition; also when there are occasional shooting pains in the chest, especially during inspiration.

DOSE.—Dissolve a drop, or eight globules, in three tablespoonfuls of water, and give a teaspoonful every three hours.

COFFEA is useful in the febrile stage, when there is

14

great nervous excitability; its use should precede that of Aconite.

DOSE.—Dissolve a drop, or six globules, in two tablespoonfuls of water, and give a teaspoonful every three hours, until the excitability is allayed.

CHAMOMILLA is also of great service in allaying the nervous excitability of the febrile stage; it is particularly applicable to this stage in children, when there are signs of suffocation, and diarrhœa with colic and vomiting, or when the disease is announced with starts or convulsions, or when in the advanced stage the nights are disturbed by convulsive cough, or tightness across the chest.

DOSE.—Dissolve a drop, or six globules, in three tablespoonfuls of water, and give a teaspoonful every two hours, until amelioration or change.

OPIUM in the eruptive stage is of great use when there are symptoms of stupor, or strong inclination to perpetual sleep.

DOSE.—Dissolve a drop, or six globules, in four tablespoonfuls of water, and give a teaspoonful every three hours, until amelioration or a change; or in alternation with Belladonna every three hours.

PULSATILLA is of great utility in confluent small pox, when the eruption is preceded by an effloresence, similar to that of measles; or else accompanies it, attended with nausea or vomiting, and an aggravation of all the symptoms towards evening.

DOSE.—Dissolve one drop, or six globules, in three tablespoonfuls of water, and give a teaspoonful every three hours, until amelioration or change.

RHUS. TOX, is of great service in confluent small pox when there are rheumatic pains in the back and extremities, which become worse at night, and are somewhat relieved by movement; and also when the fever assumes a typhoid character, attended with great prostration, and signs of putrid development.

DOSE.—Dissolve one drop, or six globules, in three tablespoonfuls of water, and give a teaspoonful every three hours, until better.

STRAMONIUM is particularly serviceable in forwarding the eruption, and in shortening its duration; that is, when some pustules appear already formed, and others appear to be forming.

DOSE.—Dissolve one drop, or six globules, in three tablespoonfuls of water, and give a teaspoonful every four hours, until the eruption begins to disappear.

VACCININ has been in clinical use in the treatment of this disease for some time. It is believed to be effectual in curing the worst forms of the uncomplicated disease, promoting the appearance of the eruption, hastening the crisis, moderating the reaction, and protecting the skin, against the disorganisation the disease is prone to inflict. It is said to prevent the pitting so commonly found to result from the affection.

DOSE.—Dissolve one drop, or six globules, in four tablespoonfuls of water, and give a teaspoonful every four hours, until better, or a change.

There are other remedies that may be called into use in treating the disease; as for instance, Tart. emetic, Ipecacuanha, and Arsenicum, when there are such symptoms as indicate their use, as follows: nausea, vomiting, excessive thirst and dryness of the mouth, the tongue being at the same time very foul and dark, with great prostration of strength.

DOSE.—Dissolve a drop, or six globules, of either in three tablespoonfuls of water, and give a teaspoonful every three hours.

When small pox is attended with pleurisy, or inflammation of the lungs, *Phosphoros* may be called into use; when there is salivation, *Mercurius; Sulphur* will be found in these complications an invaluable remedy. When complicated with laryngitis, or bronchial difficulties, *Hepar Sulph.* and *Spongia.*

DOSE.—*For Phos. or Mercurius,* when indicated, one drop or six globules, in half a tumbler of water, a teaspoonful every six hours. Sulp. Hep. Spongia, when indicated, may be repeated once in twenty-four hours.

When the eruption strikes in (repercussion) Bryonia, Sulphur, and Pulsatilla, may be resorted to; a dose of either every three hours.

DIET AND REGIMEN.—Before detailing the diet, it may be remarked, that *cool fresh air* is essential for the patient, warmth being incompatible with a healthy re-action. Children attacked with convulsions in the early stage of the disease, may be relieved by taking them into the open air, or a well ventilated room without fire.

Great cleanliness must be observed as an essential condition, and the linen ought to be changed frequently.

The room ought to be darkened when the pustules begin to form; this will be a measurable security against disfigurement from the disease. The drink should be cold water, or cold black tea. No food should be taken warm. Gruel made of barley, rice, farina, or oatmeal is all the food to be allowed until the disease has spent its force, and convalescence becomes established; when absti-nence from animal food for some length of time is required. Boiled rice, or plain rice pudding, toast, or panada, and if desired, custards or eggs boiled soft, and a slice of toast, with *cocoa* or *broma*, may be allowed.

Gout. (*Arthritis.*)

This disease is characterised by inflammation and pain in the joints; it usually begins in the great toe, and then passes to the other smaller joints. Often times when it has progressed no further than the toes and smaller joints; the stomach and digestive organs in general become sympathetically deranged; and after this the more important joints may become affected.

The disease is remarkably fugitive, flying from place

to place, first attacking one joint, and then another, which becomes painful, red and swollen; and usually at night.

The disease may be *hereditary*, or it may be *acquired*. When it is hereditary it will manifest itself at about the age of twenty-five or thirty; or if acquired, at a later period of life.

It is difficult to cure the gout, and when hereditary, this constitutional tendency must be eradicated before anything approaching a permanent cure can be effected.

It is equally difficult to effect a radical cure of acquired gout, especially where the system has been further depressed by such *abominations* as are often resorted to for relief.

A luxurious living, and habitual use of wine, are regarded fruitful sources of the disease; but other *exciting causes* may bring it on: as sudden check of perspiration, mental emotions, and sedentary, studious habits, and the use of cathartics or tonics, or any kind of stimulants, irregular habits, want of rest.

GENERAL TREATMENT.—Persons predisposed to gout should avoid all the exciting causes of the disease, as far as possible. They should use no wine, cider, or malt liquors; they should be regular in their meals, avoiding the use of coffee and stimulating condiments; they should take no more than one *substantial* meal during the day, and that at noon, and a moderate breakfast, and tea and toast in the evening. Those who have acquired the disease, should break off whatever course of life has brought it on; they should avoid aperients, or tonics, or any irregularities in eating or drinking, exposure, either in relation to sleep or rest.

MEDICAL TREATMENT.—The remedies employed are

14*

Aconite, Arnica, Arsenicum, Belladonna, Bryonia, China, Causticum, Colocynthis, Ferrum, Mercurius, Nux vom., Pulsatilla, Rhus tox.

ACONITE, when there is considerable fever, as at the commencement of the disease, redness and swelling of the joints; full and bounding pulse.

DOSE.—One or two drops, or six globules, in a tumbler of water, and give a teaspoonful every three hours, until the fever is subdued.

ARNICA, when there is great soreness, as if bruised, or as if the swelling of the joints were occasioned by a sprain, or a sense as if luxated.

DOSE.—One drop, or six globules, in three tablespoonfuls of water, give a teaspoonful every three hours.

ARSENICUM, is useful when the pain in the joints is a burning, tearing, violent suffering, relieved by warmth, and aggravated by cold.

DOSE.—Dissolve one drop, or six globules, in four tablespoonfuls of water, and give a teaspoonful every two hours.

BELLADONNA.—When the pains fly quickly from one part to another, and the redness spreads very much, and is very deep; may be used in alternation with Pulsatilla.

DOSE.—Dissolve two drops, or ten pellets, in half a tumbler of water, and give a teaspoonful every three hours.

BRYONIA.—When there is aggravation of the suffering from motion, or at night, coldness and shivering, with general perspiration or fever; and also when the patient is suffering from biliary or gastric derangement.

DOSE.—Dissolve two drops, or twelve globules, in half a tumbler of water, and give a teaspoonful every three hours.

CHINA.—When the parts affected cannot endure con-tact with any thing, or are worse from being touched.

DOSE.—The same as for Bryonia.

CAUSTICUM.—When the limbs are stiff from old gouty

swellings, and when there is a sense of laceration of the joints.

DOSE.—One drop, or four globules, morning and evening, not to be repeated oftener than once a week.

COLOCYNTHIS.—When gout has been treated with Aconite, Bryonia or Sulphur, and the joints remain stiff, this remedy may be called into requisition.

DOSE.—One drop, or six globules, in four spoonfuls of water, a spoonful every four or six hours.

FERRUM MET.—When the face is very pale and haggard, the pain stinging and tearing, worse at night, and when the limbs require to be moved from one place to another continually from a restless aching.

DOSE.—Dissolve one drop, or six globules, in four tablespoonfuls of water, and give a teaspoonful every six hours.

RHUS TOX. may follow if Ferrum does not relieve, and Bryonia if the motion aggravates instead of relieving.

MERCURIUS is suitable when there is painful swelling of the joints, without redness, very much aggravated at night, or rendered worse when turning in the bed; attended with biliary derangement and constipation.

DOSE.—One drop, or four globules, in a spoonful of water, every six hours.

NUX VOMICA is exceedingly valuable in obstinate cases, when the pains are increased by motion, and attended with weakness, fretfulness, moroseness of temper, and nausea and constipation, with cramps and throbbing in the muscles.

DOSE.—The same in all respects as for Mercurius.

PULSATILLA is decidedly beneficial when the pains are of a shifting nature, aggravated towards evening and at night in the bed, with a paralytic or torpid sensation in the part affected, and more particularly when the dyspeptic symptoms for which this remedy is so well suited are present, and also when the pain is relieved by uncovering the affected limb.

DOSE.—One drop, or six globules, in half a tumbler of water, give a teaspoonful every six hours.

RHUS TOX. may be used when there is paralytic weakness and trembling of the extremities when attempting to move them, or when the pains are worse during rest.

DOSE.—One drop, or six globules, may be dissolved in four tablespoonfuls of water, and a tablespoonful must be given every morning, noon and night.

For further insight into the treatment of gout, that for rheumatism may be consulted; for what will suit a group of symptoms in the one, will suit a similar group in the other; the inflammatory fever of the one is very much the same as that of the other; and there is some truth in the remark of the man who attempted to point out the specific difference between the two diseases, when he said "rheumatism is as if the joint were screwed up in a vice as tight as possible, and gout is one turn more;" with this view of the case, it is proper to state that nearly every remedy that has a curative effect in rheumatism, will prove very beneficial in gout.

With regard to the administration of the medicines, they do not always require to be dissolved in water; three or four pellets may be given at a time dry, and repeated as often as directed for the solution.

DIET.—In acute attacks of gout, when there is considerable fever, the same diet should be observed as in ordinary fevers; stronger food may be allowed after the abatement of the fever, such as is easy of digestion and nutritive; milk toast and black tea; poached eggs; the tender meat of chickens; mutton and beef, *broiled*.

Inflammatory Rheumatism.—Rheumatic Fever.—Acute
Rheumatism.

Inflammatory rheumatism generally commences with
the ordinary signs of fever; chilliness and heat alternately; restlessness and thirst; coldness of the extremities; constipation; after which the fever sets in and runs
very high, the skin being exceedingly hot, and the pulse
greatly accelerated, beating as high as 120 per minute;
there is from the beginning, more or less pain and stiffness in the principal joints, which increases to acute
suffering, so that any attempt to move the affected joints
causes them to be excruciatingly painful; the affected
parts are usually red, swollen, and extremely painful to
the touch; sometimes, however, the pain is excessive,
and yet there is no sign of any inflammation; the pain
is generally worse at night, sometimes an acrid perspiration accompanies the disease.

The larger joints of the extremities are usually affected
by this disease; it is seldom confined to one, sometimes
nearly all the joints of the extremities are involved,
rendering the patient unable to move hand or foot;
during the continuance of the disease it spends its force
in one joint, leaves and goes to another; during its,
absence from the joint it first affects, there is relief from
pain. This difficulty is often associated with derangement of the heart; and sometimes when it commences
in the joints the heart becomes implicated, under such
a circumstance the disease assumes a more dangerous
character; whenever a remission of pain in the joints is
followed by anxiety, jerking or feeble and rapid pulse,
and acute pain in the region of the heart, together with
the physical signs, a translation of the disease to the

heart may be inferred, and the treatment must be modified accordingly.

CAUSES.—Standing or sitting in cold, damp places;
sitting in a draught; sleeping in damp sheets, or
remaining long in wet clothes, or any other exposure
of any part of the body to cold and moisture, especially when other parts are protected or when the whole
body is in a violent perspiration. There would also
seem to be some hereditary predisposition to it in
some persons. It may also result from the suppression
of an eruption, or the striking in of measles, rash, or
chicken-pox, or other eruptions, or sudden stoppage of
dysentery.

GENERAL TREATMENT.—The room should be kept
moderately warm, and quiet; the bed should be a hair
mattrass; no draught should blow upon the bed; and
the ventilation should be had from the tops of the
windows.

The remedies employed, are Acon., Arnica, Bell., Bry.,
Cham., Chin., Hepar sulp., Lachesis, Mercurius viv., Nux
vom., Puls., Rhus tox., Sulphur.

ACONITE is mostly indicated in the commencement,
and especially when there is high fever; dry, hot skin;
thirst, and redness of the cheeks; violent shooting, or
tearing pains, worse at night; redness or shining swelling
of the part affected; the pains are aggravated by the
touch; extreme irritability of temper. The remedy may
be continued until the fever is reduced.

DOSE.—Dissolve a drop, or six globules, in four tablespoonfuls of
water; give a teaspoonful every three hours.

ARNICA.—When the joints feel as if bruised or
sprained; hard, red, and shining swelling; sensation in
the part affected, as if it were resting on some hard sub-

stance; feeling as if paralysed, and crawling in the affected part; the pains are aggravated by the least motion of the limb.

DOSE.—A drop, or six globules, in two tablespoonfuls of water; a teaspoonful every three hours.

BELLADONNA.—When the pains are seated for the most part in the joints, and are shooting or burning in their character, worse at night and on movement; excessive swelling, and shining redness of the affected part; fever, with determination of the blood to the head, and redness of the face; and the pains are aggravated by lifting the limb.

DOSE.—The same as for Aconite and Arnica.

BRYONIA.—If there are shooting or tensive pains, shifting from muscle to muscle; red, shining swelling, and rigidity of the parts affected; the pains are worse at night, and on the least movement; profuse perspiration, or coldness, or shivering; heat, with headache, and derangement of the stomach; peevish or passionate temper.

DOSE.—The same as for Aconite, and may be used in alternation with that remedy.

CHAMOMILLA.—When there are drawing or tearing pains, with a sensation of numbness, or of paralysis in the parts affected; the pains are aggravated at night; fever, with burning, partial heat, preceded by chilliness; hot perspiration; desire to remain lying down; great agitation and tossing, and general restlessness.

DOSE.—The same as for Bryonia and Aconite.

CHINA is suitable against pains that are aggravated by the slightest touch; profuse perspiration; great debility from loss of blood.

HEPAR SULPH. is useful in protracted cases, after other remedies have been tried without relief.

DOSE.—One drop, or four globules, in a tablespoonful of water, night and morning.

LACHESIS is likewise a valuable remedy when Aconite, Bryonia, or other remedies, have been indicated, but have failed of success.

DOSE.—The same as for Hep. sulph., repeated three times a day in extreme cases.

MERCURIUS VIV. is good for shooting, tearing, or burning pains, aggravated at night, or towards morning; and by the warmth of the bed, or exposure to damp or cold air; puffy swelling of the affected part; the pains seem to be seated in the bones or joints; profuse perspiration without amelioration of the sufferings; if this remedy does not relieve when indicated, Lachesis may be used afterwards.

DOSE.—Of a solution of six globules, or one drop, in four tablespoonfuls of water, give a teaspoonful every four hours, until relief, or change.

NUX VOMICA, when there are pains in the calves; swelling of the ankle-joints, and stiffness after the fever has disappeared, or after the most violent symptoms of the disease.

DOSE.—The same in every respect as directed for Mercurius viv.

PULSATILLA is serviceable when the pains are aggravated in the evening, or at night in bed, and also in a warm room, or in changing the position; pains which pass quickly from one joint to another; sensation of torpor, and paralysis in the parts affected; the pains are relieved by exposure of the part to the cold air; paleness of the face and shivering.

DOSE.—Four globules of pulsatilla, may be given every four hours, dry; or six globules, or a drop may be dissolved in half a tumbler of water, and a teaspoonful given every three hours.

RHUS TOX. when there is red, and shining swelling of the joints, with rigidity and shootings when touched;

the pains worse during rest; or when there is a sense of paralytic weakness, and crawling in the limb affected; sufferings aggravated in cold or damp weather; suitable after Aconite, Arnica, or Bryonia, or may be used in alternation with either of them.

DOSE.—The same in all respects as directed for Pulsatilla.

SULPHUR is sometimes of great service at the commencement of the disease, to be followed by such remedies as the symptoms indicate. It is also of great service when there is a translation of the disease to the heart; for this latter difficulty, Aconite, Arsenicum, and Spigelia, may be used in association with this remedy, according to symptoms.

DOSE.—Of a solution of one drop, or six globules of either, in four tablespoonfuls of water, a tablespoonful may be given twice a day.

DIET AND REGIMEN.—Crackers, or plain toast, with black tea, occasionally a boiled custard, or *Blanchemange*, or puddings made of rice, sago, tapioca, or arrowroot; cocoa, chocolate, &c.; but more stimulating food should be avoided, and all stimulating drink.

Chronic Rheumatism.

The only difference between the inflammatory and chronic form of rheumatism, is, the latter has the pain without the fever, swelling or redness, as in the former. In time, the affected limbs lose their power of motion, and lameness results; sometimes there is atrophy or emaciation of the muscles, and the limbs will diminish in size; sometimes permanent contraction of a limb may be the result, or a bony stiffness of the joint.

CAUSES.—The same as detailed for the acute or inflammatory kind, as the same influences will bring on the former as the latter.

15

TREATMENT. — The remedies employed, are Aconite, Bryonia, Calc. carb., Causticum, Dulcamara, Hepar sulph., Lachesis, Lycopodium, Phosphorus, Rhus tox., Sulphur, Silicea, Veratrum.

ACONITE and BRYONIA are more particularly applicable to the sufferings of a rheumatic subject, after taking cold; acute attacks of chronic rheumatism may be very much like the acute form of the disease, and require the same treatment so long as any fever remains; and these two remedies are suited to this condition.

DOSE.—Of either one drop, or four globules, three times a day.

CALC. CARB. for stiffness and pain in the joints, CAUSTICUM for gouty pains in the joints, as if lacerated, or paralysis of one side.

DOSE.—Of either one drop, or four globules, every twenty-four hours.

DULCAMARA.—When there is a recurrence of the suffering on every exposure to cold, or from suppressed eruption from cold; HEPAR SULF. when there is weakness of the whole spine; swelling of the knees.

DOSE.—Of either one drop, or four globules, night and morning.

LACHESIS and LYCOPODIUM are suitable where the acute form was the immediate source of the chronic difficulty. The former is of use when there remains an affection of the heart, and the latter when there are gouty twitches, or aching, lacerating pains in the joints.

DOSE.—One drop, or four globules, of either, dissolved in a tablespoonful of water, may be given every night, one hour before bed-time.

PHOSPHORUS is suitable for stiffness of the neck, paralytic weakness in the small of the back, and trembling of the extremities.

DOSE.—One drop, or four globules, may be given every day before breakfast.

RHUS TOX. is especially useful when chronic rheumatism is made worse and almost unbearable in bad weather.

SILICEA and SULPHUR are also remedies to be consulted when every change of weather occasions a relapse.

DOSE.—Of either four globules, or one drop, every twenty-four hours, at night.

VERATRUM.—When there is paralytic and pain as if bruised in the extremities; coldness of the arms and legs; violent cramps in the calves.

DOSE.—One drop, or four globules, morning and evening.

Lumbago.—Pain in the small of the back, neck, &c.

This is a kind of rheumatism confined to the small of the back and the loins, and although it is seldom accompanied by fever or swelling, as in inflammatory rheumatism, yet it is accompanied with very acute symptoms; the most excruciating suffering is induced by any change of posture, and it is difficult to move any part without exciting it.

TREATMENT.—The remedies employed are Aconite, Bryonia, Belladonna, Mercurius, Nux vom., Pulsatilla, and Rhus tox.

ACONITE is suitable for the commencement of the disease, and as it probably is accompanied by some fever.

DOSE.—One drop, or six globules, in three tablespoonfuls of water; give a teaspoonful every six hours, or four globules every six hours.

BRYONIA, when the pains in the back are exceedingly severe, compelling the patient to bend forward when he walks, aggravated by motion or by a draught, and generally associated with rigors and general chilliness.

DOSE.—Four globules, or one drop, may be given twice a day.

BELLADONNA is useful either after or in alternation with *Aconite*, when the pains are deep-seated, and cause a sensation of heaviness, gnawing or stiffness.

DOSE.—One drop, or six globules, in half a tumbler of water; give a teaspoonful every six hours, in alternation with Aconite.

MERCURIUS, NUX VOMICA and PULSATILLA are suitable when there is a sensation as if bruised in the whole lumbar region, or as if the pain was occasioned by excessive fatigue, and when aggravated by turning in bed at night, and when accompanied by weakness, constipation and irritable temper. Mercurius and Nux vomica are better suited to bilious or sanguineo-bilious temperaments. Pulsatilla is better suited to persons of mild dispositions, and females.

DOSE.—Of a solution of one drop, or four globules, of either, in four tablespoonfuls of water; give a teaspoonful every four hours.

Rheumatism of the Neck.—(*Kink of the Neck.*)

The muscles of the neck sometimes become seriously affected with rheumatism and fever. Exposure to a draught of cold air, or a sudden jerk of the head, may give rise to the difficulty.

TREATMENT. *Remedies.*—Aconite, Belladonna, Bryonia, Cocculus.

ACONITE, when there is some degree of fever, will effect a cure in a short time; Belladonna will prove useful in alternation.

DOSE.—Dissolve six globules, or one drop, of each, in two spoonfuls of water, in separate glasses, and give a teaspoonful every two hours, alternately.

BRYONIA and COCCULUS may be used in the same way as Aconite and Belladonna, after these latter remedies have been used without effect.

DOSE.—The same as directed for Aconite and Belladonna.

Sciatic Rheumatism.—(*Sciatica.*)

This form of rheumatism may be *acute* and attended with some degree of fever, or it may be, and more frequently is, chronic.

SYMPTOMS.—Severe pain in the region of the hip joint, which shoots along the course of the sciatic nerve to the ham, and sometimes it extends to the foot, and consequently the pain must be in the nerve.

CAUSES.—The same as in acute or inflammatory rheumatism.

TREATMENT.—The remedies used are Aconite, Chamomilla, Colocynthis, Ignatia, Nux vom. and Rhus tox.

ACONITE, only in the acute form, when attended with fever.

DOSE.—Dissolve six globules, or one drop, in three spoonfuls of water, and give a spoonful morning, noon and night.

ARSENICUM, when the pains are acute and dragging, with a sensation of coldness in the part affected; also when the pains are periodical. It is also useful in cases attended by emaciation.

DOSE. —One drop, or four globules, morning and evening.

CHAMOMILLA, when the pains are aggravated at night, and the limb is very sensitive. COLOCYNTHIS is especially useful when seated in the right hip.

DOSE.—Of a solution of six globules of either; give a teaspoonful three times a day, One drop, of either, may be used in half a tumbler of water in the same way.

IGNATIA, when there are cutting pains, especially on the slightest movement of the limb; Nux vomica when the pain is attended by a sensation of stiffness or contraction of the limb; also when a feeling of paralysis or torpor, with chilliness, is experienced in the affected part.

DOSE.—Of either one drop, or four globules, morning and evening.

RHUS TOX. is better suited when rest aggravates the suffering, and motion or warmth mitigates it.

DOSE.—One drop, or four globules, morning and evening.

15*

DIET and REGIMEN.—In any of the chronic forms of rheumatism, the patient may be allowed a moderately generous diet.

All condiments must be prohibited, such as vinegar, pepper, mustard, &c. Black tea, cocoa and other non-medicinal drinks are allowable. The patient must be kept warm, if this mitigates his sufferings, or moderately cold if warmth aggravates them, or he must be kept in bed if rest relieves him, or up and in motion if this contributes most to his comfort.

CHAPTER VI.

DISEASES OF THE DIGESTIVE ORGANS; OR, OF THE ALIMENTARY CANAL.

1.—Diseases of the Teeth.—Toothache.—(*Odontalgia.*)

REMARKS ON GENERAL TREATMENT.—The office of the teeth is so important in preparing the food after it is taken into the mouth, for the further action of the digestive organs, it is proper to consider the best means of preserving them, as well as the best means of relieving the suffering incident to them when diseased.

The only proper method of preserving the teeth is to keep them clean, and to avoid the contact of any disorganising agent. This may be accomplished by rinsing the mouth every morning, and after every meal; by not picking the teeth with any instrument calculated to do them violence; nor by drinking very hot drinks; or taking into the mouth very hot food, for the expansive power of heat may burst the enamel and furnish the nucleus of disease; and, on the contrary, by not subjecting the teeth to the other extreme of temperature.

The teeth may be cleansed by the aid of a brush and finely powdered sugar of milk.

It is decidedly injurious to clean the teeth with charcoal or lemon juice, or with any other acid; nearly all the tooth powders and tinctures are injurious. It is far better to cleanse the teeth with luke-warm water, with the aid of a little soap; acidulated cream may be used to whiten the teeth, provided the mouth be immediately rinsed after using it.

The teeth should not be extracted if possible to retain them, even if they are hollow from decay, unless they are ulcerated at the roots. It is always deleterious to use laudanum or kreosote to allay the toothache, for they only palliate for a brief period, when the pain returns with increased violence. It is better to obtain relief from some remedial agent that will remove the diseased condition of which the toothache is the result.

The principal remedies employed are Aconite, Arnica, Arsenicum, Belladonna, Chamomilla, Mercurius, Nux vom., Pulsatilla and Sulphur.

ACONITE.—When the toothache is accompanied with fever and heat about the head, and results from taking cold or from nervous excitement.

ARNICA.—When the pain is occasioned by any mechanical injury, as from extracting or plugging.

ARSENICUM is useful when any thing cold aggravates the pain.

BELLADONNA.—When from cold there is severe pain in the teeth involving the whole jaw, the pains extending up the side of the face and into the ear, and worse from applying any thing hot.

DOSE.—Of a solution of six globules, or one drop of either of the above remedies, in half a tumbler of water; give a tablespoonful every three hours until relieved.

CHAMOMILLA.—When the toothache is produced by drinking coffee or tea, or is attended with diarrhœa, or when there is flushed face or swelling of one cheek, or pain extending into the ears, worse when in the room than out of doors.

DOSE.—Of a solution of one drop, or six globules, in half a tumbler of water; give a spoonful every three hours until relieved.

MERCURIUS VIV.—For pains in hollow teeth, worse in the morning, extending into the head; pain in the gums, with swelling, or in the jaw-bones or ears, or swelling of the parotid gland; and also when diarrhœa accompanies these symptoms.

DOSE.—Give a drop, or six globules, three times a day, if the first dose does not relieve.

NUX VOMICA.—Toothache arising from cold, which at the same time affects the head and back; when there is chilliness and pains in the limbs; when worse after eating; or when moving the mouth; or when there is swelling of the cheeks; or when it is aggravated by taking cold drinks; and worse in the morning from drinking ardent spirits.

DOSE.—One drop, or four globules, repeated if necessary every six hours.

PULSATILLA is most suitable for persons of a mild, quiet, timid disposition; or for persons of a fretful temper; when the pain is on one side, or when it occurs in the spring with earache and headache, or when it attends the menstrual period; and when the pains are of a jerking, tearing or stinging character; or when cold air relieves the pain, or it is relieved by chewing.

DOSE.—The same as directed for Nux vomica.

SULPHUR is suitable for jumping pains in hollow teeth extending to the upper jaw and into the ear; swelling and bleeding of the gums; or when it occurs in the evening, or is made worse by rinsing the mouth with cold water.

DOSE.—One drop, or four globules, at night, and repeated if necessary in twelve hours.

Other remedies may be used under the following circumstances:—When the toothache occurs from pregnancy, *Calcarea carb.;* from nursing or from debilitating losses, *China;* from grief, *Ignatia;* for sense of elongation of the teeth, and excessive pain relieved by warmth, *Arsenicum;* for pain, with tears and excessive anguish, *Coffea,* &c., &c.

For ulceration of the gums, Mercurius, Silicea, Hepar Sulph. and Sulphur.

DOSE.—Of any of the remedies mentioned above, one drop, or twelve globules, in half a tumbler of water; a teaspoonful at a time, repeated, if necessary, every four, six or twelve hours until relief is obtained.

It is well for persons suffering from toothache to avoid holding hot acrid stimulants in the mouth, and also to refrain from the use of laudanum, creoste, oil of cloves, or any agent that interferes with the action of the remedies; and when it becomes apparent that any exciting cause will bring on the toothache, whether eating, drinking or exposure, it is always best to guard against such as far as possible; when tea or coffee invariably excites pain in decayed teeth, their use should be refrained from entirely; when there is fever, or the stomach is deranged, the DIET should be light, and great care should be exercised at all times to keep the stomach and bowels in a healthy state.

2. Quinsy.   Sore Throat.   Inflammation of the Tonsils.

SYMPTOMS.—In ordinary quinsy, there is inflammation of the throat, redness and swelling of the back part, difficulty of swallowing, alteration of the voice, fever. At first there is a sense of constriction about the throat, and soreness which becomes manifest in the act of swallowing; unless arrested, the swallowing becomes more difficult, the tonsils and tongue become swollen and red, and occasionally with a number of little yellow eminences at the back part of the throat, particularly at the tonsils; there is considerable thirst; the pulse is high, strong and frequent; sometimes the cheeks swell and become red; the eyes become inflamed; and in very severe cases, delirium is a frequent occurrence. As the difficulty increases, the tonsils frequently become the seat of suppuration, unless the disease is made to terminate by resolution; or in other words, the inflammation and swelling disappears without suppuration. When the former is the case, the pain is relieved when the abscess breaks.

Sometimes both tonsils are implicated, at other times only one; in the latter event, it frequently happens, that the inflammation and suppuration of the one, has barely passed, before the same train of symptoms has to be gone through with the other.

This disease is not regarded dangerous, if properly treated; but sometimes, it becomes of a putrid character, and is attended with febrile symptoms of a typhoid type; when this takes place, there is evidently a predisposition on the part of the patient, to become affected in this manner.

TREATMENT.—The remedies employed, are Aconite, Belladonna, Bryonia, Cantharides, Chamomilla, Dulca-

mara, Hepar sulph., Ignatia, Lachesis, Mercurius viv.
Nux vomica, Nitric acid, Sulphur, and under some
circumstances, Silicea and Arsenicum.

ACONITE, in the commencement when the disease is
attended with fever, when the pulse is full and bounding;
dry heat upon the skin; thirst; deep redness of the part
affected; painful and difficult swallowing; pricking
sensation in the throat, made worse by talking.

DOSE.—Four globules may be taken dry upon the tongue, or one drop
may be dissolved in two tablespoonfuls of water, and a teaspoonful may
be given every three hours, until the symptoms disappear.   In severe
cases, where swallowing is difficult, four globules may be given upon the
tongue every three hours, or even as often as every two hours, until a
change for the better.

BELLADONNA is one of the best remedies for inflammation of the throat, when there is congestion of the
tonsils.   And when there is swelling of the outside of
the throat; and drinking produces spasms in the throat,
the fluids returning through the nose; constant disposition to swallow, but difficult, with pricking pain,
producing spasms; sensation of a plug in the throat;
violent pressing, shooting pain in the tonsils, as if they
would burst; thirst; profuse salivation; headache, and
furred tongue.

DOSE.—Dissolve one drop, or six globules, in four tablespoonfuls of
water, and give a spoonful every four hours, until relieved.

BRYONIA is a useful remedy when the throat is painful
on being touched, or on turning the head; difficult and
painful deglutition, as if something hard were in the
throat; soreness and shooting pains, attended with a
sensation of dryness, which renders it very difficult to
speak.   The occurrence of all these symptoms, are for
the most part, after being overheated, or after drinking
very cold, or ice-water; considerable fever usually

accompanies these symptoms, sometimes with, at other times without thirst, and great irritability.

DOSE.—Of a solution of one drop, or six globules, in four tablespoon-fuls of water, give a teaspoonful every three hours; or if the swallowing is so difficult as to render it incompatible, four globules may be placed on the tongue, and repeated at the same intervals.

CANTHARIDES is useful when the throat manifests a burning and grating sensation; when there is redness and tension in the mouth, or pressure, terminating in shooting pains on swallowing; or when there is a difficulty in swallowing liquids; the taste, sour and bitter; tongue coated; with flow of saliva; violent tickling in the larynx; dry cough, followed by dis-tressing respiration, and sometimes by expectoration of bloody mucus. It is also useful at the conclusion of what is termed inflammatory sore throat, and at the commencement of that which is catarrhal.

DOSE.—Four globules may be given upon the tongue, or one drop, or eight globules may be dissolved in four tablespoonfuls of water, and a teaspoonful given every two hours, until relieved.

CHAMOMILLA is a useful remedy for children, when the complaint is caused by a cold from exposure to a draught of air, while in a state of perspiration; when the throat is red, and swollen, accompanied with fever, and swelling of the glands of the lower jaw; sensation of there being an obstruction when swallowing and bending the neck; sense of something in the throat difficult of removal.

DOSE.—Dissolve one drop, or eight globules, in half a tumbler of water, and give a teaspoonful every four hours; or three globules upon the tongue, may be repeated at the same intervals, until relieved.

DULCAMARA is useful in inflammation of the tonsils, which is occasioned by exposure to the wet; it may succeed the use of Belladonna or Mercurius, or be followed by them, when it is not sufficient of itself to

complete the cure, provided these remedies are indicated
by the symptoms.

DOSE.—The same in all respects as for Chamomilla.

HEPAR SULPH. is a very useful remedy to promote
suppuration, when it is impossible to obviate the inflammation without it; and the quinsy has progressed so far
that bursting is desirable, to relieve the painful sense of
suffocation, arising from the swollen state of the tonsils.

DOSE.—Dissolve a drop, or eight globules, in four tablespoonfuls of
water, and give a teaspoonful of the solution every two hours, until the
abscess breaks. If Hepar proves insufficient, wait three hours, and try
Silicea.

IGNATIA is particularly indicated when there is a
feeling as if a plug were in the throat, when not performing the act of swallowing; and red inflammatory
swelling of the tonsils or palate; burning pains during
the act of deglutition, as if the substance being swallowed
were passing over a raw surface, or in a measure
obstructed by something in the throat; greater difficulty
in swallowing liquids than solids; and also when lying
still, and the mouth not in motion, shooting pains in the
cheeks, thence extending to the ears; induration of the
tonsils, or the appearance of small blisters upon them.

DOSE.—Dissolve one drop, or ten globules, in half a tumbler of water,
and give a teaspoonful every two hours, or if swallowing is too difficult, four
globules upon the tongue every two hours, until relieved, or another
remedy is required.

LACHESIS is a useful remedy after *Belladonna*, or *Mercurius*, have been used without effect; if the palate is
swollen around the uvula; continual disposition to
swallow; profuse flow of saliva; undue accumulation
of phlegm in the throat; fetid and gangrenous ulcers;
spasms, which prevent drinking; great sensitiveness of
the throat on the slightest touch; unable to bear the
bed clothes; aggravation of symptoms in the afternoon

16

or immediately after sleeping in the morning. Persons who have taken much *mercury* may derive great benefit from this remedy.

DOSE.—Dissolve a drop, or six globules, in half a tumbler of water and give a teaspoonful every two hours, or three pellets, dry, at the same intervals.

MERCURIUS VIV.—After *Belladonna* has been used without effect. This remedy is often of great use, especially if the throat continues swollen, red, or merges into ulceration. When the process of ulceration is slow, or at the commencement of the disease; when the pricking pains are very violent, when swallowing, extending to the ears or to the glands of the throat, and to the lower jaw; when the burning in the throat is so severe that deglutition can hardly be performed; stitches in the tonsils, and a very disagreeable taste in the mouth; the gums and back part of the tongue swollen, and profuse discharge of saliva; chills in the evening, or heat followed by perspiration, which fails of relief; uneasiness, or an aggravation of all the symptoms at night; also worse in the air, accompanied with severe headache and twitching in the neck.

DOSE.—Dissolve one drop, or six globules, in four tablespoonfuls of water; give a teaspoonful every six hours, until better, or there is a necessity for a change. This remedy may be used in alternation with Belladonna, and the same interval should elapse between each dose of the different remedies. The remedy may be taken four globules at a time, dry, if swallowing is too difficult to take them in water.

NUX VOMICA is a remedy that may be employed after *Chamomilla* or *Ignatia* have failed of effecting a cure; when there is a sensation of lump in the throat when swallowing, and pressing pains, aggravated by swallowing saliva, and when the throat feels raw and excoriated, as if scraped, and also when the uvula is swollen and red, and the cold air affects the throat so as to occasion pain.

DOSE.—Of a solution of a drop, or eight globules, in half a tumbler of water; give a teaspoonful every two hours, until relieved, or there is another remedy required; or three globules may be given dry, at the same intervals.

NITRIC ACID.—In superficial ulcerations of the throat, after *Aconite* and *Mercurius* have been administered; when the small·white and gray ulcers refuse to put on a healing appearance, after the use of the latter remedy.

DOSE.—Dissolve a drop, or six globules, in three tablespoonfuls of water, and give a teaspoonful every three hours at first for three doses, and then every six and every twelve hours, until a cure is completed.

SULPHUR is especially indicated in the latter stage of quinsy, when it occurs in vitiated constitutions, when the healing of the cavity, after the matter has been discharged, goes on very unfavorably, and when fresh abscesses form in succession; and also when the suppuration takes place slowly; it may be used after *Hepar sulph.*, or in alternation with this remedy and *Silicea*. This latter remedy is useful in rapidly forwarding the suppurative process, and causing the ripened abscess to burst; and it generally promotes the healing more effectually than *Hepar sulph.*

DOSE.—Dissolve a drop, or six globules, of either remedy in half a tumbler of water, and give a tablespoonful night and morning in alternation, or every night singly, when indicated.

ARSENICUM is useful in gangrenous sore throat, and may be used in alternation with Lachesis; yet when the inflammation is of an erysipelatous character, or when the fever is of a typhoid character; great prostration of strength; burning heat; cold hands; great restlessness and anguish; ulceration; discharging fetid matter; it is far better to use it alone. (See malignant sore throat.)

DOSE.—A drop, or four globules, every six hours.

DIET AND REGIMEN.—The diet must be regulated according to the degree of inflammation present. Deglutition being difficult, solidified food is rarely to be recommended, unless it partakes of the character of a custard or jelly. A plain cup custard, when only one side of the throat is suppurating, may be allowed, but when the inflammation determines to both sides, and the throat is nearly closed, only thin liquids can be taken. Warm water may be used as a gargle, and when much pain is present, inhalation of vapor from boiling water will often afford much relief. All medicinal gargles are hurtful; blisters, leeches, or other topical applications, are of no use, and homœopathic treatment is all that can be relied upon for the best and most speedy relief.

Some persons are predisposed to sore throat; *Mercurius, Graphites* and *Sepia* have been found useful in overcoming this constitutional difficulty.

3.—Malignant Quinsy, or Putrid Sore Throat.

The malignant sore throat often makes a part of that awful scourge,—the malignant scarlet fever. It is usually epidemic, and generally occurs in damp and sultry autumnal seasons.

SYMPTOMS.—It begins with shivering, followed by heat and languor; oppression at the chest; nausea, vomiting, and often with purging; eyes inflamed and watery; cheeks of a deep red color; greater or less inflammation of the tonsils, and they secrete a thin, acrid discharge, sometimes excoriating the nose and lips; *pulse* weak and hardly perceptible, small and irregular; *tongue* white and moist; swallowing painful and difficult; throat of a bright red color, and much swollen. This state soon passes away, and numerous ulcers, varying in size, then manifest themselves upon the swollen part, which finally become covered with a livid coat. Sometimes these ulcerations are more extensive than at others, spreading to the back part of the mouth, over the entire arch, and down to the opening into the windpipe, &c., and assuming a sloughing appearance as they increase in magnitude. Excessive prostration of strength immediately ensues; the lips, tongue and teeth are covered with blackish incrustations, there is more or less delirium; the breath is fetid, and the patient conscious of a disagreeable odor; the countenance is sunken, and there is severe purging.

There is considerable swelling of the neck, and its color is livid. There are often livid spots upon the body (petechiæ,) which indicate in some measure the violence of the disease.

This affection carries off many children and adults, and may be regarded as exceedingly dangerous when there is the appearance of livid spots, or *petechiæ*, and other indications of a putrid character, with weak, fluttering pulse, sometimes intermittent; extreme prostration; bleedings from the nose, mouth, &c.

When there is a gentle sweat, that breaks out about the third or fourth day, and when the sloughs are thrown off in a favorable manner, leaving a clean, healthy looking bottom, and the countenance becomes lively and the respiration normal, and the pulse stronger and more equal, a salutary result may be expected.

The fever accompanying the malignant sore throat is more frequently of a typhoid or typhus character, and calls for those remedies best adapted for these fevers in their uncomplicated form.

TREATMENT.—Remedies, Aconite, Arsenicum, Bella-
16*

donna, Conium, Lachesis, Mercurius, Nitric Acid, Pulsatilla, Rhus, Secale, and Sulphur.

ACONITE is only useful in the very first stage of the
disease, when the fever appears of an inflammatory
character; and after the use of this remedy, *Belladonna*
may be called into requisition as soon as the patient
complains of dryness, with difficulty in swallowing, and
a sense of choking in the throat.

DOSE.—Of either remedy, one drop, or four globules, every three
hours.

ARSENICUM is useful when there is great prostration
of strength, rapid sinking of the patient, nausea, or
vomiting; or when the ulcers present a livid hue, and
also, when in a more advanced stage, they are covered
with dark scabs, surrounded with a livid margin; the
lips and teeth encrusted with brownish scabs; the skin
dry and parched; the tongue blackish, dry, cracked,
and tremulous; constant muttering and delirium; unable
to close the mouth; labored breathing; acrid discharges
from the nostrils, causing excoriations; the eyes dull and
glassy; thirst excessive, though but little is drunk at a
time, and swallowing is performed with difficulty; and
finally, when in addition to extreme prostration there is
a rash of livid color that breaks out in blotches, inter-
mingled with petechiæ, or livid spots.

DOSE.—This remedy is of so much importance, when indicated as
above, that it should be administered with the greatest promptness, as
follows: One drop of the dilution, or four globules, may be given in a
spoonful of water, every two hours, until three doses are given, and then,
every three hours, until amelioration, or change.

CONIUM will class very well with *Arsenicum*, for
malignant quinsy, because it is equally energetic, and
has been employed with great success, when the
diseased parts have suddenly assumed an ashy gray

color, or a blackish appearance, and the ulcerations secreting a fluid exceedingly offensive and fetid, without sensible pain, the strength and also the natural temperature of the body have suddenly declined, the spirits of the patient have become depressed and anxious, with signs of indifference, the febrile seasons irregular, sometimes commencing with chills, and concluding with heat, at others beginning with heat and chilliness simultaneously, or in rapid alternation, and concluding at night in a copious perspiration; a whitish eruption also appearing in the skin; the face grows pale, features change, and often with swelling; the tongue becomes coated with a thick dark covering, swells and is painful; the speech is difficult, and the stools are thin, watery, or bloody and involuntary. Many of these symptoms may indicate the use of *Mercurius corrosivus*, and if so, this remedy may precede the use of *Conium*. The *Mercurius corr.* should be given three times, in doses of four globules, or one drop, in a spoonful of water.

DOSE.—Of a solution of one drop, or six globules, in four tablespoonfuls of water, give a teaspoonful every two hours at first. If the patient exhibits any signs of convalescence, do not repeat the remedy oftener than once in three or four hours.

LACHESIS. This remedy is one of the polycrests in malignant ulceration of the throat, and will frequently be found useful after *Arsenicum*, should the patient complain of great pain in the throat, aggravated by the slightest external pressure; or should the scabs or sloughs seem indisposed to cast off, and the neck become much swollen and discolored; after this remedy has been used for some time, if the tendency to gangrene continues, and the patient is still affected with great prostration of strength, accompanied with debilitating sweats, *China* may be called into requisition, as there is no remedy more likely to meet the existing condition of the system; or *Arsenicum* may come in well after *Lachesis*, especially if the countenance is sunken, and the eyes appear glassy, and there is the extreme sinking for which this remedy is so remarkably adapted. After the use of *Arsenicum*, *Nux vomica* may be given with great benefit, when diarrhœa is present, and only partially checked, and numerous foul, offensive, though small ulcers, are found in the mouth and throat. This remedy, again, may be succeeded by *Carbo vegetabilis*, should a copious, fetid, thin, sanious fluid be discharged from the ulcers, attended with great prostration, and small, indistinct, or scarcely perceptible pulse.

DOSE.—Of a solution of one drop, or eight globules, in four tablespoonfuls of water, give a teaspoonful every two hours until it becomes necessary to follow with one of the other remedies, then it is necessary that whatever remedy is selected to succeed Lachesis, should be dissolved in the same manner and given at the same intervals.

MERCURIUS is more serviceable in the early part of the disease, before the ulceration has progressed so far as to present the more fetid and putrid odor; but when from the increasing size and painfulness of the ulcers, this remedy does not promise to arrest their progress or cause them to assume a healthy aspect, it will be well to call *nitric acid* into requisition.

DOSE.—Of a solution of one drop of the dilution, or eight globules, in four tablespoonfuls of water, give a teaspoonful every hour or two hours, until it becomes evident that a change is necessary.

NITRIC ACID.—This remedy is particularly required after *Mercurius* has failed of arresting the increase of the swelling of the throat, and when the ulceration has progressed so far as to present numerous little yellow or white pustules upon the tonsils.

DOSE.—Of a solution of one drop, or eight globules, in four tablespoon-fuls of water; give a teaspoonful every four hours, say every hour at first, until two or three doses are given, and then every two hours, and after-wards every three hours.

PULSATILLA is useful when the symptoms are of a mild character, or which have been in a measure subdued by the use of *Belladonna*, and an increased action of the mucus membrane supplies the place of a previous dryness, while the patient is at the same time afflicted with nausea and bilious vomiting; bloated appearance of the face; constipation of the bowels; or on the other hand, the opposite condition or diarrhœa at night, occasionally pains in the bowels, with shivering.

DOSE.—One drop, or four globules, may be given every three hours, or four globules may be given dry upon the tongue with the same frequency.

RHUS TOX. is particularly useful in extreme cases, where there is great muscular weakness with trembling of the extremities, especially on movement; sopor and other symptoms described under this remedy in the chapter where typhus fever is treated of.

DOSE.—Of a solution of one drop, or eight globules, in six spoonfuls of water; give a teaspoonful every three hours.

SECALE CORNUTUM is exceedingly useful when the stupor is long continued, or there is lethargic sleep, or involuntary diarrhœa, and when the ulceration of the throat is of a fetid or putrid character, and there is nausea and disposition to vomit.

DOSE.—One drop, or four globules, may be given every three hours.

SULPHUR is a remedy that may be called into use in the treatment of malignant sore throat, when it becomes apparent that skin difficulties have become suppressed, and when there is swelling and suppuration of the glands; or, when there is deep and fetid ulceration of the tonsils, this remedy may be given with advantage at the very commencement of the disease, and particularly if there is rough throat and loss of voice.

DOSE.—One drop, or four globules, of sulphur, may be given three times a day.

DIET AND REGIMEN.—It is not often that subjects of malignant sore throat can take much food of any description, and only such as is entirely divested of every rough property, such as rice, arrowroot, corn starch, or thin flour gruel; when the mouth becomes dry, and the sloughs become dry and hard, it is well to moisten them with a little warm milk and water, and to wash the mouth very gently with the same. The room where the patient is, must be kept free from stagnated air, and if it be over a wet, damp cellar, he must be removed. It is far better to secure a good and wholesome atmosphere at first, than to rely upon remedial measures in a bad atmosphere. And when the patient begins to recover, and his appetite becomes established, be careful about overloading the stomach, as this may prove the cause of exciting the most painful sequellæ. It is well to begin moderately with toast, black tea, cocoa, milk toast, bread and butter, and as strength is acquired to use some of the digestible meats in great moderation.

4.—Scurvy of the Mouth.—Canker of the Mouth.
(*Cancrum Oris.*)

The peculiar characteristics of this disease are sensitive gums, hot, red and spongy; sometimes they swell, and sometimes they shrink from the teeth, leave them loose and they fall out; at other times small ulcers make their appearance on the gums, the inside of the lips, the cheeks, on the palate, and even on the tongue; not unfrequently there is great offensiveness of the breath, and some.

times discharge of sanious tough phlegm and saliva from the gums; mastication becomes impaired because the teeth are so loose, and the power of swallowing becomes diminished because the throat is so sore, that the act becomes painful in the extreme; sometimes the glands of the throat swell and become painful, there appears to be great prostration, and oftentimes a torpid feverish condition of the system.

TREATMENT.—The remedies employed are Arsenicum, Carbo veg., Dulcamara, Hepar sulph., Mercurius, Natrum muriaticum and Sepia.

ARSENICUM is particularly useful when the ulceration is very extreme, with violent burning pains; and in alternation with *China*, if gangrene is threatened, the gums becoming black and the patient very much reduced.

DOSE.—Of a solution of one drop, or six globules, in four tablespoon-fuls of water; give a teaspoonful every four hours.

CARBO VEGETABILIS is in the highest degree useful when the scurvy has arisen from the abuse of mercury, or too long a subsistence on salt food, and when the gums bleed very much and smell very offensively.

DOSE.—One drop, or four globules, every six hours.

DULCAMARA may be given in the first onset of the disease, when the canker results from taking cold, and the glands of the throat are swollen and hard. This remedy is useful after *Mercurius* fails of effecting a cure.

DOSE.—One drop, or four globules, every four hours.

HEPAR SULPHUR is for the most part a collateral remedy, and never to be used in scurvy or canker of the mouth, only when *Mercurius* proves insufficient, from the fact that the disease first originated from the use of *Calomel.* This remedy may follow *Mercurius,* and also it may follow *Carbo veg.* when this remedy has failed.

DOSE.—One drop, or four globules, dissolved in a spoonful of water, twice a day.

MERCURIUS VIV. is useful in almost every case, and may for the most part be given at the commencement of the disease, unless calomel or some other form of mercury has produced the disease, in which case resort to *Hepar sulph.* and *Carbo veg.* or *Nitric acid.*

DOSE.—Of a solution of one drop, or six globules, in four tablespoonfuls of water; give a teaspoonful every three hours.

NATRUM MURIATICUM.—When the ulcers spread very slowly, and when the canker is so torpid that none of the preceding remedies seem to have any great effect in removing it. The gums appear swollen, bleeding and sensitive; every thing cold or warm, or eating or drinking affects them; when blisters and small ulcers appear on the tongue, which burn so as to render it painful to speak.

DOSE.—One drop, or four globules, two or three times a day.

DIET AND REGIMEN.—Animal food should never be taken either in the solid form or in that of broth or soup, so long as the virulence of the disease remains; food entirely of a farinaceous or a vegetable form may be used. All stimulants should be avoided, as drink. The mouth may be washed with brandy and water, or even with lemon juice in water, with a soft brush.

And also, the mouth may be washed with a decoction of sage, as this is an old domestic remedy, which experience proves to be generally useful.

The mouth may also be washed with a solution of borax in water.

5.—Inflammation of the Tongue. (*Glossitis.*)

This disease is announced by pain of the tongue, which becomes aggravated by moving it; the tongue being hot, red and swollen. At first the inflammation may be restricted to only a small part, but gradually it may extend to the other parts of the organ until the whole is involved. During 'its progress, the pain becomes more acute, burning and lancinating, and the slightest effort at motion of any kind, swallowing, speaking, spitting, &c., excites the severest suffering.

Sometimes this affection is of a very formidable character, and threatens suffocation; the tongue swells so enormously as to protrude from the mouth. When thus swollen it is usually furred with a thick coating; and the saliva flows copiously from the mouth.

CAUSE.—Mechanical injuries, or chemical agents that come in contact with the tongue, so as to disorganise, or from some other exposures not observed.

TREATMENT.—Aconite, Arnica, Arsenicum, Belladonna, Lachesis, Mercurius, Phosphoric acid.

ACONITE is one of the most useful remedies in the commencement of the disease, when it is attended with intense inflammation and fever, and acute lancinating pains.

DOSE.—One drop, or six globules, may be dissolved in four spoonfuls of water, and a spoonful may be given every four hours, until relief or change.

ARSENICUM is highly useful when the inflammation is disposed to become gangrenous, which is indicated by dark and greenish or black appearance of the tongue; such cases are highly dangerous.

DOSE.—Of a solution of one drop, or six globules, in four tablespoonfuls of water; give a teaspoonful every three hours, until mitigation or change.

17

ARNICA, when the inflammation is known to have been produced by wounds inflicted by the teeth, or external bodies, and when the inflammation is mostly confined to the locality where the wound is inflicted.

DOSE.—One drop, or four globules, every six hours, or in alternation with Aconite every three hours.

BELLADONNA is very serviceable after *Mercurius* has proved inefficient and the inflammation extends to neighbouring parts, and assumes the character of erysipelas; and also when there appears on the tongue and gums a number of pustulous sores, and also when the tongue or any part thereof becomes indurated.

DOSE.—Dissolve one drop, or six globules, in half a tumbler of water, and give a spoonful every two hours, until amelioration or change. Mercurius viv. may be used after this remedy.

LACHESIS is useful in malignant inflammation of the tongue, verging towards gangrene. It may be associated with *Arsenicum* in this disease, and when one fails the other may be called into requisition.

MERCURIUS VIV. is suitable after *Aconite* has reduced the fever and some of the more violent symptoms, or it may be used in the first commencement when there is violent pain, swelling, hardness, and flow of saliva, and also when the tongue becomes involved in ulcerations of the throat.

DOSE.—Dissolve six globules, or one drop, in half a tumbler of water, and give a teaspoonful every three hours, until mitigation of suffering, or change.

PHOS. ACID is recommended for injury done to the tongue by biting it when asleep.

When the swelling of the tongue becomes so enormous as to threaten suffocation, cutting the tongue so as to let it bleed freely may be necessary to save life or allow time for remedial measures.

DIET.—It is only in the mild forms of inflammation of the tongue, that a diet can be prescribed at all; for in the severe forms, the patient can take neither food or drink.

6.—Mumps. (*Parotitis.*)

This disease consists of inflammation and swelling of some of the salivary glands, the *parotid* and *submaxillary*, not usually dangerous, unless the patient is exposed when the disease is upon him, and they are thrown back upon the system, so as to involve some of the vital organs. Sometimes the whole neck is involved, so that chewing and swallowing are both obstructed. They increase for four or five days, and then they begin to disappear. Sometimes on the fifth or seventh day the swelling will leave the neck, and attack the breasts, or testicles, which become red and painful; and pain in the bowels, or other symptoms usually make their appearance.

TREATMENT. — The patient should be kept in a moderately warm room, and great care should be exercised to prevent his taking cold; he must have no stimulants, and no external applications, with the exception of a muslin cap or handkerchief, extending around his neck. The medicines applied are Belladonna, Carbo veg., Hyoscyamus, Mercurius.

BELLADONNA, when the mumps assume an inflammatory character, or the swelling is very red, resembling erysipelas; or when it recedes, and affects the brain, which may be known by the appearance of delirium, and sometimes unconsciousness, or the subsidence of the swelling.

DOSE.—Dissolve a drop, or four globules, in a spoonful of water, and give three times a day.

CARBO VEGETABILIS, when the patient has a torpid fever, and the swelling and induration of the glands appear more fixed, and when the swelling of the glands recedes, and the stomach becomes affected; and also when *Merc. viv.* has failed to give relief in the early stage of the disease, or the patient has been drugged with calomel.

DOSE.—One drop, or four globules, may be taken twice a day.

HYOSCYAMUS, when *Belladonna* fails of affording relief, and when it appears to be the remedy indicated. This remedy is of the greatest service, and will, very likely, produce a favorable result.

DOSE.—Dissolve one drop, or six globules, in four tablespoonfuls of water, and give a teaspoonful every four hours.

MERCURIUS is regarded the principal remedy in this affection, when the disease is uncomplicated with any other diathesis in the system, a few doses only, are required to affect a cure.

DOSE.—Give a drop, or four globules, three times a day.

Whenever the disease occurs, in connection with other difficulties, such as scald head, measles, &c., the remedies for these affections must be consulted.

DIET.—Toast and black tea, cocoa, custards without spice, and bread puddings, if the disease is not combined with some other serious malady.

7.—Affection of the Stomach.

WANT OF APPETITE is sometimes associated with an impaired condition of the stomach, which may be produced by various diseases, and which requires appropriate treatment, in order to restore the appetite, and thus enable the stomach to receive its accustomed nourishment.

Sometimes there is a disinclination to take food, when there is no perceptible cause other than an inappetency. The best remedy in such cases is *cold water*, a copious draught of which, in the morning, before breakfast, and in the evening, before going to bed, and about two hours before each meal will overcome the difficulty.

This is far better than to use artificial stimulants, barks, wine, or beer, for these only create a morbid appetite, that soon disappears, and a worse inappetency is likely to follow.

8.—Indigestion. (*Dyspepsia.*)

This difficulty is so common, and manifest in so many different aspects, that but little is required in the way of description, except an enumeration of the principal exciting causes, and the symptoms which indicate specific remedial treatment.

EXCITING CAUSES.—Irregularities in diet, over indulgence in the luxuries of the table, partaking of rich food and stimulating soups; excessive use of wine, malt liquors, and alcoholic drinks, strong tea and coffee; imperfect mastication of food; irregularity of meals; too long fasting between meals; sedentary habits; intense study; chewing tobacco: keeping late hours; severe exercises of mind, &c.

It may be stated further, that much of the disorder that prevails is fairly attributable to the injurious practice of nurses and physicians, in administering calomel and other drastic purges, for various abdominal derangements in early life. The weakening of the digestive function by such means, has continued in after life; and hence much of the complaint about dyspepsia, which literally means "difficult digestion."

17*

TREATMENT.—In adapting a treatment for the disease in question, it is proper to make a division of the subject into the *acute* and *chronic* forms.`

ACUTE FORM, frequently occurs in warm climates, and becomes developed under the influence of rapid atmospheric changes, or the use of unwholesome food.

CAUSES.—The common cause of an attack of this kind, is taking strong food into the stomach when too weak to bear it; and also drinking cold water when the system is in a heated condition; a season of debauch, or a blow upon the stomach, and sometimes the retrocession of some eruption of the skin.

SYMPTOMS.—Repugnance to food, sense of weight and fulness at the pit of the stomach, and sense of pain, aggravated by pressure, nausea, and frequent eructations, which often bring up bitter or acrid fluids, or gaseous matters, tasting like rotten eggs. Sometimes attending these local symptoms, there is pain in the back, and dull pain in the front part of the head, confusion, inability to think, and depression of spirits, and also shiverings and heat.

This form of dyspepsia is generally known under the common name of "*bilious attacks*," among most classes of people, but they are more properly regarded acute derangements of the digestive function.

The remedies employed in treating the *acute forms* are Aconite, Ant. crudum, Arsenicum, Belladonna, Bryonia, Ipecac., Tart. emet. and Veratrum.

ACONITE.—When there is fever in the commencement of an attack, with thirst, nausea, and clear water flows from the stomach, or when the patient vomits greenish bile, or mucous matter; when there is great weight at the pit of the stomach, and the breathing is difficult, and when there is a feeling of tightness in

the stomach, as if from acrid substances; and more especially when the fever is of an inflammatory character
and runs high.

DOSE.—Dissolve a drop, or six globules, in four tablespoonfuls of water,
and give a teaspoonful every three hours.

ANTIMONIUM CRUD. is indicated when the tongue is
coated with a white or yellow mucus; when there is loss
of appetite; eructation, with the taste of the food, or
acrid vomiting of mucus and bile; sense of fulness at
the pit of the stomach or epigastrium, or spasmodic
crampy pain in the part. This remedy is particularly
useful when the disease dates its origin from overloading
the stomach.

DOSE.—A drop of the dilution, or four globules, every four hours, until
relieved.

ARSENICUM is indicated if the vital powers become
prostrated, with pale, sunken countenance and cold
extremeties; when the tongue is white or of a reddish
or brownish color, dry and trembling; intense thirst;
ardent desire for cold water, acids and stimulants; complete aversion to all kinds of food; nausea and vomiting
of food after eating or drinking, or at night, or vomiting
of mucous or bilious matters of a yellowish or greenish
color; severe pain at the pit of the stomach, with tension,
and great pain on pressure; a sense of weight as from a
stone; cramps and sensation of coldness in the stomach,
and also burning; great prostration of strength; dark
circle around the eyes; pointed nose; irregular, small,
frequent and weak pulse.

DOSE.—Dissolve a drop, or six globules, in four teaspoonfuls of water,
and give a teaspoonful every hour, until relieved.

BELLADONNA is useful when in addition to the derangements of the stomach there is strongly marked symptoms

of the head being affected with dullness, loss of consciousness or delirium.

DOSE.—Dissolve one drop, or four globules, in six teaspoonfuls of water,
and give a teaspoonful every two hours, at first, and afterwards the intervals should be longer. This remedy may be used in alternation with
Aconite or Nux vomica, which may be better suited to the difficulties of
the digestive functions.

BRYONIA is very suitable after *Aconite*, when the
patient complains of dryness of the mouth, with burning
thirst; tongue covered with a white coating, or rather
dirty; loss of appetite; great demand for acid drinks;
morbid craving of food, or on the contrary, complete
aversion to all kinds of food; vomiting the contents
of the stomach, and white, glairy mucus; cutting pains
in the stomach; tensive pain when coming in contact,
with a feeling of heat or cold and shivering over the body.

DOSE.—Dissolve one drop, or six globules, in six teaspoonfuls of water,
and give a teaspoonful every two, three or four hours, according to the
intensity of the suffering.

IPECACUANHA is for the most part indicated when the
tongue is furred with white or yellowish coating; insipid,
clammy taste; no thirst; vomiting of undigested food,
or of greenish or yellowish bilious matter. It should be
used at the commencement of the disease.

DOSE.—Of a solution of one drop, or six globules, in six teapoonfuls
of water; give a teaspoonful every two or three hours.

TARTAR EMETIC is indicated when there is continued
nausea and inclination to vomit, with pain in the stomach,
as if overloaded, with considerable anguish and pressure
at the pit of the stomach, accompanied with great prostration and coldness of the extremities.

DOSE.—Dissolve one drop, or six globules, in six teaspoonfuls of water,
and give a teaspoonful every two hours, until relieved.

VERATRUM is indicated when there is extreme coldness of the extremities; sudden prostration; pale and
haggard countenance; craving of cold drinks, with

intense thirst; great weakness, amounting to faintness; violent vomiting and continual nausea; severe prostration, preceded by coldness of the upper extremities, with shuddering of the whole body, followed by or in connection with general heat, succeeded by rush of blood and heat in the hands; bitter or sour vomiting.

DOSE.—Dissolve one drop, or six globules, in half a tumbler of water, and give a teaspoonful every two or three hours, as it may be required.

DIET.—It is evident that the same rules must be observed with regard to the diet as in other acute difficulties, accompanied by any thing like an inflammatory fever. After all signs of nausea or irritableness of the stomach have passed away, the patient may begin to take the lightest forms of food, and if his stomach bear these, he may gradually increase the strength of the diet until he is able to live in his accustomed manner.

9.—Chronic Dyspepsia.

So numerous are the cases of chronic dyspepsia and so varied are the forms which it assumes, that a few preliminary remarks, with regard to the general character of the malady, as well as its numerous complications and sympathies, will not be out of place.

The chronic form may arise either from the imperfect dissolving of the aliment in the stomach, or the imperfect separation of the nutritious from the innutritious portion, after it has passed from the stomach into the small intestine.

The symptoms referable to the stomach are those which first indicate the difficulty of digestion, and they occur at some periods without awakening the alarm of the patient or causing any painful constitutional disturbance. They are often produced by the use of certain articles of diet only, or under the influence of particular circumstances, while at other times the taking of any kind of food is fraught with the difficulty. Towards the termination of the digestion of the food in the stomach, especially when the process has been difficult, the nervous and sanguiferous systems become frequently implicated, that is, they may cause neuralgia or congestions of blood in other localities, produced entirely by the struggle of the stomach to perform its function in breaking down and chymifying the food.

The truth is, there is a combined operation required in the stomach to chymify or digest the food; there must be the solvent power of the gastric fluid, and the *churning* motion of the stomach; if either of these processes is impaired, the other, however active, cannot remedy the deficiency.

The secretion of the gastric fluid may be impaired directly by influences acting upon the stomach, or by other causes which affect it through the medium of the nerves; among the former are those substances taken into the stomach, such as calomel, opium condiments, &c.; and among the latter, which are by far the most numerous, every description of mental emotion or passion, such as fear, anxiety, &c.; these first affect the nervous system, and then the stomach, through this medium.

It is a common remark that depression of spirits accompanies the dyspepsia, but the reverse of this is nearer the truth. Dyspepsia accompanies depression of spirits, for when the mind is weighed down by disappointment or anxiety, or trouble of any kind, the energies of the nervous system undergo a corresponding depression, and of course the stomach loses, in common with other organs, a portion of its vital power, and dyspepsia is the consequence.

The stomach is also known to have close sympathy with the skin; any irritation upon the skin, if kept up for any length of time, may be transferred to the stomach and impair the tone of the organ.

Pain in any part of the body, if intense and excruciating, and of long duration, impairs the nutritive function; and the stomach may be said to sympathise and become affected.

And also the urinary organs may sympathise with the stomach and *vice versâ*. It is well known that any difficulty of the kidneys may by sympathy affect the stomach. One of the attendant symptoms of inflammation of the kidneys is nausea, and sometimes vomiting.

Those causes that interfere with the mechanical power of the stomach, may include every thing that distends the stomach and thereby prevents its churning motion; for any thing of this kind will palsy the efforts of the stomach.

With regard to the difficulty in the process of digestion after the food has passed from the stomach in the *duodenum* or small intestine; the effects are not felt for some time after eating, and no oppression is felt in the stomach, but at the right side, and some puffiness is frequently perceptible in the region occupied by the intestine. Sometimes in duodenal indigestion the pain complained of affects the back in the region of the right kidney. That headache should accompany dyspepsia cannot be a matter of surprise, when we consider the close sympathy between the nerves of the stomach and the brain; either the stomach or bowels may sympathise with the brain; if the former, there will be a languid and feeble pulse, whitish, slightly coated tongue, the edges of a pale, red color; mistiness before the eyes, and general indistinctness of vision; dull weight or pain in the head, giddy and afraid of falling; but when the head-ache accompanies indigestion in the bowels, there is the appearance of occular spectres, which very much distress the patient; chilliness of the body; coldness and damp-ness of the hands and feet; severe pain in the head, attended with sensation of coldness and tightness of the scalp; slight giddiness; weight, distension and stiffness of the eyeballs; flatulency and a sensation of dryness and inactivity of the bowels. The last symptom is con-sidered as abundantly indicative of the derangement.

10.—Bilious Headache. (*Stomachic Headache.*)

This affection usually occurs in the early stage of digestion, when the operation is going on in the stomach; but duodenal or that which happens after the food has passed from the stomach, takes place at a later period.

Since headaches arise from congestion of the brain, as well as from sympathy with a deranged stomach, it may be noted that the former are distinguished from those of dyspeptic origin by plethoric symptoms, as by a full and oppressed pulse; by a difference in the character of the pain; in that which arises from fulness of blood there is a throbbing and a sense of action in the system, which sometimes is the cause of alarm; whilst the headache, arising from dyspepsia, is dull, aching or racking, often moving from one part to another, and attended with soreness of the scalp. In headache, arising from con-gestion, the eyes are red; but in that arising from bilious derangement, the eyes have a languid appear-ance.

Another result of dyspepsia is biliary derangement,

or perhaps it may be equally proper to say another cause of dyspepsia is biliary derangement; as for instance, when the secretion of the liver is deficient, the work of duodenal digestion is impeded; and when redundant, the obstruction is of a different character, when vitiated, the stomach partakes somewhat of the derangement.

But it matters but little whether we speculate or not upon the mutual injury a diseased liver and a diseased stomach might inflict; one thing is quite evident, that a simple disease of the mucus membrane of the stomach, if neglected, will certainly disease the liver, and *vice versâ;* and we have to adapt our remedies with reference to the conjoint symptoms of these two organs. The simple knowledge of the pathological condition of the organs that are prone to sympathise with each other, does not point out the precise remedy required; but if we believe in the truth of the claim set up, that medicines will cure only as their pathogenetic character corresponds with the manifestation of the disease, the remedy must in all cases be selected to correspond with a certain group of symptoms; and as dyspepsia is a disease ever varying in its manifest character, many remedies may be required to treat a single case.

TREATMENT.—The remedies employed to meet various stages and groups of symptoms, are Antimonium crud., Arnica, Belladonna, Bryonia, Chamomilla, China, Hepar sulph., Ipecacuanha, Ignatia, Lachesis, Nux vomica, Pulsatilla, Sulphur, Tartar emetic.

ARNICA is the remedy indicated when the affection is caused or proceeds from a blow, or by lifting or straining, with pain and cracking in the small of the back; by fatigue, much mental labor, and generally when it arises from over-excitement and irritability; when the patient

18

is very nervous, and has a dry tongue, or yellowish coat
ing; putrid, bitter or sour taste, with a fetid odor from
the mouth; an inclination for acids, eructations, sometimes
with a taste as of bad eggs; a sense of fulness after meals;
inclination to vomit; retching; flatulence in the bowels,
which are distended; a heaviness in all the limbs; weakness in the legs; fulness in the head, particularly over
the eyes; dull feeling and heat in the head; unpleasant
warmth; wakes frequently from sleep, and starting when
asleep; anxious dreams; after all the benefit is obtained
that can be from this remedy, and the patient is not
cured, *Nux vomica* or *Chamomilla* may be given.

DOSE.—Dissolve one drop, or six globules, in half a tumbler of water,
and give a teaspoonful every six hours.

ANTIMONIUM CRUDUM is indicated when the patient
feels sick at the stomach, and has blisters or a white
coating upon the tongue, and frequent eructations which
tastes of the food last taken; flow of saliva from the
mouth, or else much thirst, particularly at night; accumulation of mucus in the throat, or vomiting bile and
mucus; sensation of fulness of the stomach, and soreness
from contact; and also flatulency with griping, or alternations of constipation and looseness of the bowels. When
this remedy has been given according to the directions
without producing any improvement in the condition of
the patient, *Bryonia* is a suitable remedy to succeed.

DOSE.—Give one drop, or four globules, morning and evening.

BELLADONNA, when *Hepar* or *Sulphur* has been given
without producing any amelioration in the condition of
the patient, may be given and repeated once or twice, and
afterwards *Sulphur* may be administered again, with
prospect of more favorable action.

DOSE.—One drop, or four globules, may be given morning and evening,
for one day; if there is a decided improvement in the condition of the

patient, the remedy need not be repeated so long as the patient continues to improve; if there is no amelioration, follow with a dose of Sulphur, twelve hours after, and then wait for twenty-four hours and do not repeat if there is manifest improvement.

BRYONIA, when there is chilliness and coldness of the body, with derangement of the stomach; constipated bowels; white or yellow coating upon the tongue, or white blisters upon the tongue; continual thirst both night and day; dryness of the throat and stomach. This remedy is better suited to warm and damp weather.

DOSE.—One drop, or four globules, night and morning, to be discontinued as soon as the patient is evidently better. If after administering the remedy for two days, there is no amelioration, give *Antimonium* for one day, according to the directions, and wait a while for the result.

CHAMOMILLA is indicated when there is bitter taste in the mouth, immediately after eating, during an irritable or fretful state of mind; or there is, apparently, bilious eructations, vomiting of greenish mucus, or bile; or when there is restlessness and tossing about during sleep, frequently waking, pain and fulness in the head, and face red and hot, the eyes burning and red, and the mind prone to be very sensitive. If this remedy fails of relief, give a single dose of *Sulphur*, and in twelve hours recur to it again.

DOSE.—One drop, or four globules, may be given, morning and evening, for two days; if there is no sign of relief, give a dose of Sulphur the next morning, and repeat the Chamomilla in the evening, and wait twenty-four hours; if no improvement, resort to *Ant. crud.*, and if this does not produce very soon, a favorable change, in twenty-four hours, give Bryonia.

CHINA is suitable in those seasons of the year, when the weather is variable, and the air is filled with noxious vapors, and in those localities where there is much fog, and also for persons who are obliged to work where they have not a sufficient supply of fresh air. It frequently antidotes predisposition to agues, and some. times steels the constitution against them. The particular symptoms indicating the use of this remedy, are sense of having eaten to satiety, and indifference to food and drink; slow and torpid digestion; constant belchings, and vomiting of undigested food; morbid craving for something strong, sharp or sour; weakness in the body, and a disposition to lie down, but unable to remain quiet; stiffness of the limbs in the morning, which require bending and stretching; flushes of heat; chilliness after every breath of air; dark colored urine, with copious sediment; wakefulness after lying down; melancholy and morose disposition.

DOSE—One drop, or four globules, twice a day,

HEPAR SULPH. is indicated when the greatest care in eating and drinking cannot avoid derangement of the stomach; and when there is under such circumstances, a craving for acids or wine, accompanied with nausea, sickness of the stomach, and eructations, principally in the morning; at times sour and bilious vomiting, and throwing up of phlegm, which accumulates in the throat; pain in the bowels, and hard, dry stools; and when the stomach has been rendered sensitive from taking calomel or blue pills.

DOSE.—One drop, or four globules, every twenty-four hours.

IPECACUANHA is indicated in dyspepsia, when the tongue is not coated, although the patient is troubled with vomiting, and sickness at the stomach. It is particularly indicated when habitual tobacco chewers begin to loathe the sight of the weed, as well as every description of food, and are given to easy or violent vomiting, for the most part, accompanied by diarrhœa; and also, when these symptoms come on in daily or bi-daily paroxysms, at or about the same time of the day.

DOSE.—The same as directed for *Chamomilla* or *Bryonia*.

IGNATIA is indicated when a protracted period of grief has brought on dyspepsia, attended with the following symptoms: when there is hiccough after eating or drinking; nausea and vomiting of food; burning in the stomach, and an empty and weak feeling in the pit of the stomach; fulness and distension of the bowels.

DOSE.—One drop, or four globules, may be given morning and evening.

LACHESIS is indicated in cases when the difficulty is worse immediately after meals, or early in the morning; when several days pass without any evacuation. It may be called into requisition after Hepar has proved insufficient.

DOSE.—Lachesis should not be given oftener than a dose of four globules, every twenty-four hours, and great care should be exercised to discontinue its use immediately after there is a mitigation of the disease. One drop in a spoonful of water, may be administered, and then it would be well to wait forty-eight hours for the result.

NUX VOMICA is indicated when dyspepsia has been brought on by dissipation and irregular hours; by drinking wine or strong coffee, and particularly if the patient has taken cold upon this condition; or as indicated by dryness of the mouth, without thirst; white coating upon the tongue; accumulation of phlegm in the mouth; heartburn and loss of taste, or that every kind of food and drink tastes insipid; water collects in the mouth; vomiting; pressure at the pit of the stomach; distension of the bowels; small and hard evacuations or constipation; reeling, giddiness, or dullness in the head; heaviness in the back part of the head; ringing in the ears; drawing in the jaw, teeth and limbs; want of energy and inability to think; restless, fretful and sullen; sometimes heat in the face.

DOSE.—One drop, or four globules, may be given twice a day, if without good effect; follow after the elapse of a day with *Chamomilla.*

PULSATILLA is indicated when the stomach is in that condition that fat meat deranges it and produces flatulency; or when different kinds of food do not intermingle in the stomach without producing distress and flatulency; or when the dyspepsia is excited by any kind of rich food; when the taste is bitter or greasy, resembling putrid meat or tallow; and all kinds of food taste bitter, and there is a loathing of tobacco; and also when there is accumulation of phlegm in the mouth; eructations of acrid bile or acidity from the stomach; aversion to warm food; distension of the abdomen, with rolling and rumbling; slow, troublesome and scanty evacuations or diarrhœa; sensation of chilliness; weakness; fretful and silent; annoyed at trifles.

DOSE.—Dissolve one drop, or six globules, in half a tumbler of water, and give a tablespoonful morning and evening.

SULPHUR is useful in those cases of dyspepsia that have been brought on by the use of aperients containing calomel or some other form of mercury; and particularly when there are neuralgic pains in the limbs, and at times soreness and tenderness of the stomach; unable to bear external pressure; constant belching of fetid flatus, and especially when some skin difficulty or tetter has preceded the gastric difficulty.

DOSE.—Give a drop, or four globules, of Sulphur in a tablespoonful of water, and repeat in forty-eight hours, if there is not a decided improvement in the patient.

TARTAR EMETIC is particularly indicated when there is loathing of the food, and sometimes inordinate appetite and great desire for acids and fresh fruit; empty risings; eructations tasting like rotten eggs; nausea, with inclination to vomit; anguish; vomiting of mucus, and pain in the stomach, as if overloaded; colicky pains in the bowels, with great mental uneasiness, as if the bowels would be cut to pieces; papescent stools, or mucous diarrhœa.

DOSE.—One drop, or four globules, may be given twice a day.

Further indications for the use of remedies in dyspepsia from different causes, may be found in the following leading considerations :

When every thing taken causes suffering on account of the weakness of digestion, Carb. veg., Chin., Nux vom., and Sulph.

From cold water, if it should be found to disagree, Ars., Cham., Chin., Ferrum, Nux vom., Puls. and Veratrum.

If caused by beer, Bell., Colocynth., Rhus and Sep.

When produced by milk, Bry., Calc., Nux vom., and Sulph.

From animal food, Ferrum, Ruta, Silicea and Sulphur.

When caused by fat or gravies, Nat. Mur., Puls., Sep. and Sulphur.

For different ages and constitutions.—Children suffering from dyspepsia require chiefly Calc., Ipecac., Nux vom., Hyos. and Sulphur, according as the symptoms may indicate. Old people require Cicuta, Ant. cr., Carbo veg., China and Nux vom.

Hypochondrical persons require for the most part Nux vom. and Sulphur.

Hysterical females require Puls., Sep., Sulph., Veratrum and others.

When brought on by sedentary habits, Bry., Calc., Nux vom., Sep., Sulphur.

When by prolonged watching, Arn., Carb. veg., Cocc., Nux vom., Puls., Verat.

When by excessive study, Arn., Calc., Lachesis, Nux vom., Puls. and Sulphur.

When by debilitating losses, as in diarrhœa, dysentery, vomiting or bleeding, China, Ferrum.

When by sexual excesses, Calc., Merc., Nux vom., Phos. ac., Staphysagria.

When the disease is in persons of the lymphatic temperament, Chin., Puls., Sulph.

When in persons of sanguine temperament, Bry., Nux vom., Bell., Phos.

When in persons of bilious temperament, Cham., Cocculus, China, Sulph.

When in those of melancholic temperament, Aurum, Ars., Nux vom., Puls., Sep.

When in nervous temperaments, Coffea, Ignatia, Sulph., &c.

The habits or temperaments are by no means the guide in the selection of remedies, but they should for the most part be taken into consideration with the indicating symptoms.

DIET.—Sometimes persons will suffer from difficult digestion when they take any kind of food or drink, and yet their systems cannot be sustained without food; such articles, therefore, of a non-medicinal quality, as cause the least suffering, determined by the experiuce of the patient, must be taken in great moderation, but not without the most thorough mastication. Some can take a few well known articles of diet, while many other common articles disagree. Such should restrict themselves during treatment to what they know from experience is easy of digestion. Others find a larger number of kinds of food that agree— these should be governed accordingly. Any article known to disagree should in all cases be avoided. Mastication should be very thoroughly performed, and considerable time should elapse between the taking of each morsel of food into the mouth and stomach. For the most agreeable kinds of food, to be taken without seasoning, or medicinal condiments, consult the diet table of the articles allowed under homœopathic treatment.

11.—Heartburn.—Waterbrash. (*Pyrosis.*)

This disease is of common occurrence among persons suffering from disturbed digestion, and consists of burn-ing sensation in the pit of the stomach, followed in general by sour or acrid eructations or risings. In many instances the affection spreads over the whole region of the stomach, and is attended with disagreeable gnawing, anxiety, nausea, coldness of the extremities, debility, and sometimes even with faintness. It is in most cases so nearly allied to dyspepsia, that the range of remedies for that disease are to be regarded the best adapted to this.

Nux. vom., Cham., Puls., China, Carbo veg. and Bella-donna, are remedies that seldom fail of removing the difficulty, when the accompanying symptoms otherwise indicate which is to be used.

Doses.—When either of the above remedies are used in this complaint, the dose should be the same, and the repetition as frequent as prescribed for the same remedy in dyspepsia.

But in cases where there is no other gastric dis-turbance, *Belladonna* may be given when the heartburn is attended with thirst.

DOSE.—One drop, or four globules, three times a day.

China.—When it occurs after meals, and causes hic-cough and acrid risings.

DOSE.—One drop, or four globules, whenever it occurs.

STAPHISAGRIA.— When produced by smoking, and attended with hiccough.

DOSE.—One drop, or four globules, as often as relief is required.

COCCULUS is particularly indicated for pyrosis in pregnant females. Sometimes it will afford complete relief, but the irritation being kept up, the disease may often recur, and require a repetition of the remedy. Remedies used in dyspepsia, or other gastric difficulties, may sometimes afford relief in this affection, but as all remedies are to be regarded more in the light of palliatives, any simple resort that will afford relief is commended. Sugar and water drank in the morning, or cold water drank freely, or water crackers, may be taken with advantage. *But one deleterious practice must be discouraged: Chalk, Saleratus, Pearlash, Magnesia* and the like, are always hurtful resorts. They may relieve for the time, but they are likely to entail more serious difficulties.

12.—Spasms of the Stomach.—Cardialgia.—Gastralgia.

This affection is often termed *cramp in the stomach*, and consists in gnawing or contractive pains in the stomach, extending to the chest and back; attended by nausea and vomiting; faintness, and coldness of the extremities, and great anxiety. Sometimes the patient is relieved by belching wind, or by the discharge of a portion of burning, acrid, limpid fluid. The disease is sometimes attended with headache and constipation. In some cases the pain is not severe, but there are always anxiety and nausea, which may be increased by taking food. The disease originates in a diseased condition of the nerves of the stomach; is often associated with disease of the liver, spleen, or even both; cancer of the stomach or intestines. It seldom occurs before the age of puberty. It may occur from gout or any chronic irritation that deranges the nerves of the stomach.

CAUSES.—Spasm of the stomach may be brought on by persisting in the use of improper articles of diet, or by the use of stimulants. These, however, are not the only causes. Sometimes the system may gradually acquire a condition that favors the disease, and then crude, uncooked vegetable substances, salads, old cheese, new bread, sweetmeats, cherries, chestnuts, strong tea or coffee, and all other stimulating drinks, or long fasting between meals, or any indigestible food, or exposure to damp or cold, may bring on the difficulty; and when any one is aware of his predisposition to suffer from this difficulty, he should avoid all these things.

The patient must also be warned against those miserable resorts for relief that always stand in the way of a cure; laudanum, opium, morphine, brandy, Hoffman's anodyne, &c., are all hurtful, and defer a cure. Nothing can be worse, especially when it occurs in females, after the cessation of the menses, or from their interruption.

Notwithstanding the disease has been regarded incurable, under allopathic treatment, homœopathy has in many cases been effectual, *even when of long standing and of the worst kind.*

TREATMENT.—The remedies found most successful, are Belladonna, Bryonia, Calcarea, Carbo veg., Chamomilla, China, Cocculus, Coffea, Ignatia, Nux vomica, Pulsatilla.

BELLADONNA is indicated after *Chamomilla* has been tried without affording relief, especially in delicate and sensitive females. When there is gnawing pressure, or spasmodic tightness of the stomach, which obliges the patient to lean back to mitigate the pain, or keep the breath; and also when the pain returns after dinner, so violent as to deprive of consciousness, or to produce fainting; when drinking increases the pain, and the patient cannot sleep at night.

DOSE.—Of a solution of one drop, or six globules, in four tablespoonfuls of water, give a teaspoonful every six hours, until relief, or change.

BRYONIA is also a remedy that may be classed with *Chamomilla*, and when the latter remedy fails of relieving the peculiar kind of pressure for which it is indicated, the former may be called into use; and particularly when the difficulty begins during meals, or occurs immediately after; and there is swelling of the pit and region of the stomach; and when the pressure changes to contracting, pinching, or cutting pains, which are relieved by pressing against the stomach, or by the belching of wind, or when the least motion aggravates the pain; and also when the foregoing symptoms are attended with constipation, pressure in the temples, forehead, or back part of the head, as if the bones were rent asunder, and which is relieved by being pressed hard, or by tying a handkerchief around the head.

DOSE.—Of a solution of two drops, or ten globules, in half a tumbler of water, give a teaspoonful, according to the intensity of the pain, every three, four, six, or eight hours, until the patient is better or worse, or there is change of remedy.

CALCAREA is the most suitable for chronic cases, and particularly when *Belladonna* has afforded temporary relief. Its use is indicated by oppressive cutting, spasmodic pinching, choking pains, with anxious feelings, and frequently vomiting of food, worse after eating, and during the night, aggravated by external pressure. It is particularly suited for women, habituated to copious menstruation, and those who bleed much, and often from the nose.

DOSE.—One drop, or four globules, morning and evening.

CARBO VEG. is more particularly adapted to cases after *Nux vom.* has accomplished a partial cure, or has only afforded temporary relief; and when there is burning pain, or a continual, painful, agitating pressure, aggravated by touch, or when there is a contracting, spasmodic sensation, forcing the patient to bend, depriving of breath, and becomes aggravated on lying down, sometimes attended with heartburn and nausea, loathing of food, and constipation.

DOSE.—One drop, or six globules, may be dissolved in half a tumbler of water, and one teaspoonful may be given three times a day.

CHAMOMILLA is the remedy to be called into use when there is pressure at the pit of the stomach, as from a stone; and painful pressure at the region of the heart as if this organ would be crushed; flatulent distension at the same part; also in both sides of the abdomen and bowels, with shortness of breath, anxiety, and throbbing headache; mitigation of the above symptoms on partaking of coffee; a distinguishing mark between the use of this remedy and Nux vomica, is the relief which the drinking of coffee gives; on the other hand, it is indicated when the symptoms as described are liable to be brought on by a fit of passion, or by any other agitation or emotion; the pain in the stomach sometimes alleviated by drawing up and lying still.

DOSE—Of a solution of one drop, or six globules, in half a tumbler of water, ; give a teaspoonful every three hours, or if the pain is not *very* severe, give a teaspoonful every six hours.

CHINA.—When spasm of the stomach occurs in debilitated persons, or in debilitated conditions of the system which may have been brought on by using emetics or cathartics, being bled or cupped frequently, or by profuse loss of blood in any way, or by salivation or loss of

19

206 DISEASES OF THE DIGESTIVE ORGANS;

fluids by other means. When spasms occur in nursing, this remedy is of the first importance; and especially when the system is weakened by protracted nursing; when this remedy does not afford complete relief, *Bella-donna* is suitable to succeed; when, therefore, spasms of the bowels occur in females that have been nursing too long, this remedy is to be used first; and afterwards, if the milk is disposed to disappear, *Belladonna* must be used; and also, *China* is indicated when the digestion is not good, and much mucus acidity and acrid bile in the stomach; when the stomach feels sore, when meat and drink cause pressure and distension, and when the pains are worse during rest, and better when the patient is in motion.

DOSE.—Dissolve one drop in four spoonfuls of water, or eight globules in the same quantity, and give a teaspoonful every six hours until amelioration or change.

COCCULUS is a useful remedy after *Nux vomica* has been available in giving temporary relief, with recurrence of the pain again in a short time, accompanied by hard evacuations or obstinate constipation; and when there is pressing and contractive pain in both the stomach and bowels, which is somewhat relieved by the discharge of wind, and there is sickness at the stomach, and accumulation of water in the mouth without waterbrash, and when the patient is sullen without any manifestation of irritability or violence.

DOSE.—Of a solution of one drop, or six globules, in half a tumbler of water; give a teaspoonful every four hours until relieved, or there is necessity for a change.

COFFEA is sometimes useful after *Chamomilla*, when the pains are very violent, and when there is extreme restlessness and inquietude, it may be used alternately with *Chamomilla* or with *Belladonna*.

DOSE.—Of a solution of one drop, or six globules, in half a tumbler of water, give a teaspoonful every three hours if by itself, or if in alternation with either of the above named remedies, three hours should intervene between the times of administration.

IGNATIA is useful when the disease has been of two or three days' standing, after other remedies have been tried, and particularly if the pains resemble those described under *Pulsatilla* or *Nux vom.*, or when there is pressure after every meal, either in the throat or at the pit of the stomach; looseness of the bowels, and nausea and vomiting; or when the spasm occurs in consequence of scanty supply of food or starvation.

DOSE.—One drop, or four globules, every four hours.

NUX VOMICA is of the utmost importance in the treatment of those cases brought on by the use of coffee or alcoholic drinks; when there seems to be a collection of wind on the left side under the ribs, worse after eating, or early in the morning, sometimes disturbing the sleep of the patient, and also when the pain in the stomach is pressing or contracting, and when the clothes seem too tight; and particularly if these symptoms are accompanied by oppression of the chest, as if something were drawn tightly around it; sometimes the pain extending between the shoulders and to the small of the back; frequently attended with an accumulation of water in the mouth and nausea, or when there is a sour, bitter or acrid water rising in the throat; vomiting of food; sour or putrid taste in the mouth; flatulency; distension of the bowels and costiveness.

DOSE.—Dissolve one drop, or six globules, in three tablespoonfuls of water, and give a teaspoonful every four hours until mitigation or change.

PULSATILLA is particularly indicated when the pains are of a shooting character, worse when walking or making a misstep, and generally attended with nausea or vomiting, loose stools, thirst during the most violent pains; when there is great tightness of the stomach, violent throbbing with anxiety, griping pains, relieved in a measure by eating. This remedy is most useful for persons of a lymphatic temperament, and especially if the pains are brought on or aggravated by eating rich or fatty kinds of food.

DOSE.—Dissolve a drop, or ten globules, in a tumbler of water, and give a tablespoonful every six hours until mitigation or change.

This remedy may be used in alternation with *Ignatia* every four hours, until better, or there are indications of a change. The character of this disease being that of neuralgia of the stomach, it would not be amiss to observe certain rules for protection : Those subject to the affection should have the feet well protected and kept warm; flannel should be worn next to the skin.

DIET.—This should be exceedingly simple, weak black tea, cocoa, or broma, is allowable, stale bread, or crackers, the lean of well-fed meat, in great moderation.

Wines and spices should be strictly prohibited, as well as coffee and green tea. All kinds of rich food and gravies, fresh bread, or warm cakes, preserves and cheese.

13.—Sea Sickness.

For sickness of the stomach, occasioned by riding in a coach, or by the motion of a vessel at sea, and by the peculiar circumstances attending this kind of sickness, Cocculus, Colchicum, Sepia, and Staphisagria, are the chief remedies.

Cocculus is the remedy usually indicated for this kind of sickness, when unattended with other difficulties.

Sepia, when there is pain in the head, accompanied

with sickness at the stomach, resembling the sick headache.

COLCHICUM is serviceable when the odor of the food, and the peculiar smell of the vessel, produces unpleasant sensations.

STAPHISAGRIA is indicated if there is an offensive putrid taste in the mouth, and bleeding of the gums, and severe constipation.

DOSE.—Of a solution of one drop, or six globules of either of the above remedies, when indicated, give a teaspoonful every three hours, until relieved ; or four globules may be taken at a dose, and repeated, if necessary, in four or six hours.

Owing to a difference of habit and constitution, persons are differently affected by the motion of a carriage, or of a vessel at sea; hence it is necessary to adapt remedies to the peculiar constitutional habits.

14.—Vomiting of Mucus.

There is a peculiar condition of the stomach in some persons, arising from debility, that causes them to vomit mucus from the throat and stomach, which accumulates there, from some disorder or derangement of the mucous coats of these organs.

SYMPTOMS.—Insipid, sweetish taste in the mouth, weak and miserable before eating, and painful uneasiness and fulness after eating.

TREATMENT.—The remedies employed are Ipecacuanha, Rheum, and Veratrum.

IPECACUANHA is useful when there is simply vomiting of phlegm, with a disagreeable, sick feeling at the stomach.

RHEUM is useful if there is sickness and vomiting attended with slimy diarrhœa, of a sourish or musty odor.

19*

VERATRUM, when the symptoms are violent and attended with the vomiting of bile, or bilious discharges from the bowels.

DOSE.—One drop, or four globules, of either of the above remedies may be given when indicated, and repeated every four or six hours, until a change.

The appetite in this affection, is sometimes unimpaired, yet the diet should be simple, and free from irritating substances. In this affection, cold water has been found of great service, drunk copiously, several times a day. And also the washing of the mouth and throat internally, with the same, is found of great benefit.

15.—Vomiting of Blood. (*Hæmatemesis.*)

This affection proceeds sometimes from rupture of one or more of the blood-vessels of the stomach, caused by debility, produced by disease, or by poisoning, as by corrosive sublimate or arsenic, or from violent vomiting and purging, and frequently from suppression of the menses, and from a sudden check of the bleeding piles, which causes a determination of blood to the stomach. The blood evacuated is of a dark color sometimes, and at others red. In the former case, it is venous blood; in the latter, arterial.

TREATMENT.—The remedies employed, are Aconite, Arnica, Arsenicum, China, Ipecacuanha, Nux vomica, Pulsatilla and Sulphur.

ACONITE is indicated when there is the presence of strongly marked, febrile symptoms, weight, pressure, fulness or pain in the region of the stomach, nausea, and vomiting of blood, of a bright red color.

DOSE.—Dissolve a drop, or six globules, in half a tumbler of water, and give a teaspoonful, at first, every thirty minutes, and then every hour, until mitigation, or change. When the premonitory symptoms of an attack begin to appear, attended with fever, a timely resort to the use of Aconite, as here directed, may obviate an attack.

ARNICA is useful in severe cases, when the vomiting of blood occurs in persons of a full robust habit, and a choleric disposition; also when the patient complains of pains, as if bruised in the stomach and extremities.

DOSE.—Dissolve six globules, or one drop, in two tablespoonfuls of water, and give a teaspoonful every two hours, until the patient is manifestly better, or there is a change.

ARSENICUM, when the vomiting of blood is in persons of weak constitution, and when there is intense burning in the stomach, and great prostration.

DOSE.—Dissolve a drop, or six globules, in three tablespoonfuls of water, and give a teaspoonful every four hours, until a change.

CHINA is useful when a quantity of blood has already been vomited, in restoring the weakened energies of the system from the loss.

DOSE.—One drop, or four globules, may be given every four hours, until there is evident restoration of strength.

IPECACUANHA is indicated when nausea and sickness of the stomach remain after an attack, or it may be used in alternation with *Aconite* at the commencement, when there is the presence of febrile symptoms, and also when there is vomiting of bile with the blood.

DOSE.—Dissolve one drop, or six globules, in half a tumbler of water, and give a teaspoonful every three hours, until a change.

NUX VOMICA is particularly useful when vomiting blood occurs in persons of full and plethoric habit, with a strong tendency of blood to the stomach; when there is tendency to constipation, particularly arising from suppression of piles, or suppression of the menses; or from indulgence in stimulating drinks, such as wine or beer; and also when the patient is of an irritable temper.

DOSE.—One drop, or four globules, every four hours, until better.

PULSATILLA is particularly serviceable when the vomiting is from suppressed menses, and also in males of the lymphatic temperament and mild disposition it is more suitable than *Nux vom.*

DOSE.—Precisely the same in all respects as for **Nux vom.**

SULPHUR is indicated when the symptoms occur after the suppression of an eruption or piles, or when there are evident signs of the vomiting of blood being but a transfer of some other flux to the stomach.

DOSE.—One drop, or four globules, three times a day.

DIET.—The rules to be observed in adapting a diet in this affection are nearly the same as in spasm of the stomach, only greater strictness is required. No solid food should be taken; all drinks should be cold. Preparations of milk, light puddings or broths may be allowed, but not for several hours after an attack, and then very cautiously and in small quantity, observing that every article taken should be cold, or at least only tepid or lukewarm. From the very nature of the affection, rest and quietness of mind· and body must be inferred as absolutely essential.

16.—Constipation. (*Costiveness.*)

There is not, perhaps, any abdominal difficulty that occasions so much attention on the part of those wedded to old opinions and unenlightened notions, as costiveness, and it may also be remarked that there is nothing of a moderately dangerous character that more frequently baffles the efforts of allopathy. The reason is, such efforts, arising from mistaken views, are directly opposed to the operations of nature.

Constipation is generally dependent upon some other derangement of the organism, and on this account it is

frequently alluded to as a symptom of other derangements. The very means that have been resorted to
obviate this difficulty have too frequently operated to
fasten it upon the system. A cathartic only relieves
for the time being, and then the difficulty is apt to occur
in a more stubborn form. This certainly cannot have
escaped observation, and the result of this course, of
flying to a dose of Magnesia, Epsom salts, Castor oil,
or to some one of the many kinds of pills, is a weakening
of the natural force of the bowels, and constipation
becomes an habitual thing.

Mothers, acting upon the idea that the *bowels must be
kept open*, frequently give their children aperient medicines, for the purpose, as they suppose, of keeping them
from getting sick; and the result frequently is the
derangement of their delicate systems, to a degree, that
subjects them to dyspepsia and constipation throughout
life. It is far better to leave slight cases of constipation to nature, or if medicines are needed, those
which only force evacuations of the bowels are by
no means the ones that operate a cure; these at best
only remove the effect and not the cause, and this
only temporarily; but as constipation results from a
morbid condition of the system, reason would dictate
that the successful use of remedies would overcome this
condition. It is found that remedies which correct
deranged conditions of the stomach, will often remove
constipation, though they possess no cathartic property.
We must look upon constipation as the mere result
of a peculiar condition, or want of balance in the general
system; it is to the changing of this that our attention
should be directed, if we wish to cure constipation,
instead of effecting a mere temporary palliation.

CAUSES.—Constipation results from derangement of the digestive or biliary organs, secondarily, and these may be primarily operated upon, either by disease, or deleterious medicines, or cathartics.

TREATMENT.—A mere arrangement of a judicious diet will often prove sufficient to remove mild forms of constipation, provided great care is taken to masticate the food well before taking it into the stomach.

The remedies employed are Alumina, Antim. crud., Bryonia, China, Calcarea carb., Cocculus, Lycopodium, Lachesis, Nux vomica, Opium, Pulsatilla, Plumbum, Sepia, Sulphur and Veratrum.

ALUMINA is indicated when there is dry, hard fæces, evacuated with considerable difficulty and exertion of the abdominal muscles, sometimes streaked with blood, and which appears to result from want of motion or activity in the intestinal canal, such as may result from travelling.

DOSE·—One drop, or four globules, every twenty-four hours. The best time for taking it is in the evening, half an hour before retiring.

ANTIMONIUM CRUD. is serviceable when the constipation is preceded by diarrhœa, or when there is a feeling of slight derangement of the stomach, and nausea.

DOSE.—One drop, or four globules, once a day, at night.

BRYONIA is a remedy that may be employed with advantage in *warm weather*, when the affection occurs in persons of dark complexion and irritable or obstinate dispositions, with a tendency to chills and rheumatism; and further, it may be employed to remove the difficulty when it arises from a *disordered stomach*, and is attended with determination of blood to the head and severe headache.

DOSE.—Dissolve one drop, or six globules, in four tablespoonfuls of water, and give a teaspoonful morning and evening, and continue until complete relief is obtained.

CHINA is a remedy that may be called into requisition when the constipation arises from debilitating losses, as in miscarriage, or from diarrhœa, or from violent purgation, or when occurring after a protracted season of looseness and the like.

DOSE.—One drop, or four globules, in a spoonful of water, to be taken every twelve hours, until better or a change.

CALCAREA CARB. is one of the remedies to be called into use after a journey, when the constipation appears to result from travelling. It is better suited to persons of sanguine temperament.

COCCULUS is another remedy found exceedingly useful for costiveness resulting from sea-sickness, or from riding in a coach or in the cars, and especially if the affection is preceded by nausea or vomiting.

CONIUM is another of the same class of remedies, and is more particularly indicated if the constipation is accompanied with painful piles.

DOSES.—It is not necessary to repeat either of the above remedies more than once a day. *Calc. c.* may be taken at night, one drop, or four globules, in a spoonful of water. *Cocculus*, perhaps, it would be better to take in the morning in the same way; and *Conium* either at night or in the morning.

LYCOPODIUM is one of the very best remedies in chronic constipation, as proved by clinical experience, when there is determination of blood to the head, colic, flatulence, sense of weight in the lower part of the bowels.

DOSE.—One drop, or four globules, in a tablespoonful of water; to be taken every night.

LACHESIS is indicated after the use of *Nux vomica* in chronic constipation, and particularly if this latter remedy has failed of fulfilling its indications. It is especially suited to those who take wine freely as a habit, and who feel a flatulent distention after meals, and ineffectual efforts to eructate.

DOSE.—One drop, or four globules, in a spoonful of water, every evening until amelioration or change.

NUX VOMICA is, for the most part, indicated when constipation results from too heavy a meal, or from partaking of indigestible food, or wine, or other stimulating drinks, or when it has resulted from the reaction after prolonged diarrhœa, or after the use of cathartics; when persons have taken aperients until the bowels have become so torpid as not to move without them, this remedy in alternation with *opium* may sometimes overcome the difficulty. In the most obstinate cases of constipation which afflict coffee drinkers, or those who have been somewhat given to the use of wine or brandy, *Nux vom.* may be considered one of the best of remedies; it is particularly adapted to persons of irascible and vivacious temperaments, with strong tendencies of blood to the head, and headache; unfitness for exercise; disturbed sleep, and a feeling of general oppression or heaviness; frequent and ineffectual efforts to relieve the bowels, attended with a sensation of a stricture, and sometimes painful difficulty in passing urine. It is an excellent remedy for persons suffering from piles, or are subject to them.

DOSE.—One drop, or four globules, every night, until amelioration or change.

OPIUM.—It is thought that this remedy is chiefly to be selected in recent cases of constipation, which do not occur as being peculiar or habitual; but its use is by no means confined to cases of this kind; it is equally useful when the disease occurs in vigorous, plethoric, well-nourished subjects, and arising from inactivity in the intestinal canal or from sedentary habits; when it occurs in aged subjects in alternation with diarrhœa, it is also an exceedingly useful remedy; and also when there is want of power to relieve the bowels, with a feeling of constriction in the anus; pulsation and sense of weight in the abdomen; dull, heavy pain in the stomach; parched mouth, and want of appetite; *determination* of blood to the head, with redness of the face and *headache.* This remedy is highly recommended for the constipation of pregnant females, which arises from pressure of the womb or abdominal tumors upon the rectum.

DOSE.—Dissolve four globules in a tablespoonful of water, and take morning and evening.

PULSATILLA is indicated when the patient is morose, taciturn, or soured, after eating fatty substances, and when there is constipation from sedentary habits and from drinking ardent spirits, or from eating too many kinds of food at a meal, or in consequence of surfeit or after a diarrhœa; want of appetite; disagreeable taste; the tongue coated; sickness of the stomach; tightness of the abdomen, and particularly when the constipation attends difficult menstruation.

DOSE.—Of a solution of one drop, or four globules, in a tablespoonful of water; give one half at night, and the other in the morning.

PLUMBUM is indicated for the most obstinate constipation, as from palsy of the bowels; when it may be attended by agonizing colics, contraction of the abdomen about the navel, with throbbing; sensations of heat or coldness in the abdomen; ineffectual efforts to evacuate, with painful constriction of the anus; for persons of a paralytic diathesis, affected with palsy, epilepsy, dropsy or emaciation, &c.

DOSE.—Give a drop, or four globules, every six hours, until relieved.

20

SEPIA SUCCUS is particularly indicated for constipation in females, or for persons addicted to rheumatism; and in some cases it may be regarded a useful remedy after *Nux vomica* or *Sulphur*, when either of them has proved inefficacious.

DOSE.—Of a solution of one drop, or four globules, in two tablespoonfuls of water; give a tablespoonful morning and evening.

SULPHUR is useful in most cases of constipation, especially after the use of *Nux vom.*, for persons of a melancholy disposition, who are subject to piles, and also when there is frequent and ineffectual effort to evacuate, with confined flatus, distention of the abdomen, and unfitness for intellectual labor.

DOSE.—One drop, or four globules, night and morning.

VERATRUM is useful for obstinate constipation, with ineffectual efforts to evacuate, on account of deficient expulsive power of the large intestine; or torpidity of the rectum, attended with congestion of the head, and flushed face; or for nausea, with sour or bitter eructations, and tenderness of the abdomen to the touch; and also for bilious and gastric affections; for infants and young children, after having been drugged with quinine.

DOSE.—Of a solution of one drop, or six globules, in four tablespoonfuls of water; give a spoonful three times a day, until there is an amelioration or change.

DIET.—Persons afflicted with costiveness should avoid all high seasoned food, and coffee, and green tea, and bread made of superfine flour. They may be allowed bran bread, crackers, apples and other fruits, tender beef and mutton, puddings made of rice or bread, and sauce made of prunes, peaches or plums. Patients should regularly go to stool, so as to establish the habit of regular evacuations.

17.—Diarrhœa.

This disease consists of loose or watery evacuations from the bowels, brought on by various causes; sometimes by fright, fear or vexation; from sudden check of perspiration; from taking cold; from disordered stomach and bowels, and from excessive heat.

Some diseases terminate in diarrhœa, and some commence with the same difficulty; but in all cases it may be regarded a morbid state of the functions. It is not unfrequently the case that diarrhœa is connected with affections of the liver or kidneys.

As in the treatment of *constipation* the use of cathartics or aperients is discouraged on account of the prostration they occasion, as well as on account of their failure in producing any good effect other than an ephemeral palliation. So in arresting diarrhœa, astringent drinks and other artificial means should be laid aside as having a decidedly injurious effect. The sudden arrest of diarrhœa very often causes the disease to tend strongly towards the head, and not unfrequently, fatal consequences result.

The usual consequences of suppressed diarrhœa are dyspepsia, liver complaint, and other kindred difficulties, and these affections are by far more difficult to remove after suppressed diarrhœa than before, because impurities that would have passed off are retained and thrown back upon the system. It will therefore be regarded in the utmost degree dangerous to thus throw back upon the system what may prove so injurious, by suddenly arresting a diarrhœa; besides arresting a diarrhœa is by no means curing it; it is only changing the disease into another form which may prove much more formidable than the diarrhœa itself.

Many have supposed that the alimentary canal is a tube smooth on its inner surface, through which can be forced whatever it contains without injury or violence, but this is an erroneous idea; the intestinal tube is a living organ and needs no activity to speed its contents on their way; no force can be applied with impunity. Its very structure indicates that nature is averse to forcible evacuations of any kind, either from disease or drugs, and *there never is* diarrhœa only when some *diseased action, opposed* to nature, is operative. When diarrhœa is produced by aperient medicines, in the attempt to rid the body of the poisonous materials, even if accomplished, it leaves the intestines very weak and relaxed. If the purgative were not a poison it would not purge at all, for only such things as the body cannot suffer, but ejects, acts as aperients. The poisonous effects of these medicines become most evident when they remain in the body; for when the body has not the power to reject them they show their whole force as a poison. You will be told that it is the disease which produces these symptoms, but do not believe it, it is false; more persons die of magnesia or castor oil, or more children die of rhubarb, than of arsenic, of which every one is afraid. With costive evacuations the action of the intestines is greater, or the excrements could not be ejected, and consequently nothing can remain behind; for the hard excrements we find always to fill the intestines completely, which is never the case in diarrhœa. When the action of the intestine stops, it is true the contents remain stationary, but it can easily be excited again, as has been shown under *"constipation."* Doctors who dissect thousands of bodies almost always find impurities in those who have had diarrhœa, but never in those who have been constipated.

When loose evacuations relieve a patient suffering from some complaint, wait awhile ___ore giving him medicine, and resort to it only in case of its continuing so long as to be injurious. Although diarrhœa affords evidence of disordered action in the system somewhere, yet it does occur when it should not be meddled with, because it is nature's method of affording relief, and this obtained, the diarrhœa passes away without requiring any medical aid. Such is the case with children when teething, and it is always better to wait a day or two when it occurs before giving any medicine. With respect to the treatment of the various kinds of diarrhœa, it is partly general and partly medicinal.

MEDICAL TREATMENT.—The remedies used, are Arsenicum, Antimonium crud., Bryonia, Calcarea carb., Chamomilla, China, Colocynthis, Dulcamara, Ipecacuanha, Mercurius, Nux vomica, Phosphoric acid, Pulsatilla, Rhus tox., Secale, Sulphur, and Veratrum.

ARSENICUM is indicated when the diarrhœa is watery or slimy, whitish, greenish, or brownish, taking place principally at night, after midnight, or towards the morning, or else after eating or drinking, with griping, burning, or tearing pains in the abdomen; violent thirst, anorexia with nausea, or else vomiting; excessive emaciation; great weakness; sleeplessness and anxiety at night; distension of the abdomen; coldness of the extremities; paleness of the face, with sunken cheeks and hollow eyes, surrounded by a livid circle.

DOSE.—One drop, or six globules may be dissolved in half a tumbler of water, and a teaspoonful may be given every two hours, and in some violent cases, every hour, until a reaction, or change.

ANTIMONIUM CRUD. may be successfully employed when there is watery diarrhœa, with disordered stomach;

20*

tongue covered with a white coating; loss of appetite; belching and nausea. It is particularly adapted for aged persons, and for *females* during pregnancy, or when lying in; and in some cases of diarrhœa, during dentition in children.

DOSE.—Of a solution of one drop, or six globules, in half a tumbler of water, give a teaspoonful every two hours; or if the disease is not very violent, give a teaspoonful every three or four hours, until amelioration or change.

BRYONIA may be used in diarrhœa that occurs during the heat of summer, and more particularly when it is caused by cold drinks; or when it is brought on by vexation or fright, or a fit of passion, It is a valuable remedy to call into requisition after *Chamomilla* has proved inefficient.

DOSE.—Dissolve one drop, or six globules, in half a tumbler of water, and give a teaspoonful every three hours, until amelioration or change.

CALCAREA CARB. is a useful remedy in diarrhœa of long standing, and especially if it occurs in scrofulous children, and seems to be attended with weakness emaciation, paleness of the face, and keen appetite. It is useful after the ineffectual employment of *Sulphur*.

DOSE.—One drop, or four globules, night and morning.

CHAMOMILLA is a most effectual remedy for watery slimy, bilious diarrhœa, of a greenish or yellow color, mingled frequently with undigested food, rumbling in the bowels, want of appetite, thirst, coated tongue, tearing colic, or griping fulness in the stomach, distension and hardness of the bowels, frequent eructations or bilious vomitings, bitter taste in the mouth. It is a useful remedy for children, and in young children, when attended with crying, agitation, tossing, constant desire to be carried in the arms.

DOSE.—Children may have two globules every three hours, until relieved. Adults may require a drop, or four globules, every three, four, or six hours, until better, or a change.

CHINA is indicated in profuse, watery, and brownish diarrhœa, mingled with undigested portions of the food; at night, or soon after eating, with violent pressive constrictive colic. It is also useful in painless diarrhœa, and great weakness in the abdomen; rumbling in the bowels; eructations; burning pains in the arms; want of appetite; violent thirst; and general debility.

DOSE.—Of a solution of one drop, or six globules, in four tablespoonfuls of water, give a teaspoonful every four hours, until amelioration, or change.

COLOCYNTHIS is more particularly useful in bilious or watery diarrhœa, with violent spasmodic colic, especially when caused by vexation or fits of passion, and when Chamomilla has previously been used with only partial success. *Chamomilla* is also a good remedy to be employed after *Colocynthis*, when the latter has proved insufficient.

DOSE.—Dissolve one drop, or six globules, in half a tumbler of water, and give a teaspoonful every three hours, until mitigation, or change.

DULCAMARA is indicated when there are liquid, yellowish, slimy, or bilious evacuations; or when there are evacuations at night, composed of slimy matter, and crude undigested particles of food, with colic and griping, especially around the navel; want of appetite, and violent thirst; nausea, or else vomiting; paleness of the face; great lassitude and uneasiness; and particularly when the diarrhœa has been brought on by a cold.

DOSE.—One drop, or six globules, may be dissolved in half a tumbler of water, and a teaspoonful may be given every four hours, until relief is obtained, or there is necessity for a change.

IPECACUANHA is a useful remedy when nausea, and vomiting of whitish or greenish mucus, attends a watery or slimy diarrhœa, of greenish or yellowish appearance; tearing colic, or cuttings in children, with cries, tossing and restlessness; accumulation of saliva in the mouth; distension of the bowels; weakness, with desire to continue lying down; paleness of the face, with livid circle round the eyes; coldness; irritability, and irascibility.

DOSE.—Dissolve one drop, or six globules, in half a tumbler of water, and give a teaspoonful every three hours, until amelioration, or change.

MERCURIUS is called into use when the evacuations are principally at night, and are of a bilious, slimy, or frothy appearance; or sanguineous stools of a greenish, yellowish, or whitish color, sometimes attended with straining; burning and itching, and excoriation of the anus; violent colic, or griping; heartburn, nausea, and eructations; shivering, and shuddering, and perspiration, sometimes cold, with trembling and great lassitude.

DOSE.—Dissolve one drop, or six globules, in half a tumbler of water, and give a teaspoonful every three hours, until amelioration, or change.

NUX VOMICA is more particularly useful when there are frequent but scanty evacuations, of watery, whitish, or greenish stools, with colic, and straining, or bearing down pains in the rectum; and also if there is nausea and vertigo, on rising up.

DOSE.—Dissolve one drop, or six globules, in half a tumbler of water, and give a teaspoonful every three hours, until mitigation, or change.

PHOSPHORIC ACID is useful when the evacuations are involuntary, and of a dark, dirty, painless character; or when they are watery or slimy, with particles of undigested matter.

DOSE.—Of a solution of one drop, or six globules, in half a tumbler of water, give a teaspoonful every three hours, until amelioration, or change.

PULSATILLA is indicated when the evacuations are of a pap-like consistence, or slimy, bilious or watery, and of a whitish, yellowish, or greenish color, or else which change their character; and also when they are liquid and fetid, with excoriations of the anus; bitter taste in the mouth; white coating upon the tongue; nausea; disagreeable eructations, or else slimy, bitter vomiting; colic and cutting pains, especially at night.

DOSE.—Of a solution of one drop, or six globules, in three tablespoonfuls of water, give a teaspoonful every three hours, until a change.

RHUS TOX. may be successfully employed against diarrhœa that takes place principally at night, with pains in the limbs, headache, and colic which seems to be invariably aggravated after eating or drinking.

DOSE.—Dissolve one drop, or six globules, in four tablespoonfuls of water, and give a teaspoonful every four hours, until complete relief is obtained, or there is mitigation, or else a change.

SECALE is particularly indicated in painless evacuations, attended with great weakness, or watery fæces, or yellow or greenish, expelled promptly and with great violence, and frequently involuntarily; and also when there are evacuations of undigested matters, attended with colic and griping, especially at night; mucous coating upon the tongue; clammy taste; frequent rumbling in the bowels, and much flatulency, with fulness and distension of the abdomen.

DOSE.—Dissolve one drop, or six globules, in half a tumbler of water, and give a teaspoonful every three hours, until mitigation or change.

SULPHUR is certainly a valuable remedy in many cases of the most obstinate diarrhœa, and is especially indicated when the evacuations are frequent, and principally at night with colic, straining, distension of the bowels, oppression of the chest, shivering, and great weakness; slimy or watery; frothy or putrid evacuations of a whitish or greenish color, mingled with undigested matters; or when the evacuations are sour or bloody; and also when a slight cold invariably aggravates the diarrhœa or brings it on; and also when there is rapid emaciation.

DOSE.—One drop, or four globules, night and morning.

VERATRUM is particularly indicated when the evacuations are of a thin watery appearance, attended with great prostration; nausea and vomiting; rapid sinking of the system and emaciation; and also when there is rice water evacuations, attended with cramps in the stomach and bowels.

DOSE.—Of a solution of one drop, or six globules, in four tablespoonfuls of water, give a teaspoonful every hour in violent cases, until relief is obtained, or there is amelioration or change.

GENERAL TREATMENT AND DIET.—Whenever a diarrhœa commences, the patient should abstain from acids, coffee, tea, and every thing highly seasoned with salt; and also from fruit, either fresh or dried; eggs; chickens; but very little drink should be taken, and this should be restricted to mucilaginous drinks made of rice, barley or gum arabic, oatmeal or hominy.

When the patient has an appetite for food, he may be allowed mutton broth, thickened with flour, oatmeal or rice; and also milk fresh from the cow, in moderation, if the patient is fond of it.

18.—Dysentery. (*Bloody Flux.*)

SYMPTOMS.—Constant straining and desire to evacuate the bowels; violent pains and burning in the lower bowels; more or less fever; and the stools are either of mucus or blood, and sometimes of both.

The disease is generally preceded by loss of appetite; chilliness and fever; nausea or vomiting, or costiveness; this state is soon succeeded by dull pains in the abdomen; increase of the fever; loose evacuations, generally of

mucus at first, then mucus mixed with blood, and sometimes of pure blood, with intense pains and almost incessant desire for a stool, with violent straining; under some
circumstances the disease comes on without any previous
warning.

The disease may occur during any season of the year,
but its occurrence is most frequently in the *autumn*,
and very likely it is brought on by a change of the
temperature of the weather during the nights, which
causes a check of perspiration, and the fluids are driven
inward upon the mucus surfaces; or it may be brought
on by indulging in unripe fruits or vegetables, drinking
cold water when the system is either in a heated state
or in profuse perspiration; it frequently occurs in the
autumn as an epidemic or endemic, in particular regions
of country, and more particularly in low marshy situa-
tions.

TREATMENT.—When the patient first experiences any
of the premonitory symptoms of the disease, he should
avoid all cold drinks, unless prepared with barley or
mucilage; and, in fact, the less he drinks the better; his
apartments should be well ventilated, and he should rest
as much as possible.

The remedies employed are Aconite, Arnica, Arsenicum, Belladonna, Bryonia, Chamomilla, China, Colocynth,
Mercurius corr., Nux vomica, Pulsatilla and Sulphur.

ACONITE is particularly indicated in the commencement of dysentery, when it is accompanied with tearing,
cutting pains, resembling rheumatism in the upper and
lower extremities, neck and shoulders; violent chills;
excessive heat and thirst; bilious or thin watery evacuations, sometimes mixed with mucus slightly tinged with
blood; dull or cutting pains in the bowels; it is a remedy

often used in autumnal dysenteries, when there are warm days and cold nights.

DOSE.—Dissolve one drop, or six globules, in half a tumbler of water, and give a teaspoonful every three hours, until there is a change in the symptoms, and some other remedy is required.

ARNICA is useful in autumnal dysentery, when the disease makes its appearance by pains and aching in the limbs and lumbar region, as if they had been bruised or beaten; and when there is a soreness remaining after straining at stool; and also when there is an ineffectual straining and urging to stool, and contusive pains in the sides of the abdomen.

DOSE.—Dissolve one drop, or six globules, in four tablespoonfuls of water, and give a teaspoonful every three hours, until there is a change of symptoms demanding another remedy.

ARSENICUM is indicated when the stools have a putrid smell, and when they pass involuntarily; when the urine becomes offensive, and there is great loss of strength and benumbing of the faculties, with a fetid odor from the mouth; and when there are red or blue spots that make their appearance here and there upon the surface of the body; and also when there is tossing about in great agony, as if there was no rest to be had; the spirits sunken,, the patient looks for death, and when at the same time the breath is cool or else burning; *Carbo veg.* may be used after *Arsenicum*, if this remedy should produce no amelioration; when it aggravates, *Nux vomica* should be given; if the putrid smell still remains after having given *Carbo veg.*, give *China*, allowing an interval of two or three hours between the employment of the different remedies.

DOSE.—If alone, give one drop, or four globules, in a spoonful of water every four hours, allowing the same interval to elapse between the use of different remedies.

ARSENICUM and CARBO VEG. may be given in alternation every three hours, or with *Nux vom.* in the same way; but it is decidedly best to give each remedy by itself, until there is amelioration or indication for a change.

BELLADONNA is indicated when there is frequent small evacuations of blood, attended with severe pain in the front of the head, and chilliness extending down the back, or when there are involuntary stools.

DOSE.—Dissolve a drop, or six globules, in half a tumbler of water and give a teaspoonful every three hours, until amelioration or change.

BRYONIA is of great service in the incipient stage of dysentery, when it occurs in warm weather, and is brought on by partaking of unripe fruit, and when it is worse after drinking or eating the smallest quantities, and when there is nausea and yellow or dark colored coating upon the tongue, and bile mixed with mucus and blood in the stools. It is an excellent remedy to follow *Aconite*, after this remedy has reduced in some measure the febrile symptoms.

DOSE.—Dissolve one drop, or six globules, in four tablespoonfuls of water, and give a teaspoonful every three hours, until mitigation or change.

CHAMOMILLA is very suitable after *Aconite*, if there is still some fever and thirst and rheumatic pains, particularly in the neck and head; or when there is nausea, foul tongue, bilious stools, bitter taste, &c., and particularly if the disease succeeded immediately after a sudden check of perspiration, or if accompanied with great agitation and tossing.

DOSE.—One drop, or four globules, may be given every four hours.

CHINA is indicated for those dysenteries that appear in marshy districts afflicting many persons at a time,

21

and particularly when the disease is of an intermittent form, or worse every other day.

DOSE.—Dissolve one drop, or six globules, in four tablespoonfuls of water, and give a teaspoonful every three hours, until amelioration or change

COLOCYNTH. is indicated when there is extreme pain in the bowels, as if the intestines were pressed between hard substances; the patient writhing with pain; slimy stools, sometimes mixed with blood; the bowels much distended, sometimes like a drum; fulness and pressure of the bowels; shuddering, commencing in the abdomen and extending over the whole body; white mucus coating upon the tongue.

DOSE.—Dissolve one drop, or six globules, in half a tumbler of water, and give a teaspoonful every two hours, until some relief, and then every four hours.

MERCURIUS VIVUS is particularly useful when there is an urgent desire to evacuate, accompanied by a sense as if the intestines were being pressed out; after much straining a discharge of light blood, or greenish, broken up matters, mixed with blood, and the straining augmented after the evacuation. This remedy is very useful for the disease in children, when accompanied with crying and screaming. *Mercurius corr.* is the chief remedy resorted to by some physicians in autumnal dysentery, and is particularly useful after *Aconite*, when attended by much straining and colic, and also when in the commencement, there is considerable discharge of mucus, bile and blood; *Colocynth.* is useful after *Mercurius corr.*, provided it has failed of affording relief.

DOSE.—Of a solution of one drop, or six globules, of either, as indicated; give a teaspoonful every three hours, until the patient is better, or a change of remedy is required.

NUX VOMICA.—Small, frequent evacuations of bloody slime with tenesmus, violent cutting about the umbilical region, heat and thirst. Particularly useful when the dysentery occurs during the heat of the summer, and particularly when *Arsenicum* only aggravates the putrid smell of the evacuations.

DOSE.—One drop, or six globules, in half a tumbler of water; give a teaspoonful every hour.

PULSATILLA is of service when the stools are chiefly mucus, streaked with blood; nausea and coated tongue; bitter taste in the mouth; and in other respects when the symptoms may indicate the use of *Nux vom.*

DOSE.—One drop, or six globules, in four tablespoonfuls of water; give a teaspoonful every two hours, until amelioration or change.

SULPHUR is of great use when the disease seems protracted, and also when any of the remedies employed in the disease fails of affording entire relief.

DOSE.—One drop, or four globules, of Sulphur, may be given twice a day.

DIET.—During the febrile stage of the disease give barley water as a drink, and avoid the use of cold water. No solid food will be required.

Boiled milk, diluted with water, may be allowed in moderation, and also weak mutton soup after the fever has subsided, but no solid food should be taken until the cessation of the dysenteric stools, and then such as is of easy digestion and of a nutritive quality.

19.—Cholera Morbus.

SYMPTOMS.—Violent vomiting and purging; pain in the stomach and abdomen; thirst, and sometimes cramps and coldness of the extremities; before the attack there is generally some indications of its approach. Some. times shivering, pain in the stomach, and nausea; but there are occasionally attacks of the disease, without any premonition whatever; violent vomiting and purging setting in at the same time. The contents of the stomach are first ejected, and afterwards bile. It is in the very severe forms of the disease that cramps in the muscles, paleness of the surface, pinched features, sunken eyes, cold and clammy skin, and great anxiety and depression seem to characterize the disease.

The disease is of so short duration that attacks frequently come on at night, and by morning the patient may be entirely relieved, and nearly if not quite well.

The disease is common to warm climates, and warm seasons, and occurs the most frequently in the latter part of summer or early part of autumn.

CAUSES.—Improper diet, unripe fruits, or cucumbers, are generally considered as among the exciting causes; eating too much at a time, and indulging in too great a variety of luxuries, at a meal, and then exposing oneself to the heat of the weather, are also to be avoided as inducing the disease; sudden changes of temperature, great fatigue, the too free use of ice, or ice water, or ices of any kind, may also be reckoned among the exciting causes.

TREATMENT.—The principal remedies are the following: Arsenicum, Chamomilla, China, Cuprum, Ipecacuanha, Nux vomica, Veratrum.

ARSENICUM is indicated when the disease commences with violence, and is attended with rapid prostration of strength; insatiable thirst; excessive anxiety, with fear of approaching death; burning sensation in the region of the stomach; almost constant discharge from the bowels; or recurrence of the evacuations after drinking anything. When there is suppression of urine, or scanty discharge, followed by burning sensation; violent pain, and vomiting; tongue and lips dry, cracked, and of a dark or blackish appearance; hollow cheeks; pinched appearance of the nose; small, weak, trembling, and sometimes nearly imperceptible pulse; severe cramps in the extremities, and clammy perspiration.

DOSE.—Dissolve two drops of the dilution, or twelve globules, in half a tumbler of water, and give a teaspoonful every half hour, until some mitigation of symptoms, and then, every hour until the disease appears to be further reduced, and then, one in two, three, or even four hours, until complete convalescence is established.

CHAMOMILLA is useful when the attack is induced by some severe mental emotion, or fit of passion; or if indicated by the following symptoms: severe colic; heavy pressure in the region of the navel, sometimes extending to the heart, with excessive anguish; bilious diarrhœa; cramps in the calves of the legs; yellow coating upon the tongue, and sometimes vomiting of acid matter.

DOSE.—Dissolve a drop, or six globules, in half a tumbler of water, and give a teaspoonful every hour, for three or four times, and then, if there is the slightest amelioration, give a teaspoonful every two or three hours, until completely relieved.

CHINA is not so much indicated during the attack, as after it, to obviate the weakness which remains. Sometimes, however, it is of use during the course of the disease, particularly when there is vomiting of food, and frequent watery and brownish evacuations, containing portions of undigested food; and when there is oppression at the chest, with eructations which afford temporary relief; Severe pressure in the abdomen, especially after partaking of the smallest portion of food; great exhaustion, sometimes amounting to fainting. This remedy is particularly marked when the disease has been excited by crude, indigestible substances, such as unripe fruit, &c.

21*

DOSE.—Dissolve one drop, or six globules, in half a tumbler of water, and give a teaspoonful every three hours, if the attack has subsided; but every two hours if given during the attack.

CUPRUM is requisite when there are violent cramps in the extremities, especially in the calves of the legs, fingers and toes; it is useful also when the evacuations are very frequent and whitish, with intense pains in the bowels, bluish appearance of the skin, &c.

DOSE.—Dissolve one drop, or six globules, in half a tumbler of water, and give a teaspoonful every half hour or hour, according to the severity of the case.

IPECACUANHA is sometimes useful after *Chamomilla*, in the treatment of this affection, should the vomiting continue or become aggravated; or it may be given as the principal remedy when vomiting predominates, or at least exists in as great a degree as the diarrhœa. *Nux vomica* is exceedingly useful after *Ipecacuanha*, should there be anxiety, pain in the abdomen, frequent small evacuations, and straining, with headache.

DOSE.—Of a solution of one drop, or six globules, in half a tumbler of water, give a teaspoonful every two hours, until amelioration, or change.

NUX VOMICA is exceedingly useful when the disease comes on suddenly, with vomiting and purging, simultaneously, with much anxiety, and pain in the bowels; evacuations frequent and small; or ineffectual urging to stool; or cramps.

DOSE.—One drop, or four globules, every three hours, dissolved in a spoonful of water.

VERATRUM is a very useful remedy to succeed *Nux vomica*, provided there appears to be any increase of the disease, and particularly if there is violent vomiting, with severe diarrhœa; excessive weakness, and cramps in the calves of the legs; eyes hollow or sunken; countenance pale, and expressive of acute suffering; coldness of the extremities; violent pain in the region of the stomach, and about the navel; tenderness of the bowels˙when touched; pains and cramps in the fingers; shrivelled appearance of the skin, or the palmar surfaces.

DOSE.—Of a solution of one drop, or six globules, in half a tumbler of water, give a teaspoonful every half hour, until amelioration of the disease, and then every hour, or two hours, &c., according to the violence of the disease.

20.—Asiatic Cholera.

This formidable disease, so much dreaded in the community, is generally preceded by certain sufferings, or premonitory symptoms, which have continued for several days before the more certain phenomena of the disease appears; or these premonitory symptoms may not have made their appearance three hours before the attack.

These premonitory symptoms are great debility, as if the patient had suffered great loss of blood; dimness of vision, with giddiness and noises in the ears; and also much thirst, loss of appetite, and distension of the bowels. The principal symptoms are vomiting and purging; the purging commencing generally sometime before the vomiting.

If the disease is not soon checked the evacuations become frequent, ultimately assuming a copious liquid, watery and inodorous character, resembling rice water, and on this account the evacuations are generally termed rice water discharges; the patient becomes very restless as these evacuations continue; cramps attack the calves of the legs, fingers and toes, and sometimes even the muscles of the abdomen.

If the disease is not arrested in this stage, a still more formidable character will soon develope itself; for the constant watery discharges must soon exhaust the body so as to bring on *collapse* or the blue stage; the pulse almost imperceptible; coldness of the extremities, and thence of the body in general, including the face; the countenance seems pallid and sunken; eyes very much sunken in the sockets; and the thirst almost unquench-able, and the restlessness so excessive as to defy all efforts to obviate it; the breath becomes cold, and the skin over the hands and body become shrivelled and shrunken; the urine is suppressed; the nose becomes cold, and in some cases gangrenous; the voice husky; the breathing becomes slower and slower; hiccough precedes death. This is the course when the disease terminates fatally; but when it terminates favorably the pulse rises, the blue-ness disappears, warmth is restored to the body, and gene-ral reaction indicated by heat, fever and headache takes place; the reaction in some cases is so great that the utmost efforts of the physician are required to save the patient from the fatal efforts of congestion of some of the internal vital organs.

CAUSES.—The nature of the malaria from which cholera originates, is unknown; but we may reckon among the exciting causes,—living in filthy, crowded and badly ventilated places; errors of diet; extreme changes of habits; excessive or habitual use of intoxi-cating drinks or purgative medicines; severe mental emotions; excesses of any kind; and even debility may act as exciting causes.

When the disease prevails epidemically, many seem to predispose themselves to become its victims through fear and anxiety. The best security against the disease when it prevails, is to live on unconcerned in the regular dis-charge of the uses of life, partaking of the regular ordi-nary diet, keeping free from excitement or any thing that depresses the spirits; in short, the best prevention of the cholera is a fearless discharge of duty, without regard to the future, and a clear conscience before God and man.

TREATMENT.—The remedies which have been the most successful in grappling with this scourge of mankind, are Arsenicum, Carbo veg., Camphor, Cuprum., Ipecacuanha, Phosphorus, Phos. acid, Sulphur and Veratrum.

It is probable that several remedies will be required in curing any single case; some will be found useful in the first stage, some in the second, others in other stages, &c.

ARSENICUM is particularly indicated after Ipecacuanha, when the purging and vomiting become very frequent; and when the evacuations from the bowels become very thin, watery, brownish or blackish color, and of a putrid smell; or like rice water and nearly void of smell, but accompanied by cramps in the stomach and bowels; and burning pains in the stomach, with violent thirst and great prostration of strength; also burning in the anus and rectum, with tenesmus. This remedy is also worthy, of attention in the last stage of the disease.

DOSE.—Dissolve a drop, or six globules, in half a tumbler of water. and give a teaspoonful every twenty or thirty minutes, until amelioration or change,

CARBO VEG. is indicated when the disease has progressed to a stage of collapse or asphyxia; the pulse scarcely perceptible; the surface cold and bluish; .the breath cold; or when the evacuations and cramps have ceased, and congestion of the chest takes place, if reaction should ensue after this remedy has been given, and the cramps, vomiting and purging ensue, it will be necessary to recur to *Veratrum* or some other remedy suited to a prior stage.

DOSE.—The same in all respects as for *Arsenicum*.

CAMPHOR is of great service in the early stage of the disease, both as a curative and preventive of a more serious stage.

DOSE.—One drop, or four globules, may be given every hour until amelioration or change; when taken as a preventive it may be repeated three or four times a day.

CUPRUM is very suitable after *Veratrum*, or it may be useful as an alternating remedy; when the latter has failed to remove the cramps, which are violent, and extend over the whole body, or change to spasms or convulsions, with constriction of the chest and difficult respiration.

DOSE.—Dissolve one drop, or six globules, in two tablespoonfuls of water, and give a teaspoonful every fifteen minutes at first, until there is a change in the symptoms.

IPECACUANHA is indicated in the first stage of the disease, when there is nausea and sickness of the sto-mach, slight diarrhœa, and is very effectual in arresting the disease in the first stage.

DOSE·—Dissolve two drops, or twelve globules, in four tablespoonfuls of water, and give a teaspoonful every thirty minutes, until amelioration or change.

PHOSPHORUS is indicated for the looseness of the bowels and diarrhœa, which results from the irritability or weak-ness, that often occurs after an attack of cholera.

DOSE·—One drop, or four globules, three times a day.

PHOSPHORIC ACID is of great service in the diarrhœa which generally precedes cholera. So certain and salu-tary is its effect that some regard it a specific, particu-larly if the evacuations are frequent, loose and slimy, or of a whitish gray color, or if they consist of undigested substances.

DOSE·—Dissolve one drop, or six globules, in half a tumbler of water, and give a teaspoonful every hour or two hours, according to the severity of the symptoms, until amelioration or change.

SULPHUR is reckoned among the best remedies for the *cholerine*, or diarrhœa preceding cholera, especially when there is but little sick stomach, and when the patient complains of dimness of vision, giddiness, ringing in the ears and want of appetite, with tumid abdomen; the stools watery, frothy or mucous, and sometimes of a whitish or greenish color, occurring oftener at night.

DOSE.—Dissolve one drop, or six globules, in half a tumbler of water, and give a dessertspoonful every six hours, until amelioration or change.

VERATRUM is a very useful remedy in cholera when it becomes fully developed; when there are rice-water discharges almost constant, with cramps in the calves of the legs, fingers, toes, and sometimes of the muscles of the abdomen and chest; great restlessness and anxiety, and cold extremities.

DOSE.—Of a solution of two drops, or ten globules, in half a tumbler of water; give a teaspoonful every fifteen minutes, until several doses are taken, or there is a decided change in the symptoms. It may sometimes be used in alternation with *Arsenicum,* especially when the pains are of a burning character, and when the thirst is unquenchable, and the evacuations increased by taking cold water.

VERATRUM, CUPRUM and CAMPHOR are highly recommended as preventives of the disease; to be taken three times a day during an epidemic.

DOSE.—One drop, or four globules, of either.

During the treatment of cholera the patient should be kept in a warm room, and the external heat of the body should be kept up as much as possible by the application of friction and bottles of hot water to the abdomen and feet.

Salt, heated, and put in small bags, may be placed around the patient and over the limbs. *Oats,* heated, and applied in the same manner, is a very good way of keeping up artificial warmth.

To quench the intense thirst, small pieces of ice may be placed in the mouth of the patient from time to time.

Cramps in the intestines, or colic, may sometimes be relieved by injections of cold water.

The manner and indications for using the principle remedies in cholera, are embraced in the foregoing, but nevertheless it may be well to give an example of their use in a single case.

A.—— B.——, aged 25; first felt nausea and sickness at the stomach; had slight diarrhœa; was given *Ipecacuanha* every thirty minutes, as directed. The nausea merged into vomiting, and the diarrhœa, instead of abating, became aggravated; the remedy was discontinued, and *Veratrum* substituted in its place, and given as directed for the use of that remedy; but in spite of this, the patient merged into a state of collapse, and then *Carbo vegetabilis* was given. It will be seen from this that a remedy must invariably be discontinued when it becomes apparent that it does not meet the case, and one better adapted to cover the symptoms must be selected.

Often in the commencement, *Sulphur* may be used, but if it fails of success, perhaps *Cuprum* may be called into requisition, and if this fails, *Arsenicum*, if indicated, may be used, and so on.

DIET AND REGIMEN.—As soon as cholera passes off, the patient needs nourishment to aid the recuperative energies of nature in restoring strength; but during the time the disease is raging there is no food required, and it would be decidedly better for the patient if he would take very little drink, if any; but after the disease has spent its violence, and the patient has been left in a prostrated condition, the greatest care should be exercised in the selection of diet, at first, when the stomach is yet weak. *Arrow root* gruel may be given, or in its stead gruel made of groats, rice flour, corn starch, and then a little plain toast, and then the same with butter, and then mutton soup, not very strong; thus gradually strengthening the food as the condition of the patient can bear it, until he is able to eat and drink regularly. Care should be taken to provide suitable clothing, and to guard against the extremes of temperature.

21.—Cholerine.

It may have been noticed that an affection bearing this name is treated of in the books, but it is to all appearance the beginning of cholera, and usually prevails in all places where the epidemic cholera is prevailing at the same period. The remedies suitable for this affection may be found under Diarrhœa, of which *Sulphur, Nux vomica, Phosphoric acid*, &c., are among the best.

22.—Colic. *(Enteralgia.)*

This disease consists of greater or less degree of pain; griping, cutting, tearing, gnawing pain in the abdomen, more particularly about the region of the navel; generally occurs in paroxysms; sometimes the abdomen is drawn in, at other times it is distended like a drum; pressure generally relieves the pain, as the bowels are seldom painful to the touch. Sometimes the pains are accompanied with costiveness and sometimes by vomiting or diarrhœa.

Colic may be distinguished from inflammation of the bowels by the character of the pulse, which is soft and yielding; whereas it is febrile and sometimes accelerated in the latter disease.

22

It may be distinguished from *hernia* or *rupture* by the tumor which is always present in the latter difficulty.

CAUSES.—Errors of diet; constipation; flatulent food; grief; dissipation; cold, and whatever produces inaction of the bowels, or derangement of the digestive organs.

It may arise from any obstruction in the intestinal canal, from *cancer* or *intus-susception*, or stricture of the intestine.

FLATULENT OR WIND COLIC frequently occurs in children, fed on an improper diet, and in persons suffering from dyspepsia, particularly those fed upon improper food, or who are addicted to the use of ardent spirits.

BILIOUS COLIC generally occurs when the patient has been suffering under symptoms of disordered stomach and intestines, such as bitter taste, yellow fur on the tongue; nausea and vomiting; severe cutting or writhing pain, with thirst and anxiety; after suffering a while from the pain, vomiting supervenes, the bowels are freely moved with bilious stools, under proper treatment, the pain abates gradually, and the patient recovers.

Painter's or Lead Colic. (*Colica pictonum.*)

This disease is brought on by being exposed to the action of lead, and is a common affection among painters, who use the white lead, and among those who work in lead mines, or lead factories, in smelting ores.   The *symptoms* of this difficulty, are loss of appetite, restless nights, and disturbance of the nervous system. This is followed by vomiting, pain in the abdomen, at first in paroxysms, but generally increasing until it becomes continuous. There is but little fever, but there is con-

siderable headache, pain in the limbs, obstinate consti-
patiou, and sometimes paralysis of the extremities.
When a bluish line, extending along the edge of the
gums, it may be regarded a symptom of lead colic.

GENERAL TREATMENT. — A warm bath will often
produce speedy relief. Hot water sweetened with
molasses, may frequently relieve flatulent colic, for a
time, taken internally; placing the patient in a warm
bed, or in a position to be surrounded by heat, will
often afford salutary relief. Warm clothes placed over
the abdomen, is a resort that frequently affords relief.

The remedies employed, are Aconite, Belladonna,
Chamomilla, China, Cocculus, Colocynthis, Ignatia,
Mercurius viv., Nux vomica, Pulsatilla and Sulphur.

ACONITE is indicated when in addition to violent colicky
pains, and griping, rumbling, and heat of the abdomen,
and pains in the small of the back, there is an affection
of the bladder, with pain, and a perpetual inclination
to make water, without being able to pass urine ; and
also when there is accompanying the difficulty of the
bladder, nervousness and uneasiness, and the abdomen is
excessively sensitive.

DOSE.—One drop, or six globules, in two spoonfuls of water, to be
given four hours apart; then follow with some other remedy that may be
indicated.

BELLADONNA is indicated when there is redness of the
face, and tendency of blood to the head, and the pains in
the abdomen, are so violent as to render the patient
almost distracted; and also when there are pains under
the navel, and griping, as if produced by taking hold of
the parts with the finger nails, and accompanied by
pains in the small of the back.

DOSE.—Dissolve one drop, or six globules, in half a tumbler of water,
and give a dessertspoonful every half hour, for several times, and then

every hour, or two hours, or follow with some other remedy indicated, if necessary.

CHAMOMILLA is useful when there are pains in the stomach, and abdomen, attended with great restlessness and anxiety, with blue circles under the eyes, and much saliva in the mouth, tearing pains around the navel, and sensation as if the back were broken in the lumbar region. This remedy is suited for colic in children, and adults when attended with the above symptoms.

DOSE.—Dissolve one drop, or six globules, in half a tumbler of water, and give a teaspoonful every half hour; in severe cases. *Pulsatilla* is a suitable remedy to follow, when *Chamomilla* fails.

CHINA is very suitable for *flatulent colic* in debilitated persons, when it comes on after heavy sweats, or in females when nursing, or when there appears to be a contraction of the intestines in the lower part of the abdomen, and tensive pains and tension under the short ribs, as if there was an incarceration of wind.

DOSE.—Dissolve one drop, or six globules, in half a tumbler of water, and give a spoonful every hour until relieved, or there is necessity for change.

COCCULUS is indicated when the colic is attended with constipation and sense of weight in the abdomen, with rolling and rumbling with great heat, and particularly when there is a contraction in the bowels downward, attended with nausea; or when there is accumulation of wind in the stomach and intestines causing distension of the upper portion of the bowels, and pain with rattling in the stomach and pressure under the ribs, which seve-rally become relieved when the wind is dislodged and passes off upwards.

DOSE.—Dissolve one drop, or eight globules, in half a tumbler of water, and give a teaspoonful every half hour for two or three times, and then at longer intervals, until complete relief is obtained.

COLOCYNTHIS is particularly indicated when the pains are intense and constant, or cease only for a short time, and then commencing of more intensity than ever; and when the most violent pain is confined to a small spot about the navel, and returns periodically about every five or ten minutes; or when it commences with a slight drawing pain tending to the centre, which gradually augments, and finally changes to a boring or tearing pain, so violent as to cause the patient to cry out and shriek aloud, and to twist about; is covered with perspiration; and is disposed to press against something for relief, or to press the abdomen with the hands.

DOSE.—One drop, or four globules, dissolved in a spoonful of water, may be given every hour.

IGNATIA is useful for colic produced by any emotional excitement or grief, and for that which awakens the patient out of sleep; when there are shooting pains, which extend into the chest and sides, when the wind is discharged with much difficulty, and after which the pains become less acute; it is suitable for sensitive females; when the colic commences in the evening, and the flatulency causes nausea and vomiting, *Pulsatilla* is better.

DOSE—Of a solution of one drop, or six globules, in half a tumbler of water; give a teaspoonful every half hour until relieved, or there is necessity for change of remedy.

MERCURIUS VIV. is particularly indicated when there is violent writhing colic, and hardness around the navel; jerking pain in the muscles of the abdomen, which is inflamed and hard; when there is crawling in the throat; hiccoughing; voracious appetite; dislike for sweet things; nausea, with water rising in the throat; straining evacuations; secretion of slime; great debility; severest attacks occur about midnight; when this remedy is indicated and fails, and the patient has an itching of the nose, take *China;* and if this fails after one or two doses, try *Sulphur,* which, without doubt, will effect a cure.

22*

DOSE.—Dissolve one drop, or six globules, in four tablespoonfuls of water, and give a teaspoonful every hour, until amelioration or change.

NUX VOMICA is indicated when there are costiveness, sensation of weight in the abdomen, with rolling and uneasy feeling, and great heat; when the pains are pinching, drawing, compressing, as if the intestines were severely pressed in various parts; oppression in the pit of the stomach; the abdomen is painful when touched; the breath short and difficult; a general feeling of distension; the parts under the ribs feel as if stuffed; during the most violent paroxysms of pain the hands and feet are cold; sometimes the patient is deprived of consciousness; pain and incarcerated flatus deeply seated in the abomen; a strong pressure on the bladder and rectum, as from a blunt knife; the pain makes the patient double himself up, and is worse at every step; better when at rest, when sitting and lying; when generally attended by violent headache and pain in the small of the back; a number of these symptoms are attributed by ignorant persons to the want of an evacuation, and hence they often resort to some laxative or cathartic, but this is highly pernicious.

DOSE.—Dissolve one drop, or six globules, in four tablespoonfuls of water, and give a teaspoonful every half hour at first, and afterwards every hour or two hours.

PULSATILLA is indicated when there are stinging pains in the bowels, and throbbing at the pit of the stomach; a disagreeable tightness in the abdomen, as if it were too full; rumbling; incarcerated wind; irritation and heat of the abdomen, which is inflated; general heat and swelling of the veins on the hands and forehead; heat and tightness so disagreeable as to cause the patient to remove his clothes; the bowels are sore when touched; sensation as if bruised; all the symptoms are aggravated when lying down; but partially relieved when up and walking about; when in attempting to rise up there is pain in the small of the back, as if bruised; and also when there is tearing and shooting pains above the navel; uneasiness; heaviness in the belly, with painful tension; when there is weakness of the stomach, white frothy saliva in the mouth, and diarrhœa; and when there are violent pains in the stomach; pale face; blue circles around the eyes, and contractions of the whole body; pressive headache, caused by overloaded stomach. If *Pulsatilla* proves insufficient for the relief of these sufferings, give *Belladonna,* which is very suitable to follow.

DOSE.—Dissolve one drop, or six globules, in half a tumbler of water, and give a teaspoonful every hour until some relief, and then every two hours.

SULPHUR is very suitable after *Mercurius,* and may be resorted to under all circumstances where *Mercurius* has been tried, according to indicating symptoms, and failed. It is also useful after *China.*

DOSE.—One drop, or six globules, in four tablespoonfuls of water, and give a teaspoonful every three hours, until a change is required.

In some violent cases of colic, when there appears to be some obstruction, or excessive costiveness; injections may be necessary. If so, to a pint of tepid water add a teaspoonful of salt, and with a good syringe adapted to the purpose, inject it into the bowels. If the first trial does not produce motion of the bowels, the second may be tried.

DIET.—It must be apparent to every one that food easy of digestion is required, when suffering from this disease. All articles of diet of a flatulent character must be carefully avoided, and so must any article of food which the patient has found to disagree with him. Mutton soup may be allowed if there is tendency to diarrhœa, and if there is not, chicken broth with rice in it would be better.

21.—Flatulency.

This condition of the abdominal organs may take place when there is no colic, although there may be great uneasiness from a collection of wind in the intestines, attended with heat and fulness of the abdomen, that interferes with respiration. This inconvenience may be felt after drinking beer or water, and after eating flatulent food or fat meats; when the latter is the case, give *China*, or if it occur in choleric persons, give *Nux vomica*. To quiet, mild persons, give *Pulsatilla*, or if caused by fat meat or pork, give *Pulsatilla;* should it return, frequently give *Sulphur*.

DOSE.—Of either of the above remedies, dissolve one drop, or four globules, in a spoonful of water, and give three times a day.

Inflammation of the Stomach. (*Gastritis.*)

SYMPTOMS.—Constant burning, and constrictive pain in the stomach; shortness of breath, and the pain aggravated by breathing, pressure or contact; intense thirst, and desire for cooling drinks, which when taken are immediately vomited; small, wiry pulse, often intermittent and scarcely to be perceived; scanty urine and stools. These symptoms are uniformly present in the severer forms of the disease, but the milder forms are characterised by less degree of pain, and vomiting not so frequent.

Inflammation of the stomach is regarded a dangerous disease, on account of the relative position of the organ implicated, and should receive prompt and careful treatment.

In the severe forms of gastritis, there are great anxiety and prostration; small, thread-like pulse; cold extremities, and often fainting fits and convulsions. When the disease does not terminate in health, it may terminate in *gangrene*, or *nervous paralysis*, and consequently death.

CAUSES.—Inflammation of the stomach máy result from mechanical injuries, corrosive poisons, as the acids. The use of cold drinks when the stomach is heated; sudden stoppage of bilious diarrhœa and suppression of eruptions; inflammation of adjoining organs, and metastasis or transfer of inflammation of other organs to the stomach.

TREATMENT.—For the treatment of inflammation of the stomach caused by poisons, see Poisons and their Antidotes. The remedies employed in ordinary gastritis, are Aconite, Arnica, Arsenicum, Belladonna, Bryonia, Chamomilla, China, Hyoscyamus, Ipecacuanha, Mercurius viv., Nux vomica, Pulsatilla, Sulphur and Veratrum.

ACONITE is indicated at the commencement of the disease in nearly all cases, and particularly when the pain and fever are very violent, and there is great difficulty in breathing, with accelerated pulse.

DOSE.—One drop, or six globules, in half a tumbler of water; give a teaspoonful every hour, until the patient is better, or there is an aggravation of the sufferings, then select another remedy according to indications.

ARNICA is indicated when the pains are of a pressing or shooting character, and render the respiration painful and difficult; when the pains resemble those of nervous fever, or when the patient is indifferent, dull and stupid, and does not appear to realize his suffering, but on the contrary insists that there is nothing the matter with him.

DOSE.—Of a solution of one drop, or six globules, in half a tumbler of water, ; give a teaspoonful every hour, until the patient is relieved, or the symptoms indicate the use of another remedy. *Nux vomica* may be given when *Arnica* affords no relief.

ARSENICUM may be regarded a very important remedy in the treatment of inflammation of the stomach, when there is rapid prostration of strength, accompanied with burning pain, vomiting, pale, sunken countenance, and coldness of the extremities.

DOSE.—Dissolve one drop, or six globules, in ten spoonfuls of water, and give a spoonful every hour, until some relief is obtained, or tnere is an aggravation of symptoms, and a call for another remedy.

BRYONIA may be indicated after the use of *Aconite*, when the fever is intense and the pain violent, and especially if the disease was brought on by cold, or by taking cold drink in an overheated state of the system. it may be administered after *Ipecacuanha* when that remedy fails of removing the symptoms for which this remedy seems adapted.

DOSE.—Dissolve one drop, or six globules, in half a tumbler of water and give a teaspoonful every hour; after repeating several times without effect, *Nux vomica* may be given; but if *Bryonia* ameliorates, it should be resorted to as often as an aggravation of symptoms become apparent, until it ceases to have a mitigating effect. If stupor and mental aberration attends the disease, *Hyoscyamus* may be administered several times in succession; if this does not give relief, *Belladonna* may follow, give one or two doses, and wait a day, if practicable. If the extremities become cold, give *Veratrum*, especially if the patient seems to be sinking; or *Arsenicum* may be given if *Veratrum* seems inefficient.

CHAMOMILLA is indicated if the pains are of a dull character, and do not become increased by external pressure, or by exercise, or drawing in the breath; and if there is pressure on the stomach, tension under the ribs, difficulty of breathing, a yellow tongue, bitter taste, yellowish skin, and seasons of oppression and restlessness. When these seasons come on frequently during the night, attended with green, slimy diarrhœa, and sickness of stomach, *Pulsatilla* may be used in alternation with this remedy. If, on the contrary, the bowels are costive, and the chest more affected, *Bryonia* may be a useful alternating remedy.

DOSE.—One drop, or six globules, in half a tumbler of water, give a teaspoonful every half hour, observe the same rule with each of the remedies, whether used singly, or in alternation.

CHINA is indicated when the pain is worse, on the left side under the ribs, whence it extends downwards; and when in the beginning, there is vomiting of blood, and violent fever.

DOSE.—One drop, or six globules, may be dissolved in three table-spoonfuls of water, and give a teaspoonful every hour, until a change.

HYOSCYAMUS is indicated when the gastritis is attended with stupor, and the patient is insensible of his sufferings; and also when the patient speaks unconnectedly, this remedy is indicated.

DOSE.—Of a solution of one drop, or six globules, in half a tumbler of water, give a dessertspoonful every hour, until better, or a change.

IPECACUANHA is especially indicated when the pains are worse in the front part of the bowels, and extend under the ribs on the left side, and thence towards the back, with swelling in the region of the stomach, great agitation and vomiting.

DOSE.—One drop, or four globules, in a spoonful of water, may be given, and repeated in two hours, if efficacious.

MERCURIUS VIV. is particularly indicated when there is pressing pain, that forbids the patient lying on the right side, with bitter taste in the mouth and throat, constant chilliness, yellowness of the eyes and skin.

DOSE.—Dissolve one drop, or six globules, in four spoonfuls of water, and give a teaspoonful every hour, when given alone. It may be alternated with *Belladonna*, and in some cases of a critical character, it may be alternated with *Lachesis*, at intervals of one hour.

NUX VOMICA is especially indicated for acute pain, frequently attended with throbbing and stitches, and sensitiveness of the part affected, to contact; and also when there is sour, bitter taste in the mouth, with nausea and vomiting; shortness of breath, as if the clothing were too tight; and also when the removal of the clothes aggravates the sufferings; thirst; highly colored, or red urine; and oppressive headache.

DOSE.—Of a solution of one drop, or six globules, in four tablespoonfuls of water, give a teaspoonful every hour, for two or three doses, and then change, unless the patient is relieved.

PULSATILLA is particularly useful after *Ipecacuanha* or *Bryonia*, when the inflammation of the stomach arises from indigestion, or a chill in the stomach, from ice-water or ice.

DOSE.—Of a solution of one drop, or six globules, in half a tumbler of water, give a teaspoonful every hour, until amelioration or change.

SULPHUR is of great service after *Nux vomica*, if this remedy should prove of little effect in removing the symptoms for which it is indicated, and the stinging pains continue without amelioration. It is also of service after other remedies recommended, when they afford little relief.

DOSE.—One drop, or four globules, every six hours, until three doses are given, and then it is better that several days should elapse before any other remedy should be given, and then, if the disease has been worse, every other day give *China* as directed for the use of this remedy.

VERATRUM is indicated in gastritis, when there is vomiting; severe pain in the stomach; sometimes cramps or spasms; prostration of strength; and coldness of the extremities.

DOSE.—Dissolve one drop, or eight globules, in four tablespoonfuls of water, and give a teaspoonful every hour, until three doses are given, and then every two hours, until amelioration or change.

The above embraces the principal remedies employed in the treatment of this disease, *Opium* and *Camphor* and *Hyoscyamus* are sometimes called into requisition, when the indication for their use requires them.

DIET.—When the disease is in its most active stage, nearly everything taken into the stomach is vomited. A little cold water, or toast water is all that the patient can take. .After the violence of the disease has subsided rice, or barley gruel may be given in small quantities, as the patient can bear it; or gruel made of arrow root or farina, may be substituted, if the patient has a preference.

25.—Inflammation of the Bowels. (*Enteritis.*)

This disease is very similar to the preceding, exceedingly painful and rapid in its progress. It rarely happens that enteritis sets in by itself, as it is more frequently the sequel of some other disturbance, such as the various forms of fever.

SYMPTOMS.—Inflammation of the bowels, when the peritoneal coat is involved, is characterised by intense burning pain in the region of the navel, aggravated by the slightest pressure or movement, with tightness, heat, and distension of the abdomen like a drum; sobbing; anxiety; violent thirst, with aggravation of suffering from cold drinks; obstinate constipation, and great difficulty in procuring a movement of the bowels; violent vomiting, sometimes slimy at first, and afterwards of a bilious character, and sometimes of excrementitious matter, and even urine; small and contracted pulse; inflammatory fever; flatulence, and frequently obstruction of the urine.

23

When the peritoneal coat is not primarily the seat of the suffering, the pain is not so severely felt. It is more diffused, and consists of soreness, which is generally made worse by pressure. Indigestible food or cold drinks almost invariably cause an aggravation of pain; the tongue is often very red, smooth and glossy; and generally speaking, the tongue is red at the tip and margins, however dirty or foul the centre may be. There is also loss of appetite; difficult digestion; nausea and vomiting in a greater or less degree, mainly dependent upon the portion of the intestinal tube affected. The vomiting is always greater when the seat of inflammation is near the stomach. That inflammation of the bowels which is remote from the stomach and near the large intestine, often gives rise to mucous diarrhœa, mixed with blood, and in some cases consisting of pure blood, when the inflammation and pain is severe; when the large intestine, and particularly the rectum, is implicated, there is considerable straining; rapid pulse; frequently excessive thirst; variable degree of fever and extreme prostration.

Sometimes inflammation of the bowels terminates by resolution, or in other words, passes off without any disorganization, and the intestines resume their accustomed state of health.

When the peritoneal coat is involved it often terminates in dropsy, (ascites,) suppuration or gangrene.

When the lower portions of the intestinal tube are involved, it often terminates in induration or hardening the intestines, and lays the foundation for chronic constipation.

CAUSES.—Among the exciting causes may be reckoued the frequent use of cathartics; mechanical injuries;

errors in diet; abuse of ardent spirits; suppressed crup-
tion; cold; worms; prolonged use of acids; highly
stimulating diet, &c.

GENERAL AND PREVENTIVE TREATMENT.—In order to
guard against the disease, it is necessary to lead a regular
course of life; to avoid a deteriorating atmosphere; to
subsist on digestible food, and to avoid the extremes
of temperature. This is especially requisite for those
who are predisposed to difficulties of the kind.

MEDICAL TREATMENT.—The remedies employed are
Aconite, Arsenicum, Arnica, Belladonna, Bryonia, Chamomilla, China, Cantharis, Colocynth, Colchicum, Lachesis,
Mercurius viv., Nux vomica, Nitric acid, Pulsatilla, Rhus
tox., Silicea, Sulphur, Tartar emetic and Veratrum.

ACONITE is uniformly indicated when the accompanying fever is intense, and the skin hot and parched. (See
Bryonia.)

DOSE.—Dissolve one drop, or six globules, in three tablespoonfuls of
water, and give a teaspoonful every two hours until the fever abates.

ARSENICUM is indicated when there is severe vomiting; intense burning pain around the navel; severe prostration, and constipation of the bowels. This remedy
may be given alone or in alternation with Veratrum.
For more full indications see the indications for the use
of these remedies in gastritis.

DOSE.—If used alone, dissolve one drop, or six globules, in half a
tumbler of water, and give a teaspoonful every hour, until the violence
of the symptoms becomes modified, and then every three hours, until
amelioration or change. If in alternation, dissolve the remedies separately
as above, give a teaspoonful of each one hour apart, at first, and afterwards
every two hours, until there is amelioration or indications for other reme.
dies.

ARNICA may be administered without hesitation, when
the exciting cause of enteritis is some mechanical injury.

DOSE.— Dissolve one drop, or six globules, in three tablespoonfuls of water, and give a teaspoonful every two hours until there is amelioration of symptoms or change.

BELLADONNA is indicated when the tongue is red and smooth, or coated with a white or yellowish fur in the centre, with intense redness of the tip and margins, and inflammatory redness of the papillæ; skin hot and dry; great thirst; face hot and flushed; giddiness and occasioual delirium at night; sensation of soreness or of excoriation in the region of the naval, or over the entire abdomen, with tenderness on pressure, and sometimes distension like a drum.

DOSE.—Dissolve one drop, or six globules, in half a tumbler of water, and give a teaspoonful every hour, until the violence of the symptoms cease, or there is no indication of relief. *Lachesis*, administered in the same manner, may follow the use of *Belladonna*.

BRYONIA may be employed after the use of *Aconite*, when the patient complains of severe headache, with constipation and acute pain in the abdomen, aggravated by movement and after meals. It is also indicated after *Aconite*, when there is redness of the tongue, or yellowish coating; parched mouth and throat; loose evacuations after taking food or drink, and nausea and vomiting after eating.

DOSE.—One drop, or four globules in a tablespoonful of water may be given three times a day, to allay the immediate symptoms, and then morning and evening, until permanent amelioration, or change.

CHAMOMILLA is indicated when the disease manifests itself in children, or in nervous and excitable persons, extremely sensitive to pain; when there is sensation of soreness in the abdomen, as if arising from internal excoriations, and painful tenderness on slight pressure, and slimy, whitish, watery, or greenish diarrhœa, of an offensive, or fetid smell.

DOSE.—One drop, or four globules, in a tablespoonful of water, every three hours, until the acute suffering is removed, and then night and morning. until there is decided amelioration, or change.

CHINA is often found of great service after the use of *Aconite*, or any of the remedies used in the incipient stage; when there is great distension of the abdomen; diarrhœa, with portions of undigested food, or aggravation after a meal; intense thirst; great debility, and extreme weakness of the digestive function.

DOSE.—Dissolve one drop, or six globules, in three tablespoonfuls of water, and give a teaspoonful every three hours, until there is relief, or indications of change.

CANTHARIS is indicated in severe cases, when there is discharge of pure blood at stool, and inability to pass urine; and also in advanced stages of the disease, when there are mucus evacuations; or of solid substances, like shreds of membranes.

DOSE.—Dissolve a drop, or six globules, in half a tumbler of water, and give a teaspoonful every three hours, until there is a modification of symptoms, and then every six hours, until a further change.

COLOCYNTHIS is indicated when the large intestine is the seat of inflammation, attended with distension of the abdomen like a drum, with soreness, and sensibility to the touch; sense of burning, and diarrhœa, with increase of pain, followed by urgent desire to go to stool after eating or drinking; nausea, or vomiting of bilious matter, and frequent discharge of urine.

DOSE.—One drop or four globules, in a tablespoonful of water, every three hours, until the acute suffering has passed away, and afterwards, night and morning, until complete amelioration, or change.

COLCHICUM is particularly useful in advanced stages of the disorder, when there is a drum-like distension of the bowels; diarrhœa, the stools consisting of white or transparent mucus, or of blood, mixed with substances of a pseudo-membranous appearance.

DOSE.—One drop, or four globules, in a tablespoonful of water, three times a day, until the symptoms against which it is directed, are overcome, and then morning and evening, until permanent amelioration, or change.

23*

LACHESIS is particularly useful when there is burning, aching, cutting pain; oppressed respiration; tense, distended abdomen, with painful sensibility on pressure over the affected part, and inveterate constipation. *Belladonna* is sometimes of service after *Lachesis*, if indicated; and the same is true with regard to *Sulphur*, *Nux vomica*, *Bryonia*, and other remedies.

DOSE.—One drop, or six globules, may be dissolved in half a tumbler of water, and a teaspoonful may be given every four hours, until the immediate symptoms abate, and then give a teaspoonful every night and morning, until decided amelioration, or change; recourse may be had, however, to *Belladonna* and other remedies, if remaining, and distinct indications super-exist.

MERCURIUS VIV. is indicated in the most serious cases of *enteritis* after the use of *Aconite*, and other remedies. When there is foul tongue, dry, and with white or brown coating, or covered with mucus; intense thirst; hard, distended abdomen, tender to the touch; bilious and watery stools, of a fetid odor; or constant urging to stool, followed by *severe straining*, and meagre evacuations of mucus, tinged with blood, or of pure blood, in considerable quantity; great debility and prostration; chilliness and shivering, with tendency to perspire at night, which, however, is unattended with relief. This remedy may, in some cases, be used in alternation with *Belladonna* or *Lachesis*.

DOSE.—Dissolve one drop, or six globules, in four tablespoonfuls of water, and give a teaspoonful every four hours, until the immediate symptoms are relieved, and then every twelve hours until a positive mitigation, or change. After two days' treatment of twelve hour doses, if the disease should remain stationary, rest for twenty-four hours, and then select another remedy according to indications.

NUX VOMICA is for the most part indicated when there is redness of the margin of the tongue, with whitish or yellowish coating upon the centre of the tongue; feeling of soreness with burning heat in the abdomen; loss of appetite; indigestion, attended with vomiting, after partaking of food, and aggravation of the abdominal pain after drinking; flatulence; costiveness; and sometimes alternating with looseness; *stools* watery, mucus, or scanty, and frequently tinged with blood, and attended with straining. When the above train of symptoms has been brought on by sudden check of the bleeding piles, this remedy is of the greatest service, and *Sulphur* is of great value to follow.

DOSE.—Dissolve one drop, or six globules, in half a tumbler of water, and give a teaspoonful every three hours, until amelioration or change. It may be used in alternation with *Sulphur*, every six hours, after suppression of the piles.

NITRIC ACID is indicated if there is a group of symptoms, such as those described for the use of *Mercurius*, and therefore it may be used in connection with this latter remedy, when necessary to complete a cure. It is more useful in chronic cases, attended with abdominal tenderness, and pains as in dysentery. It is also indicated when the disorder occurs in mercurialized patients.

DOSE.—Dissolve a drop, or six globules, in six teaspoonfuls of water, and give a teaspoonful every night and morning, for a week ; after which, wait for a day, or perhaps two, and if the patient gradually improves, do not give any more, but if stationary, resort again to the remedy, as before directed, and so on, until convalescence is established.

PULSATILLA is to be prescribed when acute inflammatory symptoms result from suppression of the catamenia, or bleeding piles, or occuring as the sequel of measles: provided *Aconite* proves insufficient, and particularly if the tongue is loaded with white, grayish, or yellow coating, without thirst, or on the contrary, with intense thirst; disordered digestion; loss of appetite; nausea and vomiting, after partaking of the smallest quantity of nourishment; and also if the abdomen is sensitive to touch, pressure, or movement and flatulence.

DOSE.—One drop, or four globules may be given three times a day.

RHUS TOX. is indicated when eruptions break out around the mouth, and there is redness of the tongue, with pain, as if from soreness or ulceration in the abdomen, and sensitiveness to contact or pressure; slimy, frothy, bloody, or watery stools; *slow fever*, with delirium at night; and therefore it will be seen that *Rhus* is better adapted to enteritis, when it is symptomatic, as in typhus fever.

DOSE.—Dissolve one drop, or six globules, in six teaspoonfuls of water, and give a teaspoonful every four hours, until amelioration, or change.

SILICEA is indicated when the disorder has been excited by sudden suppression of perspiration of the feet, or the too sudden healing up of some sore or ulcer; or when there is dryness of the mouth; coated tongue; intense thirst; loss of appetite; and frequently disgust for animal food, or any kind of warm food; constant desire for cold food and drinks; hardness and tensely distended abdomen, hot, and painful to the touch; costiveness, or on the contrary, watery and fetid stools; rumbling in the bowels, especially on movement; skin dry and parched during the day, and covered with sweat towards morning; pulse quick and hard.

DOSE.—One drop, or four globules, in a spoonful of water, night and morning.

TARTAR EMETIC is indicated when there is nausea and vomiting, or constipation, with painful tenderness of the abdomen, and burning and heat around the navel; and also when there is a wiry pulse and quick; cold extremities; great prostration and anxiety.

DOSE.—Dissolve a drop, or six globules, in four tablespoonfuls of water, and give a teaspoonful every three hours, for three doses, and then if there is mitigation of suffering, wait for several hours, and even a day; if not, give a teaspoonful every six hours, until amelioration or change.

VERATRUM is one of the principal remedies in enteritis, and should be used with great care with *Arsenicum*, when there is coldness of the extremities; great prostration; severe burning in the hypogastrium, and around the navel; and also when there is nausea and vomiting; furred tongue; great thirst, &c.

DOSE.—Dissolve one drop, or six globules, in half a tumbler of water; give a teaspoonful every hour until amelioration or change, or in alternation with *Arsenicum*, as directed under *Arsenicum*.

26.—Chronic Inflammation of the Bowels.

This is only a degeneration of the usual form of the disease, and is denoted by fixed pain and a habitual fulness or uneasiness and oppression in the lower part of the abdomen, increased after meals or after *cold drinks;* appetite habitually impaired, or capricious; thirst usually after dinner, and at night; bowels constantly relaxed, or in the opposite condition, alternating with diarrhœa; skin hot, dry, harsh, and of an unhealthy hue; pulse rather quick; furred tongue, with redness of the lips and margins, and sometimes a slimy redness of the whole tongue; tendency to emaciation, weakness and languor.

Among the remedies already considered under inflammation of the bowels, may be found those well adapted for the chronic stage, as Nitric acid, Sulphur, Arsenicum, Silicea, to which we may add Phosphorus. Each of these remedies may be employed in the chronic stage, if indicated.

DOSE.—One drop, or four globules, night and morning, of the remedy that may be indicated.

DIET.—In acute cases of inflammation of the bowels the regimen must of course be the same as described in *fever*, and in the chronic stage the food should be very light and given in small quantities; raw fruit, green vegetables, and even potatoes are injurious, and are prohibited; toast water, barley water, and rice gruel, &c., must constitute the drink.

27.—Inflammation of the Peritoneum. (*Peritonitis.*)

There is a membrane that lines the cavity of the belly and invests the stomach and bowels, which sometimes becomes the seat of inflammation, and as this membrane is called Peritoneum the disease is called Peritonitis.

SYMPTOMS. — Painful tension and swelling of the abdomen, with a sensibility to the touch, even more acute than in enteritis, so much so that the patient cannot bear even the pressure of the bed clothes or the slighest covering; in other respects the symptoms are like enteritis.

CAUSES. — External injury; parturition in females; chill of the abdomen, are the general causes of the inflammation.

TREATMENT.—The remedies employed are Aconite, Arnica, Belladonna, Bryonia, Cantharides, Chamomilla, Colocynthis, Lycopodium, Nux vomica, Rhus, &c.

ACONITE is the chief remedy in the commencement of the disease, until there is a mitigation of the fever and inflammation; and in many cases this remedy has proved sufficient to master the disease, and in all cases it materially modifies its violence.

DOSE.—Dissolve one drop, or six globules, in half a tumbler of water, and give a teaspoonful every two hours, until the fever is more or less reduced, (a few doses generally proving sufficient,) after which consider the remaining medicines that make up the group, if further treatment is required.

ARNICA is indicated when the cause of *Peritonitis* is an external lesion, and it may be used internally and externally at the same time.

DOSE.—The same as for *Aconite.* If used as a lotion, add a teaspoonful of the Tincture of *Arnica* to a tumbler of water, and saturate linen bandages and cover the affected part; frequently wet them as they become dry.

BELLADONNA is a useful remedy to follow *Aconite*, when the inflammatory fever is high, with excessive local tendency.

DOSE.—The same as directed for *Aconite*.

BRYONIA and NUX VOMICA are both indicated when the vomiting and other symptoms clearly resemble those of inflammation of the bowels; while at the same time there is extreme tenderness of the external part of the belly.

DOSES, and administration.—The same as in inflammation of the bowels.

ACONITE and BRYONIA can be employed in alternation when the disease implicates the pleura and lungs.

DOSE.—One drop, or four globules, of either, in a spoonful of water, may be given, and followed by the same dose of the other in six hours, or in very acute cases every three hours.

CANTHARIDES may be employed when there is an implication of the bladder and stranguary. *Colocynthis* and *Chamomilla*, when there are violent colicky pains; and *Lycopodium*, when there is inveterate constipation, and *Rhus* and *Arsenicum* when symptomatic of *puerperal fever*.

DOSE.—Of either medicine, as selected, dissolve six globules in half a tumbler of water, and give a teaspoonful every three hours.

DIET AND REGIMEN.—The same as observed in inflammation of the bowels.

28.—Worms. (*Helminthiasis, Invermination.*)

The existence of worms in the intestines frequently arises from a peculiar constitutional taint, which diseases the lining membrane and gives rise to worms; infants and children are more frequently affected than adults, and this arises from the excessive nutrition in early youth.

When children have been fed upon sweet things, pap or cakes, and similar articles of a hurtful nature; or when mothers overload their stomachs when nursing with meat and fat things, or pies, their children become predisposed to worm difficulties.

And when children are dosed with *vermifuges* and purgatives, the worms will increase and come away; but this is a pernicious practice and more frequently increases the difficulty than otherwise.

The appearance of worms is often the symptom of derangement of the alimentary canal, which must be relieved before the worms will cease to prosper and increase; a simple regulation of the diet is frequently all that is required to cause them to diminish, and if symptoms of their presence remain, the resort to remedies will prove effective.

It is true that *pink root, spirits of turpentine, worm seed,* and other nostrum vermifuges may kill the worms, but these things will often kill the children also, or so derange the abdomen as to be the source of disease and difficulty long afterwards.

Under homœopathic treatment the various kinds of worm difficulties are easily cured without endangering life.

There are three species of worms met with in the human subject, viz.:—*The pin worms* (ascarides); *the long round worm* (lumbrici); and the *tape worm* (tænia), which can be removed by appropriate treatment.

The existence of *ascarides* or *pin worms* is indicated by itching of the anus, though sometimes the itching is produced by other causes; to determine whether it is produced by the worms or not is an easy matter, for the worms will show themselve in some way, as in the stools. *When the Lumbrici* or *long round worms* are at work, there are certain symptoms that usually indicate their presence, especially in children, such as picking the nose, inordinate appetite, distension of the bowels, sometimes colic and inclination to vomit; parts around the navel are hard, and frequent ineffectual straining to evacuate, and nothing but slime passes.

When persons are suffering from *Tænia* or *tape worm*, many symptoms are present that may characterise other difficulties, and therefore it is only when there is in connection with these symptoms portions of the worm discharged from time to time that we have any sure indication of its existence, and it has been observed that these portions usually pass away about the new and full of the moon.

GENERAL TREATMENT.—Children who have worms should have enough to eat, but not too much bread; they should not be allowed cakes or confectionary, or pastry, unripe fruits, or sweatmeats, or raisins. The diet will be stated at the close of the *medical treatment*.

MEDICAL TREATMENT.—The remedies found most useful are Aconite, Belladonna, Carbo veg., Chamomilla, China, Cina, Calcarea carb., Ipecacuanha, Lachesis, Mercurius viv., Nux vomica, Pulsatilla, Sulphur and Silicea.

ACONITE is indicated when there is considerable febrile irritation, with restlessness at night; fever and irritability of temper; continual itching and burning at the anus, and at times a sense of crawling in the throat.

DOSE.—One drop, or twelve globules, in six teaspoonfuls of water, and give a teaspoonful every six hours, until there is a mitigation of the symptoms or an evident modification of them. When the fever has abated

24

some under the use of this remedy, but not broken up, consult some other remedy.

BELLADONNA is indicated when there is disturbance about the head; great nervous excitement; delirium at night; starting during sleep; easily started or frightened by merely trivial causes.

DOSE.—Dissolve one drop, or six globules, in half a tumbler of water, and give a tablespoonful three times a day, until there is apparent amelioration or change. Should Belladonna fail of removing the symptoms for which indicated, recourse may be had to other remedies according to indications.

CARBO VEG. is indicated when children are habitually passing long round worms, and when the tongue is heavily coated and there is a fetid odor from the breath.

DOSE.—Dissolve a drop, or eight globules, in half a tumbler of water, and give a teaspoonful every six hours; if this should not prove sufficient in removing these symptoms, *Pulsatilla* is a suitable remedy to follow.

CHAMOMILLA is a useful remedy for childhood, either at the time of teething, or at a more advanced period when worm difficulties seem to occur as symptomatic of checked perspiration; it is particularly indicated when the evacuations are watery, slimy, bilious, green or yellow, or fetid, resembling the odor of rotten eggs, accompanied with fulness or distension of the stomach and bowels; severe colic or spasm; pain in the bowels; bitter taste in the mouth; foul tongue; thirst; want of appetite; bilious vomiting and flatulency, particularly in infants, with restlessness; screaming and drawing up of the limbs towards the stomach.

DOSE.—Of a solution of ten globules, or one drop, in half a tumbler of water; give a teaspoonful every time the bowels are moved, until positive amelioration or change; if in debilitated constitutions this remedy proves inefficient, *Sulphur* may be called into requisition; and even if *Chamomilla* partly relieves, *Sulphur* may be indicated to effect a cure.

CHINA is indicated in worm difficulties when there is looseness in consequence of indigestion, particularly if occasioned by partaking of fruit or flatulent food, such as vegetables; profuse stools frequently attended with but little pain, for the most part occurring soon after partaking of food, or during the night; watery and brownish evacuations, sometimes containing portions of undigested food; it is sometimes indicated when considerable spasmodic or griping pain is present, accompanied with want of appetite, thirst, flatulence and great weakness; it may be found useful after improper treatment or protracted cases of this affection, when considerable debility remains.

DOSE.—Dissolve one drop, or ten globules, in six teaspoonfuls of water, and give a teaspoonful every time the bowels are moved, until there is amelioration or change; this direction is better suited to casual adult cases. In similar cases for children, a double quantity of water may be employed, and given in the same manner.

CINA.—This is an eminently useful remedy in worm diseases, when there is boring of the nose; obstruction of the nose; great waywardness of the temper; bashfulness; heat and irritation; continual inquietude and restlessness; and in children, a desire for things which are rejected when offered; fits of crying when touched; paleness of the face, with livid circle round the eyes; constant inclination to take food, with craving appetite, even after meals; griping; distressive heat, and hardness in the abdomen, with discharge of thread and round worms; costiveness; constipation, or loose evacuations; fever; chills towards evening; hard, quick pulse; little sleep, restlessnes, or turning about; startings; talking, or calling out suddenly during sleep; transitory paroxysms of delirium; heaviness of the limbs; changing of color, the face being at one time cold and pale, at another, red and hot; pupils dilated; tongue covered with tenacious mucus; disagreeable eructations; vomiting; itching in the anus, and crawling out of thread worms;

involuntary passing of the urine, which is white and
turbid; occasional convulsive movements in the limbs;
weakness and lassitude. This remedy is also indicated,
when there is colic, produced by worms.

DOSE.—Dissolve one drop, or six globules, in six teaspoonfuls of water,
and give a teaspoonful night and morning until the six teaspoonfuls are
consumed; after which, pause for two days, and then suspend or continue
treatment, with the same, or other medicines, according to circumstances.

CALCAREA CARB. is regarded one of the remedies
indicated for the *tape worm*, and when there is any
ground for apprehending the existence of *tænia* in the
body. This remedy may be administered with advan
tage. Sometimes the *tape worm* is discharged after taking
a few doses.

DOSE.—Of a solution of one drop, or ten globules, in four tablespoon
fuls of water, give a tablespoonful morning-and evening. Should this
prove efficient, it is well, but if not, prepare *Sulphur* in the same manner,
and administer it in the same way.

IPECACUANHA is only indicated when there is little or
no certainty of the difficulty being from worms; when
there is vomiting at frequent intervals, and no nourish
ment seems to yield due support to the system, and the
child seems to become emaciated.

DOSE.—Dissolve one drop, or six globules, in ten teaspoonfuls of water,
and give a teaspoonful every time the child vomits. If the tongue has a
thick coating upon it, give *Carbo veg.* after, or else *Pulsatilla.*

LACHESIS is indicated when there is much thirst,
sudden starting and fright. It may be used after
Belladonna, in very bad cases.

DOSE.—One drop, or four globules, may be dissolved in a spoonful of
water, and given every morning and evening.

MERCURIUS VIV. is indicated when, in addition to the
common symptoms of worms, there is especially a constant inclination to go to stool, and diarrhœa, with tenesmus; distension and hardness of the abdomen, and profuse
flow of saliva.

DOSE.—Of a solution of one drop, or six globules, in half a tumbler of water, give a teaspoonful three times a day, for two days, after which pause for two days, and if the patient is better, suspend the treatment altogether, or continue if otherwise.

NUX VOMICA is indicated in worm affections, after *Chamomilla* or *Cina*, if there is considerable derangement of the digestive functions; irritability of temper and constipation; or great distension of the stomach and bowels, with sensibility and tendency of heat to the abdomen; inclination to vomit; increase of symptoms early in the morning.

DOSE.—Dissolve one drop, or six globules, in half a tumbler of water, and give a teaspoonful every night at bedtime, for three days, then miss three and begin again, unless the patient is better.

PULSATILLA is for the most part indicated when there has been want of success attending the use of other remedies, especially if *Ipecacuanha* or *Carbo veg.* have not had a beneficial effect when apparently indicated.

DOSE.—Dissolve a drop, or six globules, in six teaspoonfuls of water, and give a teaspoonful every hour until vomiting ceases, and the fetor from the breath begins to disappear.

SULPHUR and SILICEA are indicated when there are vermicular difficulties in lymphatic children, who become frequently affected with attacks of cold, and in the head; bitter, slimy taste; aversion to meat; irresistible longing for sugar; variations of appetite, sometimes voracious, at others the reverse; frequent regurgitation of the food, together with heartburn or waterbrash; hiccough; vomiting and rumbling in the stomach and bowels; and also soreness and itching of the anus. The *Sulphur* may be used first, and afterwards the *Silicea*, and even after this latter remedy *Calcarea carb.* may be administered, after allowing sufficient time to elapse after either of the others.

DOSE.—One drop, or six globules, in six teaspoonfuls of water; give a teaspoonful on retiring every night, until there is an evidence of improvement, then wait for the result.

24*

The symptoms must of course be our guide in the
selection of a remedy, and moreover in the treatment
of the different varieties of worm difficulties, we find
nearly the same group of symptoms produced by the
thread, long, or tape worms. Therefore we have some
remedies that will be adapted to cure either variety, but
in general, Aconite, Mercurius, Nux vomica, Sulphur,
will be found the most suitable in removing (ascarides)
or pin worms.

Belladonna, Chamomilla, China, Cina, and Spigelia,
for removing (lumbrici) long round worms.

Calcarea carb., Sulphur, Lachesis and Silicea, against
tape worms. In chronic cases of worms, (or invermi-
nation,) great success has attended the use of Nux
vomica, Mercurius, Sulphur and Calcarea.

DOSE.—One drop, or four globules, of each, in a spoonful of water,
taken as follows: a dose night and morning of *Nux vomica*, to be followed
the next night with *Sulphur*, the next with *Mercurius*, the next with *Calcarea*, &c.

REGIMEN.—The food in vermicular difficulties ought
to be wholesome and nutritious, to consist mostly of
meat, such as roast or boiled beef or mutton, sometimes
chicken, and occasionally a light pudding; vegetables
and fruits are not allowed, neither is milk, pastry or
sweetmeats of any kind, and the utmost care should be
exercised to prevent children from eating raw herbs,
roots, &c., which they are prone to do in their rambles.
Exercise in the open air is essential, and must on no
account be neglected.

29.—Itching of the Anus.

This vexatious and troublesome affection arises from
some peculiar state of the system, and often indicates

the incipient stage of piles, or the presence of seat worms, (ascarides.)

If caused by ascarides, which can only be ascertained by discovering them, Aconite, Nux vomica, Sulphur and Silicea are the remedies to be employed.

ACONITE is indicated when the difficulty occurs in children, and renders them very uneasy during the night, and is attended with fever.

NUX VOMICA is especially indicated when the itching is seated either internally or externally, and is worse after taking stimulating food and drink, attended with costiveness, and is caused by *ascarides.*

SULPHUR and SILICEA are remedies that may be employed after *Aconite* or *Nux vomica,* when these reme-dies prove inefficient, and also when the trouble returns again after having been once removed by the use of *Aconite* and *Nux vomica.*

DOSE, and administration.—Of *Aconite*, dissolve one drop, or six globules, in half a tumbler of water, and give a teaspoonful every six hours, if partially relieved, or not al!; after two days, resort to *Nux vomica*, pre-pared the same way, and give a teaspoonful every six hours, until com-pletely relieved. If a return of the disorder, dissolve one drop of *Sulphur* or six globules, in three tablespoonfuls of water, and give a spoonful every night, until cured, or there is necessity for the use of another remedy. Prepare and administer *Silicea* in the same way.

When the itching is caused by dry piles, or moist and bleeding piles, or strong liquors or beer, or coffee, or in people of sedentary habits. The remedies are Nux vomica, China, Sulphur or Ipecacuanha, and sometimes in connection with other remedies.

ACONITE may be employed when there is fever attend-ing the itching, and when there is pain in the funda-ment.

DOSE.—The same as before.

NUX VOMICA is indicated when there is burning and

pricking sensation, and the anus appears to be so contracted that the natural discharges are effected with
difficulty, accompanied by dull, shooting pains, and
jerking in the small of the back, and around the anus,
at every evacuation; or pain in the small of the back
as if from a bruise, which makes the patient cry out
and bend forward when walking or sitting. *Ignatia*
is a good remedy to follow *Nux vomica*, if necessary,
after an elapse of one or two days.

DOSE.—Of a solution of one drop, or six globules, in half a tumbler
of water, give a teaspoonful three times a day, at intervals of six hours.
If after two days there should not be decided relief, give *Ignatia* in the
same way, after waiting twenty-four hours.

SULPHUR is a grand remedy in this complaint, after
Nux vomica, and it may be used in alternation with this
latter remedy.

DOSE.—Of *Sulphur* alone, one drop, or six globules, in six tablespoonfuls of water, and give a tablespoonful every morning for several mornings.
Calcarea carb. may follow *Sulphur*, if necessary, and particularly if there
is a return of the disorder after *Sulphur* has apparently removed it, or alternately with *Nux vomica* every morning.

IPECACUANHA is indicated after the use of *Aconite*
when in addition to the itching there is thick coating
upon the tongue, nausea, and sometimes sickness at the
stomach and vomiting.

DOSE.—Dissolve one drop, or six globules, in half a tumbler of water,
and give a teaspoonful every six hours, and continue as long as necessary.

GENERAL TREATMENT. — It often happens that this
disorder is the occasion of so much annoyance to the
patient, that immediate measures are necessary for relief.
Under such circumstances such means should be employed as comports well with the remedial agents.

Sweet oil may be applied externally and internally
to allay the itching, or a piece of fat bacon may be cut
of suitable size to introduce into the rectum, attached to

a string; allowed to remain, however, only about fifteen minutes, and then to be removed.

Cold water injections may be resorted to every evening in many cases, when there is not speedy abatement of the itching from the medicines; applications of this kind are not at variance with the remedies.

Salt water injections, in small quantities, may be allowed when all other means fail, as may be the case in children who have an hereditary tendency to the disorder.

Vinegar and water, in the form of a weak injection, has sometimes proved efficacious in allaying the itching.

Lemon juice in water, in the form of an injection, has also proved efficacious, and may be resorted to twice a day.

URTICA URENS, given every morning, one drop, or four globules, in a tablespoonful of water, and continued for several days, is believed to be one of the best remedies for children.

When the itching is caused by piles, swollen, red or bluish tumors in the anus, resort must be had to *Nux vomica* and *Sulphur*, which may be used in alternation. *Sulphur* at night, and *Nux vomica* in the morning, until complete relief is obtained.

It is affirmed by some that eating asparagus in its season, which is usually the season when ascarides prove the most troublesome, is of great advantage, and often removes the disorder; and undoubtedly there is truth in the statement.

DIET AND REGIMEN.—The same as stated for vermicular diseases.

30.—Determination of Blood to the Abdomen.
(*Congestio ad abdomen.*)

The symptoms that characterise this derangement are a disagreeable or painful sensation of weight, heat and burning, with hardness and tension in the lower portion of the bowels.

CAUSE.—Sedentary habits, or piles; torpidity of the bowels; hypochondriacs are very often afflicted with the difficulty.

The remedies found of service in removing the difficulty are Arsenicum, Belladonna, Bryonia, Chamomilla, Pulsatilla, Nux vomica, Rhus tox., Sulphur and Veratrum.

ARSENICUM is indicated when there is determination of blood to the lower bowels, attended with diarrhœa and extreme prostration.

DOSE.—One drop, or six globules, in three spoonfuls of water, give a spoonful every six hours, until the three doses are taken, then cease for twenty-four hours, and repeat again, prepared in the same way, every twelve hours, until amelioration, or change.

BELLADONNA and BRYONIA are indicated, the former when there is flushed appearance of the countenance; sensation of heat and burning in the stomach; hardness and tension, accompanied by dull pain in the bowels; and the latter when there is biliary derangement and dull pain in the lumbar region accompanying the usual symptoms, and considerable debility.

DOSE.—One drop, or six globules, of either, dissolved in three tablespoonfuls of water, give a teaspoonful every three hours, until relief is obtained, or a change is necessary.

CHAMOMILLA is suitable for children when they are prone to looseness of the bowels, and there has been a sudden check and constipation, and especially if there has been flatulency and other signs of indigestion.

DOSE.—One drop, or four globules, in a spoonful of water, every four hours.

OR, OF THE ALIMENTARY CANAL. 275

PULSATILLA is indicated for congestion of the bowels in females when the usual symptoms are present, and particularly when there is difficult or suppressed menstruation.

DOSE.—Dissolve one drop, or six globules, in six teaspoonfuls of water, and give a teaspoonful every four hours, until relieved. *Sepia* may follow *Pulsatilla*, if there is nausea and uncomfortable fulness and dull pain remaining.

NUX VOMICA is particularly indicated, and is one of the most frequent sources of relief to those of sedentary life, or who are much addicted to indulgence of the pleasures of the table, and particularly when there is hardness, tension and fixed pain in the abdomen; sense of great weakness or prostration, and difficult or almost impossible to walk about; constipation; pain in the loins; depressed spirits and irritability.

DOSE.—One drop, or four globules, in a spoonful of water every night at bed-time, until there is some manifest improvement, then cease for three or four days and repeat as at first; should there be little or no improvement after four days, resort to *Sulphur* as directed below.

RHUS TOX. is indicated when there is much hardness, burning and fulness of the abdomen, attended with great debility.

DOSE.—The same as directed for *Nux vomica*.

SULPHUR may be regarded in connection with *Nux vomica*, one of the principal remedies, and will be found of great service in effecting a cure after *Nux vom.* has produced amelioration; and in cases of long standing it may be selected in preference, when there are dull pains and disagreeable sensation of distension in the bowels; constipation; tendency to obstinate attacks of piles; extreme digestion.

DOSE.—One drop, or four globules, in a spoonful of water every morning for a week, or until there is perceived some general change, then wait for five or six days, and repeat again in the same manner, and continue as before until there is manifest improvement or change.

VERATRUM may be administered when the indications are the same as for *Arsenicum*, when the latter remedy should fail of producing the desired relief.

DOSE.—The same in all respects as for the use of *Arsenicum*.

DIET AND REGIMEN.—When it is practicable the patient should take daily exercise in the open air, and should be very careful to abstain from all food of difficult diges- tion, and subsist upon farinaceous gruels or toast and black tea, or weak cocoa.

31.—Piles. (*Hemorrhoids.*)

SYMPTOMS.—Discharge of blood from the anus every four or six weeks in small quantities, usually preceded by more or less sickness, and followed by a sensation as if relieved.

The flux may often be regarded favorable, as prevent- ing more serious or dangerous diseases.

Tumors are frequently formed in the anus; which become very painful when no blood is discharged; some- times when there is discharge it ceases in part or entirely, and at others the discharge is so profuse that it becomes alarming; very often when the bleeding from the tumors is suddenly arrested, disease of a more serious character takes its place.

To relieve all these unpleasant symptoms requires a judicious treatment, both of a medicinal and dietetical character; the living should be such as to prevent the disease from assuming the dangerous form; the patient should take moderate exercise, not allowing himself to sit much on cushions, except when the tumors protrude.

Persons afflicted with piles should abstain from all alcoholic drinks, wine, cider, porter, ale or coffee; water should constitute the only beverage to be indulged in freely.

The resort to the scissors for the purpose of excising the tumors can only be regarded with distrust, as it is evidently done through ignorance of the nature of the disease, although such an operation is easily performed; yet it is frequently attended with dangerous consequences; inordinate hemorrhages often result which cannot be arrested without recourse to the actual cautery or by the use of some powerful styptic, productive of incurable ulcers; and the only use that can under any circumstances result is temporary relief from pain, for the tumors almost universally reappear in a short time higher up in the rectum, when the pain is more violent than before, and when it is more difficult to excise them, and if the attempt is made the rectum is liable to sustain incurable injury; every operation causes their reappearance higher up till there is no possibility of reaching them, then the patient is obliged to be left in a worse condition than if no operations had been attempted.

It is a matter of rejoicing that in homœopathy there is for the most part a more safe and sure method of procuring entire relief, without the scissors; but not for those cases which have been frequently operated upon, because by the operations they have been made to assume a more obstinate and incurable character.

Injections of cold water are sometimes a source of relief when the tumors are painful, but do not bleed; these may be resorted to once or twice a day, but cautiously when the tumors are in a bleeding condition, inasmuch as the discharge may be suddenly arrested by them; though when they bleed too freely the water may be applied, provided proper care is exercised with regard to the administration of appropriate remedies at the same time.

Syringes with gum-elastic tubes should be used in giving the injections, as these will be less liable to do violence to the affected parts; the water should not be too cold, and water of moderate warmth even under many circumstances is preferable.

Washing the parts with cold water, or tepid water, is sometimes of service, and particularly when the tumors are too painful to allow of injections. Sitting over the steam of hot water when the tumors are much swollen, and painful; and also the sponge saturated with tepid water, may be used with advantage; and sometimes the application of moderately warm fomentations.

REMEDIAL TREATMENT.—The remedies most employed are Aconite, Antimonium crud., Arnica, Belladonna, Carbo veg., Chamomilla, Colocynthis, China, Hamamelis, Ignatia, Mercurius viv., Nux vomica, Pulsatilla, and Sulphur.

ACONITE is indicated, and frequently affords relief, when the blood is discharged, and there are shooting pains and pressure on the anus; fulness of the abdomen, with tension, pressure, and griping, and the small of the back feels as if it was broken.

DOSE.—Dissolve one drop, or six globules, in half a tumbler of water, and give a teaspoonful every four hours, until amelioration or change.

ANTIMONIUM CRUD. is indicated when there is a discharge of mucus from the anus, that stains the linen. It may sometimes be given alternately with *Pulsatilla*.

DOSE.—The same in all respects as directed for the use of *Aconite*.

ARNICA is particularly useful when the tumors are swollen and sore; and when there is pain in the small of the back, as if bruised.

DOSE.—The same as directed for *Aconite* or *Antimonium crud.*

BELLADONNA is chiefly employed against bleeding piles, with intense pain in the lumbar region, as if the back were breaking.

DOSE.—One drop, or four globules, may be taken morning and evening, if insufficient after three doses, give *Hepar sulph.* in the same way, and after an elapse of four days, *Rhus tox.* may be given without hesitation, and repeated twice, and then it is better to wait for the result.

CARBO VEG. is indicated when there is discharge of mucus with burning pain, and particularly when there is bleeding from the nose, and great determination of blood towards the head, especially in patients who are very weak; if this remedy proves inefficient, it should be followed with *Arsenicum*, or the remedies may be used in alternation.

DOSE.—Dissolve one drop, or six globules, in four tablespoonfuls of water, and give a tablespoonful every morning and evening, or if in alternation, give *Arsenicum* in the morning, and *Carbo veg.* in the evening, for two days.

CHAMOMILLA may be used when the blood flows freely, with contractive pains in the bowels, and frequent straining to evacuate; occasional diarrhœa, particularly when attended with smarting and burning, with tearing pain in the back, especially at night.

DOSE.—One drop, or four globules, may be given in a spoonful of water, every night and morning, until amelioration or change.

COLOCYNTHIS is indicated if the piles are accompanied with colicky pains, very severe, and there are signs of determination of blood to the abdomen.

DOSE.—Dissolve a drop, or six globules, in two tablespoonfuls of water, and give a spoonful at night, and the other in the morning; and after twenty-four hours, if the patient is not decidedly better, repeat again, and so continue until amelioration, or change.

CHINA is indicated when there has been profuse bleeding from the tumors, followed by great weakness. It is useful after either *Aconite, Ipecacuanha,* or *Sulphur* has been employed in the first stage.

DOSE.—Dissolve one drop, or six globules, in four spoonfuls of water, and give a spoonful morning and evening, or in alternation with *Aconite*, three times a day. If *Sulphur* is employed, give the *Sulphur* at night, and the *China* in the morning.

HAMAMELIS is one of the most useful remedies in bleeding piles, and may be used also when there is merely a varicose condition of the hemorrhoidal veins, and particularly, if in females subject to varicose condition of the veins of the lower extremities.

DOSE.—One drop, or four globules, in a spoonful of water, may be given morning and evening, until amelioration, or change.

` IGNATIA is indicated in piles, against violent stitches which pass upwards, with itching, and crawling in the anus; when much blood is discharged; or there is protrusion of the rectum at each evacuation; or when, after an evacuation, there is painful soreness and contraction, particularly when accompanied by ineffectual straining to evacuate; or a discharge of blood and mucus.

DOSE.—Dissolve one drop, or six globules, in three spoonfuls of water, and give a spoonful three times a day, at intervals of six or eight hours, until amelioration, or change.

MERCURIUS VIV. is particularly indicated when patients have been injured by taking *Sulphur*, or other drugs or nostrums, to rid themselves of the suffering consequent upon piles; but if patients have taken much *Calomel* and *Sulphur*, *Lachesis* may be given, first once or twice, and then if the symptoms seem to be aggravated again, *Nux vomica* may be given, two doses twelve hours apart, and then after a pause of twenty-four hours, *Sulphur* may be administered, and perhaps in alternation with *Sepia*, at intervals of twenty-four hours.

DOSE.—Dissolve one drop, or six globules, in four spoonfuls of water, and give a spoonful every morning and evening, and if necessity requires a resort to the other remedies, prepare, and use them in the same manner, according to the directions above given.

NUX VOMICA is useful when there is burning, pricking pain in the tumors; the symptoms resembling those mentioned of the same remedy under "Itching of the anus," when there is much light colored blood discharged after each evacuation; or where there is constant inclination to evacuate; also in constipation, and during pregnancy. If *Nux vomica* proves of little avail, or does not afford complete relief, give *Ignatia*, and afterwards if the complaint returns, give *Sulphur*. This latter remedy, given at night, and *Nux vomica* in the morning, will prove of service in a majority of instances, when patients are suffering from piles.

DOSE.—Dissolve one drop, or six globules, in four spoonfuls of water, and give a spoonful every morning, fasting, and every evening before retiring to rest. Or when there is alternation with *Sulphur*, give a spoonful of *Nux vomica* in the morning, and one of *Sulphur*, prepared in the same manner, in the evening before retiring.

PULSATILLA is of service when there is blood and mucus discharged with the fæces, with painful pressure on the tumors; pains in the back; pale countenance, and disposition to syncope. *Mercurius* is a suitable remedy to follow *Pulsatilla*, if the latter remedy proves inefficient, and afterwards *Sulphur*.

DOSE.—The same in all respects as directed for *Nux vomica*.

SULPHUR, as before remarked, is one of the principal remedies for bleeding piles. It is particularly indicated when there is constant urging to stool, with ineffectual straining; when there is an acute, sore pain in the anus, internally and externally; when the tumors burn, are moist, protrude considerably, and are pressed back with much difficulty; with violent shooting pains in the back and in the small of the back, with a feeling of contraction, and burning or smarting pain on passing urine.

DOSE.—One drop, or four globules, may be dissolved in a spoonful of water, and given every twenty-four hours on retiring to rest at night, until

25*

amelioration or change. It may be used in alternation with *Nux vomica* or *Pulsatilla,* as directed above.

There are other remedies that have been advanta- geously employed in this painful affection.

CONIUM may be given with advantage, when the tumors protrude and are swollen and painful, disabling the patient from walking about, but the remedy should not be repeated oftener than once in three days.

DOSE.—One drop, or four globules, dissolved in a spoonful of water.

When in a case of excessive *hæmorrhage* from the tumors, threatening life, there is call for immediate remedial measures, give *Aconite;* if this - does not arrest the discharge at once, give *Ipecacuanha* in twenty minutes ; and if this also fails of relief, in ten minutes, give *Sulphur.*

DOSE.—Of each.   One drop, or four globules, in a spoonful of water.

Or in a similar case, *Aconite, Belladonna* and *Calcarea carb.* may follow each other in rapid succession.

DOSE.—The same as above.

DIET AND REGIMEN.—As "the piles" seem to be a difficulty mainly dependent upon derangement of the digestive function, the diet and habits should be regu- lated in accordance with the injunctions which have been explicitly set forth respecting derangements of the digestive functions in general.   Bread made of superfine flour is not so good as that from the unbolted; and persons subject to piles should never take coffee or stimulating food or drinks of any kind.

32.—Protrusion of the Intestine. (*Prolapsus ani.*)

This affection is sometimes termed by mothers and nurses, "the falling of the bowels," and consists of the protrusion of the mucus membrane of the rectum through the anus. It occurs much more frequently in children than in adults, and invariably takes place from straining at stool, or when urinating. The reduction of the protruded portion is easily effected by pressing it gently with the thumb and fore finger, which have been softened with lard.

TREATMENT.—The principal remedies in effecting a cure of this difficulty and of removing a tendency to the same, are Calcarea, Ignatia, Mercurius, Nux vomica, Lycopodium, Sepia and Sulphur.

CALCAREA is to be regarded a remedy for *prolapsus ani* in obstinate and inveterate cases where other remedies have failed, especially after *Sulphur* has proved inefficient.

DOSE.—Dissolve one drop, or six globules, in four tablespoonfuls of water, and give one of the spoonfuls every morning, and another every evening, until the four are taken. Give half the quantity to children under twelve years of age.

IGNATIA is particularly indicated when the difficulty occurs in children or persons of mild, sensitive temperaments, and is attended with constipation.

DOSE.—One drop, or four globules, in a tablespoonful of water, (half the quantity for children,) every twelve hours, until amelioration or change.

MERCURIUS is well suited to children in whom the disease is attended with hardness and swelling of the abdomen, and great distension.

DOSE.—Dissolve one drop, or six globules, in three tablespoonfuls of water, one to be taken every morning until amelioration or change.

NUX VOMICA is more particularly indicated for persons of irritable or lively disposition, and addicted to high stimulating diet, with a tendency to hæmorrhoids and constipation.

DOSE—Dissolve one drop, or six globules, in three tablespoonfuls of water, give a teaspoonful night and morning, until better, or a change.

LYCOPODIUM and SEPIA are amongst the remedies that are important in treating obstinate cases, when other remedies have not effected a cure, and particularly after a course of *Sulphur.*

SULPHUR is regarded as one of the best remedies to effect a cure.

DOSE.—One drop of either of the above remedies, or six globules, may be dissolved in six teaspoonfuls of water, and a teaspoonful may be given every morning, or the same quantity may be dissolved in twelve teaspoonfuls of water, and a teaspoonful may be given every morning, for children under twelve years of age.

DIET AND REGIMEN.—As this disorder is often the result of derangement of the digestive organs, or piles, the same restriction as to diet should be observed as in derangements of the digestive function in general.

33.—Liver Complaint.

Under this head is comprised the different diseases to which the liver is subject, both *chronic* and *acute;* the former is what is usually termed liver complaint, a careful discrimination will often disclose the fact that the real disease is a deranged condition of the stomach and bowels; the liver however is often implicated, and in itself deserves considerable attention; when the disease has been unchecked for a long time, and a torpid inflammation becomes deeply seated in the substance of the liver, an abscess frequently forms, bursting either internally or externally; in the former case it often proves critical, and is attended with hectic fever in most cases.

34.—Acute Inflammation of the Liver. (*Hepatitis.*)

This disease is comparatively of rare occurrence in temperate regions, being much more common in tropical climates; and even in these regions a luxurious manner of living, and exposure to the tropical heat by day, and to damps and dews of evening, may be recorded among the principal exciting causes; but even in our climate it may arise from violent mental emotions, stimulating drinks; suddenly suppressed evacuations; frequent use of the *blue pill*, or strong emetics or cathartics, or gall stones or injuries of the brain.

SYMPTOMS.—The principal symptoms of the acute form are pain in the right side under the ribs, sometimes acute and lancinating, and at others dull and heavy, often extending to the chest and under the shoulder blade of the right side; the pain is increased by coughing, draw- ing in the breath, and by pressure, or by lying on the left side; relief is often obtained by lying on the affected side; the stools are of a grayish or ash color, resembling clay, but for the most part the bowels are constipated, the urine high colored, and tinges the linen yellow; the skin and whites of the eyes are yellowish; there is gene- rally a high fever, with a full bounding pulse and hot skin; thirst; bitter taste in the mouth; yellow furred tongue; vomiting; pain and tension in the stomach; when the inflammation is seated in the convex surface of the liver, which lies against the right wall of the abdominal cavity; the pain is acute and lancinating, and increased by coughing, drawing in the breath, and pres- sure; when the convex surface is more effected, the pain is deeper situated and not liable to be at all augmented by pressure, and greatly aggravated by efforts at vomiting.

TERMINATION.—Acute inflammation of the liver may terminate in resolution, suppuration or gangrene, or it may merge into the chronic form; when it terminates in resolution, the symptoms gradually disappear; when it terminates in suppuration, the fever usually becomes hectic, and the patient suffers from increased sense of weight in the region of the liver; the enlargement of the organ may be distinctly felt, and if the abscess is about to make its way to the surface, a sense of fluctuation with pointing may be perceived; when the abscess is not discharged externally, or through the stomach or intestines, it usually proves fatal; the termination of the inflammation in gangrene is by no means of frequent occurrence, when such is the case it rapidly proves fatal; such a misfortune may be readily recognised by the sudden cessation of the pain; sinking of the pulse; cold, clammy sweats; coldness of the extremities, and rapid change in the appearance of the countenance.

TREATMENT.—The remedies employed are Aconite, Bryonia, Belladonna, Chamomilla, China, Mercurius viv., Nux vomica and Lachesis.

ACONITE is indicated in the commencement when the fever is high, with hot skin, with much thirst and whitish furred tongue, accompanied by moaning; great restlessness, and dread of death; shooting pains in the region of the liver.

DOSE.—Dissolve one drop, or six globules, in three tablespoonfuls of water, and give a spoonful every three hours, until amelioration or change.

BRYONIA is indicated when the pains are pressive, and when there is a sense of tension in the region of the liver, and when breathing, coughing, or movement of any kind aggravates the pains; when there is violent oppression of the chest with rapid and anxious respiration; thick yellowish coating on the tongue; constipation.

DOSE.—The same as directed for *Aconite.*

BELLADONNA may be employed against pains in the region of the liver, which extend to the chest and shoulder, particularly of the right side; swelling and tightness at the pit of the stomach; oppressed and anxious respiration; congestion to the head; with giddiness; dimness of vision, and occasional fainting; intense thirst; restless-ness, sleeplessness and anxiety, It may be used in alter-nation with *Aconite*, at intervals of three hours, or it may be used after *Aconite* has been tried.

DOSE.—One drop, or six globules, may be dissolved in six teaspoonfuls of water, and a teaspoonful may be given every three hours.

CHAMOMILLA is indicated when the pains are of a dull character, neither susceptible of aggravation, by respiration, pressure or movement; with a sense of pressure in the stomach; tension in the right hypo-chondrium; oppression of the chest; yellow skin; and yellow coating upon the tongue; bitter taste in the mouth; and intense anxiety at times.

DOSE.—Dissolve one drop, or six globules, in half a tumbler of water, and give a spoonful every three hours, until relieved, or there is necessity for a change.

CHINA is indicated when the disease appears to come on in paroxysms; or in other words, becomes manifest periodically, and is worse every other day; with shooting and pressive pains in the region of the liver; swelling, and hardness of the hypochondria, and epigastrum; pressive pain in the head; thickly coated tongue, and bitter taste in the mouth; yellowish eyes and skin.

DOSE.—Dissolve one drop, or six globules, in four tablespoonfuls of water, and give one of the spoonfuls every six hours until all are given, then wait for the result; if no better after three days, repeat the same, and so on, until amelioration or change.

MERCURIUS VIV. is of great service in hepatitis, when there are pains under the ribs of a pressive character, which do not allow the patient to lie long on the right side; bitter taste in the mouth; want of appetite; thirst; continued shivering, followed sometimes by clammy perspiration; yellowness of the skin, and the whites of the eyes; also in enlargement and hardening of the liver; or after the formation of abscesses. This remedy may be profitably used after *Belladonna*, or in alternation, at intervals of three hours between the doses.

DOSE.—The same as directed for China.

NUX VOMICA is to be employed against shooting, or pulsative pains; with great tenderness of the region of the liver when touched; nausea or vomiting; sour or bitter risings which leave the same taste in the mouth; shortness of breath; and sense of pressure under the short ribs of the right side, and upper portion of the stomach; pressive pain in the head; thirst; high colored urine; giddiness, and paroxysms of anguish; constipation.

DOSE.—Dissolve one drop, or six globules, in half a tumbler of water and give a teaspoonful every three hours, until amelioration or change.

LACHESIS is particularly serviceable in cases in which *Mercurius viv.* and *Belladonna* seem to be indicated, but afford but partial relief; and also in obstinate chronic cases, occurring in drunkards.

DOSE.—One drop, or six globules may be dissolved in half a tumbler of water, and a teaspoonful given every six hours, until amelioration or change.

SULPHUR is a most valuable remedy after any of the preceding remedies, whenever they fail of producing a favorable effect, or when the improvement is but temporary, and the disease still continues, though some-what diminished in violence.

DOSE.—One drop, or four globules, dissolved in a spoonful of water, may be given every night and morning.

DIET.—The same as under fevers; modified of course, according to the violence of the disease.

35.—Chronic Inflammation of the Liver. (*Liver Complaint.*)

There are many symptoms, in the chronic and acute forms of liver affections, that have a close resemblance in every particular, except their duration. In *liver*. *complaint*, or chronic inflammation of the liver, there is continued pains, and uneasiness in the right side, which seldom leave the patient, who gradually becomes weakened in point of strength, and lean in flesh; not unfrequently there is cough, with expectoration, resembling very much, such as we find in pulmonary difficulties. By inspection of the right hypochondrium, we may see signs of considerable enlargement of the liver, which frequently remains for considerable time; or is continuous; or comes and goes periodically, attended with dyspeptic symptoms; high colored and red urine; yellow tinge of the skin and eyes; sometimes febrile symptoms; the pulse generally quick, but regular, except during these attacks.

The causes are chiefly those of the acute form of the disease, that perhaps as frequent as any other, may be found in the use of intoxicating drinks, and mercurial preparations, such as *Calomel* and the *Blue pill.*

TREATMENT.—The remedies employed are Aurum, Alumina, Calcarea carb., China, Lycopodium, Nux vomica, Silicea, and Sulphur.

AURUM is particularly indicated, when the patient has taken much *Blue pill*, and has been frequently salivated, and there are pains in the bones, and soreness of the flesh, when pressed against the bones, and there is melancholy, and propensity to suicide.

DOSE.—One drop, or four globules, night and morning in a spoonful of water.

ALUMINA is particularly indicated when there are uni.

26

formly pains in the liver, when stooping, which become relieved on assuming the erect posture.

DOSE.—The same as for *Aurum.*

CALCAREA CARB. is indicated when there are pains in the liver, mostly stitching, or tensive aching, and distension of the abdomen.

DOSE.—The same as for *Alumina* and *Aurum.*

CHINA is adapted when the pains are worse every other day. (See acute Hepatitis.)

LYCOPODIUM is indicated when there is great torpidity of the bowels attending continuous pain of the right side. (See Constipation.)

DOSE.—One drop, of either of the last two remedies mentioned, or six globules, may be taken every morning before eating.

NUX VOMICA AND SULPHUR are among the best remedies employed in liver complaint. For the indications which require their administration, see the use of these medicines under "Acute Inflammation of the Liver."

DOSE.—One drop, or four globules, once a day.

SILICEA is only indicated in certain cases, when the formation of abscess is the characteristic mark of the disease.

DOSE.—One drop, or four globules, every night.

DIET AND REGIMEN.—The diet should be light, veal or chicken broth, with stale bread, roasted apples, also French beans, sago or tapioca made into plain puddings. The drink should be confined mostly to water; and bacon, butter, eggs, milk, wine, spirits, malt liquors, should, except in rare cases, be prohibited.

36 Jaundice. (*Icterus.*)

The main features of this disease are yellow color; whitish fæces; orange-colored urine; deranged digestion; sometimes pain in the region of the liver. Generally preceding an attack there is loss of appetite; giddiness; nausea; vomiting; flatulence, and some degree of tension in the region of the liver. There is also greater or less depression of spirits and loss of strength.

There is for the most part but little fever attending the mild forms of this disease, but in bad cases there may be an unusual degree of fever, which more or less affects the brain, producing a sort of stupid sleep from which it is difficult to be aroused; when the disease assumes this form it is regarded dangerous, and death may follow in a short time from oppression of the brain.

Sometimes the color of the skin changes from a yellow to a dark brown or black, giving rise to the appellation of "*black jaundice.*" There is frequently a disagreeable itching or tingling before the discoloration of the skin appears. When this disease arises from some undue emotion of the mind, it may come on suddenly, but generally it makes its appearance in a gradual and often in an unobserved manner.

CAUSES.—These are various. It may arise either from the acute or chronic inflammation of the liver, or from diseases of the stomach and bowels, or from fevers. Blows upon the head, or on the region of the liver, often produce the disease; as may also moral emotions or inveterate fits of passion; we may enumerate also among the causes, the inordinate use of quinine, rhubarb or calomel, in certain fevers, because these agents sometimes obstruct the biliary duct.

TREATMENT.—The remedies the most frequently found

useful are Aconite, Belladonna, Chamomilla, China, Digitalis, Mercurius viv., Nux vomica, Pulsatilla and Sulphur.

ACONITE will be indicated when the jaundice is accompanied with symptoms of acute inflammation and pain in the region of the liver, and also in the incipient stage of the fever attending the disease. It may be advantageously followed by *Belladonna* or *Chamomilla.*

DOSE.—One drop, or four globules, may be dissolved in a spoonful of water, and given every four hours, until amelioration or change; but if after taking three or four doses, there is only a partial removal of the symptoms, wait three hours, and give *Belladonna,* as directed for *Aconite.* After four doses of *Belladonna,* if the symptoms still remain, proceed with *Chamomilla* four hours after, as directed for the *Aconite* and *Belladonna,* until amelioration or change.

CHINA is indicated when the inflammatory symptoms have abated, and also in case of there being little or no fever at the commencement, and especially if *marsh* miasm is the cause, or if the fever is intermittent, or if the appetite is impaired, or there is general derangement of the digestion, and if the patient has been weakened by vomiting blood or by diarrhœa.

DOSE. —One drop, or six globules, in two tablespoonfuls of water, and give one at night and the other in the morning, provided the disease is anti-periodic in its character. This course may be pursued until there is a positive change for the better, or there is indication for the use of another remedy; but if the disease be accompanied by a fever of an intermittent character, the same doses should be given every six hours during the respite, observing that the last dose should be given one hour before the expected attack. The remedy may be given in alternation with *Arsenicum,* if necessary, observing to give a dose of the former in the morning, and of the other in the evening, or *China,* soon after the paroxysm, and *Arsenicum* about an hour before the anticipated attack.

DIGITALIS is a useful remedy when there is nausea, retching or vomiting; tongue clean, or coated with a white fur; pressure at the pit of the stomach and region of the liver; sluggish state of the bowels, and clay-colored evacuations; alternate flushes of heat and chills.

DOSE.—Dissolve one drop, or six globules, in three tablespoonfuls of water, and give a teaspoonful every two hours, until there is some modification of the violence of the symptoms, and then every four hours, until there is decided improvement, or indication for change of remedy.

MERCURIUS VIV. is indicated when the disease appears to have arisen from derangement of the digestive organs, or from obstructions of the biliary duct, that have not been occasioned by the abuse of this drug, in which case *China* is preferable, and this in obstinate cases may be followed by *Sulphur.*

DOSE.—Of a solution of one drop, or six globules, in half a tumbler of water; give a tablespoonful every six hours, and *China* in the same way, and *Sulphur* every twelve hours.

NUX VOMICA is indicated for persons of an irritable temperament, when the disease arises from a fit of passion, and when there is constipation, or alternately, costiveness and looseness of the bowels; and also when sedentary habits, protracted study, or over indulgence in stimulants appear to be the predisposing or exciting causes; and in alternation with *Chamomilla.*

DOSE.—Dissolve one drop, or eight globules, in half a tumbler of water, and give a tablespoonful every four hours, for two days, and then every eight hours, or in alternation with *Chamomilla*, at intervals of six hours between the remedies.

PULSATILLA is especially indicated when there is great weakness and anxiety and lassitude towards evening; obscure pressure, and sometimes shooting or pricking pains in the region of the liver, occasionally extending upwards towards the right shoulder; and when the stools are clay-colored or white.

DOSE.—Precisely the same as directed for *Nux vomica.*

SULPHUR is indicated in inveterate cases, when other remedies have failed. It may be used in alternation with *Nitric acid,* or *Calcarea,* or *Lachesis,* according to indications.

26*

DOSES.—One drop, or four globules, may be given in a spoonful of water night and morning, for a week, or if in alternation with either of the other remedies, at intervals of twelve hours between each remedy.

DIET.—The diet should be light and free from condiments or stimulants of any kind. Chicken or veal soup, with stale bread, tapioca or sago, or rice, and gruels made of arrow-root, corn starch or farina. The chief drink should be water, and all stimulating or tonic bitters made of cider, and barks or wine; and above all, avoid any indigestible food, and eggs, butter, fat meats, milk, &c.

37 Inflammation of the Spleen. (*Splenitis.*)

The spleen is situated on the opposite side from the liver, near the spine, and immediately under the ribs on the left side. Aristotle termed the spleen the *bastard liver*, because it is perhaps associated with the liver in purifying the blood. When this organ becomes the seat of disease, the symptoms that become manifest are all that we can rely upon by which to judge of its nature. Inflammation of the spleen has the following symptoms, viz:

SYMPTOMS.—Sharp, pressing or shooting pains in the region of the spleen, with, in most cases, a high degree of fever; general derangement, and sometimes enlargement and tumefaction of the organ; and when the disorder is very severe there is vomiting of blood.

The disease is not of frequent occurrence in temperate regions, appearing sometimes in hot seasons, and frequently mistaken for other affections. It may sometimes arise in individuals of debilitated constitutions, and in children in consequence of marsh miasms, and particularly when added to this exposure there is continual mental disquietude; improper nutriment and insufficient clothing, and confinement without proper exercise. From the fact that we possess but a limited amount of knowledge concerning the physiology of the spleen, it is somewhat difficult to discriminate between what is properly a disease of the organ, and some of the contiguous parts, unless the disorder is presented in the most tangible form. The best indications we can have are tenderness or sensibility on pressure in the region of the organ, with general debility, paleness of the complexion; whites of the eyes remarkably free from blood; languid circulation, and tendency of the extremities to become cold.

TREATMENT.—The principal remedies employed in this disorder are Aconite, Arnica, Arsenicum, Baryta carb., Bryonia, China, Calcarea carb., Carbo veg., Ferrum, Lycopodium, Nux vomica, Plumbum, Platina, Rhus tox., Stannum and Sulphur.

ACONITE.—If there is fever present during the affection, this remedy will prove of service.

DOSE.—Dissolve one drop, or six globules, in two tablespoonfuls of water, and give a teaspoonful of the solution every two hours, when the febrile symptoms run high, or in less urgent cases, it may be given every six hours, until the fever abates ; then pause four hours, and proceed with such of the subjoined medicines as may appear the best indicated.

ARNICA is indicated when there is pressive pain in the left side under the ribs, causing difficult respiration, and when the vomiting of blood is excessive, and particularly when any external violence has given rise to the difficulty. (See *Rhus tox.*)

DOSE.—Dissolve one drop, or six globules, in half a tumbler of water, and give a teaspoonful every three hours, at first, and during the severer stage, for four doses, and then every six hours, until amelioration or change.

ARSENICUM is indicated when there is an inflammation of the spleen accompanying the ague, and also when the patient complains of violent burning pain in the region of the spleen, and a constant pulsation at the cardiac portion of the stomach, attended with great anxiety; also vomiting a dark-colored fluid; watery or sanguinous diarrhœa, and burning at the anus; excessive weakness and swelling of the feet. (See *China and Arsenicum under Intermittents.*)

DOSE.—Dissolve one drop, or six globules, in half a tumbler of water, and give a tablespoonful once in twelve hours, if the disease presents no positive periodical character, and the symptoms do not appear violent. But if the symptoms are severe, the dose may be repeated every six hours. If the disease comes on at regular periods, the medicines should be administered one hour before an anticipated paroxysm.

BARYTA CARB. is particularly indicated in *splenitis*, when the mesentery is affected, or the mesenteric glands become involved.

DOSE.—One drop, or four globules, every twelve hours, until amelioration or change.

BRYONIA is indicated in very mild cases, when an aching, shooting pain is felt in the region of the spleen, that becomes aggravated by movement; or when the patient complains of a constant stitch in the side, or the left side under the ribs, and general gastric derangement with constipation.

DOSE.—One drop, or six globules, may be dissolved in three tablespoonfuls of water, and one spoonful may be given night and morning, until amelioration or change.

CHINA is requisite as being indicated when the inflammatory symptoms have passed away; or it may be indicated at the commencement, particularly if the disease owes its origin to marsh miasm; or if the accompanying fever presents an intermittent type, in which case it should be administered between the paroxysms, or when the fever is not present; and also if there is impaired appetite and general derangement present. It is also particularly useful when the patient has been weakened by vomiting blood, or diarrhœa. If the abuse of *Quinine* has been the cause of this disease, resort to *Arsenicum*, or *Carbo veg.*

DOSE.—One drop, or four globules, may be dissolved in a spoonful of water, and given night and morning, twelve hours apart; if the disease appears to sustain nearly the same character from the commencement, and the symptoms are not violent; but if severe, give the medicine every six hours. If attended with paroxysms of fever, coming on at regular periods, give a dose one hour after each paroxysm, and one hour before an anticipated return; in either case, continue the medicine, until amelioration, or change.

CALCAREA CARB. AND CARBO VEG. are both indicated when there is a chronic enlargement of the spleen, or if there are indurations.

DOSE.—One drop, or four globules, of either, every morning for a week, and wait the result, if not favorable, proceed with the other.

FERRUM, LYCOPODIUM, AND SULPHUR may also be consulted for enlargement and indurations, when the mesenteric glands are implicated.

DOSE.—Precisely the same as for *Calcarea carb.* and *Carbo veg.*

NUX VOMICA is indicated when there is inflammation of the spleen, accompanied by symptoms of deranged digestion, constipation, &c., which remain after the more threatening symptoms are removed.

DOSE.—Dissolve one drop, or four globules, in a spoonful of water, and take, every night, half an hour before retiring,

PLUMBUM, PLATINA, AND STANNUM may be consulted in chronic enlargements, or chronic inflammation and induration, and particularly if the mesenteric glands partake of the difficulty.

DOSE.—The same in all respects as directed for *Calcarea carb.*

RHUS TOX. is indicated when severe corporeal exertions have been the cause of the disease, and there is difficulty of breathing.

DOSE.—Dissolve one drop, or six globules, in three tablespoonfuls of water, and give a teaspoonful every six hours, until amelioration or change.

But if vomiting of blood occur, give the same dose every three hours. (See *Bryonia* and *Arnica*.)

DIET.—Similar rules should be observed, with reference to food and drinks, while under treatment for diseases of the spleen, as were given for liver complaint.

CHAPTER VII.

DISEASES OF THE URINARY AND GENITAL ORGANS.

The urinary and genital organs embrace the kidneys, the bladder, the urethra, (the penis, the testes, and the scrotum in the male;) and the female organs of generation, the ovary, the uterus, and the vaginum.

1.—Inflammation of the Kidneys. (*Nephritis.*)

SYMPTOMS.—Pressing, pungent pain in the back, each side of the spine in the lumbar region, shooting along the ureters to the bladder; difficulty in passing urine; a complete stoppage, or suppression of the urine; when both of the kidneys are involved; the urine hot, and highly colored red; swelling of the testicle on the affected side; numbness, and spasmodic difficulties about the foot of the affected side; nausea; vomiting; colic and straining; motion aggravates the pains; and also lying on the affected part.

CAUSES.—Blows, falls, or strains, or other external injuries; immoderate use of wine, or alchoholic drinks; lying for a great length of time upon the back; abuse of *Cantharides*, or deleterious drugs; suppressed piles, or menstruation.

TREATMENT.—The chief remedies in this affection, are Aconite, Arnica, Belladonna, Cannabis, Cantharides, Cocculus, Colchicum, Hepar sulph., Mercurius, Nux vomica, and Pulsatilla.

ACONITE is always useful in the febrile or inflammatory stage of this affection, and should be repeated frequently in the same manner as in inflammatory fever.

DOSE.—Dissolve one drop, or six globules, in three tablespoonfuls of water, and give a teaspoonful every three hours, until the pulse becomes reduced in frequency, and the skin moist, or covered with profuse perspiration, or until a change.

ARNICA is indicated if the kidney inflammation is produced by mechanical injuries of any kind, but more particularly such as continuous or severe concussions. It should be employed at first, whatever be the remedies indicated by after development of the symptoms.

DOSE.—Dissolve one drop, or six globules, in four tablespoonfuls of water, and give a teaspoonful every three hours, until amelioration, or change. But if only partial relief should ensue, in the course of twelve hours, it is better to seek an affiliation of other remedies.

BELLADONNA may be indicated when shooting pains are experienced in the kidneys, extending to the bladder; and also when the disease is attended with colic, and pain around the region of the heart; heat and distension in the region of the kidneys; scanty emission of urine of an orange color, or bright red; depositing red sediment, or sometimes thick whitish sediment; anxiety; restlessness, and periodical aggravation; constipation.

DOSE·—Dissolve one drop, or eight globules, in two tablespoonfuls of water, and give a teaspoonful every three hours, until decidedly better, or a change.

CANNABIS is more particularly indicated when the pain is of a dragging, aching, or pressive character; or a sensation, as if from excoriation, is experienced, extending from the region of the kidneys down towards the groin, accompanied by painful and difficult urination.

DOSE.—As directed for *Belladonna*.

CANTHARIDES may be employed with advantage at the commencement of the attack, even when the accompanying fever is considerable, particularly when the urine passes off in drops, or is tinged with blood; or when it is exceedingly painful to pass the urine on account of the burning pain in the urethra; when there are general symptoms of shooting, cutting, and tearing pains in the region of the kidneys, and in the loins; or in cases of complete suppression of the urine.

DOSE.—The same as directed for Belladonna and Cannabis.

COCCULUS and ARSENICUM are remedies that may be required to complete a cure after other remedies have produced an amelioration, or *Cocculus* may be used alone after *Nux vomica*. If both are employed, three doses of one should be given, and after an elapse of one day, a single dose of the other.

DOSE.—Dissolve one drop, or four globules, in a spoonful of water, and give every six hours, or one half every three hours, until there is decided improvement or change. If both remedies are used, twelve hours at least should elapse between the last dose of the first and the first dose of the last; if the patient is not relieved by the employment of these remedies, give *Sulphur* in the same way.

COLCHICUM is indicated when in addition to the usual symptoms of this disease, there is excessive nausea with drum-like distension of the abdomen; painful urination, or scanty emission of urine of a bright red character.

DOSE.—Dissolve one drop, or six globules, in half a tumbler of water, and give a teaspoonful every three hours, until amelioration or change.

HEPAR SULPH. is indicated in chronic inflammation of the kidneys, and particularly when there is induration of the glands as a consequence.

DOSE.—One drop, or six globules, may be dissolved in six teaspoonfuls of water, and a teaspoonful may be given night and morning for a week, until there is some appearance of improvement or change, then pause for three days, resuming the former course again at the expiration if necessary.

MERCURIUS VIV. is also indicated in chronic inflammation of the kidneys, when in a similar condition as noted under *Hepar* is present, and particularly if there is diarrhœa and tenesmus.

DOSE.—The same as directed for *Belladonna*.

NUX VOMICA is especially useful when the difficulty can be traced to a suppression of a hemorrhoidal discharge; determination of blood to the abdomen; excess of stimulants and sedentary habits; and where we find constipation; feeling of faintness; nausea; vomiting; distension of the abdomen, and drawing up of the testes and of the spermatic cord.

DOSE.—The same as directed for *Bellad.nna.*

PULSATILLA is of great service when this disease occurs in females of lymphatic temperament, when the complaint is connected with suppression of the menses or irregularities of them.

DOSE.—Dissolve one drop, or six globules, in six teaspoonfuls of water, and give a teaspoonful every three hours, until complete relief is obtained or change.

DIET.—The same restrictions as to diet as in inflammatory fevers during treatment. Persons predisposed to the affection should strictly avoid wine, malt liquor, spirits, and also oysters and other stimulating food; good wholesome nourishment is by far the best for predisposed persons, but it must be free from condiments, except salt.

2.—Inflammation of the Bladder. (*Cystitis.*)

This affection is attended with pain in the bladder, with tension, heat, and swelling externally; and also severe pains when pressed or touched; frequent and painful discharge of urine, or suppression or frequent ineffectual efforts and straining to pass urine; fever and vomiting usually attend the affection, as in *Nephritis.*

27

CAUSES.— The sources of this painful difficulty are the same as Nephritis. Females may become affected with the difficulty more frequently from parturition.

TREATMENT.—The chief remedies are nearly the same as in Nephritis, Aconite, Arsenicum, Cantharides, Digitalis, Hyoscyamus, Nux vomica and Pulsatilla.

ACONITE is ever requisite in the initiatory treatment of this disease, if there be a considerable degree of fever, with hot dry skin, rapid pulse, bounding or hard.

DOSE.—Dissolve one drop, or six globules, in six teaspoonfuls of water, and give a teaspoonful every two hours, until the pulse becomes reduced and the skin moist, and there are other indications of relief; to complete the cure, consult other medicines with which to continue treatment.

ARSENICUM is indicated when there is severe scalding of the urine during micturation, intense thirst and restlessness.

DOSE.—Dissolve one drop, or four globules, in four spoonfuls of water, and give a spoonful every three hours, until there is a change of the symptoms for the better. then every four or six hours according to the degree of mitigation, until complete relief is realised.

CANTHARIDES is more frequently indicated in this painful difficulty than any other remedy; it almost always follows *Aconite*, if the disease commences with a high fever; and when such is not the case, *Cantharides* may be used from the commencement.

DOSE.—Dissolve one drop, or six globules, in four tablespoonfuls of water, and give a teaspoonful every two hours, until amelioration or change that calls for another remedy.

DIGITALIS also is valuable when in addition to the suppression of urine, a constrictive pain is felt in the bladder, (Laurie.)

DOSE.—One drop, or six globules, dissolved in six teaspoonfuls of water, and give a teaspoonful every three hours, until amelioration or change.

HYOSCYAMUS is indicated when it is difficult to pass urine in the early stage of the disease, particularly when we have reason to apprehend that the difficulty originates from spasmodic constriction of the neck of the bladder, and when in fact the difficulty is more characteristic of a spasmodic difficulty than of inflammation.

DOSE.—One drop, or six globules, dissolved in three tablespoonfuls of water, give a spoonful every three hours.

NUX VOMICA is especially indicated when the affection is fairly attributable to habitual indulgence in wine, malt or spirituous liquors. There is no article of drink more pernicious on account of the peculiar properties of its composition than the *lager beer*, so much used as a common beverage, and which is productive of more bladder and kidney difficulties than almost any other form of malt liquors. (*Nux vomica* is the best remedy that can be employed to antidote the pernicious effects of this beverage); when inflammation of the bladder springs from this difficulty, a timely administration of this remedy will arrest it; and also when it results from suppressed hemorrhoids or other habitual discharges, or from dyspeptic derangements.

DOSE.—Dissolve one drop, or six globules, in four tablespoonfuls of water, and give a teaspoonful every three hours, until amelioration or change; but if within six hours after the fourth dose the improvement should cease to progress, consult some other remedies.

PULSATILLA is of great service in checking the affection or of preventing its development when it arises from suppressed menstruation, and moreover it is indicated in cases arising from whatever cause in lymphatic temperament, with the following symptoms:—Frequent desire to urinate; painful and scanty emission of slimy or sanguinolent urine, which deposites a purulent looking sediment; burning and cutting pains in the lower parts of the bowels, with external heat and tumefaction; suppression of urine.

DOSE.—One drop, or six globules, in four tablespoonfuls of water; give a teaspoonful every six hours, until amelioration or change.

3.—Chronic Inflammation of the Bladder.

This difficulty is accompanied by an extremely irritable condition of the bladder, together with a profuse secretion of mucus which is discharged along with the urine ; from the latter circumstance the designation of catarrh of the bladder, has commonly been given to this complaint.

The most appropriate remedies for this complaint are Dulcamara, Pulsatilla and Sulphur.

DULCAMARA is indicated when the catarrh returns on the slightest exposure to cold.

PULSATILLA, when it is produced in females at every menstrual period, and also in both sexes of phlegmatic constitutions when there is constant desire to urinate, or when every exposure seems to affect the bladder and produce pain.

DOSE.—Dissolve one drop, or six globules, in half a tumbler of water, and give a teaspoonful every morning and evening; both *Dulcamara* and *Pulsatilla* may be prepared and administered in this way, and which ever is selected, continue until amelioration or change.

SULPHUR is very useful in chronic irritation of the bladder or catarrhal inflammation of the neck of the bladder, causing a frequent inclination to urinate, and also when there is discharge of mucus from the uretha.

DOSE.—One drop, or four globules, every twenty-four hours, at night; independent of chronic inflammation of the bladder, there may be what is termed "*irritability of the bladder*" in aged persons; this is attended with some pain in the region of the bladder, which apparently darts in various directions to the back of the anus, thighs, and along the urethra; and whenever the urine accumulates in the bladder the pain is aggravated, and the patient is obliged to urinate several times during a night, and frequently through the day, and not unfrequently it is accomplished with difficulty, usually drop by drop; this irritability constantly draws upon the health, the appetite becomes impaired, the spirits depressed, and all the functional processes seem to become more or less impaired, and the patient loses flesh and becomes emaciated.

When the irritation and pain becomes so acute as to cause a spasmodic constriction of the bladder and complete retention of the urine, it may become necessary to evacuate the bladder by means of a *catheter*, or else the straining will give rise to more formidable symptoms; great anxiety; restlessness and clammy perspiration, but without fever or soreness on pressing upon the region of the bladder.

Sometimes spinal irritation may give rise to this difficulty, as also may disease of the prostate gland.

For this condition of things in aged persons: Sulphur, Pulsatilla, Calcarea and Conium, may be useful.

DOSE.—Of either, one drop, or four globules, may be given twice a day, one dose in the morning, fasting, and one in the evening at bed-time; consult also *Cannabis, Cantharides, Dulcamara, Hepar, Mercurius* and *Nux vomica;* according to indications, doses and repetition the same as *Sulphur,* &c.

4.—Gravel. (*Urinary Calculus.—Stone.*)

Gravel is the formation of concretions in the kidneys, for the most part, of a calcareous character, from whence they pass along the ureters into the bladder, and when they are incapable of being discharged with the urine, they remain in the bladder, a nucleus for the depositions of a similar-character.

The foundation or nucleus for the formation of stone in the bladder, may also be a drop of blood, or some extraneous substance lodged there, which receives the calculus concretion in successive accumulations, till it becomes the size and character of *a stone.*

The chemical composition, as well as the size and color of urinary calculi, are various; some are rough, others are smooth on the surface. The greater number are of an oval shape; some are round and some of other shapes. Their size may be from that of a pea, to a hen's egg; sometimes they are white, like chalk; sometimes

27*

red, or of a chocolate color; or of a yellowish brown tint; some are easily crushed by the slightest force, others resist the stroke of the hammer.

These formations may exist in the kidneys, ureters, bladder, prostate gland and urethra. But they are most commonly met with in the bladder, where they lie loose in the most pendant part of the organ. Sometimes there is only one, at other times there are a number; hundreds have been taken from a single individual.

Sometimes a stone of considerable size may form in the kidney, without occasioning any serious inconvenience to the patient; at others it may occasion severe irritation, and even suppuration of the gland.

When a calculus passes along the ureter, there is frequently the most excruciating pain, causing the patient a frequent desire to urinate, with ability to pass but a few drops at a time, and these, for the most part, high colored, and mixed with blood.

Sometimes the pain is so great when the calculus is passing the ureter, that the patient is unable to leave the bed, and for the purpose of gaining temporary relief, he is obliged to bend himself double.

Attending the difficulty, there is commonly more or less fever, nausea, vomiting, eructation, and retraction of the testicle ; as soon as the stone is passed into the bladder, these distressing symptoms subside. There is even in some instances an intermission of the pain for a few hours before the stone leaves the ureter, but a relapse afterwards.

SYMPTOMS.—Of the group of symptoms denoting the presence of stone in the bladder, one of the first is frequent desire to pass urine, and severe pain towards the last that is passed; attending which, is itching of the glans penis, and the penis itself; in order to relieve the itching, the patient acquires the habit of pulling the prepuce. Another symptom, is the sudden stoppage of the stream of urine, this is owing to the stone being carried to the inner opening of the urethra into the bladder, and blocking it up; a proof of which, is, that the flow of urine may return on lying down, or by a change of position. After a while, these symptoms continuing, there is bearing down pains in the rectum, attended with prolapsus of the intestine, which is induced by constant straining to evacuate the bladder. When there is considerable roughness of the stone, there is frequently a mixture of mucus and blood discharged with the urine.

CAUSES.—The causes of stone are obscure, it occurs most frequently in dyspeptics, who live in variable climates, moist and cold. It appears in some instances to be hereditary, and it seems to be a peculiar affection of some families.

TREATMENT.—The most frequent remedies called into requisition in the management of this difficulty, are Cantharides, Calcarea carb., Cannabis, Nux vomica, Nitric acid, Lycopodium, Phosphorus and Sarsaparilla.

DOSE.—Dissolve one drop, or six globules, of the first named remedy in three tablespoonfuls of water, and give a teaspoonful every three hours, until amelioration, or change. If little or no relief is obtained, after two days, proceed with the next remedy, and so on.

DIET.—Persons afflicted with stone, should subsist upon farinaceous food, and mucilaginous drinks, as much as possible.

5.—Retention of Urine. (*Ischuria.*)

When an interruption of the flow of urine occurs, and the secretion of the kidneys goes on, the bladder becomes so filled and distended with the fluid, that it rises up above the pubis, and forms a perceptible swelling in the hypogastric region. The bowels also become somewhat swollen, and tender to the touch. There is always considerable fever present. The inclination to pass water, frequent and urging, but painful and ineffectual; inflammation, and consequent mortification will ensue, when this difficulty continues for any great length of time; under such circumstances, the bladder will become ruptured, and the urine will find an outlet into the abdomen, and death will be the result.

CAUSES.—Inflammation of the urethra, or stricture; suddenly suppressed piles, or enlargement of the hemorrhoidal veins. Over-distension of the bladder may in some instances close the internal orifice of the urethra, as also may spasm of the neck of the bladder; paralysis of the bladder as well as inflammation and hernia of the organ.

Sometimes fatal retention of the urine has been the result of intoxication, or habitual use of wine, sometimes by the abundant use of fly blisters, which yield their poison to the system, and sometimes from the lodgement of indurated fæces, or difficulties of the uterus, tumors on the neck of the bladder, swelling of the prostate gland, urinary calculi lodged in the neck of the bladder, or in the urethra.

TREATMENT.—The remedies ordinarily the best adapted to afford relief, are Aconite, Belladonna, Arnica, Camphora, Arsenicum, Sulphur, Pulsatilla, Cantharides, Dulcamara, Nux vomica, Opium, Staphysagria, Phosphorus, &c.

ACONITE is decidedly indicated when there is considerable pain with burning heat in the region of the bladder, externally manifest to the touch. When the difficulty occurs in children, and there is also distension of the bowels, with complete interruption of the urine, and feculant discharges, this remedy is also indicated.

DOSE.—Dissolve one drop, or six globules, in half a tumbler of water, and in urgent cases give a teaspoonful every half hour, until the symptoms yield.

BELLADONNA is indicated when retention of urine results from distension of the uterus, in consequence of congestion of that organ, or of an accumulation of the menstrual fluid, or from retroversion of the uterus, or from any cause that produces the difficulty but the enlargement of this organ, causing it to press against the urethra or the neck of the bladder. This remedy may be used in connection with *Sepia*, *Pulsatilla* or *Nux vomica*.

DOSE.—Dissolve one drop, or six globules, in a tumbler one-third part filled with water, and give a teaspoonful every three hours, until ameliora- tion or change. If it should fail of relief, proceed with the other remedies as indicated.

ARNICA is indicated when the retention has been caused by some mechanical injury done to the bladder by the use of the catheter, or when the bladder has been distended from want of opportunity of emptying it while travelling, thereby causing the difficulty.

DOSE.—Dissolve one drop, or six globules, in six teaspoonfuls of water, and give a teaspoonful every hour until relieved, or if it becomes necessary to empty the bladder by means of a catheter. The remaining effects may be alleviated by the use of this remedy.

CAMPHORA is indicated when the retention arises from spasmodic action, and is also a valuable remedy when it is difficult to assign any particular cause of the dis- order. This remedy may be used even when there is a burning heat in the abdomen and urethra, with shivering coldness of the surface, and shivering succeeded by a hot fit; but as soon as fever sets in, *Aconite* is decidedly preferable. The spirits of camphor smelled simply will often relieve the difficulty in children and persons very susceptible to impressions. In other cases, one or two drops on a small lump of sugar, repeated, if necessary, once or twice, or, until relieved, every half hour.

When the retention of urine has been caused by the excision of piles, either by the knife or ligature, which is sometimes the case, the urine should be drawn off by the catheter, and the pain relieved by the alternate use of *Aconite* and *Sulphur*, or *Nux vomica;* if the patient has been addicted to the habitual use of intoxi- cating liquors, or in case of severe burning, *Arsenicum.*

The repeated application of cold water to the stomach may also prove of service in relieving the sufferings that remain after emptying the bladder by the catheter. But when no assistance of the kind is at hand, *Camphora* or *Aconite* ought to be tried first, and it will be found that these remedies will often supercede the necessity of mechanical means at all.

The application of hot fomentations over the region of the bladder, or injections of tepid water, or a hip bath of moderately warm water, may sometimes prove serviceable in procuring a relief.

ARSENICUM may be used with advantage when in conjunction with the difficulty there is a burning pain in the bladder, and even after the urine is drawn off. This remedy may be employed to remove the pain- ful burning that remains, especially when the difficulty has been caused by an operation for piles.

DOSE.—Dissolve one drop, or six globules, in half a tumbler of water, and give a teaspoonful every hour, until relieved or change.

SULPHUR, PULSATILLA and CANTHARIDES, PHOSPHO-
RUS, LYCOPODIUM and STAPHYSAGRIA are severally indicated when retention of the urine is caused by distension of the uterus in consequence of an accumulation
of the menstrual fluid, or from tumors pressing against
the neck of the bladder. *Phosphorus* is also another
remedy to be consulted.

DOSE.—Of the selected remedy, dissolve one drop, or six globules, in
half a tumbler of water, and give a teaspoonful every hour, but if no relief
is manifest after twelve hours, proceed with the next remedy, and so on.

NUX VOMICA, and OPIUM or PLUMBUM are remedies
that may be used when the difficulty is caused by severe
constipation and an accumulation of hardened fæces in
the rectum.

ACONITE and PULSATILLA are indicated if the difficulty
be occasioned by the swelling of the prostate gland.

HYOSCYAMUS and DULCAMARA, if caused by paralysis
of the bladder.

DOSE.—Of the selected remedy, dissolve one drop, or six globules, in
half a tumbler of water, and give a teaspoonful every hour, and if relief
is not obtained in twelve hours, proceed to select from the other remedies.
But if the remedies seem to prove inefficient, it is necessary to resort to
mechanical measures for relief. The catheter should be resorted to with
great caution, to prevent injuring the urethra, or doing violence to the neck
of the bladder.

6.—Difficulty in discharging Urine. (*Strangury. Dysuria.*)

This difficulty may arise from a variety of causes,
such as inflammation of the urethra, arising from gonorrhœa, or the employment of acrid injections in inflammation of the kidneys or bladder; spasm in the neck
of the bladder; enlargement of the hemorrhoidal veins;
a collection of hardened fæces in the rectum; excess in
drinking intoxicating beverages; tumor or other diseases of the prostate gland; the suppression of some
habitual discharge, or an eruption, or exposure to cold,

particularly in those of gouty habits; the lodgement of particles of gravel at the neck of the bladder, or in the urethra; and the abuse of cantharides, either as an internal remedy or in the form of blisters applied externally, &c.

SYMPTOMS.—This difficulty is attended with frequent desire to urinate; smarting pain; heat, and difficulty in voiding urine, and a sense of distension or fullness in the region of the bladder. The disease is usually termed *strangury*, when the urine passes off only in drops, or in minute quantities. For a further account of the disease, as induced by the presence of calculus in the kidney or urethra, see *Gravel*, &c.

TREATMENT.—The remedies found useful are Aconite, Belladonna, Hepar sulph., Mercurius viv., Nux vomica, Pulsatilla and Sulphur.

ACONITE is useful when there is frequent inclination to make water, with great pain and difficulty in voiding it; the discharge being at the same time very small in quantity, often passed only in drops, and presenting a dark, red, muddy appearance; the symptoms will generally yield by this remedy, or become essentially relieved, in which case some other remedy may be called into use to effect a cure.

DOSE.—Of a solution of one drop, or six globules, in four tablespoonfuls of water; give a teaspoonful every hour, until complete amelioration or change.

BELLADONNA is particularly indicated when there is a pricking, darting pain, extending from the lumbar region to the bladder, and when there is general agitation and colic.

DOSE.—Dissolve one drop, or six globules, in three tablespoonfuls of water, and give a teaspoonful every three hours, until there is relief of the prominent symptoms, and then wait about six hours, and if improvement continues, there will be no necessity for other remedial agents.

HEPAR SULPH.—When *Belladonna* has given only temporary relief, this remedy has been called into requisitiou with decided good effect.

DOSE.—In all respects as for *Belladonna.*

MERUCURIUS VIV. is a remedy that may be used in alternation with *Hepar sulph.*, or it may be used if *Hepar sulph.* fails of affording the desired relief.

DOSE.—Dissolve one drop of each, as directed for *Belladonna*, or six globules, and give a spoonful at a time, alternately, at intervals of two hours, at first, afterwards every three hours, until amelioration or change.

NUX VOMICA, PULSATILLA and SULPHUR, are each useful when the strangury has resulted from the too free use of ardent spirits or wine.

DOSE.—Of the selected remedy, one drop, or six globules, in six teaspoonfuls of water, and give a teaspoonful every two hours, and in severe cases every hour, until relieved.

PULSATILLA is also useful when there is a sense of fulnes in the hypogastric region, together with a cutting, burning or aching pain.

DOSE.—The same as directed for *Belladonna.*

GENERAL TREATMENT.—As a general remedial measure, resort may be had to spirits of camphor, when the strangury is bad; and at the commencement of the difficulty, when but little fever is present, it uniformly proves of service, and particularly when poisons have occasioned the difficulty. After *Camphora, Aconite* and *Pulsatilla* may be required, and in general terms we may remark that *Aconite* will have the preference when a chill, or the prolonged application of cold, is the cause of the strangury. And intimately associated with these remedies are *Belladonna, Dulcamara, Nux vomica, Pulsatilla, Mercurius viv., Sulphur, Calcarea carb., Sarsaparilla.* When inflammation of the prostate gland, *Thuja,* and *Pulsatilla* in particular, have the preference. The age,

28

sex, and temperament of the patient have to be taken into consideration in selecting a remedy. Thus, *Lycopodium* and *Opium* are suited to the treatment of the disease in old men, perhaps in connection with other remedies. In disordered or in pregnant females, *Pulsatilla*, *Calcarea carb.*, *Phosphoric acid*, *Conium*, *Sulphur* or *Nux vomica*. In decidedly bilious temperaments, *Mercurius viv.* and *Sulphur*. In sanguine, *Aconite* and *Belladonna*, and also in children, *Aconite*, *Belladonna*, *Nux vomica* and *Pulsatilla*, are the medicines which have hitherto produced the best effects.

DOSE.—We may remark at the conclusion of these general directions, about the treatment of this difficulty, that any of the above remedies may be selected according to the indications given, and one drop, or six globules, may be dissolved in four tablespoonfuls of water, and a teaspoonful may be given every hour, two hours, or even at longer periods, according to the severity of the case.

DIET.—The diet in acute cases must be sparing, consisting in some instances, entirely of demulcent drinks, such as gruel, especially if there is great severity of the pain. Warm fomentations and injections of tepid water, sometimes give much relief. In this difficulty, it will be well to abstain from the use of anything very salt, and there must be a complete abstinence from all acids. It has been remarked, that cold water drunk frequently through the day, affords relief in chronic cases. It is requisite to avoid all exposure to currents of air, for this is a frequent cause of bringing on the difficulty, in subjects predisposed.

7.—Suppression of Urine.—(*Anury.*)

This difficulty often occurs in fever and dropsy, and in inflammations of the various organs. It may arise in consequence of the loss of the secretory power by the kidneys,—and indeed the term *"Anury,"* or suppression, is now almost exclusively confined to the latter form of the complaint, and we shall so consider it, in this article.

The disease usually occurs with those past the middle age of life, but it is occasionally met with, at a less mature age, and sometimes, even, it is met with, in quite young children.

Subjects of gout, appear to be the most susceptible to the difficulty, and particularly after being exposed to cold and wet, or on the suppression of an eruption or some accustomed discharge, such as hemorrhoids, and generally speaking, there is no inclination to make water, and moreover there seems to be no occasion, for there appears to be no tumefaction in the region of the bladder, indicating an accumulation of the urine, and therefore, the only inference to be drawn is, that there is a defective secretion of the kidneys, which may be further confirmed by the introduction of the catheter.

SYMPTOMS.—In addition to the suppression, there may be nausea, constipation, and an occasional sense of sinking. Sometimes a series of other distressing symptoms, such as frequent fits of vomiting, severe hiccough, pain in the back, intense headache, and restlessness. The pulse does not appear, for some time, to indicate any disturbance, but after awhile it becomes slower,—then it indicates danger. The skin, generally, presents a normal appearance, but profuse sweating sometimes supervenes, and the perspiration not unfrequently, or at least sometimes, exhales a strong urinous odor.

Sooner or later, the suppression of the urine will lead to serious consequences; for if the secretion does not go on, the blood is not properly defecated and cerebral difficulties will ensue, and the life may terminate in coma.

TREATMENT.—The chief remedies employed in promoting the healthy function of the kidneys, are
Aconite, Camphor, Cantharides, Nux vomica, Pulsatilla, Belladonna, Opium, Lycopodium, and Sulphur.
The leading indications for the use of any one of these
remedies, are the same or similar, to those which have
been given under the head of "*retention of the urine,*"
or "*difficulty in passing urine.*" But in selecting a
remedy, it is necessary to bestow particular attention
to the causes of the difficutly, and select accordingly.
Thus, if suppression of an eruption, is followed by
suppression of urine, give Sulphur. If suppressed piles
has caused the difficulty, give Nux vomica, Pulsatilla,
Calcarea carb. or Sepia, &c. But better information may
be obtained with regard to the treatment of this disease,
by consulting the preceding article on diseases and difficulties pertaining to the urinary organs.

DOSE.—Of the selected remedy, dissolve one drop or six globules in
six teaspoonfuls of water, and give a teaspoonful every hour. If no relief
takes place in twenty-four hours, pause four hours, select from the other
remedies, and proceed in like manner.

8.—Incontinence of Urine. (*Enuresis.*)

This disease consists in some debility that disables one
from holding the urine in the bladder, or in other words,
that deprives the will of any power to exercise control
over the organ, and consequently, the urine passes off
involuntarily. The difficulty may proceed from relaxation or paralytic affection of the bladder, in consequence
of the secretion of acrid urine, the presence of gravel,
or a diseased state of the organ itself.

The TREATMENT of this difficulty, has to be with reference to the causes that produce it, and hence the remedies

employed may be, China, Nux vomica, Opium, Calcarea carb., Sulphur, and many other remedies.

CHINA is indicated, if the incontinence of urine proceeds from debilitating losses; as from diarrhœa or hemorrhages, or if it occurs after inflammatory fevers.

DOSE.—One drop, or four globules, may be given, three times a day.

NUX VOMICA, will of course be indicated, when the incontinence proceeds from relaxation, brought on by a too free use of *vinous* or *spirituous liquors*. Considerable relief, if not a radical cure, will, in most instances, be effected by this remedy. *Opium, Calcarea carb.* and *Sulphur*, may also be used in similar instances, provided little relief is obtained from *Nux vomica*.

DOSE.—Of *Nux vomica*, dissolve one drop, or six globules, in three tablespoonfuls of water, and give a spoonful every two hours until a change. If either of the other remedies are selected, prepare and use in the same manner as directed for Nux vomica.

We may remark in general of the treatment, that if caused by self-pollution, producing a relaxed condition of the sphincter or mouth of the bladder, *Sulphur, China, Phosphoric acid, Muriatic acid.*

If from paralysis of the bladder, which may be the only organ involved or only attendant on a greater paralytic derangement, *Cicuta, Conium, Nux vomica, Sepia* and *Sulphur*.

If inflammation about the neck of the bladder and urethra give rise to the difficulty, *Camphora, Belladonna, Aconite, Pulsatilla, Ignatia, Conium* and *Cina*.

If from the secretion of acrid or highly acidulated urine produces an involuntary flow of urine, *Mercurius viv., Arsenicum, Graphites, Iodium, Tartar emetic*, and by drinking profusely of cold water.

If the presence of gravel or sand create irritation
28*

and consequent involuntary emission of urine as fast as secreted, *Cannabis* and *Phosphorus* are the remedies.

It may be remarked further that almost any disease attacking feeble constitutions may give rise to urinary difficulties, hence it is always best to select the remedies according to the general groups of symptoms.

DOSE.—If any of the remedies above mentioned be selected, dissolve one drop, or six globules, in four spoonfuls of water, and give a spoonful every two hours, or even oftener, if the accompanying symptoms are acute.

9.—Wetting the Bed at Night. (*Nocturnal enuresis.*)

This difficulty is observed to be of frequent occurrence among children under ten or twelve years of age, and in some instances adults become afflicted with the same difficulty; the difficulty may exist in children without any very apparent derangement of the general system, appearing to arise wholly from weakness of the bladder, which gives rise to the difficulty when the power of the will is withdrawn as in sleep.

TREATMENT.—The remedies employed are Carbo animalis, Cina, Kreosotum, Belladonna and Sulphur.

CINA is idicated if the child is troubled with worms, as is *Mercurius viv.*, *Graphites*, *Sulphur;* and also the same remedies may be used with adults when the difficulty arises from the same cause.

CARBO ANIMALIS may be consulted for the ordinary practice of wetting the bed, when no perceptible cause can be assigned.

KREOSOTUM may be used with great advantage when the emission takes place only during sleep.

BELLADONNA is indicated when the difficulty appears to occur from cerebral difficulty or irritation.

But in the most troublesome and protracted forms of

the difficulty a variety of remedies may be consulted: *Pulsatilla, Sulphur, Sepia, Silicea, Carbo veg.,Hepar Sulph., Graphites, Arnica, China,* &c.

DOSE.—Of the remedy selected, give a drop, or four globules, every night and morning.

GENERAL REMARKS.—For incontinence of urine, the remedies may sometimes be aided by the use of the flesh brush, or sponging with cold water.

And in the case of children, if the emission takes place towards the morning, nurses or mothers ought to get into the habit of taking the child up before the time occurs for the mishap; when children are thus predisposed, it will be well to keep them from the use of acid fruits, water-melons or cantelopes; and also from the use of any kind of drinks calculated to stimulate the urinary organs; if the difficulty occurs in young boys ten or twelve years of age, it will be well for parents to ascertain, if possible, if their solitary habits are good; for too often, even at this early period of life, the habit of masturbation is taught these young lads by older offenders; when this difficulty gives rise to wetting the bed, *China* is one of the best remedies that can be employed.

DOSE.—Dissolve one drop, or six globules, in half a tumbler of water, and give a tablespoonful three times a day.

10.—Immoderate Secretion of Urine. (*Diabetes.*)

This disease is the *diabetes mellitus* of medical critics, and consists of an immoderate secretion of urine, containing a large proportion of saccharine matter; there are some instances however when the sweet principle is wanting, and this latter variety has been termed *diabetes insipidus.* The immoderate secretion of the sweet variety is regarded by far the most dangerous and fatal. The

disease for the most part comes on slowly and unperceived; intense thirst and voracious appetite, which are
found difficult to satisfy; and these symptoms generally
remain throughout the disorder, and sometimes they
afford the only indications of the 'disease making its
appearance at the commencement; in other cases the
patient complains of great lassitude, and a tendency to
perspire after any trivial exertion; the appetite, although
keen, is generally accompanied by deranged digestion;
sometimes pain of a very severe character is complained
of in the lumbar region, and a sense of distressing weakness is generally experienced in that part of the body;
as the disease progresses, especially that form called
diabetes mellitus, the body becomes emaciated and pale,
the thirst continues excessive, but the quantity of urine
voided exceeds in quantity that of the fluid and aliment
taken into the system; there is a sense of great prostration; the pulse becomes rapid and weak; the breathing laborious, and dropsical inflation takes place in the
lower extremites.   It has been remarked that this difficulty oftener occurs in males than in females, and frequently attends sympathetically a mild form of hysteria,
hypochondriasis, dyspepsia and asthma; those who are in
the decline of life or have a shattered constitution, resulting from intemperance in eating, drinking or exposure,
or from the prolonged abuse of diuretics or cathartics, or
other powerful depleting measures, such as bleeding, &c.,
are observed to be the more frequent victims of the
disease; there are, however, many instances where no
obvious cause can be assigned, sometimes the termination
of the disease may take place in five or six weeks, sometimes in as many months, and even in as many years,
before it terminates fatally.

TREATMENT.—The remedies found the most serviceable are Kali carb., Muriatic acid, Mercurius, Veratrum, and Staphysagria.

KALI CARBONICUM is indicated when there are jerking pains in the region of the kidneys, especially on sitting down, and in the left kidney, dull stitches, somewhat protracted; frequent and violent desire to urinate; very troublesome at night; the urine of a pale green color; burning sensation in the urethra during evacuations; sharp, drawing pains through the penis; pains on motion in the inguinal region; cold feeling in the bowels, as if water were being dropped upon them; burning heat in the stomach; ulcerated gums; dry mouth; violent thirst; fetid breath; languor; very pale and sunken countenance; sunken eyes; irritable, surly state of mind; easily alarmed; uneasiness, and wakefulness; great prostration; feeling of emptiness in the whole body; drawing pains in the back, frequently proceeding from the sacrum.

DOSE.—One drop, or four globules, may be given every morning, noon and night, until there is a radical change, or amelioration of symptoms.

MURIATIC ACID is indicated in preference to all other remedies in cases where there is an entire absence of thirst, and when the urine has a milky appearance; also in cases of drunkards, where it has proved efficacious.

DOSE.—Dissolve one drop, or six globules, in two tablespoonfuls of water, and give a teaspoonful every hour; and if no improvement takes place, after two or three days, try other remedies.

MERCURIUS VIV. is indicated when there is incessant desire to make water night and day; swollen, moist prepuce and glans penis; both of them painful; drawing, squeezing sensation in the testicles; a cutting, tearing pain in the left kidney; painful swelling of the gums; white coating upon the tongue; constant dryness of the mouth; a bad, fetid breath; constant hunger; insatiable thirst; burning, acid, scraping eructations; burning pain in the pit of the stomach; wakefulness in consequence of the perpetual desire to urinate; sunken countenance; slow, languid pulse; general weakness and debility, and swelling of the glands.

DOSE.—Dissolve one drop, or six globules in three tablespoonfuls of water, give a teaspoonful every hour, or two hours, until amelioration or change; if, after twelve hours, there is no perceptible improvement, proceed to try other remedies.

VERATRUM is indicated when there is great alteration of the countenance; cadaverous appearance; swelling of the gums; looseness of the teeth; sticky dryness of the mouth and fauces, which cannot be removed by any liquids; great nausea and thirst; painful hunger; drawing pain in the region of the navel; inordinate flow of urine, even involuntary; soreness of the prepuce; extreme prostration and weakness, especially of the extremities; trembling of the whole body; inclination to faint; weak, almost imperceptible pulse; and great emaciation.

DOSE.—Dissolve one drop, or six globules, in half a tumbler of water, and give a tablespoonful every hour. If no improvement occurs in twelve hours, recur to *Mercurius* or *Kali carb.*

STAPHYSAGRIA may be called into requisition when diabetes is symptomatic of dyspepsia, asthma, &c., and particularly if there is any predisposition to lung complaints lurking in the system.

DOSE.—Dissolve one drop, or six globules, in four tablespoonfuls of water, and give a teaspoonful every hour, until amelioration or change. If after twelve hours there appears to be no improvement, resort to the other remedies indicated. For the symptomatic character of diabetes, see Asthma, Dyspepsia, Hysteria, &c.

THE DIET.—In cases of diabetes it is requisite to adopt a safe or nutritive course of diet as possible. The food should be wholesome and nutritive; that which contains the greatest amount of nutritive matter in the smallest bulk is by far the most preferable. Potatoes and fruits cannot be taken with impunity by *diabetes* patients. All kind of fluids that directly or indirectly exert an effect upon the kidneys should be strictly avoided. Milk should in general be abstained from; animal food is better for patients of this class. Beef, mutton, venison, are severally useful, if properly cooked; broiled would be preferable. Meats of a digestible quality are preferable to vegetables.

11.—Hæmorrhage with the Urine. (*Hæmaturia.*)

Various causes may give rise to the passage of blood with urine, as anything that ruptures any of the minute blood-vessels connected with the urinary aparatus may give rise to the difficulty; as for instance, falls, blows, bruises, violent exertion, leaping, jumping, running, hard riding; the lodgement of a stone in the kidney or ureter; or by inflammation of the kidney. Irregular menstruation may also occasion the difficulty, as may also the piles, or at least a suppression of them; and also excessive and habitual indulgence in spirituous drinks; the frequent use of certain vegetables, &c., such as asparagus, &c.; venereal excesses; and by the abuse of blisters of Spanish flies.

In most instances the blood is completely intermixed with the urine, but when it emits, from the lacerating effects of a rough stone, it is generally discharged in streaks and clots, and deposits a dark brown sediment in the urine, like coffee grounds. The act of urination is generally performed with some difficulty under such circumstances, and accompanied by straining efforts. When the blood proceeds from the kidneys, that part of the urine expelled first looks muddy and high colored; is usually

very copious, and attended with severe pain in the lumbar regions; anxiety; numbness in the thighs; drawing up of the testicles; constipation and derangement
of the bowels.

When the blood comes from the ureter the indicating
symptoms are nearly the same as for that which proceeds
from the kidneys, with the exception that the pains
extend from the lumbar region along the course of the
ureter, down into the pelvis, with retention of urine,
and sometimes nausea and vomiting. In hæmorrhage
coming from the bladder, there is generally spasm;
retention of urine, sometimes severe burning and other
pains in the lower and posterior portions of the stomach,
penis and anus during and subsequent to the act of
passing urine; and also when the difficulty in making
water is considerable; and anxiety; cold sweats; shivering chills; debility and fits of syncope. The blood is
not so extremely combined with the urine as in the
immediately preceding cases; generally deposits a cohe-
rent sediment, and is sometimes passed in a free state.

Whenever there is the voiding of bloody urine, it is
safe to regard it in a serious light, especially when it
is commingled with purulent matter. A variety of circumstances, however, must be taken into account, in
order for us to form a tolerable judgment concerning
the final result. For instance, we must consider the
active and passive nature of the discharge; the age and
constitution of the patient; the duration of the recur-
rences of the affection; the collateral symptoms, and the
occasional or accidental causes, &c.

TREATMENT.—Nearly the same remedies are required
for the treatment of this difficulty as for retention of
urine or gravel.

CANTHARIS forms one of the best remedies in use for this difficulty, and in almost all cases it may be resorted to, especially when we are uncertain as to the exciting cause of the disorder, and especially when there is considerable difficulty in making water; scalding in the urethra during its passage, or violent spasmodic pains in the whole region of the bowels; the blood discharged being either pure and discharged in drops, or copiously mingled with the urine, or in streaks or clots. Even when the presence of purulent matter is ascertained in the urine, the use of *Cantharides* may be attended with useful results.

DOSE.—One drop, or six globules, in half a tumbler of water; give a teaspoonful every two hours, or even every hour, until relieved.

CAMPHOR is evidently indicated, when the disorder has originated in the employment of Spanish fly-blister, or tincture, after the allopathic method.

DOSE.—One drop of the spirits every hour, until relief is obtained, Should there be any unpleasant after effects, such as burning in the urethra. employ *Carbo veg.* and *Arsenicum.*

MEZEREUM has been recommended as an excellent remedy, in hemorrhage from the bladder, or passing blood with the urine, more particularly, when the blood passed does not appear to be in large quantity, and the accompanying pains not very severe; further, when the blood is rarely, if ever, found in a clot after standing.

DOSE.—Dissolve one drop, or six globules, in three tablespoonfuls of water, and give a spoonful every hour.

ARNICA is particularly indicated when the disorder has resulted from external violence, and if the patient is of a plethoric, robust habit, *Aconite* will be requisite in conjunction with this remedy.

DOSE.—Dissolve one drop, or six globules of each in separate glasses, in four tablespoonfuls of water, and give alternately, a teaspoonful every hour, until mitigation or change.

29

Nux vomica is indicated, when the cause is over indulgence in wine and spirituous drinks, or sudden check of the piles, and there is painful aching in the back, with smarting in the urethra.

DOSE.—Dissolve one drop, or six globules, in four tablespoonfuls of water, and give a teaspoonful every hour until relieved.

Sulphur is certainly a good remedy after *Nux vomica.* Calcarea carb. may succeed *Sulphur.*

DOSE.—The same as directed for *Nux vomica.*

China, Pulstilla, Sabina, Ipecacuanha, Lycopo- dium, Uva ursi, are severally regarded essential, when purulent matter is detected in the sanguinolent urine.

DOSE.—Of either remedy: one drop, or six globules, in a half-tumbler of water, give a teaspoonful every hour, for twelve hours; but if twelve hours' trial should show the remedy to be ineffectual, select again.

Pulsatilla is very serviceable in females affected with irregular menstruation, when there is blood passed with the urine. It has also been found equally service- able to males, when the passage of blood with the urine, or bloody urine, has been attended with constriction and cutting pains around the navel, extending with great violence to the lumbar region, or when spasmodic pains were experienced in the lower extremities, particularly in the right knee, and from thence upwards, to the groin, with spasmodic retraction of the scrotum and penis, and burning pain at the orifice of the *urethra.*

DOSE.—One drop, or six globules, dissolved in half a tumbler of water, may be given, a teaspoonful every hour, until amelioration or change.

Sulphur and Calcarea carb. are useful remedies also, to follow *Pulsatilla.*

China is indicated, if the apparent cause of discharg- ing bloody urine be venereal excesses;—and *Nux vomica. Sulphur, Calcarea carb.* and *Phosphorus* may be used, as the subsequent remedies.

DOSE.—The same in all respects as for *Pu'satilla.*

When this disease occurs, the patient should seldom drink any cold water, on account of its liability to produce an aggravation of the irritation already existing. Barley-water should in most cases be drank, in considerable quantities. Sometimes, this affection occurs, as a secondary disorder merely, in connection with Nephritis and Cystitis. (See these disorders as treated of.)

12.—Inflammation of the Urethra.—Clap.—Gleet.
(Urethritis, Gonorrhœa, Blenorrhœa.)

This disease varies very much in its character; sometimes it is very trifling, at others it is severe and even dangerous. It consists of an inflammation of the mucous membrane of the urethra, resulting from impure connection, and attended with a discharge of puriform matter.

There is a kind of urethritis, however, that occurs in some instances, in the husband, by a common leucorrhœa in his wife.

That which results from impure connection, where the patient knows he has incurred the risk, commonly occurs about ten days after. In some cases, however, it begins in two or three days, and in others, again, there is no appearance for as many weeks. According to the extent and intensity of the inflammation, is the severity of the disease. In the most severe forms, it implicates the entire course of the canal, and even affects the mucus membrane of the bladder.

SYMPTOMS.—The first symptom of clap, consists of tittilation or itching at the orifice of the urethra, which sometimes extends over the whole of the glans penis, and is accompanied by a frequent inclination to make water. In a short time, some uneasiness is experienced in passing the urine, and the orifice of the urethra is observed to be red and swollen, and perhaps a small quantity of discharge is observed. It now becomes more and more painful to urinate, sometimes almost insupportable, while the stream becomes diminished and broken, notwithstanding the increased expulsive efforts exerted by the patient. A somewhat copious discharge of puriform matter, thick, white or yellowish, soon takes place from the urethra. As the inflammation advances, or when it has been intense from the commencement, the discharge becomes greenish, acrid, and sometimes mixed with blood. The glans and prepuce frequently become red and tumefied, involuntary and painful erections often occur, particularly during the night, and there is some-times considerable restlessness, headache, and other symptoms of fever.

This is the acute stage of the disease, and continues with unaltered violence for eight or ten days, or even longer, if unchecked, or suffered to be aggravated by the thoughtlessness of the patient, in committing errors, in diet, exposing himself to cold, and sexual excitement.

When the acute stage begins to subside, its decline is marked by a diminution of the pain, and scalding sensation in making water, and in a month or six weeks, none of the symptoms may remain. It frequently occurs that the acute form disappears, leaving a chronic discharge of puriform matter, which would seem to indicate that there resulted a chronic inflammation.

Women afflicted with the same difficulty, are not generally afflicted so severely with pain as men. Some-times, however, the inflammatory action affects the mucus membrane of the vagina, and even of the womb itself. The discharge takes place from the secreting surfaces of the labia, nymphae, and clitoris, as well as from the lining of the urinary opening and vagina, in severe cases.

In subjects of a healthy constitution, and when the disease is of a mild character, a cure is soon effected, and very easily, provided the patient has resorted to no deleterious agents, and when he applies before the second stage sets in.

TREATMENT. — The disease has not unfrequently yielded in the outset, by the alternate use of *Aconite* and *Cannabis*, when the following symptoms are present, viz: redness and fulness of the orifice of the urethra; disagreeable itching in the tube; frequent desire to make water; and considerable pain in voiding it.

DOSE.—One drop, or four globules, of one in the morning, and of the other, in the evening, until relieved, or change.

And even when the disease has progressed so far as to be marked by a disposition to urinate frequently, together with lessening of the stream, although the strongest efforts to force it through the urethra, still *Cannabis* is decidedly the best remedy that can be used.

DOSE.—In this stage, a drop, or four globules, may be given every four hours.

MERCURIUS VIV. is indicated in gonorrhœa, when the prepuce is extended and swollen; and also in the commencement of the second stage, when there remains a muco-purulent discharge of a white, greenish, yellow color, and in passing the last drop of water there is felt some degree of pain; and also when there is a swelling of the lymphatic glands.

DOSE.—Dissolve one drop, or ten globules, of *Mercurius* in three tablespoonfuls of water, and give a teaspoonful every three hours for an entire day, *Silicea* or *Hepar sulph.* may be used as subsequent remedies.

SULPHUR is indicated after the inflammatory stage is over, particularly when the discharge becomes serous,

29*

and a feeling of uneasiness alone remains in the urethra when voiding urine.

DOSE.—One drop, or four globules, in a spoonful of water, and do not repeat, wait four days, and see the result.

SILICEA, MERCURIUS VIV., and SULPHUR are the remedies to be called into use in painless gonorrhœa.

DOSE.—One drop, or four globules, of either, every night.

The severe forms of gonorrhœa are met with the following remedies: Aconite, Cantharides, and Cannabis.

ACONITE is useful for most cases occurring in young persons, vigorous and healthy, attended with headache, restlessness, and febrile symptoms; but it is almost indispensable when the inflammation is severe and extensive; the pain during the passing of urine is most excruciating, the glans and entire penis much swollen, and the suffering greatly aggravated by frequent and almost constant erections.

DOSE.—One drop, or four globules, in a spoonful of water, every three hours, until three doses are taken. It is rarely necessary to take more, the first dose often relieves.

CANTHARIDES is generally required after *Aconite* when the intensity of the pain and febrile irritation which may have been present, have yielded, but the difficulty in discharging urine proves obstinate, and other distressing symptoms, such as intense desire to urinate, and chordee remain.

DOSE.—One drop, or four globules, every three hours, until amelioration or change. But when used after *Aconite*, it must not be administered for eight hours after the last dose of this remedy; but it may be employed without the previous use of the *Aconite*, when there is no marked degree of constitutional disturbance; but the scalding during the passing of urine, and chordee, is very severe, and the discharge is greenish, tinged with blood. It would be better, perhaps, to give one drop, or four globules, under such circumstances, every six hours.

CANNABIS in severe gonorrhœa is requisite sometimes after *Cantharides*, when the difficulty of passing urine proves obstinate. These two remedies in alternation, three hours between the administration of each remedy, will suffice, in general, to remove the most obstinate sufferings during the passage of urine. *Mercurius* and *Sulphur* are not unfrequently called into use to complete a cure.

DOSE.—Of either of these remedies, give one drop, or four globules, from one hour to four or six hours apart, according to the urgency of the symptoms.

DIET.—Persons under treatment for this disease, must abstain from eating any stimulating food, such as oysters, &c., and from drinking any stimulating drinks. It is better to partake but lightly of animal food; fat and gravies avoid; and avoid exposures, and particularly sexual excitement, and cold, damp weather.

13.—Inflammation of the Glans Penis.
(*Balanitis. Balano. Blennorrhœa.*)

In connection with inflammation of the urethra, the glans penis sometimes becomes involved, after an impure connexion; but it by no means follows that it is always dependent upon this cause, for it may occur from mechanical injury, or from deleterious applications to the part, as sometimes happens after the patient has been handling poisonous plants.

When the inflammation of the urethra extends so as to involve the glans in the difficulty, and also the prepuce,

ACONITE may be given in two doses, four hours apart, and *Mercurius viv.* is a suitable remedy to follow *Aconite*, four hours after; *Cannabis* may also be given when *Mercurius* fails.

DOSE.—The same as for the same remedies in gonorrhœa.

NITRIC ACID is indicated when small superficial ulcerations form on the glans penis, in neglected or protracted cases.

DOSE.—One drop, or four globules, in a spoonful of water, given morning and evening.

ARNICA is indicated if the difficulty be from a bruise, but it would be well if there is much swelling and inflammation to alternate with *Aconite.*

DOSE.—One drop, or six globules, in four tablespoonfuls of water; give a teaspoonful every two hours.

RHUS TOX. is indicated when the *blennorrhœa* is produced by being in contact with some poisonous material, and likewise *Belladonna* and *Bryonia* may be consulted for the same purpose. *Rhus tox.* may also prove beneficial when the disease springs from mechanical injury.

DOSE.—Of either, dissolve one drop, or six globules, in four teaspoonfuls of water, and give a teaspoonful every four hours, until amelioration or change.

14.—Inflammation of the Testes. (*Swelled testicle.*)

This difficulty often arises from mechanical injury, but oftener it is sympathetic with irritation of the urethra. The inflammation and swelling come on suddenly, and as abruptly subside, or pass from one testis to the other.

In the incipient stage of the attack, the testicle is tumefied, soft, and sensitive to the touch; after a short period it becomes hard and excruciatingly painful. The spermatic cord becomes thickened and tender, and the veins in some instances become varicose. There is pain in the loins; colic; sickness; more or less fever; depression of spirits, and occasionnally a difficulty of making water, although these symptoms are not always present.

TREATMENT.—The medicines chiefly employed are Aconite, Arnica, Aurum, China, Graphites, Lycopodium, Mercurius viv., Nux vomica, Pulsatilla and Sulphur.

ACONITE is indicated when the accompanying fever runs high, and there is considerable heat and redness attendant upon the swelling.

DOSE.—Dissolve one drop, or six globules, in four tablespoonfuls of water and give a teaspoonful every hour or every two hours, until the fever is reduced.

ARNICA is indicated when the swelling arises from an external injury.

DOSE.—The same as for *Aconite.*

AURUM is indicated when the swelling of the testicle arises from the abuse of mercury, and when there are indurations.

DOSE.—One drop, or four globules, morning and evening.

CHINA is also indicated, if from the abuse of mercury, and may be given one drop, or four globules, every two hours.

GRAPHITES and LYCOPODIUM are useful for long standing indurations.

DOSE.—Of the remedy selected, a drop, or four globules, every six hours.

MERCURIUS VIV., NUX VOMICA and PULSATILLA, are severally indicated when inflammation and swelling of the testicles take place by *metastasis* from mumps.

DOSE.—Of the selected remedy, one drop, or four globules, every two hours.

SULPHUR is useful if the difficulty has proceeded from the abuse of mercury, and may be employed to complete a cure, when produced by other causes, especially after other remedies have been tried with only partial success.

DOSE.—One drop, or four globules, every twelve hours, until relieved, or there is necessity for change.

15.—Dropsy of the Scrotum. (*Hydrocele.*)

Dropsy of the scrotum is a pear-shaped swelling of the same, and is generally associated with dropsy in other parts. It is elastic, free from pain, and rarely occurs on both sides, but more on the left than on the right.

TREATMENT. The remedies employed are Pulsatilla, Sulphur and Silicea.

DOSE.—One drop, or four globules, in a spoonful of water, may be given of the first-named remedy every morning. If no relief is obtained within three days, proceed with the next remedy. For the same difficulty in newly-born infants, put six drops of *Arnica* in half a tumbler of water, and bathe the affected part four times a day ; in older children, one drop, or four globules, may be dissolved in two tablespoonfuls of water, and a teaspoonful may be given twice a day, and bathe the affected part as before with the *Arnica,* until amelioration or change.

16.—Venereal Disease. (*Syphilis.—Chancre.*)

There are certain symptoms produced by venereal disease termed PRIMARY, and others termed SECONDARY.

Primary syphilis consists in ulceration, sometimes followed by a swelling of the absorbient glands, which results from a direct application of a peculiar virus to the parts.

Chancre is an ulceration situated on the organs of generation.

A bubo is a glandular swelling. The ulcer may be on the prepuce, the glans penis at the angle formed by the junction of the two former at the frænum, the orifice of the urethra, the body of the penis, or even on the scrotum or perinæum.

In the female, the ulcers generally form on the labia, nymphæ, clitoris, and not unfrequently in the urethra or the vagina.

The first symptoms of the chancre become manifest from three to six days after the impure connexion, and their appearance is announced by itching, which upon examination is found to proceed from a small pimple or pustule having an inflamed base, which feels hard to the touch. Soon after, an elevated point is observed on the minute cone, and from an opening in this there is a discharge of a limpid fluid, which is followed by a more or less rapid development of ulceration.

The primary venereal sore wears a different appearance and intensity in different individuals, depending in a great measure on the habit of body, age and temperament of the patient. The most frequent varieties are the *chancre;* the superficial ulcer with raised edges; the phagedenic, and the sloughing ulcer.

The chancre commences in the way we have described. As soon as this sore is manifest, it exhibits a tendency to assume a form somewhat circular, becomes deep seated and spreads, and is covered with a tough, adherent matter, which has a hard, cartilagenous base and margin. It has been met with in every part of the genital organs before alluded to.

When the ulcer is on the glans it is more inclined to bleed, but is less painful than when found upon the prepuce or frænum.

The *superficial ulcer* is considerably elevated at its edges, and sometimes it is spongy, but not attended with induration. It is sometimes associated with two or three sores of the same kind, and has its seat very often on the outside of prepuce; but it is not unfrequently met with, attended with the other sores, on the crown of the penis, under the prepuce, or around its orifice; when located at the side of the *frænum,* it usually destroys the fold of the reflected skin.

The *phagedenic ulcer* is destitute of any hard margin

surrounding it or any granulations, but presents a livid-colored circumference, spreading rapidly and alarmingly, especially when badly treated with external irritating applications, or by excessive doses of *mercury.*

The *sloughing ulcer* has no marked degree of hardness surrounding it, and may be distinguished at first as a black spot, which extends and then casts off, displaying a corroding surface; after the slough has come away, the ulcer that remains is of a painful character, and has a dark blue or crimsom margin; a vitiated habit of body in connection with intemperance or unwholesome diet, together with a residence in an unhealthy atmosphere, may be reckoned among the principal *causes*, to which may be added abusive treatment with *mercury* or irritating local applications.

If this course of maltreatment is persevered in, or the spreading of the ulcers is not checked, they will go on sloughing and ulcerating until the destruction of the whole of the external sexual organs is completed.

TREATMENT.—The principal remedies in Syphilis are Mercurius vivus and Mercurius corrosivus, but Nitric acid, Arsenicum and Sulphur are called into requisition.

When *mercury* has not been employed in any of the various forms of the diseases, it is safe to resort to it homœopathically; for, notwithstanding the sad consequences resulting from its use in the massive doses in the hands of allopathic physicians, no fear is to be apprehended of such results in the hands of the *homœopath*, for if he restricts himself to homœopathic practice, there can be none of the dangerous aggravations predicated of its use in the hands of those who use it empirically as *the remedy.*

MERCURIUS VIV. is indicated where the health of the

patient has been remarkably good and the sore has not been of long duration, and where it has not been aggravated by previous treatment, and with it a cure can often be effected in two or three weeks.

DOSE.—One drop, or four globules, in a spoonful of water, may be given every three hours, for two days, and then night and morning, until the ulcer exhibits a healing aspect, and then only once in two days.

MERCURIUS CORROSIVUS is indicated in torpid constitutions.

DOSE.—One drop, or four globules, may be given every morning and evening, until a copious discharge of healthy pus supervenes, or the excavations of the ulcers begin to fill up with healthy granulations; as soon as either the one or the other takes place, discontinue the remedy for several days, and then commence again, a few more doses will effect a cure where granulation has taken place; but if otherwise, which is rarely the case, a dose or two of *Sulphur* may produce a favorable effect.

NITRIC ACID is indicated if pale and flabby granulations of a prominent character, that do not appear to exhibit the firm and florid appearance of the healthy granulations spoken of above.

DOSE.—One drop, or four globules, in a spoonful of water, may be given night and morning, until amelioration or change.

ARSENICUM is indicated after *Mercurius* has produced some improvement in the sore, when it becomes less contagious at its base, and fills up with florid and to elevated granulations, and remains hard at the margin, and painful irritable and bleeding at the slightest touch, and secretes a thin acrid offensive discharge.

DOSE.—One drop, or four globules, in a spoonful of water, may be given three times a day, at intervals of six hours; if this does not effect a cure after four days' trial, *Sulphur* or *Nitric acid* may be employed in the same doses to complete the cure; *Nitric acid* in the same dose may be employed after *Arsenicum*, especially when the ulcer has spread rapidly and attained a large size at the commencement, from four to eight weeks generally elapse, a cure can be established in these cases.

DIET.—While under homœopathic treatment for *venereal disease*, it is requisite for the patient to abstain from

30

all heating drinks, such as wine, gin or brandy; coffee, beer and condiments, except salt in great moderation; the diet should be light, consisting of farinaceous gruels, stale wheat bread, or plain toast and black tea; the patient should exercise but little, and should avoid all ex-posures to damp and cold, and above all, avoid keeping late hours or eating oyster suppers, and keep as free as possible from sexual excitement; and lastly, let the mind be preserved in a calm state, avoiding all unnecessary excitement, or dwelling in despondency upon the disease, or hasty resort to topical applications.

CHAPTER VIII.

DISEASES OF THE SKIN.—CUTANEOUS AFFECTIONS.

WE have already under the head of eruptive fevers, considered a number of diseases, that are attended by some. kind of eruption upon the skin, viz: *nettle rash, scarlet rash, scarlet fever, measles, erysipelas, (St. Anthony's fire, or rose,) chicken pox, varioloid* and *small pox.* We will now treat of such other diseases as are usually comprehended in cutaneous affections.

1.—Boil. *Furunculus. Abscessus Nucleatus.*

The boil is a tumor somewhat conical in shape, which is hard, inflames slowly, and suppurates. The matter which it first discharges, is for the most part mixed with blood, but afterwards it is pus, or morbidly altered cellular membrane, a portion of which formed into a round hard mass, constitutes what, in common parlance is termed the *core;* the same may form the nucleus of other prominances, after those which first appeared have healed.

CAUSES.—Some persons are constitutionally predisposed to boils. They may also follow acute fevers, other eruptive diseases, itch, &c.

TREATMENT.—The remedies employed in the treatment of boils, are Arnica, Aconite, Belladonna, Hepar sulph., Mercurius, and Sulphur.

ARNICA is indicated in a majority of instances, and will speedily cause an abatement of the swelling and inflammation, and frequently prevent others from making their appearance; but to accomplish this latter purpose, *Sulphur* may be required to thoroughly eradicate the affection. The use of the two remedies may have the best effect, if used in each attack. *Arnica* may reduce the swelling and soreness, but as soon as the tumor begins to heal, it is better to resort to *Sulphur,* to prevent others from appearing from the nuclei remaining from the first.

DOSE.—One drop, or four globules may be given in a spoonful of water, night and morning, until amelioration, or change. If the acute symptoms yield readily, pause for three days, and proceed to administer *Sulphur,* one drop, or four globules, every twenty-four hours.

ACONITE is indicated when the boil presents an intense inflammatory appearance, and the affection is attended with fever and restlessness. After it has subdued these symptoms, another remedy more specific may be resorted to, for the purpose of eradicating the remaining features of the disease.

DOSE.—Dissolve one drop, or six globules, in three tablespoonfuls of water, and give a spoonful three times a day, until the acute symptoms disappear.

BELLADONNA is of service when the boil has an inflamed, fiery, or erysipelatous, red appearance, or moreover, should it, if located on the extremities, be attended with swelling and tenderness of the glands, under the armpit, or upon the groin, with dry, hot skin, thirst and headache.

DOSE.—Dissolve one drop, or eight globules, in three spoonfuls of water, and give a spoonful night and morning, until amelioration, or change; but if the swelling should remove after the use of this remedy, pause twenty-four hours, proceed with the use of *Mercurius viv.*

MERCURIUS is especially indicated after *Belladonna* has subdued the inflammatory redness, and has failed of removing the swelling.

DOSE.—The same as directed for *Belladonna.*

HEPAR SULPH. is indicated when the matter has formed, to bring the tumor to a head, so as to curtail the suffering.

DOSE.—The same as directed for *Belladonna* and *Mercurius.*

SULPHUR is more particularly serviceable in obviating an attack after *Arnica* and other remedies have subdued the symptoms for which they are indicated; but if this remedy in connection with the foregoing is not found sufficient, *Lycopodium, Nux vomica, Nitric acid,* or *Phosphorus* may be consulted.

DIET.—The same as directed in acute fevers.

2.—Carbuncle. (*Anthrax. Furunculus Malignans. Pustulo Nigra.*)

The carbuncle differs from the boil, in having no central *core*, but in some respects, it resembles it. It is a deep-seated, circumscribed, hard, and excessively painful swelling, of a livid hue, and attended with great itching and burning heat. The carbuncle does not suppurate like the boil, but terminates in sloughing. It is usually accompanied by inflammation at the commencement, but these are soon succeeded by vesications, having an acrid, offensive fluid, which is discharged through numerous apertures occupying every part of the tumor, and communicating with cavities readily running into gangrene, and sometimes proving fatal, from the extension of mortification.

The disease is usually attended with fever, nausea, loss of appetite, great prostration of strength, and inability to sleep; in some cases, to such a degree, as to destroy the patient.

Sometimes recovery takes place from this affection, after the patient has experienced a great deal of suffering; but when seated upon the head, it is exceedingly doubtful if the patient recovers.

TREATMENT.—The most useful remedies are Arsenicum, Hepar sulph., Lachesis and Silicea. ·

ARSENICUM is indicated, when there is great prostration, and the disease exhibits symptoms of gangrene.

DOSE.—One drop, or four globules, in a spoonful of water, three times a day.

HEPAR SULPH. is the remedy best adapted, when extensive cavities are formed, and the discharge is profuse and purulent.

DOSE.—The same as directed for *Arsenicum.*

LACHESIS is particularly indicated, when the carbuncle is of a bluish or livid complexion, and is rapidly extending.

DOSE.—One drop, or six globules, in three spoonfuls of water; give a spoonful three times a day, at first, for two days; afterwards night and morning, until progressive improvement or change ensues.

SILICEA may be employed, from the commencement of the disease, and it will frequently effect a cure. It may also be used after *Hepar sulph.*

DOSE.—Four globules, night and morning, or one drop of the dilution may be dissolved in two spoonfuls of water, one of which may be given at night, and the other in the morning.

DIET and REGIMEN.—As this disease is more frequently manifested in the aged and infirm, it is requisite to provide a judicious diet. Meat-broths, and other articles easy of digestion may be resorted to, for the purpose of providing for the processes of nutrition.

3.—Chilblains. (*Perniones.*)

This affection is of an inflammatory character, and results from cold, or a sudden transition from cold to heat, or *vice versâ*. It generally attacks the feet, but sometimes, it affects the hands, ears, nose, &c.

When the chilblains burst and become ulcerated, they constitute an exceedingly painful suffering.

When chilblains become thus painful, it indicates some constitutional taint, that should receive the proper treatment, in accordance with the indicating symptoms and the temperament of the individual.

The difficulty is most prevalent, in moist and temperate climates, and often disappears spontaneously in summer, and regularly returns in the winter, and those who once suffer from the affection, are very liable to its recurrence.

TREATMENT.—This must be divided into *external* and *internal*. The remedies employed *internally* are, Arsenicum, Chamomilla, Nux vomica, Pulsatilla, Phosphorus, and Sulphur.

ARSENICUM and CHAMOMILLA may be used in alternation, for the acute, burning pains, and also for the irritable, ill-conditioned ulcers, which sometimes occur as the result,—or either of the remedies may be used alone. The *Chamomilla*, when there are acute pains in the affected part, and *Arsenicum* after the use of *Chamomilla*.

DOSE.—Of either, when used alone, one drop, or six globules, may be dissolved in four tablespoonfuls of water, and a spoonful may be given every six hours, or if used in alternation, *Chamomilla* should be given in the morning, and *Arsenicum* in the evening, until amelioration or change.

NUX VOMICA is particularly indicated when the inflammation is of a bright red color; if this remedy proves insufficient, proceed with the use of *Sulphur*.

DOSE.—As directed for *Chamomilla* or *Arsenicum*.

PULSATILLA is required when the skin assumes a deep red, or bluish or livid hue, and is accompanied by intense burning and itching.

DOSE.—Dissolve one drop, or six globules, in three spoonfuls of water, and give a spoonful three times a day six hours apart.

PHOSPHORUS is useful after *Pulsatilla* has proved inefficient, and also after ulceration makes its appearance. This remedy is of great use, and frequently operates a speedy cure.

DOSE.—As directed for *Pulsatilla*.

SULPHUR is a valuable remedy when the inflammation and itching are very severe, and the affection has failed to yield to the other remedies employed in this affection.

External Treatment.

The application of cold or iced water to mild forms of the complaint, will often effect a cure, but this application must not be used by delicate females or gouty persons, nor with those suffering from or predisposed to pulmonary difficulties.

Covering the affected part with cotton will sometimes prove salutary in curing the disease.

TINCTURE OF CANTHARIDES may be used externally in recent chilblains produced by exposure to intense cold; it operates against the formation of blisters, and aids in subduing the congestive action. It may be applied by adding four or five drops to half a tumbler of water, and bathing the parts three times a day, until relieved.

TINCT. ARNICA is useful, while the same remedy is administered internally, provided the indications are such as to require this remedy. Add a teaspoonful to a tumblerful of water, and bathe the parts with the lotion three times a day.

RHUS TOX., in external use, sometimes effects a cure when there is smarting, itching, and irritation. Add ten drops to half a tumbler of water, and bathe the parts affected three times a day, until relieved.

TINCT. CAUSTICUM may be called into requisition when the chilblains become broken, or deep ulceration has taken place. ' Add five drops to half a tumbler of water, and bathe as directed for *Rhus tox.*

4.—Corns. (*Clavipedis.*)

Some persons are prone to suffer more readily than others from these troublesome excresences, being more susceptible to the exciting causes. Some can wear tight boots or shoes without inconvenience, while others are obliged to exercise the greatest precaution, and still they are made to suffer severely. It is therefore evident that some inherent constitutional taint may often be the predisposing cause, which internal remedies may be required to eradicate.

TREATMENT.—The remedies employed to eradicate the inherent predisposition, are Antimonium crud., Ammonium carb., Bryonia, Calcarea, Ignatia, Lycopodium, Phosphorus, Sepia, Silicea and Sulphur.

ANTIMONIUM CRUD., SEPIA, SILICEA AND SULPHUR.— Either one of these remedies may be employed as found indicated, to eradicate the predisposing cause, or to overcome the irritation from which the general system suffers.

DOSE.—Of *Antimonium crud.*, give four globules, or one drop, every day, for a week, or until corns cease to form; if there appears to be an indication of a good result, but if after three weeks' trial there is not much amelioration, proceed to give the other remedies in the order which they are given, in the same manner as the first mentioned.

AMMONIUM CARB., CALCAREA, BRYONIA, IGNATIA, RHUS TOX. and LYCOPODIUM, are also remedies that may be employed in the effectual eradication of the predisposition to the formation of corns. ·

DOSE.—Of *Bryonia, Rhus tox.* or *Ignatia,* give a drop, or four globules, every morning, for a week, then wait for a week and proceed again as before. The other remedies to be used in the same way.

External Treatment.

TINCT. OF ARNICA.—After the corn has been soaked in warm water, prepare a lotion of one teaspoonful of this tincture to half a pint of water, and bathe the corn three or four times a day, scraping the corn down with great care during the time of making the application.

In case of redness and swelling of the heel, resembling a chilblain, which may have been produced by the boot or shoe, *Nux vomica* may be given internally three times a day.

DOSE.—One drop, or six globules, in three tablespoonfuls of water, one of which may be given in the morning, another at noon, and another at night, and the Tinct. of Arnica may be employed, as above.

5.—Abscess. (*Lymphatic tumors.—Disease of the Conglobate glands.*)

By the the term *abscess* is understood a collection of matter, resulting from diseased action, which is contained in a sac or cyst of organized lymph, furnished with absorbent and secreting vessels.

There are in general two classes of abscesses: the *acute* and *chronic*. *Acute abscesses* are always preceded by sensiblility in the affected part, and this is soon followed by suppuration. When the suppurative process commences, there is a change in the appearance of the skin, and the description of the pain. Before, the skin is usually red, but becomes livid when it begins to suppurate, and the pain becomes more obtuse and throbbing. There is also augmentation of the swelling, and when matter is formed, there is perceptible fluctuation of the part, especially when the abscess is not too deeply seated; lastly, in persons hereditarily predisposed to abscess, there is always fever and chills attending the inflammatory stage, by no means regular, though each chill is succeeded by fever and heat, until the violence of the whole subsides, in consequence of the suppurating process.

When the abscess is ripe, there is presented somewhat of a conical shape in its centre; over this the skin becomes livid and thin, and ere long bursts and allows the contents of the cavity to escape.

Chronic abscesses, on the other hand, are not usually preceded by any apparent inflammation or disorder in the system, until it begins to approach the surface of the skin, and forms an external swelling.

The matter which is secreted is unhealthy, thin, serous, and contains flaky substances resembling curds; when the pus is evacuated, and the air admitted into the cavity, inflammation of the cyst arises, and is productive of a good effect, if the abscess be small; but if it be large, great constitutional disturbance takes place; the cavity instead of contracting and filling up under the process of healthy granulation or incarnation, goes on discharging copiously, and results in the production of hectic fever.

TREATMENT.—The suppurative process of *acute* abscesses may be hastened by the application of warm fomentations and unmedicated poultices. The internal remedies employed are Calcarea carb., Hepar sulphur, Lachesis, Mercurius, Phosphorus and Silicea.

CALCAREA CARB. may be employed, as soon as the matter is discharged from the abscess. The remedy may be used in alternation with *Phosphorus*, in chronic cases.

DOSE.—One drop or four globules, may be administered night and morning, until amelioration or change. In alternation with *Phosphorus*, the *Calcarea* may be used one day, and the *Phosphorus* the next; or in long standing cases, two or three days may intervene between the remedies.

HEPAR SULPH. is of great use, in forwarding the suppurative process in acute abscesses.

DOSE.—Dissolve one drop or six globules, in four tablespoonfuls of water, and give a teaspoonful every four hours for one day, and then every six hours, until a change ensues.

LACHESIS is required after the use of *Hepar sulph.*, and sometimes at the commencement, when a large portion of the skin is much distended, and presents a deep red, or bluish appearance, or when the structure of this portion has been destroyed by the magnitude of the abscess.

DOSE.—Dissolve one drop or six globules, in four tablespoonfuls of water, and give a spoonful every four hours, until amelioration or change.

In ordinary cases of the *acute abscess*, the use of the lancet is rarely necessary, but in cases where the extensive diffusion or pressure of the pus, is liable to injure important parts,—as when situated under expanded ligaments and tendons. The use of the *lancet* is apparent, and also, when abscesses are so situated as to afford a reason for apprehending their discharge into some of the internal cavities,—they should be opened by the lancet, to avoid an occurrence of the kind.

When such cases occur, the artificial opening with the lancet ought to be made at the most dependent part, when this can be readily accomplished. When this is impracticable, in consequence of the great thickness of the parts between the purulent matter and the skin, then it is better to select the most prominent, or pointed part.

But if this point manifests itself upon the upper portion of the abscess, it is far better to dispense with the lancet, and to promote the spontaneous opening of the abscess, by the use of such remedies as have been found useful for the purpose.

Hepar sulph., *Silicea* and *Lachesis*, are severally adapted to promote this desirable termination; the particular indication for each, is to be determined.

It has been regarded a useful course, to make an outlet in a *chronic abscess* as early as possible, in order to prevent its large accumulation, and thereby to avoid the alarming constitutional disturbance, which is so prone to occur in such cases, from the extent of the inflammation, after the rupture of the abscess. The lancet should be inserted near the base of the abscess, and only large enough to admit of the exit of the matter. Sometimes, after the matter is evacuated, it collects again; and this is when the collection in the first place is extensive. On this account, it has been recommended to heal up the opening immediately, and make a new one when necessity requires it, and this should be done before there is a great accumulation, as before.

In the TREATMENT of CHRONIC ABSCESS, Mercurius viv., Hepar sulph., Silicea, Calcarea, and Phosphorus, are the chief remedies. One or more of these should be employed, as soon as the matter has been withdrawn from the abscess.

DOSE.—One drop or four globules, may be dissolved in a spoonful of water and be given every six hours, until some indication of a healing process commences. But if, after two days' trial, there appears to be no indication of the salutary effects of the remedy, and there appears to be some threatening of the re-formation of other abscesses in succession, wait for twelve hours, and then proceed with the next remedy and so on.

HEPAR SULPH. should be given twelve hours after the fourth dose of *Mercurius viv.*, should the latter prove inadequate to effect a cure, and if fresh matter begins to form.

DOSE.—Dissolve one drop, or six globules, in four tablespoonfuls of water, and give a spoonful every four hours; when, however, in cases of *open abscess*, the parts betraying a tendency to chronic ulceration, proceed with one or both of the next medicines, *Calcarea* and *Phosphorus*, but not for three or four days after the use of *Hepar sulphur* is discontinued.

CALCAREA AND PHOSPHORUS.—Either of these medicines may be administered by itself, alternately with the other, or in succession, according to the distinctive characteristics of the abscess or combination of the symptoms.

DOSE.—If either be given alone, dissolve one drop, or six globules, in six teaspoonfuls of water, and give a teaspoonful every night and morning, until amelioration or change; if in alternation, give two doses as just directed of the one, at intervals of twelve hours, then wait four days and give two doses of the other, and so on in rotation until the abscess indicates a change for the better.

SILICEA AND SULPHUR.—One or both of these remedies may be required, sometimes singly, sometimes in alternation, and at other times in succession; they are useful in those severe and protracted cases, associated with deep-seated and constitutional taint, in which the continued suppuration seems to exhaust the system, and hectic fever and considerable emaciation supervenes.

DOSE.—If either of the medicines be given by itself, dissolve one drop, or six globules, in six teaspoonfuls of water, and give a teaspoonful night and morning for a week, or until the first appearance of amelioration or change, then discontinue for four days, and repeat again the same course as just directed, then wait again four days, and in this way continue the treatment until permanent improvement of the abscess or change. If in

31

alternation, give one remedy one week as directed above, and the other the next week, and so on alternately until ameliotation or change.

DIET.—In acute abscess, and particularly when there is considerable fever present during the first stage, nearly the same diet is requisite as in acute fevers; but in chronic abscess, the diet may be in accordance with the patient's appetite; if he crave food, he should have such as will nourish and sustain him and prove easy of digestion; rice and barley gruel; meat broths; toast and black tea; broiled mutton chops; and sometimes a poached egg may be allowed.

6.—Itch. (*Scabies.—Psora.*)

This disease consists in an inflammatory condition of the skin, characterised by a peculiar eruption of pointed vesicles, transparent at the top, and filled with thin matter, sometimes these pimples or vesicles terminate in pustules or blisters; this eruption appears all over the body, except the face, very frequently about the hands between the fingers, and at the bend of the joints, &c., and is attended with constant and almost insupportable itching, but without fever; this disorder does not uniformly sustain the same character as to the kind of eruption, but it is exceeding difficult to point out any difference in other respects.

TREATMENT.—The remedies principally employed in the treatment of this annoying disease, are Sulphur, Calcarea, Hepar sulph., Lycopodium, Sepia, Sulph. acidum, Stramonium and Rhus tox.

SULPHUR is unquestionably one of the best remedies that can be employed in this troublesome complaint. The remedy is indicated by the main feature of the disease, the itching; it is more particularly indicated for persons of a nutritive temperament, full habit, robust and fleshy; this remedy may be followed by *Lycopodium*.

DOSE.—One drop, or ten globules, may be dissolved in four tablespoonfuls of water, and a teaspoonful may be given three times a day. If after using this remedy three days the itching does not disappear, five drops may be dissolved in a tumbler half filled with water, and with a clean sponge the whole surface of the body may be wet with the lotion.

CALCAREA is better suited for females of irritable constitutions, and particularly when the itching seems to come on or is excited by some internal derangement of the digestive or uterine functions.

DOSE.—The same as for *Sulphur*.

HEPAR SULPHUR is indicated for neglected cases, when the vesicles have spread so as to acquire the appearance of ulcers that have discharged their contents.

DOSE.—The same as for *Sulphur*.

LYCOPODIUM is also one of the remedies for neglected cases, particularly when *Sulphur* proves inefficient.

DOSE.—As directed for *Sulphur*.

SEPIA is also a remedy that is useful in the treatment of neglected cases in females, and in persons of delicate constitution.

DOSE.—As directed for *Sulphur*.

SULPHURIC ACID is particularly indicated when the breaking of the pustules, together with their discharge, should occasion extensive incrustation.

DOSE.—One drop, or six globules, may be dissolved in half a tumbler of water, a teaspoonful may be given every six hours, for a week, and then discontinue for another week, and commence again, and continue for another week, and then discontinue as before, and so on until a cure is effected.

STRAMONIUM and RHUS TOX are of great service when the pustules are large, and coagulate to form patches or blotches, and sometimes ulcerate to a greater or less extent.

DOSE.—One drop, or six globules of either, in half a tumbler of water, give a teaspoonful every six hours, until the itching subsides, and the skin begins to heal, and there appears to be a permanent improvement.

SILICEA AND MEZEREUM are remedies that may be employed when the papular appearance is very strongly marked.

For the DRY ITCH, Mercurius, Hepar sulph., Sepia, and Sulphur are the remedies.

For the HUMID ITCH, Sulphuric acid, Rhus tox., Graphites, Mercurius, Carbo veg.

When the itch assumes the pustular form, and the pustules are globular, of a yellowish or bluish color, *Lachesis* has been proved to be the most salutary remedy.

DOSE.—Dissolve as directed for *Stramonium* and *Rhus tox.*, and administer the same.

When the itch is of a *watery character*, (scabies lymphatica,) and seems to present the appearance of vesicles of considerable size, without an inflamed base, much the same treatment may be resorted to, as has been detailed under *Sulphur, Hepar sulph., Lycopodium*, &c.

Sometimes the disease becomes materially altered by the use of *Sulphur*, in an allopathic way; in such an event it is necessary to have recourse to *Mercurius, Sepia, Rhus tox., Staphysagria, Nitric acid*, &c., &c.

An exceedingly attenuated solution of *Kreosotum*, used both as an internal remedy, and as a lotion, may be found useful in some obstinate cases of this annoying difficulty.

When the itch has been suppressed by powerful external applications, Arsenicum, Carbo veg., Sulphur, Calcarea, and Silicea, are remedies to be employed.

When larger boils make their appearance during the course of the disease, or in consequence of the disease, or on its disappearance, *Silicea* is the remedy.

DOSE.—Of whatever remedy selected, dissolve one drop, or six globules, in half a tumbler of water, and give a teaspoonful every six hours during the day, and if no relief is obtained from the first selection, after a day's trial, try another.

DIET AND REGIMEN.—It is necessary that persons afflicted with scabies should have good wholesome food, free from irritating condiments, or medicinal properties; that they should sleep in well ventilated apartments, and should pay strict attention to personal cleanliness, and changes of clothing.

The itch is not an affection that can be cured in a moment. It can be driven from the skin in a very short time, by the use of external agents, or *unguents;* but this course is detrimental to the prospects of the constitution, for the enjoyment of good health afterwards, for what is suppressed from the surface, may fall upon the more vital organs of the body, and after a lapse of years, fatal disease may break out as the consequence. It is, therefore, better to cure the disease without recourse to external agents, although it may require more time, patience, and perseverance to do so.

7.—Whitlow. (*Panaris Paronychia.*)

This term is used to denote a kind of abscess, that makes its appearance near the end of the finger, sometimes surrounding the nail. It is usually attended with considerable pain and swelling. It has a great proneness to reappear in persons that have once suffered from them, and this fact alone argues the importance of treating the affection as a constitutional disturbance, and not merely as a local affection.

TREATMENT.—We may have recourse to the following medicines in the treatment of whitlow. Mercurius, Hepar sulph., Rhus tox., Lachesis, Silicea and Sulphur.

MERCURIUS is useful, when the affection is in the incipient stage, and when the redness of the abscess and pain first begin to make their appearance.

31*

DOSE.—Dissolve one drop or six globules, in three tablespoonfuls of water, and give a teaspoonful every six hours, for two days, and afterwards, every twelve hours, until relief is obtained, or there is necessity for another remedy.

HEPAR SULPHUR, is an excellent remedy with which to follow *Mercurius*, if under the use of this latter remedy, there has been no abatement of the swelling, or if the pain should become intense and throbbing.

DOSE.—Dissolve a drop, or six globules, in half a tumblerful of water, and give a tablespoonful every six hours until the whitlow discharges.

RHUS TOX. is indicated, when the constitution is tainted with erysipelas, so as to impart to the whitlow considerable degree of its character during the inflammatory stage.

DOSE.—As directed for *Hepar sulphur.*

LACHESIS is sometimes of service in whitlow, and particularly, when the affected part is of a dark red or bluish hue, and the pains extremely violent; when this remedy is not sufficient to give relief, it may be followed by *Arsenicum* and *Carbo veg.*, and particularly if the whitlow is of a black, or gray appearance, attended with a burning pain.

DOSE.—The same as for *Hepar sulphur* or *Rhus tox.*

SILICEA. This remedy is preferable to *Hepar sulphur*, in a corresponding stage of treatment, but in severe forms of whitlow, and when the pus is deep-seated and the swelling, heat, and tenseness considerable, and attended with excruciating pain, or more especially, when there is reason to apprehend that the bone is affected.

DOSE.—Dissolve a drop, or six globules, in half a tumbler of water, and give a tablespoonful every six hours until the whitlow discharges. If this result should not take place in twenty-four hours, proceed with the use of *Sulphur.*

SULPHUR should be called into requisition after *Silicea*, but not for twelve hours after the last dose of the latter remedy has been given. It may be used in alternation with *Silicea*, when this remedy does not speedily promote suppuration.

DOSE.—Four globules, in a tablespoonful of water, repeated after the lapse of twelve hours, or one drop may be given in a spoonful of water in the same way. After twelve hours, if the *Sulphur* has not produced the desired effect, *Silicea* may be again employed.

EXTERNAL APPLICATIONS.—Poultices made of bread and milk, or slippery elm, or linseed meal, may be employed to hasten suppuration, so as to relieve the pain; and moreover, it is said, that the north pole of the *magnet*, held a minute or two to the affected finger, will relieve the pain.

8.—Itching of the Skin. *(Irritation of the Skin.—Prurigo.)*

This disease is not of the same character as *scabies*, although there is intense itching. It usually accompanies other diseases, and has to be treated accordingly. In some cases, however, prurigo exists by itself, and is generally caused by scarcely perceptible colorless elevations under the cuticle, which, however, are quite large, soft, and smooth, and without desquamation, or any peculiar eruptive appearance.

TREATMENT.—Sulphur, Conium, Ignatia, Mercurius, Pulsatilla, Rhus tox., Hepar sulph., and Nux vomica.

SULPHUR is the best remedy to be directed against this distressing malady, and it is frequently specific, particularly when the itching comes on in the evening, or when the body is warm in the bed; but in other, and more ordinary cases, other remedies may be employed.

DOSE.—Dissolve one drop, or six globules, in half a tumbler of water, and give a teaspoonful morning and evening for a week, after which, if the itching is not gone, begin again, and proceed as before, until relief or change.

CONIUM is of great service in this affection, when the itching is partial, confined particularly to certain localities, as the backs of the hands, arms, and the scrotum and skin of the penis.

DOSE.—The same in every respect as directed for *Sulphur*.

IGNATIA is indicated when the irritation and itching is most severe on going to bed, and resembles flea-bites all over the body, but shifts from part to part, which scratching relieves.

DOSE.—Dissolve one drop, or six globules, in four tablespoonfuls of water, and give a teaspoonful three times a day for one day, and then discontinue for two days; if not perfectly relieved, recur to the remedy again.

MERCURIUS VIV. is indicated when the irritative or itching continues through the whole night. It is particularly useful after *Pulsatilla;* and also when the parts bleed easily after scratching.

DOSE.—One drop, or four globules, every night and morning for three days, then discontinue for three days, and if necessary recur again. *Sulphur* may follow if the remedy appears not to suffice.

PULSATILLA is more particularly serviceable when the irritation comes on in the warmth of the bed, and is aggravated by scratching.

DOSE.—As directed for *Ignatia*. But if only partial relief is the result, within two days after the second course resort to *Mercurius*.

RHUS TOX. is of service when the itching is attended with violent burning sensation, and followed by smarting when scratched.

DOSE.—Dissolve one drop, or six globules in two tablespoonfuls of water, and give a teaspoonful night and morning, every other day, until four days elapse, and then discontinue four days, and if symptoms still continue, proceed with the use of *Hepar sulph,*

HEPAR SULPH. If their ritation should continue to be more or less troublesome, this remedy may be given four days after the last dose of *Rhus tox.*

DOSE.—One drop, or four globules may be given night and morning, and then discontinue for three days; if the itching is not subdued, commence again, and proceed as before.

NUX VOMICA when the itching appears on removing the clothes at night. This remedy may be used in alternation with *Arsenicum*, when the itching commences on undressing.

DOSE.—Give one drop, or four globules of *Nux vomica* at night, and after three days, if the itching continues, give the same of *Arsenicum*, and so on in rotation, until permanent amelioration or change.

9.—Ring-worm. (*Herpes Circinnatus. Herpes Serpigo.*)

This is a form of herpes that breaks out in a spot, and spreads in a circular form. It is a common affection of children, and believed to be contagious from the fact that many children attending the same school, or members of the same household, become affected with it at the same time; although there is doubt upon this subject. When it exists without being complicated with other diseases, it is not attended by any marked constitutional derangement.

The disorder breaks out in rings, the vesicles only occupying the circumference; these are small, and have a red colored base. About the fourth or fifth day the vesicles become turbid, and then discharge, when brownish scales form over them.

The skin embraced within the enclosure, is sometimes healthy, at other times rough and of a reddish hue, and falls off in scales as the eruption dies away.

The duration of the affection is various, sometimes the rings come, and die away in two weeks after their first appearance, and then they appear in succession on other portions of the face, neck, arms, and shoulders. This frequently happens in warm climates, or during hot weather, in the country, and on this account is more stubborn, and often proves quite protracted.

TREATMENT.—The principal remedies found salutary in this affection, are Sepia, Natrum muriaticum, Nux vomica, Calcarea carb., Rhus tox., and Sulphur.

SEPIA will prove specific for a majority of cases.

DOSE.—One drop, or four globules, may be dissolved in two spoonfuls of water, one drop may be given at night, and the other in the morning, and then wait four days, and repeat in the same manner. Should there be any indication of other rings making their appearance, try the next remedy.

RHUS TOX. and SULPHUR will be found serviceable in obstinate cases.

DOSE.—Give one drop, or four globules of *Rhus tox.*, and wait four days, and then give a similar dose of *Sulphur;* in each case dissolve the remedy in a spoonful of water; and if no new symptoms appear, this course may be repeated until permanent amelioration or change.

NATRUM MUR., NUX VOMICA and CALCAREA, may be called into requisition in case the fore-mentioned remedies have not produced the desired effect; they may be used alternately.

DOSE.—One drop, or four globules, of each in alternation, as directed for *Rhus tox.* and *Sulphur.*

There is great proneness to resort to external applications in this affection, but such should not be the case, it is always attended with bad results.

10.—Ring-worm of the Scalp. (*Pustular Ring-worm.*)

This affection is sometimes called *Porrigo, Scutulata, Tinea capitis, Tinea annularis, Favus confertus.*

Ring-worm of the scalp is, without doubt, a highly contagious disease, communicating itself readily among children who use the same comb, or brush, or even the same towel for any length of time; it is a baffling disease, and often proves serious in its character when it is dried up, or made to disappear from the surface by external applications; these should never be used except in connection with a judicious course of internal treatment at the same time, and even then, some remedies employed internally, should constitute the external lotion to be applied.

SYMPTOMS.—At the commencement of the affection there are colored irregular circular patches, on which appear numerous small yellowish points or pustules, which do not rise above the level of the skin, and are generally traversed in the centre by a hair; these pustules are more thickly studded in the circumference than in the centre of the circular patches, and they soon break and form thin scabs, which frequently unite with the adjacent patches and assume a regular and extensive appearance of a circular shape, though often irregular in this respect.

The incrustations become thick and hard by accumulation, and are detached from time to time in small pieces, which bear a close resemblance to crumbling mortar.

When the scabs are removed the skin underneath appears red and glossy, studded with slightly elevated pimples, in which there is sometimes minute globules of matter; they immediately collect again thicker than before; the areas of the primary patches extend until they become so blended together that the whole head becomes involved.

The circular character of the original groups is still manifest on the margin of the larger incrustation, which seems circumscribed by partially formed arcs uniting their extremities together. When these clusters spread, the hair covering them begins to disappear, either broken off or thrown out by the roots, until at length there appears only a belt of hair around the head; it is only when the hair follicles become destroyed that the baldness remains permanent.

Scrofulous children are more liable to the disease, and those of an emaciated habit, flabby or feeble, especially if they are not supplied with proper food or sleeping apartments, and are uncleanly and deprived of good and wholesome exercise in the open air.

There are few diseases more stubborn than this affection, even under homœopathic treatment, but in many cases the disease is rendered more stubborn from maltreatment, and also in some cases the disease becomes obstinate from culpable neglect.

TREATMENT.—This, to be successful, must be from the administration of internal remedies mainly; in some cases the same remedy administered internally may be applied externally. The remedies found the most serviceable are Arsenicum, Hepar sulphur, Dulcamara, Bryonia, Rhus tox. and Staphysagria.

ARSENICUM is indicated when the discharge is thin and acrimonious and productive of an extension of disease, or of formation of ulcers; it is useful after some of the other remedies have been used without success.

DOSE.—Dissolve one drop, or six globules, in six teaspoonfuls of water, and give a teaspoonful every night and morning for three days, then wait three, and recur again to the remedy, and pursue the same course; at the expiration of which, if the patient is no better, proceed with some other remedy.

HEPAR SULPHUR may be employed when the eruption is not confined to the head, but appears on the face and forehead, and the eyes and lids become inflamed and weakened, and soreness or ulceration breaks out on or behind the ears.

DOSE.—Dissolve one drop, or six globules, in six teaspoonfuls of water, and give a teaspoonful every morning and evening for three days; if there is no change on the side of improvement by this time, after waiting two days, proceed with the use of *Rhus tox.*

DULCAMARA is more particularly indicated when the

glands of the throat are implicated, become inflamed and tender.

DOSE.—Dissolve one drop, or six globules, in six teaspoonfuls of water, and give a teaspoonful three times a day, for three days, and then discontinue for the same length of time, and then, if there is no perceptible change for the better, proceed again with the remedy a second course, and still if there is no amelioration, proceed with the use of *Bryonia.*

BRYONIA. This remedy may be employed at the onset, in such cases as call for *Dulcamara;* three days after the use of the latter remedy, if the glands of the neck are inflamed and tender, this remedy may be proceeded with.

DOSE—Dissolve one drop, or six globules, in six teaspoonfuls of water, and give a teaspoonful every six hours until amelioration or change. If, however, after the use of *Bryonia* for four days, the predominant symptoms should remain the same, after the immediate indications for the use of *Bryonia* have been subdued, proceed with the use of *Staphysagria.*

STAPHYSAGRIA should be administered, two days after the last dose of the preceding remedy if there is an offensive discharge, breaking out, attended with very violent itching without much redness.

DOSE.—In all respects as directed for *Bryonia.* But if such symptoms should be manifest as call for any of the other remedies, proceed with the use of such as are indicated.

RHUS TOX. will, for the most part, be found most useful, while the patches exhibit an irritable and inflammatory aspect.

DOSE.—Dissolve one drop, or six globules, in six teaspoonfuls of water, and give a teaspoonful morning aad evening ; at the same time, the solution may be applied externally.

SULPHUR should be administered, if the eruption presents a dry, scaly appearance, that exfoliates and forms anew.

DOSE.—One drop, or four globules, in a spoonful of water, may be given every morning for a week ; then discontinue for a week, and then if there is not a permanent amelioration or change, pursue the same course again ; but if there should be a change of symptoms, calling for either of the other remedies named, proceed with the use of the remedy indicated.

32

DIET AND REGIMEN.—When adults are suffering from this affection, or other cutaneous diseases, they should avoid the use of salt meat, mackerel, or other kinds of fish. Children should be restricted, so as to avoid their taking heating, farinaceous food. Regular attention should be paid to cleanliness, and the hair should be removed at an early period of the disease.

11.—Ulcers. (*Ulcera.*)

By an ulcer is understood, a sore of some continuance, which may result from a bruise, burn, or abscess. It may arise from gross or otherwise unwholesome living, —from a bad habit of body, in connection with sedentary habits. When an ulcer arises from this source, its formation is preceded by pain, heat, redness, and swelling of the part. Very frequently small pustules appear, which on bursting, expose gaps or breaches in the skin.

Sometimes there is at the commencement, only a single excavation; at others, there are several contiguous, ulcerated spots, which become blended together and form an ulcer of considerable size.

When an ulcer does not heal, it always presents an excavation or hollow, the margins of which are red, sharp, sometimes thick, rounded, prominent, or callous, and often jagged and irregular, while on the other surface, it is usually covered with, and discharges a thin, watery *humor* or *sanies*, frequently tinged with blood, and sometimes so acrid, as to produce inflammatory excoriation of the skin. When ulceration is taking place, the adjacent skin becomes inflamed and painful; but when it evinces a tendency to heal, this inflammation disappears, and healthy granulations exhibit the appearance of minute cones of a pointed shape, of a firm consistence, and a florid color.

The matter secreted is altered to a bland, thick, and whitish or cream-like fluid, which is denominated "healthy pus," and does not adhere to the granulated surface. These granulations do not rise higher than the surrounding skin, and generally when they have risen to a level with it, those at the edges of the sore become covered with a smooth skin, which at first is semi-transparent, but soon changes to opaque when thoroughly converted into new skin.

TREATMENT. — The principal remedies used in the treatment of ulcers in general, are Arsenicum, Carbo veg., Lachesis, Lycopodium, Mercurius viv., Silicea, Sulphur, Sepia and Nitric acid.

ARSENICUM is indicated when the ulcer looks bloody, and bleeds at the slightest touch, presenting a livid appearance, and instead of healthy pus, secretes an acrid discharge, mixed with blood; the margin at the same time is hard and irregular, and the patient complains of much pain of a burning character.

DOSE·—Dissolve one drop, or six globules, in six teaspoonfuls of water, and give a teaspoonful night and morning, for one week, then discontinue for the same length of time, and then repeat again. Continue this course until amelioration or change.

CARBO VEG. is very useful for similar cases, and is a valuable remedy to use in alternation with *Arsenicum*, especially when the discharge from the ulcer is very offensive, and the burning pains become more aggravated towards evening, and at night, when the ulcer rapidly extends, or is surrounded by numerous pustules, and when there is much swelling and discoloration of the surrounding parts; and if situate on the leg, the ulcer presents a dark blue or purple appearance, and mottled.

DOSE.—As directed for *Arsenicum*, whether used by itself, or as a succeeding remedy, or in alternation, until amelioration or change.

LACHESIS is one of the best remedies when the ulcer is large or seems inclined to spread rapidly, or when surrounded by many small ulcerations or pustules, or much swelling and discoloration of the surrounding parts, and the leg, if implicated, presenting the same appearance as described under *Carbo veg.*

DOSE.—In all respects as directed for *Arsenicum.*

LYCOPODIUM is indicated when the pus is of the color of a citron and the edges of the ulcer are callous or inverted, and an itching almost unendurable; sometimes attended with burning pain at night, in bed. The remedy is also very serviceable in superficial chronic ulcers.

DOSE·—Dissolve one drop, or six globules, in six teaspoonfuls of water, and give a teaspoonful night and morning, for a week. Then discontinue for a week, after which recourse may be had to the same remedy again, and so on until there is permanent amelioration or change.

MERCURIUS VIV. is indicated when the ulcer is deep, and secretes a thin and offensive discharge.

DOSE.—Dissolve one drop, or six globules, in six teaspoonfuls of water, and give a teaspoonful night and morning, or if used in alternation with any of the other remedies, give *Mercurius* in the morning, and the other remedy in the evening, observing that both remedies are to be prepared for administration in the same way.

SILICEA is indicated when the secretion is thick and discolored, and also when the discharge consists of a thin, acrid and offensive sanies, or matter mixed with blood, and particularly in sores with imperfect granulations.

DOSE.—Dissolve one drop, or four globules, in a tablespoonful of water, and give every morning fasting, for a week, then discontinue for the same length of time, and then if there is no improvement, proceed with another remedy.

SULPHUR is one of the chief remedies in almost all ulcers of long standing, and of itself proves salutary in effecting a cure in many chronic cases. It is particularly indicated when there is excessive itching, burning or gnawing; and smarting pains are experienced in the ulcer, which is prone to bleed when dressed, presents no distinct granulations, secretes a fetid sanies, or thick, yellow, unhealthy pus, and has its margins elevated and surrounded by groups of pimples, which increase the irritation of the sore; also when there is a dropsical condition of the legs.

DOSE.—Dissolve one drop, or six globules, in half a tumbler of water, and give a spoonful every twenty-four hours, for three days, then wait a week and repeat, provided there has not been a positive change for the better, in which case it would be better not to give medicine, so long as convalescence seems to be going on. This remedy may be used in alternation with *Mercurius*, giving three doses of the former one week, and three of the latter the next, twenty-four hours between each dose.

SEPIA AND NITRIC ACID.—One or both of these remedies may sometimes be indicated in alternation with *Silicea*, in very intractable cases.

DOSE.—After *Silicea* has been given, according to directions, dissolve one drop, or six globules, of *Sepia*, in six teaspoonfuls of water, and give a spoonful every twenty-four hours, for three days, and afterwards, if necessary, *Nitric acid*, observing not to commence with the last-mentioned remedy until three days have elapsed, after the last dose of either of the former remedies.

GENERAL TREATMENT.—Any ulcer, highly inflamed and painful, may be soothed by saturating soft linen in warm water, and applying it to the sore.

When the ulcer is on the leg, the limb should be kept at rest, and not even in a depending position.

The application of lint dipped in cold water, kept perpetually wet with the same, is a very useful form of dressing, and frequently more effectual than when wet in warm water, more especially when the ulcer presents sharp, jagged edges, with no distinct formation of granu. lations, but exhibits a surface consisting of a whitish spongy substance, covered with a thin discharge of acrid matter, and bleeds from the slightest disturbance.

32*

The application of a moderately tight bandage, will prove of service, when the granulations are sufficiently developed, provided it be properly applied, and particularly when they exhibit a pale color, often large and flabby, with a smooth and glossy surface, the edges of the surrounding skin, being at the same time thick, rounded and prominent; thin and watery pus, mixed with flakes of coagulating lymph, which adheres closely; trifling pain, and the sore by no means sensitive.

External application of the same remedies, used for internal administration, may be found of great service in promoting healthy granulation and cicatrization; but in other cases it will be found sufficient to keep the bandage wet with cold water, giving, however, at the same time, the appropriate internal remedy.

When only external applications are made, to effect a disappearance of the ulcers, their absence will only be temporary, in a majority of instances, for the sole reason that the inherent taint in the system has not been eradicated.

In the treatment of healthy or healing sores, it is better to dress them no oftener than due regard to cleanliness will absolutely require, for it is well to avoid all unnecessary irritations, these will for the most part, retard the healing process, already established; dry lint may be used for the dressing, and change every forty-eight hours, unless the secretion of pus should be so much as to moisten the lint in a shorter period.

Varicose Ulcers.

These ulcers that arise from varicose veins, are, for the most part, obstinate, and difficult to heal, particularly when it is inconvenient, or impossible for the patient to keep at rest. Under such circumstances, great advantage may be found from wearing the lace stocking.

To effect a cure of this kind of ulcerated leg, the main dependence is upon remedies to be taken internally.

ARNICA AND PULSATILLA.—These two medicines, either singly, or alternately, are of great service in effecting a permanent cure. If administered in an early stage of the disease, and even if the varicose ulcer has existed for a long time, these remedies may be regarded of the first importance.

DOSE.—Dissolve, of either, if given singly, one drop, or six globules, in six teaspoonfuls of water, and give a teaspoonful every night and morning for a week, then discontinue for four days, after which, if necessary, the same course may be repeated, and so on, until a change ensues. If the remedies are given in alternation, twelve hours should elapse between them, or perhaps it would be better to give *Arnica* for two days, and then *Pulsatilla* for two days, alternately, until amelioration, or change.

LACHESIS, SULPHUR, SILICEA, ARSENICUM, and CARBO VEG., are respectively of considerable service, when there are indications for their use, and particularly if *Arnica* and *Pulsatilla* have proved insufficient. One or more of these remedies may be called into requisition in completing the healing process.

DOSE.—*Lachesis*, *Arsenicum*, or *Carbo veg.* may be employed in the same way as *Arnica* and *Pulsatilla*. Of *Sulphur* and *Silicea*, give one drop, or four globules, in a spoonful of water every twenty-four hours.

DIET AND REGIMEN.—The diet should be nutritious, avoiding all manner of condiments; salt meats; old fish; old cheese, &c.; and all stimulating or unhealthy beverages.

There are other common affections of the skin, that take the form of *rash*, not clearly characterised. In all such cases when there is fever, the patient must be careful not to take cold, neither should he keep himself too warm; either state may prove injurious.

12.—Hives. (*Or Rash in Children.*)

When hives make their appearance on children, it is better to keep them moderately warm, and give them *Chamomilla*, twice a day, until the disease disappears; or if the child is sick at its stomach, give *Ipecacuanha* or *Bryonia*. (*For further particulars see Eruptive Fevers.*)

DOSE.—Dissolve, of either of the remedies selected, one drop, or six globules, in six teaspoonfuls of water, and give a teaspoonful every three hours, until amelioration or change.

CHAPTER IX.

ORGANS OF RESPIRATION, AND THEIR DISEASES.

1.—General Description of the Organs of Respiration.

THE organs of respiration are the mouth and nose, the throat, the windpipe and its branches, and the lungs, to which might also be added the pleura, diaphragm, and in some sense the ribs, the muscles of the thorax and abdomen.

The organs most immediately concerned in respiration are the windpipe, larynx and trachea, its branches, the bronchia, and the lungs, (*often called the " lights."*

Respiration itself is the act of inhaling and expiring, (*drawing into the chest, and throwing out from it*) the air or atmosphere.

All the organs of respiration are to a high degree capable of expansion and contraction, that is they can be stretched out or drawn in, spread out or puckered up, as may be necessary for the performance of their several offices.

Upon this expansive and contractive power m$_{uch}$ of their usefulness is dependant. If it be in any way interfered with, their usefulness is to that extent diminished. If it be interrupted their usefulness is lost.

The use of the act of respiration, the function performed by those organs, is to impart life to and take away impurities from the blood.

It is supposed to impart life by supplying oxygen, which is one of the constituents of atmospheric air, and to take away impurities by carrying off carbonic acid, which is one of the principal ingredients of all dead or decaying substances.

If "life is in the blood," and is conveyed to it by every inspiration of air, if death is in the carbonic acid which is conveyed out at every successive expiration, it will be seen how essential is this function to the continuance of life and health.

Upon the perfect expansive and contractive power of the organs of respiration, the life and health of the body is constantly dependant. If these are to any extent interrupted, all the other parts must suffer. If they are lost, the other organs perish.

The organs by which so important a function is performed would afford an interesting theme for years of study and research, whilst the diseases to which these organs are liable, already form no inconsiderable portion of the science of medicine.

When it is remembered that nearly one-third of the whole number of deaths which occur in a community are from diseases connected with the respiratory system, it will be seen how highly important is a more perfect knowledge of the functions and the disorders of that system, to all those who would in any way administer to the relief of the sick.

In their external appearance the organs immediately concerned in respiration, namely, the windpipe and lungs, might not inaptly be compared to a small tree or shrub, having two large and numerous small branches, densely set with leaves or foliage. The roots of this tree will be found in the throat or larynx, extending upwards around the roots of the tongue and the cavities of the nose and mouth. The trunk is the windpipe. The branches of the windpipe (*bronchial tubes,*) are the limbs and the substance of the lungs, constitutes the leaves of the tree, rolled up into little cells, (*air cells of the lungs,*) exceedingly minute, but capable of immense expansion and contraction. These air cells or leaves are surrounded and connected together by a peculiar yielding, elastic and compressible substance, for which I know no other name than parenchyma, which like a net-work encloses each little cell, and connects and encloses the whole together, giving to the lungs their shape or form.

From the comparison I have just made, it is easy to form a conception of the location of these organs, or the place they occupy in the body. This tree, it will be perceived, has its roots upward, its trunk and limbs extending downwards into the chest. The wind-pipe or trachea, extends from the throat or larynx, to the upper part of the breast-bone, just below the pit of the throat, where it divides into two large branches,—one passing towards the right, and the other towards the left side. These branches afterwards divide and subdivide continu-ally, until they are lost in the air cells of the lungs, and have received the name of bronchia or bronchial tubes.

The lungs, properly speaking, that is, the air cells, connected together by the net-work or parenchyma with which they are always invested, spring out from, and envelope the bronchia, or branches of the windpipe, somewhat like the leaves of a tree from its branches, each small cell being so connected with its parent stem, that the one seems actually to run into and to pervade the substance of the other.

The lungs extend from the breast bone, a short distance below the throat pit, towards the right and left side, occupying the upper and back parts of the chest, pressing upward towards the shoulders, and when they are full and strong, occupying all the cavities between the bony structures around what are popularly termed the shoulder and collar bones, and so filling up the chest, as to give that peculiar round and plump appearance, which is at once an element of beauty, and an indication of health. Or, to keep up the comparison of the tree, branches of the lungs appear to extend upward and outward, towards the windpipe and towards the shoulders, as the branches of a tree, sometimes hang downwards and outwards towards the trunk, and towards the earth, upon which, the branches of a tree are sometimes even found reclining.

The lungs extend downward along the spine, to the region of the angle of the shoulder-blades, where they are separated from the liver, by a large and thin muscular sheet called the diaphragm, which extends downwards and forwards, to the lower attachments of the ribs, and to the breast bone. This sheet or membrane, divides the chest into two cavities or apartments, the upper one of which, called by physicians the thorax, is completely filled with the heart and lungs, which consequently press constantly, as it were, upon the diaphragm, as they do also, upon the walls of the thorax, all along the region of the ribs in front, (except a portion of the left side, which is occupied by the heart,) and above the shoulder-blades, behind or along the back.

It will be perceived that the diaphragm, from its peculiar location alongside the lungs, may be affected with, disease, which will create cough and difficult respiration. These diseases will be considered in their proper place.

The lungs, in addition to their own proper tissue and covering, are separated from the walls of the thorax, and from the heart, by an additional covering which is called the pleura, and is the seat of the disease called pleurisy. This covering is divided into two parts,—one for the right, and one for the left lung, forming two large sacks, which investing each lung, have a common union along the spine, from which they are reflected upon the walls of the chest, and upon the diaphragm.

From the intimate connection which exists between all these organs, it will be seen how diseases of the one, will necessarily affect the other, and how necessary is a knowledge of their exact locations, connections, and dependance, each upon the other, to anything like a true and just understanding of the disease or diseases, with which any one of them may be affected. Hence, the more knowledge we give to the world, or to mankind at large, of themselves, and of the delicate structure of their own organism, the more likely they are to apply to some intelligent physician, in every emergency, or for any disease with which they may be affected, whilst ignorance is the support of mountebanks and quacks.

Having taken a hasty glance at the organs of respiration from without, or an external view, our next object will be to view them from within. Without, we find organs and tissues, within cavities and tubes. From the cavities of the mouth, nose and throat, if we descend within the wind-pipe, larynx and trachea, we find a tube of considerable size, several inches in length, and about an inch in diameter, though varying according to age, size, or idiosyncrasies of the subject, which extending the whole length of the trachea, and opening into each of the bronchia, stretches through all their divisions and ramifications, to the remotest air cells of the lungs, of which tubes, these air cells themselves seem to be only continuations and expansions.

Or to continue the figure of the tree. Our tree, we find, is a hollow tube; all its branches are hollow; every twig is hollow, and contains in itself a tube; all its leaves are cavities; and each part is possessed of an expansive and contractive power, adapting it to its peculiar function, the reception and expulsion of air.

Thus far I have considered the organs of respiration in regard to their anatomical relations, and functional use, it remains to consider the various tissues or structures, of which these organs are composed, with the usefulness, the connections, and dependencies of each; from which we can pass with ease, to a consideration of the various diseases to which they are subject.

And first. Of the skins or coverings of the respiratory organs. All the parts of the body are covered with a skin, or membrane. The body itself is covered; all its internal organs are covered, each with its own skin; every muscle has a covering; all the cavities are coated or clothed; every vein, artery, nerve, or other organ, however minute, is enveloped by its own separate sheath, covering, or skin, which serves to protect it from contact with external objects, as well as to secrete some

33

peculiar fluid, adapted to some particular want or necessity of the organ itself.

Passing from the external to the internal parts of the
body, if we enter the mouth, we find the external
covering or skin of the body is continued within that
cavity, but so altered in its nature, as to secrete
constantly from its surface, a peculiar fluid, which lubri
cates all its parts, gives to the organs contained in the
mouth, a soft and pleasant feel, and enables each organ
contained therein, to perform its office without unduly
infringing upon the repose of any other organ. This
skin is continuous through all those tubes, pipes, cells, or
other cavities, which open into, and therefore may be
said to be exposed in any degree to the influence of the
atmosphere. It differs from the external skin, or the
skin of the body, but little more than different parts of
that skin differ from each other. It lines, of course, not
only the mouth and nose, but the throat, the larynx, the
windpipe, the bronchia, and all the minutest air cells of
the lungs. It is usually the first, and from its exposed
situation, usually the most liable, to be affected with
disease, and its diseases, if duly arested, are most easy of
repair. It is the only tissue connected with the organ
of respiration, for which it is safe for an uneducated
physician or nurse, for any length of time to continue to
prescribe, and even in these diseases, if they do not
yield promptly to the medicines prescribed, it is better
to seek the aid of wisdom and experience. When it lines
any internal cavity, tube or cell, it is called mucus membrane, mucus coat, &c., and its secretions are termed
mucus secretions.

Exactly opposed to the mucus coatings, which line
the internal parts of the respiratory organs, and are

adapted to defend these organs from injury by too close contact with the atmosphere or with any other external objects, is the serous coat, which lines the external parts. This coat completely covers all these organs, wherever they lie along side of, or come into proximity with, any other organs or parts of the body. It is frequently reflected or doubled in, so as to form a kind of medium or middle line between different parts of the same organ, and whenever it is in health, it secretes from its free surface, a slimy, tenacious, oily-feeling substance, called serum. This substance, to any one who examines the system as a machine, appears to lubricate each organ, to render its motion more easy and free, or in other words to prevent friction. This serous coat, being exceedingly smooth in itself, when it is also lubricated by this healthy secretion from its own surfaces, presents the least possible resistance to the free motion of any and every portion of the organ with which it is connected, and consequently renders it eminently adapted to that constant activity which pervades the lungs, pleura, diaphragm, and other parts of the respiratory aparatus.

Between the mucus and serous coatings (or if in any portion the serous coat be wanting, its place is generally supplied by a substance called areola or cellular tissue of a nature very similar to the serous coat) is found the substance or tissue of which the organ itself is composed, which in the organs of respiration is generally either muscular or cartilagenous. This tissue is to the highest degree elastic and compressible in the lungs themselves, whilst in some of the other organs as the windpipe and its branches, the throat and nose, it is more firm, unyielding and dense, bearing an affinity to the softer bones, and is called cartilage.

We thus find in the respiratory organs four distinct varieties of substance, and two entirely different secretions, liable to be affected with different forms of disease; and it may be well to remark, that these substances are liable to considerable modification in the different organs where they occur, as are also the diseases to which they are subject.

All the parts of every organ are of course supplied with two distinct sets of blood vessels, the arteries and veins, by means of which they are themselves supported and nourished; and with two distinct sets of nerves, by which sensation is produced, and in which, to a considerable extent, the power of motion rests. In addition to this, the lungs are pervaded in every part by another distinct set of blood-vessels, the pulmonary arteries and the pulmonary veins, by means of which all the blood of the whole body is conveyed through the lungs, for the purpose of being brought into such proximity with atmospheric air as to become both enlivened and purified.

These organs are also subject to the disorders incident to their use or function, and are to be carefully regarded in determining the diseases with which any of the organs of respiration may be affected.

2.—Diseases of the Respiratory Organs.

From the description already given of the organs of respiration, it will be inferred that they are liable to a variety of diseases. The mucus membrane, having so close an affinity with the skin, might be expected to be affected with similar diseases to those to which the skin is subject, with such variations and modifications as might arise from the peculiar conditions and functions of each organ. The serous coatings, will, of course, be more exposed to that class of diseases which usually affect serous surfaces, whilst the muscular, vascular, and other tissues, will each one of them be more liable to the diseases usually affecting those tissues in other parts of the body.

To prescribe intelligently and well for the diseases of any of these organs, it is therefore necessary to consider, not only the organ which is affected with disease, but the tissue or tissues upon which the disease is located; observing that this is always to be discovered by the symptoms, provided all the symptoms are taken into consideration, and not by any particular theory or theories, which may be involved in such terms as pneumonia, catarrh, cold in the head, cold on the breast, &c., or the more fashionable terms, Bronchitis, Laryngitis, Stomatitis, &c., terms much more frequently resorted to as a cloak for ignorance, than as a means of expressing anything definite or certainly known.

These names of diseases, or rather the confidence that has been reposed in them, has been a constant source of injury, both to the profession of medicine and to the public at large. If a case of bronchitis, for instance, has been cured by a given remedy, that remedy has been afterwards lauded and relied on, not only by the public, but too often by the physician, to cure every case which could be called bronchitis, not considering that the bronchia are a series of organs, composed of various tissues, and that an injury, irritation, or a lesion of one of these tissues, might arise from very different sources, and require very different treatment from that which would be requisite for the relief or cure of another.

It is not my purpose, in a work designed only for domestic use, to illustrate at length every subject of this

33*

nature, to which it may appear to be duty to refer. It is as important for the uneducated, non-professional practitioner, to know when to stop his ministrations, and why he should go no further, as it is to know how far he may proceed with safety; and I would here caution every practitioner, whether professional or non-professional, educated or uneducated, against attributing his lack of success, to any lack of efficiency in the remedies employed. It is much more probably to be attributed to his ignorance of the nature of the disease he has to combat, and consequently, of the adaptedness of any given remedy or class of remedies, to the specific purpose he wishes to accomplish. The intelligent layman who uses this work, will, whenever he finds himself at a loss, repair at once, to the more intelligent, because better educated physician, and the physician himself, if in any case his ministrations fail, will read and re-read the chart which nature has given, viz., the symptoms, in order to discover whether he has indeed, so affiliated his remedies, that he ought to expect a cure. Without this care, all medical practice is little better than empiricism, and the practitioner of medicine, whether professional or otherwise, is only an ignorant charlatan or quack. With it, medicine is exalted to a science, and the practice of the profession to a rank among the most liberal and humanizing arts.

3.—Of Cold in General.

It should be borne in mind that diseases of the organs of respiration frequently either originate in or are excited and made to manifest themselves by a cold, a term which is used to designate the effects produced upon the system by sudden changes of temperature, or by too long exposure to dampness, wetting the feet, &c.

These effects are usually first manifested upon the skin and upon the mucus surface, and produce smartings, stingings, burnings, swellings, irritations, or sense of rawness, sneezing, coughs, pimples, vesicular eruptions, salivation or watery discharge from the mouth and throat; running at the nose, first of a thin watery fluid, second of thick mucus, phlegm, or thick mucus from the mouth, throat and lungs; stoppage of the nose; stoppage of the throat; painfulness of the parts; soreness; sensitiveness to touch; oppression and other sufferings.

The attentive observer cannot but be struck with the similarity of the effects produced by a cold upon the internal parts, to those effects which are perhaps still more plainly seen upon the external parts, and it is but reasonable to draw from this analogy some reflections upon the treatment most effectual for a common cold.

This more commonly commences in the internal surface (mucus lining) of the nose, though at times it may appear first on the lips, skin, mouth, throat, or any of the other organs, especially if by any chronic weakness those organs are more subject to irritation than they would be in a healthy state.

Hence we shall first treat of cold in the head, and afterwards shall proceed to consider cold on the chest and the other organs of respiration.

4.—Cold in the Head.
(*Coryza. Catarrh. Catarrh in the Head, &c.*)

The first symptoms in their natural order, or when uncomplicated with other-diseases, are tingling, itching, with a sense of dryness, and partial, though perhaps slight obstruction of the nose; sneezing; running of a watery secretion; and as the symptoms progress, accumulation of thick mucus in the nose, more especially in children; entire obstruction of one or both nostrils; hawking, tickling of the throat, coughing, &c.

At this stage it may perhaps always be arrested by the use of appropriate remedies and care; but if not arrested, it may ultimately involve the throat, windpipe, lungs and chest.

Whilst it is confined to the nose and the external parts, it is but slightly dangerous, and is hardly thought to be of sufficient importance to demand medical treatment, which it assuredly is not, if that treatment must involve such a routine of harsh remedies as is usually prescribed by the allopathic school.

In this appears the superiority of homœopathy. It meets disease in its incipient stages no less than in its later developments. It prescribes for its earliest symptoms, and by an appropriate use of specifics, the use of which it teaches with scientific accuracy, and with the most absolute certainty it cures most safely, most pleasantly, and most surely. Hence in these early manifestations of disease, the attentive student of nature need never be mistaken, and a truly homœopathic prescription will never disappoint his reasonable expectations.

The medicines usually called for in this case, are Aconite, Arsenicum, Belladonna, Bryonia, Chamomilla, Causticum, Euphrasia, Hepar sulph., Lycopodium, Mercurius viv., Nitric acid, Nux vomica, Phosphorus, Pulsatilla, Rhus tox., Sambucus, Silicea and Sulphur.

ACONITE is indicated for persons of florid complexion, lively character, sanguine temperament, especially if the cold be the result of exposure to a dry north-west wind, and attended with erysipelatous tumefactions of the lips, nose or face; violent sneezing, with pain in the abdomen and left side; coryza, with catarrh; pain in the head; buzzing in the ears, and colic; or with burning and ' pricking in the throat, especially when swallowing.

DOSE.—One drop of the dilution, or six globules, in six spoonfuls of water; give a spoonful every two hours, until amelioration or change. After *Aconite*, give *Phosphorus, Mercurius viv., Belladonna* or *Hepar sulph.*

ARSENICUM is indicated for persons of leucophlegmatic constitution, with tendency to dropsical complaints, or for those of lymphatic constitutions, with tendency to eruptions, tetter, or bleeding or burning ulcers, especially if the burning pains are in the interior parts, and if the skin be dry, with pricking itchings, and if there be profuse bleeding at the nose, with swelling and dryness of the nostrils; but especially if with the stoppage of the nose there be abundant secretion of thin and corrosive mucus, and burning in the nostrils; sense of debility or prostration; weakness. After *Rhus tox., Belladonna, or Nux vomica.*

DOSE.—One drop of the dilution, or six globules, in ten spoonfuls of water, a spoonful to be given every four hours, until amelioration or change,

BRYONIA.—Temperament dry, meagre, bilious; complexion dark, with brown or black hair and eyes; irritable. If the nose be swollen and painful to the touch, with frequent bleeding; stinging in the forehead; obstinate dry coryza; hard mucus drying in scabs; lips swollen and cracked, or dry eruptions, with burnings and smartings; sensation as if the ears were stopped; worse in the evening; and also if the cold extends to the chest, with cough and bursting headache.

DOSE.—One drop of the dilution, or six globules, in six spoonfuls of water, give a spoonful every two hours, afterwards give *Mercurius viv.* or *Rhus tox,* according to the symptoms.

BELLADONNA.—Pains in the nose, aggravated by touch or by movement; swelling, redness, and burning of the nose; nose very cold; smell at times acute, at times diminished, offensive or putrid; coryza of one nostril, or stoppage of the nose, especially with pains in the head, aggravated by movement; or with vertigo, swelling of the veins, and pulsations of the arteries.

DOSE.—One drop of the dilution, or six globules, in ten spoonfuls of water, give a spoonful every four hours, in alternation with *Aconite*, *Mercurius*, or some other indicated remedy.

CHAMOMILLA.—Obstruction of the nose; inflammation or ulceration of the nostrils, with very acute smell; dryness of the mouth and tongue; blisters or aphthæ (canker) in the mouth; putrid smell from the mouth, especially for children.

DOSE.—One drop of the dilution, or six globules, in ten spoonfuls of water, give a spoonful every two hours, until amelioration or change.

CAUSTICUM.—Dry, chronic coryza, with eruption on the point of the nose; blowing of blood, or discharge of fetid mucus from the nose; loss of smell; worse in the morning;

DOSE.—See *Hepar*.

EUPHRASIA.—Profuse flowing coryza by day, with obstruction of the nose at night; corrosive tears, with redness of the eyes; painful sensibility of the nostrils; confusion in the head.

DOSE.—The same as *Belladonna*, *Hepar sulph.*, *Sulphur*.

HEPAR SULPHUR.—When one nostril is implicated, or with headache, aggravated by slight movement; inflammatory swelling of the nose, with pain as from a bruise when touched. After *Belladonna* or *Mercurius viv.*

DOSE.—One drop of the dilution, or six globules, in ten spoonfuls of water, give a spoonful every four hours.

LYCOPODIUM.—For chronic or acute choryza; entire obstruction of the nostrils, especially at night; respiration through the mouth only; dryness of the nose, mouth and tongue, with excessive acuteness of smell; nostrils ulcerated, scabby, obstructed with mucus; confusion in the head; burning pain in the forehead, worse at night. After *Belladonna* or *Mercurius viv.*

DOSE.—One drop, of the dilution, or six globules, dissolved in ten spoonfuls of water, give a spoonful every four hours, until a change is effected.

MERCURIUS VIV.—Dry or flowing coryza, with frequent sneezing; swelling, shivering, redness and itching of the nose; or with discharge of corrosive serum, or fetid, acrid pus; obstinate headache, and pains, even in the bones; swelling of the bones of the nose; scabs in the nose. After *Belladonna* or *Nux vomica.*

DOSE.—One drop of the dilution, or six globules, in ten spoonfuls of water, give a spoonful every four hours, until amelioration, or change.

NUX VOMICA.—Coryza, when attended with inflammation; dry coryza, with heat and heaviness in the forehead, and obstruction of the nose; flowing coryza in the morning; dryness and obstruction at night; insupportable itching, scraping in the nostrils, and burning, with frequent sneezings; great acuteness of smell; offensive smell.

DOSE.—One drop of the dilution, or six globules, to be dissolved in ten spoonfuls of water, give a spoonful every four hours, until amelioration, or change.

PHOSPHORUS.—Nose red and swollen, with dry and hard scabs in the nose; ulcerated nostrils; constant discharge of yellow mucus from the nose; acute sense, or entire loss of smell; obstruction of the nose, especially in the morning. After *Bryonia* or *Rhus tox.*

DOSE.—One drop of the dilution, or six globules, in ten spoonfuls of water, give a spoonful every four hours, until amelioration or change.

PULSATILLA.—Loss of taste and smell; shivering, if relieved in the open air, and worse in a warm room;

tickling; frequent sneezing; with obstruction and dry coryza, worse in the evening, and heat of room; painful pressure, as if an abscess at the root of the nose; ulceration of the nostril, with discharge of fetid or yellowish pus; and if there be shooting, sharp, drawing pains, extending into the ears and sides of the head, and especially if the pains are changing from place to place.

DOSE.—One drop of the dilution, or six globules, in ten spoonfuls of water, give a spoonful every four hours, until amelioration, or change.

RHUS TOX.—Swelling and redness of the nose, or around the lips; violent spasmodic sneezings; dryness, with pain, as if the nose were raw; burnings, crawlings, and shootings; painful crawlings in the nose and head; bleeding at the nose, especially at night, or when stooping; all the symptoms being aggravated by rest, especially for persons subject to erysipelas.

DOSE·—One drop of the dilution. or six globules, in ten spoonfuls of water, give a spoonful every two hours, for twelve hours, after which, give *Arsenicum* or *Mercurius viv.*

SILICEA.—Chronic coryza, with disposition to take cold in the head; gnawing pains high up, or in the bones of the nose; long continued, dry coryza, with loss of smell, or with constant sneezing.

DOSE.—Give a spoonful of the dilution, every twelve hours.

GRAPHITES or SILICEA, for frequently recuring colds.

NATRUM MUR., for cold in the head, with obstruction of the nose every second day.

LACHESIS, if with much swelling, there be a watery secretion.

SULPHUR, in many obstinate cases.

It will be seen that for all the varieties of affections of the nose and head, called coryza, or cold in the head, homœopathy has no lack of properly adapted remedies. These remedies should be prescribed with care as well as with confidence, and implicitly relied on. They will seldom disappoint us, whilst they will much more frequently surprise us, by the rapidity, the certainty, and the ease, with which they remove the most troublesome symptoms, and prepare the wav for the restoration of health.

5.—Cold on the Chest.—Catarrh.—Catarrh on the Breast. Catarrhal Fever, &c.

This disease appears at times to prevail as an epidemic, when its symptoms are in general, more severe, and it has received the name of Influenza, Grippe, or Epidemic Catarrh.

It usually commences with similar symptoms to a cold in the head, such as sneezing, stoppage of the nose, &c., to which is added oppression across the breast, tickling in the throat, sense of rawness or burning in the throat, cough, at first dry, afterwards with more or less abundant secretion of mucus; sputa, at first thin and watery, afterwards becoming more thick and opaque; slight febrile symptoms, such as chilliness, difficult breathing, and pain, especially in the head, aggravated by coughing.

In severe cases, the cough is violent, occurs in paroxysms, accompanied by severe pain, with sense of soreness or laceration, extending along under the breastbone, nearly to the stomach pit, or with shooting pains to the back and sides: more oppression and prostration of strength, with fever; at times, the fits of coughing occasion vomiting, or they may be accompanied with pain in any portion of the chest,—even in the lowest portion of the bowels or in the loins. Whilst the disease progresses, the sputa becomes more viscid, ropy and stringy: but as it terminates in health, it assumes a

34

yellowish or whitish aspect, is more easily expectorated, and loses its viscid, ropy character.

The sputa of a common catarrh, if uncomplicated, will always be suspended in water.

When the disease prevails as an epidemic, the above symptoms are generally more severe, accompanied with great prostration of strength, sleepiness, giddiness, aching pressive pains, which seem to pervade the whole system, even to the bones; dry, burning heat of the skin, or offensive sweats, when it receives the name of Influenza, or Grippe.

The remedies are Aconite, Arsenicum, Bryonia, Belladonna, Chamomilla, Camphor, Conium, Causticum, Dulcamara, Hepar sulph., Mercurius viv., Phosphorus, Pulsatilla, and Rhus tox.

ACONITE is indicated at the commencement of an attack, particularly, if from exposure to severe cold, or to a dry cold wind: and if there be dry, hot skin, or shivering and heat, with thirst, dryness, roughness, excoriation, or scraping in the throat or chest, with short, dry cough, restless sleep, confused dreams, rapid pulse, pains in the head, abdomen, and left side, with violent sneezing, coryza, and bleeding at the nose.

DOSE.—One drop, or six globules, in ten spoonfuls of water; give a spoonful every two hours, until amelioration or change. After *Aconite, Hepar sulph., Mercurius viv.,* or *Phosphorus* may be indicated.

ARSENICUM. If there be marked remissions and exacerbations, with great prostration, or sense of weakness, and desire to lie down; burning pains, especially in the head, and dryness of the mouth and throat; dry, fatiguing cough, with mucus which clings to the throat so as to be raised with difficulty, worse in the evening or at night, and after drinking; or if the cough be excited

by a stifling sensation in the throat, with sense of constriction in the chest, short breath, anguish and anxiety ;
corrosive burning and sanguineous mucus from the nose,
or from the mouth and throat, with offensive breath;
burning sensations in the mouth, throat or nose; pain in
the limbs with shivering. After *Aconite, Nux vomica* or
Rhus tox.

DOSE.—One drop of the dilution, or six globules, in six spoonfuls of
water ; give a spoonful every four hours, until amelioration or change.

BELLADONNA may be indicated, at any period, if the
cough be spasmodic, with sore throat, insupportable
throbbing headache, as if the head would burst, aggravated by talking or movement, by light and exposure to
air. It is appropriate after *Aconite*, or in alternation
with or after *Hepar sulph.* or *Mercurius viv.*, but may be
given in alternation with any other remedy, should the
symptoms appear to require it.

DOSE.—One drop of the dilution, or six globules, dissolved in ten
spoonfuls of water, a spoonful to be given every two hours, until amelioration or change.

BRYONIA will be found useful, if the cough be dry,
with tickling in the throat, hoarseness, sensibility or
soreness to the touch of the throat and nose, with discharge of a watery secretion ; or if the cough be cramp-
like, suffocating, with tenacious, slimy mucus in the
throat; stinging in the sides of the chest; pains in the
head as if it would burst; pressure towards the forehead, or pulsative pains, aggravated by every movement; or if the cough appears to proceed from the
stomach, or is attended with pain at the stomach pit, or
pain in the right or left hypochondria. *Bryonia* is useful at the onset, or after *Aconite*, and may be followed
by *Nux vomica,* or *Phosphorus*, according as the condition of the patient shall require.

DOSE.—One drop of the dilution, or six globules, in ten spoonfuls of water; a spoonful to be given every two hours, until amelioration or change.

CAMPHOR will be found useful if there be a sense of chilliness or coldness over the body, or if the catarrh be caused or preceded by a chill, with symptoms of approaching fever, as shivering, weariness, uneasiness, heaviness, with burning heat in the throat, and tendency to èrysipelatous inflammation of the face, and coldness of the skin.

DOSE.—Take a drop of the spirits of camphor on sugar every half hour, for two or three hours, then select some other remedies for the remaining symptoms,

CHAMOMILLA is indicated for hoarse, catarrhal cough, and cough resulting from a chill, with sore throat; obstruction of the nose; redness of the skin of the face, mouth or throat, with miliary éruption, or with aphthæ in the mouth; pains in the stomach, face, teeth, ears or head, especially in children, with fretfulness, restlessness and anxiety; chilliness from slight causes, or burning heat in one part and chilliness in another; also if the cough be worse at night.

DOSE.—One drop of the dilution, or six globules, dissolved in ten spoonfuls of water, may be given every three hours, a spoonful until amelioration or change. After *Chamomilla, Mercurius,* or *Hepar sulph.,* if indicated.

CONIUM, especially for epidemic catarrh, or influenza, or if the cold be accompanied by fever, with internal heat and thirst; great debility; scrapings or creeping, itching, sensations in the throat, which produce incessant cough; impatient of the slightest noise; unrefreshing, restless sleep; anxious dreams; obstruction of the nose; buzzing in the ears; and especially if with the cough there be pains in the abdomen or in the side, with rumbling of wind.

DOSE.—One drop of the dilution, or six globules, dissolved in ten spoonfuls of water, give a spoonful every four hours. After *Nux vomica* or *Arsenicum,*

CAUSTICUM.—If there be obstinate hoarseness, with loss of voice; spasmodic or convulsive cough, worse in the night or towards morning; great sensibility to cold; tightness in the head, with shooting pains, and sensation of a gauze or mist before the eyes; rumbling or buzzing in the ears and head, with obstruction of the nose or ears, especially if there be also an accumulation of mucus in the throat, which can only be expectorated by hawking or gagging; and a sense of excoriation, with stinging pain when swallowing; or a short, dry cough, excited by tickling in the throat, with burning pains in the throat and chest.

DOSE.—One drop of the dilution, or six globules, dissolved in six spoonfuls of water; a spoonful to be given every four hours, until amelioration or change. After *Hepar sulph.* or *Chamomilla.*

DULCAMARA.—If the sufferings are worse at night, and have been caused by exposure to wet or dampness; in obstinate catarrh, with hoarseness, moist cough, like hooping cough, with reddish colored expectoration; especially if there be sensation of heaviness in the head, with buzzing in the ears, and pains in the limbs aggravated by rest, and accompanied by coldness or numbness. It is suitable before or after *Causticum*, or after *Hepar sulph.* or *Mercurius viv.*

DOSE.—One drop of the dilution, or six globules, may be given in ten spoonfuls of water, a spoonful every two hours, until amelioration or change.

HEPAR SULPH. will be found useful if there be a sensation in the throat as if there were a tumor or a plug in it, with hawking up of mucus, or sense as if there were much mucus in the throat, with ringing and pain in the head as if it were going to burst; also pain with stinging

34*

and soreness, extending even to the ears, especially if the patient be subject to herpetic or scrofulous affections, or if there be symptoms of tuberculous ulceration, swelling of the glands, and shooting pains, the parts being painful when touched, worse by exposure to cold air and motion.

DOSE.—One drop of the dilution, or six globules, may be put in ten spoonfuls of water, a spoonful to be given every four hours, until amelioration or change. *Hepar sulph.* is especially useful after *Mercurius viv.*, or it may be alternated with *Bryonia, Aconite* or *Phosphorus*, to advantage.

MERCURIUS VIV. is indicated for a dry fatiguing shaking cough, excited by a tickling dryness in the throat, impeding speech, worse at night and in bed; or cough with febrile shivering and heat; swelling of the throat; profuse lacrymation and salivation; running or obstruction of the nose, with sensation of a tumor in the throat, and constant disposition to swallow; offensive smell from the mouth; bitter or offensive taste; much thirst; pains in the limbs and in the joints, and especially if there be profuse sweat which affords no relief. To persons subject to suffer from cold, affected with swelling of the glands, sore throats or lymphatic abscesses, it may be given in the onset of the disease, either alone or in alternation with *Belladonna*, and followed by *Hepar sulphur*, should the symptoms appear to require it. For persons subject to hepatic complaints, it is especially efficacious after *Bryonia* or *Chamomilla*, and in persons subject to rheumatism before or after *Dulcamara*.

DOSE.—One drop of the dilution, or six globules, may be dissolved in half a tumbler of water, a spoonful to be given every four hours, until amelioration or change.

NUX VOMICA is one of the most prompt and efficacious remedies for a cold, especially if there be constipation or costiveness, or if the patient be subject to hemorrhoids, of a dry and bilious, or of a lymphatic and exhausted constitution, sanguine, or nervous and excitable temperament, and especially for persons addicted to the use of wine, spirits, coffee, or narcotic drugs. It is especially indicated if there be a dry cough in the morning, and occasionally during the day, with little or no cough at night. After a fit of coughing, a small quantity of adhesive mucus is with difficulty expectorated; if at every fit of coughing there be bursting headache, sore pain at the stomach pit, or in the abdomen and around the umbilicus, or if there be wandering fever, chills, worse during movement, alternating with flashes of heat, pains as from a bruise in the hypochondria and back; nausea or want of appetite; confusion in the head, with giddiness. It is also of great utility for persons subject to chronic gastritis, or hepatitis, in which case the cold is likely to be complicated with gastric or hepatic complaints, such as a sense of weight at the stomach pit, tensive feeling across the hypochondria, perhaps with nausea and vomiting. This remedy has an extensive range of action in all diseases of this nature, and is generally adapted to the earlier stages of catarrh to subdue the more prominent symptoms, after which *Mercurius viv.*, *Hepar sulph.*, *Arsenicum*, *Bryonia* or *Phosphorus* may be indicated. It is useful after *Aconite* or *Bryonia*, and may occasionally be given in alternation with or after almost any other remedy, should the symptoms manifestly require it.

DOSE.—One drop of the dilution, or six globules, in half a tumbler of water, a spoonful to be given every four houis until amelioration or change. It is often useful to give *Nux vomica* in the after, and some other remedy, in the fore part of the day.

PHOSPHORUS, especially if there be great sensibility to cold air, and coryza with fever, shiverings, and headache; hoarseness, loss of voice; cough, with dryness in the throat; and stingings, with sense of constriction; or with pains in the stomach and abdomen. The pains in the throat are tensive, and burning, or smarting and stinging, often as if the chest were raw. Also pressure in the throat, and constrictive, pressive sensation in the chest, or with symptoms of congestion of the throat, chest, and-lungs; pulse quick and hard; disturbed sleep; tossing about with startings and fright, or with lamentations, and moaning during sleep. *Phosphorus* may follow *Bryonia* or *Rhus tox.*

DOSE.—One drop of the dilution, or six globules, may be dissolved in ten spoonfuls of water, a spoonful to be given every four hours, until amelioration or change.

PULSATILLA is considered specific for colds, with cough, worse at night, with evening chills; sneezing; loss of smell and taste; pain in the forehead; with fulness, expectoration, thick, yellowish, or green, tenacious, and bitter, constriction in the throat, with shaking cough, worse at night, and when lying down; and if there be shooting or sharp drawing pains, which change rapidly from place to place; also if the sufferings affect one side only; or are accompanied with leucorrhœa.

DOSE.—Dissolve one drop of the dilution, or six globules, in half a tumbler of water, give a teaspoonful of the solution every two hours.

RHUS TOX. is especially indicated when there is redness of the skin, with tendency to erysipelatous eruptions around the nose and mouth; with burning itching in the throat; sensation of contraction in the throat, with difficulty in swallowing; pressure and shootings; great anxiety, and restlessness, with drawing, pressive sensations, especially at night; crawlings, creepings, or shiverings, with thirst.

DOSE.—One drop of the dilution, or six globules, in half a tumbler of water, give a spoonful every three hours, until amelioration, or change.

In epidemic catarrh, or influenza, the medicines should

always be selected according to the foregoing indications, and if promptly and wisely administered, the disease will always be found to yield, much more readily, and certainly, than has ever been seen, under allopathic administration.

It will be remembered that cold, coryza, or catarrh, is a usual precursor, if not a producing cause, of nearly all the diseases of the respiratory organs. Its treatment, therefore, will be found to run into, and connect itself to a greater or less extent with the treatment which will be necessary in those diseases. In the natural order of those diseases, the next subject to be considered, is

6.—Cough. (*Tussis.*)

A cough is always a symptom of some other disease. Although it might, at first view, be regarded as a disease in itself, it is, in fact, only an effort of nature to rid itself of a diseased condition, or to throw off accumulations which disease has created. It is nonsense to call it "*a forcible and violent expiration without fever.*" A man can make a great number of such expirations, and not cough. It is only that peculiar effort of nature, which is made for the purpose of expelling from the respiratory organs, offensive matter, which can be denominated a cough. This offensive matter may or may not be already exuded upon the internal surface of the organ. Whether it exists in the form of an exudation, of a congestion, of an eruption, or of a simple irritation, it is still there, and nature gets up an excitement to rid itself of the diseased condition. The result, or rather the manifestation and combination of the results, is cough.

Let no physician then, and certainly no homœopath, ever boast of curing a cough. It is not the cough he wishes to cure, but the disease which causes it; and unless. he can discover, with at least some degree of certainty, the cause, let him be very cautious how he prescribes, for the effect.

A cough is always accompanied with fever. This fever may be general or local, severe or slight, perceptible in the pulse, skin, &c., or imperceptible. All these circumstances must be carefully noted, and will influence the treatment.

Coughs with febrile or inflammatory symptoms, have either been noticed under the article colds, or will be considered each in a separate article, according to the organ or organs implicated in the subsequent pages of this work.

It remains to consider a cough where the inflammatory symptoms are so slight as to be nearly imperceptible, or where, after the inflammation appears to have been subdued, either by time or by the administration of appropriate remedies, the cough still remains. This would not improperly be termed a *chronic cough.*

Tussis chronica, or a continued cough, that is, a cough continuing after the other acute symptoms of disease have subsided.

In this condition, some one of the following remedies will usually be found appropriate: Aconite, Antimonium crud., Arsenicum, Belladonna, Bryonia, Chamomilla, Causticum, Carbo veg., Calcarea carb., Dulcamara, Drosera, Hepar sulph., Hyoscyamus, Ignatia, Lachesis, Lycopodium, Mercurius viv., Nux vomica, Pulsatilla, Rhus tox., Sepia, Silicea, and Sulphur.

ACONITE, if the patient be of a nervous, sanguineous temperament, and if the cough be attended with constriction, pressure, or pricking sensations, with sense of numbness or paralysis; cough, short and dry, or convulsive, hoarse and choking; expectoration white or bloody, or with spitting of blood.

ANTIMONIUM CRUD.—Dry cough in the morning, especially if attended with heat and burning in the throat, involuntary and copious discharge of urine, sensation of sóme foreign body in the throat, which cannot be expectorated; great weakness or entire loss of voice.

ARSENICUM.—Cough, excited by a sensation of dryness in the throat, worse in the evening, or attended with heat and burning; periodic, dry cough, or cough with tenacious mucus, difficult to expectorate, and sense of suffocation, especially of old people; bloody expectoration, with burning.

BELLADONNA.—Cough, with headache, redness, and heat in the face,—afternoon or evening, and in bed, excited by movement, especially if it be short, dry, and at times convulsive; shootings as if from knives, spasmodic contractions, cuttings in the abdomen, or pain in the nape of the neck, and especially in phthisical persons, or tendency to consumption.

BRYONIA.—Spasmodic, suffocating cough, after eating or after midnight; dry, or with dirty, reddish or yellowish expectoration; aching pains in the head, as if it would burst, and with stingings or prickings in the chest and sides; excoriating pain at the stomach-pit, or pains in the region of the liver or spleen; cough, with palpitation of the heart; can lie only on the back; shootings under the left shoulder-blade as far as the heart, aggravated by movement.

CALCAREA CARB.—Hacking cough, with vertigo or trembling of the limbs, or dry, with violent beatings of the heart and pulsations of the arteries, shootings in the head, from without inwards, or bursting, shaking pains, as if the head would fly open, with yellowish, sweetish, or saltish and viscid expectoration.

CAUSTICUM.—Hacking cough, with tickling in the throat, or as if something like a wedge in the throat, and rattling in the chest, or with abundant secretion of mucus, difficult to expectorate.

CARBO VEG.—Dry cough, with flushes of heat and sweat, roughness in the throat, pains above the left hip, or painful stitches through the head, or in mucus consumption of old people ; spasmodic cough, with vomiting, especially in the evening ; expectoration, if mucus, greenish,—if pus, yellowish or bloody ; expectoration with burning. See also *Arsenicum*.

CHAMOMILLA.—Tickling itching in the throat-pit, extending under the sternum; tenacious mucus in the throat; suffocative cough after midnight.

DULCAMARA.—Cough, with copious secretion of mucus, or with expectoration of bright colored blood; barking, shaking cough, stinging in the chest, anxiety and fulness in the præcordial region.

DROSERA.—Early morning cough, if the expectoration be bitter and nauseous; or dry, spasmodic cough, with inclination to vomit, or with bleeding from the nose and mouth.

HEPAR SULPH.—Dry, hollow, suffocative cough, with anguish and weeping; or cough with wheezing respiration and danger of suffocation when lying down; cough, with weakness of the organs of speech; emaciation; hectic fever and sleeplessness; hoarse, hollow cough.

HYOSCYAMUS.—Cough when lying down; cramp-like cough; dry, shaking cough, with pains in the abdomen; convulsive cough; expectoration greenish or bloody.

IGNATIA.—Cough, as if a feather were in the throat, or tickling above the stomach pit; spasmodic dry cough, or with fluent coryza; cough and constriction at the throat pit, and also of the chest.

LACHESIS.—Fatiguing cough, with tickling in the throat, chest or stomach pit, and dryness of the throat; cough always after sleeping, often when sleeping, or soon after lying down; contractions and constrictions with sense of swelling, or with swelling and tension.

LYCOPODIUM.—Cough, dry, night or morning, affecting the head, stomach and chest, or with pains through the chest, even to the back; cough of long standing, with obstinate constipation; cough with greenish or bloody, or yellowish-grey expectoration.

MERCURIUS VIV.—Dry, fatiguing, shaking cough, with tickling and dryness in the chest, worse when in bed at night, and aggravated by speaking; pains in the head and chest when coughing; catarrhal cough, with diarrhœa, or with watery secretion from the mouth and nose.

NUX VOMICA.—Nervous, spasmodic cr catarrhal cough, worse in the morning, in paroxysms through the early part of the day, attended with entire loss of appetite, and inability to take food in the morning; or cough, with severe headache, or with pain as from a blow or bruise at the pit of the stomach, or with oppression across the chest, and in the upper portion of the abdomen; especially for persons subject to constipation or hemorrhoids; or if the cough be accompanied with tickling in the throat, or with itching and sensation of roughness, and followed by stinging pains; expectoration bloody, or of tenacious mucus.

PHOSPHORUS.—Dry cough, with tickling, or with

35

stingings in the throat and chest, and sensation as if the chest were raw; aggravated by motion and by cold, and with sense of weight, oppression, or constriction and anguish, with lancinating or burning pains; purulent, saltish expectoration, or slimy, bloody mucus, or pure blood.

PULSATILLA. — Cough severe, shaking, or nervous, spasmodic and suffocating; or if followed by vomiting, soreness in the abdomen, or with shooting pains in different parts of the body, or pains changing rapidly from place to place; expectoration white and tenacious, or thick and yellowish, or of clotted blood; worse in the evening.

RHUS TOX.—Cough excited by tickling in the chest, with constriction, anxiety and sense of suffocation, or with shooting pains in the chest and sides, and sense of exhaustion; expectoration of viscid mucus or bright blood; bitter taste in the mouth; worse on lying down at night, or on waking in the morning.

SEPIA.—Dry, spasmodic suffocative cough, with nausea and bitter vomiting; cough with constipation, or with lancinating pains in the chest and back; expectoration yellowish, greenish, pus-like or bloody, putrid or salt; aggravations morning and evening; chronic coughs.

SULPHUR.—Cough with painful stitches through the chest to the back; weakness in the chest; sensation as if the chest were contracted; spasmodic pains; shortness of breath, and inability to speak; pain mostly on the left side; expectoration whitish or yellowish, or fetid, and of a salt or sweetish taste; worse when lying down.

SILICEA.—Chronic cough in persons subject to ulcerations, or to unhealthy condition of the skin, or to great nervous debility, and tendency to suffer from chills, especially if there be aggravation of the sufferings at the new and full moon; expectoration of transparent mucus or pus; aggravations by movement and at night.

ADMINISTRATION.—Select the remedy with great care, dissolve two drops, or twelve globules, in half a tumblerful of water, give a teaspoonful every four hours, (or if there be recent cold with fever, in addition to the chronic cough, every two hours,) for two days, or until some manifest effect is produced. Then omit all medicine one day. After this, continue the same, or some other carefully selected remedy, at intervals of twelve or twenty-four hours, according to the severity of the symptoms, and the idyosincracies of the patient. In coughs of long standing, and if an amelioration of the symptoms has been produced by one or two weeks' treatment, omit all medicine every alternate week, and the patient will recover with more certainty and safety.

NOTE.—In case any difficulty arises from administering medicine in water, it may be taken, one or two globules at a dose, in a little pure, refined, white sugar; or in the case of infants, or adults, if necessary, the pellets themselves may be carefully placed upon the tongue, taking care that the mouth be free from all noxious or impure substances.

DIET.—In cases of cough, as in most other chronic diseases, articles of food should be selected, which are found by experience to agree with the patient. This rule is of the first and highest importance. Next to this is the rule, avoid all narcotic or other stimulants, all opening or relaxing medicines, foods, or drinks; all articles having a strong or pungent taste or smell; all ginger, pepper, spices, nutmegs, cloves, vinegar, strong acids, beers, mineral waters, strong drinks, &c., &c.; and all use of loosening drinks, infusions, &c.

Use good bread, one day old; sweet, fresh butter, or milk, if it agree; puddings of indian, wheat, rye, or oatmeal; potatoes, turnips, peas, beans, and tomatoes, apples, peaches, strawberries, raspberries, grapes, &c., but avoid plumbs and gooseberries.

Use all food well prepared, without any flavor but a

little salt, milk, eggs, or sugar, from arrowroot, tapioca, farina, sago, salep, oatmeal, barley, &c.

Let the food be taken moderately warm, or cold, but not too hot. Meat should be taken in moderate quan-tities, the lean parts of beef, mutton, poultry, venison, game, &c., and usually but once each day.

REGIMEN.—A light, dry, and airy room, out of the way of the steam or gas from the kitchen, or cook room, should always be selected, with a good chimney draught, and good ventilation.

The whole body should be thoroughly sponged with pure, clean water, of a temperature which is found to agree, at least two or three times each week. This sponging should be done rapidly, the skin afterwards dried rapidly, with a towel, and then rubbed with the hand to a glow, after which it should be warmly covered. This may be done either at night, or in the early morning, never during the day.

A moderate drink of cold water on retiring at night, and another on rising in the morning, having previously given the mouth a thorough washing in the same, will also be useful.

The morning air, frequent, long and deep inspirations during a morning walk, and avoiding night air, all crowded assemblies, and all damp or confined air, will render the cure more easy and certain.

Drawing in large quantities of air, into the lungs, and then beating the chest with the hand, or with the doubled fist, will frequently be found useful.

If a careful attendance to the foregoing rules, and the administration of remedies, according to the directions given, do not suffice to cure any cough in a few weeks, or at least to materially diminish its severity, it is best to apply to some educated and skilful physician. The case is of too serious a nature, to be treated longer by the aid of books alone, or by the usual routine of domestic practice. Do not, on that account, allow yourself to fall into the devouring jaws of allopathy, nor be led astray by the never-ending recommendations of specifics, whether of domestic, or of patent-right medicines. Place yourself at once in the care of some educated homœopath. If it is possible for life to be preserved, you are the safest in his hands.

7.—Hoarseness. (*Raucitas.*)

This affection is also rather a symptom than a disease, and arises from some irritation or congested condition of the upper portion of the windpipe or throat. It often occurs in the progress of a common cold, or it may also be an accompaniment of several other diseases. When it is an accompaniment of a cold, the cold must first be treated according to the directions given in the article on that subject; if the hoarseness still remain, or recur by itself, the idyosincracies of the patient, and any other complaints to which he may be subject, must be carefully studied, and the remedies selected according to the following indications:

ARSENICUM.—If the voice be rough, the hoarseness periodical, the patient restless, uneasy, and especially in persons subject to dropsy or eruptions, with burning pains.

BELLADONNA.—If with the hoarseness there be spasmodic constriction; soreness; sense of a lump in the throat; suffocation; weak, squeaking, nasal voice.

CAUSTICUM.—Hoarseness from weakness of the muscles of the throat, with weak and stifled voice, and if the

35*

hoarseness be long continued, sense of roughness even when vomiting, worse morning and evening.

CUPRUM.—Hoarseness with dry cough and fits of suffocation, desire to lie down in persons subject to asthma, or for women during the catamenia.

CAPSICUM.—If with dryness, crawling and tickling in the nose, pressure in the throat and ears, worse at night, aggravated by cold.

HEPAR SULPH.—Hoarseness, acute or chronic, with stingings in the throat as if from splinters, extending even to the ears, with dryness and sensation as of a lump in the throat; weakness; great sensibility, especially for persons who have suffered from large doses of mercury.

IODIUM.—Hoarseness, long continued, insupportable, with crawlings in the throat, swellings, contractive sore pain, especially in tuberculous scrofulous subjects, and if early in the morning; after Mercurius, especially large doses. '

KALI CARB.—If the hoarseness be attended with violent sneezing, or with choking sensations, as if there were a plug in the throat, with loss of voice, especially in persons subject to urinary affections, with dry skin and tendency to take cold, or for women with deficient monthly secretion, or with leucorrhœa.

LACHESIS will prove useful if there be a sensation as if there were something in the throat which could not be detached, with a disposition to swelling, or to bloatedness of the skin; weak, hollow and nasal voice; suffocative sensations; and for women with deficient catamenia.

MERCURIUS VIVUS. — Hoarseness, attended with thin coryza; burning, tickling sensations, and disposition to profuse sweatings, especially at night.

PULSATILLA may be useful for females, especially if

there be suppression of the catamenia, or if there be a thick cream-like leucorrhœa of long standing, or if there be a thick yellowish discharge from the nose

RHUS TOX., if there be tickling, burning, with sensation as if the chest were raw, or sensation of coldness when drawing in the breath, for persons subject to erysipelatous eruptions or to rheumatism.

SULPHUR, particularly in obstinate cases, voice nearly extinct, roughness, scraping in the throat, and after *Rhus tox.* or *Pulsatilla*, especially in cold, damp weather.

SILICEA, if there be also expectoration of thick puslike matter from the throat, with prickings, excoriation, oppression, constriction, and paralytic sensations.

STANNUM.—Painful drawings or dryness and shootings; continued swallowing when speaking; sensation of excoriation, with weakness even in the chest as if it were empty; voice embarrassed, and low; red tongue and sore throat.

There are many other valuable remedies in chronic hoarseness, the indications for some of which have been given under the article colds, catarrh, coryza, &c., among which are Phosphorus, Calc. carb., Carbo veg., Drosera, Nitric acid, Phosphoric acid, Ammonium carb., Aurum mur., Baryta carb., Opium, Sambucus and Zincum; but it is confidently believed the above indications will be amply sufficient for all ordinary cases. For extraordinary ones, always consult a physician.

DOSE.—Any one of the above remedies may be administered in water, by dissolving twelve globules, or infusing two drops of the dilution, in half a tumbler of water, and giving a teaspoonful of this dilution every two or four hours, according to the nature of the case and the condition of the patient; if in forty-eight hours there be no improvement, it is better to select another remedy, sometimes two remedies which harmonise may be given in alternation, the one being a vegetable, and the other a mineral remedy.

8.—Laryngitis. (Frequently called *Sore throat.*)

Inflammation of the throat, or if chronic, consumption of the throat.

That part of the throat which can be easily seen by depressing the tongue and opening the mouth sufficiently, is called the pharynx. Immediately below and partly in front of the pharynx, can be seen the entrance into what is commonly termed the windpipe. The windpipe is divided into two parts. The lower portion or the windpipe proper, the office of which is to convey air to the lungs, is called the trachea. The upper portion and below the pharanx, is called the larynx, and its office, in addition to serving as a channel for the passage of air to the lungs, is to form and modify, or give tone and compass to the voice. Besides the ordinary tissues which compose the throat and mouth, the larynx is enclosed by a series of rings, of a firm, tough, unyielding substance, somewhat intermediate between India rubber and bone, called cartilage, which is also continued around the trachea and bronchia, until they enter the lungs. When from any cause the larynx takes on inflammation, it is called laryngitis, which means neither more nor less than inflammation of the larynx, as inflammation of the trachea would be called trachietis, inflammation of the bronchi, bronchitis, &c. All these diseases are frequently spoken of by the uneducated, and sometimes even by physicians, under the general name bronchitis, under which term is frequently embraced nearly all the chronic diseases of the respiratory organs.

At the upper part or entrance of the larynx, is a circular flap-like rim, forming, as it were, a hem or edging to the larynx, and connecting it with, or separating it from, the pharynx. This rim is called the glottis, and immediately in contiguity with this and above it, is the epiglottis.

All these parts or organs, viz., the pharynx, the larynx, the glottis and epiglottis, the trachea and the bronchia, from their locality, as well as from their similarity of function and structure, might be expected to be subjected to similar forms of disease, and although there may be characteristic differences, which indeed to some extent there are, yet we shall find both the symptoms and the treatment of these diseases continually running into and interlapping one another; and in studying the symptoms of the diseases of any one of these organs, it is of quite as much importance to understand upon what particular tissue or tissues the disease is seated, and the nature or character of the morbid influence with which it is assailed, as it is to know the name of the disease itself, which is in fact only determining that some particular part of the system is in a diseased condition.

Continuing, however, the nomenclature which custom has established, we shall treat first of laryngitis, second of pharyngitis, third of trachietis and bronchitis, and afterwards proceed to the consideration of the other diseases of the respiratory organs in their order.

Laryngitis acute, or acute inflammation of the larynx, is characterised by the following symptoms: hoarseness; sense of soreness in the larynx, with a sense of tightness; or voice very hoarse, and sounding as if issuing from some narrow aperture, and at length almost or quite suppressed; inspiration difficult, tightly sounding or wheezing; sensation of distressing constriction in the throat, and of inability to breathe, accompanied with pain, severe or moderate, especially increased by external pressure, if made in the region of the Adam's apple, and upon the cartilages of the windpipe. If there is a cough attending it, as is usually the case, it may be simply a hoarse, muffled cough, as if to remove some obstruction from the larynx; or it may be spasmodic, paroxysmal and convulsive, dry or with tough, adhesive mucus; paroxysms of great oppression and difficulty of breathing, with spasms of the muscles of the glottis, occasionally occur; sensation of a foreign body or a lump in the throat. If the inflammation extend to the pharynx, there will be difficulty in swallowing, which it is supposed may sometimes occur also from motion or pressure upon the larynx while swallowing. It is usually attended with a greater or less degree of fever, and so far as can be seen with redness and swelling of the internal surface of the diseased organ.

All the above symptoms will generally yield readily to the administration of the appropriate remedies. But if in addition to the above symptoms, the sense of constriction, pressure, soreness and hoarseness, commences with a distinct chill, and if, with a painful, harsh, and whistling or closely sounding, distressing cough, nothing is expectorated, or only a little mucus, viscid and ropy, and if chilliness alternate with flashes of heat, followed by fever, with the pulse full and strong, skin hot, and face flushed, great difficulty of breathing, with prolonged, whistling, wheezing, and sonorous inspirations, whilst the expirations are more easy and free, you have reason to apprehend a case which will need the utmost care to avoid a dangerous crisis.

The patient may experience much difficulty in swallowing, from the swollen condition of the parts above the larynx, and around the roots of the tongue, and the glottis and epiglottis on examination, may be found of a bright red color and much swollen.

Should the disease continue to progress unchecked, all the above symptoms are aggravated; the voice becomes nearly extinguished; the cough 'can scarcely be heard, though it is agitating, convulsive, and very painful; the breath is drawn in with the most violent efforts, with great anxiety, as if about to suffocate; extreme restlessness, starting up suddenly, walking about the chamber with his hands to his throat, eager for air, anxious, apprehensive and distressed, unable to sleep from constant effort to get breath; the lips assume a purplish blue color, the face a livid paleness, with a dark circle around the eyes, which are sometimes protruded and watery; the skin is cool, the pulse feeble, irregular, and frequent; the patient appears nearly exhausted, but still makes the most violent efforts for breath: his shoulders rise, his whole chest heaves, his expression is ghastly and staring; perhaps after a cold sweat or delirium, he sinks into a drowsy or comatose state, which is usually followed by death.· A patient may die suddenly, from strangulation, or gradually, from an insufficient supply of air, or perhaps from the imperfect action of the air upon the blood. When fatal, the disease is generally very rapid. Death has been known to occur in seven hours, and from that to five days, is probably the most common period.

The diseases for which it might be mistaken are aneurism, or enlargement of one of the large arteries of the neck; croup, which is itself essentially a laryngeal affection, and spasm of the rim of the glottis. If a careful examination does not render the case certain, it is better to consult à physician.

TREATMENT.—Nearly all the remedies indicated for a common cold and for hoarseness, will be found more or less useful in this affection. In the early stages, whilst the skin is cool and the pulse unaffected, a few drops of Camphor on sugar, administered at frequent intervals, about every half hour, for two or three hours, may be sufficient to arrest an attack. Aconite, Hepar sulph. and Spongia, are however, most frequently called for, next to which, perhaps, is Lachesis: these remedies appearing to correspond to nearly all the symptoms of laryngitis, as they do also to croup, and to nearly all complaints accompanied with choking, hoarseness, and loss of voice. Laurie recommends the early administration of Aconite, to be followed by Spongia, if the voice be shrill, with painful sensibility of the larynx, hoarseness, and loss of voice, and afterwards Hepar sulph., to complete the cure. Or if Aconite do not arrest the febrile symptoms, or there be burning heat of the skin, give Hepar sulph. first, and Spongia afterwards, to be followed by Lachesis if necessary. The following remedies are believed to be the most reliable: Aconite, Antimonium crud., Arsenic, Belladonna, Cantharis, Hepar sulph., Iodium, Lachesis, Mercurius cor., Phosphorus, Rhus tox., and Spongia.

ACONITE should commonly be given in the early stages of this complaint. It is especially indicated for those severe febrile symptoms, which precede a dangerous attack, or if there be a distinct chill, with heat, or chilliness, alternated with flushes of heat; rapid pulse; sense of numbness or paralysis; tickling in the throat, with constant desire to cough; cough, hoarse croaking, or convulsive, with sense of suffocation or constriction; voice croaking; throat painful; with choking sensations. It will frequently require to be followed by *Hepar sulph. Spongia*, or some other indicated remedy, so soon as the febrile symptoms yield, or usually in four or six hours, after commencing the treatment.

DOSE.—One drop of the dilution, or six globules, in ten spoonfuls of water, a spoonful every half hour. If little change takes place in four hours, give *Hepar.* If there be improvement, give *Spongia.* Afterwards, combat the remaining symptoms with the indicated remedy, not forgetting *Belladonna* and *Lachesis.*

ANTIMONIUM CRUD.—If the loss of voice be attended with great weakness, or with sensation of heat in the throat, and involuntary passing of urine, when coughing or sneezing, and if the symptoms are aggravated by heat; or if there be violent spasms, as if the throat were filled with a plug, or as if something were hanging in the throat which could not be expelled, especially if there be a sensation of something alternately thicker and thinner, extending down the throat; and if there be perceptible swelling at the root of the tongue, and around the windpipe.

DOSE.—One drop of the dilution, or six globules, may be dissolved in ten spoonfuls of water, a spoonful to be given every hour, until amelioration, or change.

ARSENICUM.—If there be a sensation of constriction, and stifling, as if from the vapor of sulphur, extending even to the pit of the stomach, with difficulty of breathing, and choking; and if the pains are burning, the voice trembling, unequal, at one time strong, at another weak, rough and hoarse, with sense of dryness; constrictive and burning pains, with dryness and thirst, drinking little at a time; tongue dry, cracked, and trembling. After *Aconite, Belladonna, Lachesis*, or *Rhus tox.*

DOSE.—One drop of the dilution, or six globules, in ten spoonfuls of water, a spoonful to be given every hour, or every two hours, according to the urgency of the symptoms.

36

BELLADONNA.—Hot skin; much thirst, with inability to drink; spasms in the throat, especially when drinking; throat swollen, red, inflamed; painfulness of the throat; danger of suffocation from movement or pressure, as in coughing, speaking, or turning the neck; loss of voice; constriction; spasms; soreness of the larynx, especially to pressure; cough, as if there were something in the throat, or at the stomach pit; pain in the nape of the neck; worse in the evening, or at night, in bed, and aggravated by movement; and especially if the pains extend upward, into the upper part of the throat; with swelling of the tonsils, or of the parts around the throat; with constant desire, and inability to swallow. After *Aconite*, before or after *Hepar Sulph., Arsenicum,* or *Lachesis;* after *Belladonna, Mercurius viv.*

DOSE.—One drop, or six globules, in ten spoonfuls of water, a spoonful every half hour, in severe cases, in those less imminent, every two hours, until amelioration, or change.

CANTHARIS. — Burning pain, with contraction, and constriction, or with hoarseness and rattling of thick or stringy mucus, which seems to come up from the chest, and with pain, along the course of the windpipe; cuttings and shootings; weakness of respiration; voice feeble and trembling; especially if there be retention or difficult and painful emission of urine, and if there be severe general or local inflammation.

DOSE.—One drop of the dilution, or six globules, in ten spoonfuls of water, a spoonful to be given every hour, until amelioration, or change. Often useful after *Aconite.*

HEPAR SULPH.—Painfulness and great sensibility in the upper portion of windpipe or in the throat, aggravated by speaking, by pressure, by coughing, and even when drawing in the breath; suffocative cough, hoarse and violent, or dry, deep and dull, excited by difficulty of breathing; voice weak and rough, with a feeling of weakness in the chest, and difficulty of speaking; sensation as of a lump in the throat, and rattling of mucus in the throat; worse at night, and if any part of the body be exposed to cold. After *Aconite, Belladonna*, or *Mercurius;* and before or after *Spongia* and *Lachesis.*

DOSE.—One drop of the dilution, or six globules, in ten spoonfuls of water, a spoonful to be given every hour, (or in extreme cases much oftener, every ten minutes if necessary,) until amelioration or change. When the dangerous symptoms are manifestly abated, give the medicine less frequently, every two hours, or every four hours, until complete recovery. This medicine is often useful when *Aconite* has been given with but little manifest effect.

IODIUM is useful, if there be copious secretion of mucus in the windpipe, with hawking; dry, morning cough, pains in the chest and fever; cough, with a kind of a whoop, excited by tickling in the chest; hoarseness, sensation of crawling and inflammation of the windpipe and throat, especially with tendency to ulceration. (See Chronic Laryngitis.)

DOSE.—Two drops of the dilution, or twelve globules, in ten spoonfuls of water, a spoonful every two hours, until amelioration or change.

LACHESIS.—Extreme sensibility to the slightest pressure, either on the windpipe or on the parts of the neck around; danger of suffocation, even on stretching back the head; hoarseness, contraction, and constriction, with dryness, and with burning pains; sensation of a ball in the throat, or of some foreign body which prevents speech; choking sensations in the windpipe and chest, or with feeling of a weight or of fulness in the chest and throat; sensations, as if swollen, or actual swelling of the throat, or of the adjacent parts; large and small tumors in the throat; pains, burning or excoriating, violent and pressive, intermittent, with rapid failure of strength, pallid face, cold sweat, difficulty of breathing, and danger of suffocation; constant tickling in the throat, with dryness, or with dry, short, suffocative cough, or with expectoration of tenacious mucus, or of water from the mouth; inflammatory, erysipelatous, or dropsical swellings of the throat; loss of voice, or voice indistinct, and as if speaking through the nose; mouth and tongue dry, or filled with a watery saliva, and swollen; tongue red, cracked, dry and stiff, with sensation of paralysis, or swollen and brownish or blackish; redness of the mouth and throat.

DOSE·—One drop of the dilution, or six globules, in ten spoonfuls of water; give a spoonful every hour, in desperate cases much oftener, until amelioration or change. After *Belladonna* or *Hepar sulph.*, give *Lachesis*, or it may be useful after *Rhus tox.*, *Arsenicum*, *Spongia*, &c.

MERCURIUS VIV. is useful in acute laryngitis, more especially when the inflammation of the larynx is complicated with inflammation of the pharynx and the structures contiguous to the mouth, as the tonsils, palate, and the glands about the throat and mouth, and especially for persons subject to ulcerations and swellings, such as quinsy, sore throat; it may be given either alone, or in alternation with, or before or after *Belladonna*, when that remedy appears to be indicated, and will exert a great influence in preventing future attacks of diseases of this nature.

DOSE·—One drop of the dilution, or six globules, in ten spoonfuls of water, give a spoonful every four hours, until amelioration or change.

PHOSPHORUS.—If there be smarting, stinging, and burning, with constrictive pains; prolonged hoarseness, with partial or entire loss of voice, or very painful sensibility of the windpipe or larynx, which does not permit one to speak; dryness and pressure in the throat, dry tongue, white, or coated blackish or brown, or accumulation of saliva, or viscous mucus in the mouth, with hawking up of mucus, especially in the morning.

DOSE.—One drop of the dilution, or six globules, in ten spoonfuls of water, a spoonful to be given every four hours until amelioration or change.

RHUS TOX. for persons subject to erysipelatous affections, and to rheumatism; aggravated by changes of weather, when at rest, or during attempts to sleep, or after sleeping; difficulty, pain, pressure, and shootings, when swallowing, especially solid food; coldness in the throat when drawing in the breath, with hot breath; constriction in the throat-pit, with hoarseness and roughness, and sensation as if the chest were raw.

DOSE.—One drop of the dilution, or six globules, in ten spoonfuls of water, a spoonful to be given every two hours, until amelioration or change. *Arsenicum* may be given after *Rhus tox.*

SPONGIA is generally considered a reliable remedy in the most dangerous forms of acute or chronic laryngitis, if with hoarseness, dryness and burning in the throat, and painfulness in the larynx on touching it or turning the head, there be a dry hollow barking or whistling cough, with burning pains extending the whole length of the windpipe, and spasmodic constriction or burning sensations in the whole chest, or sensations of heat as if the blood were mounting upwards; or if there be a sensation of obstruction in the throat, with wheezing respiration, and rattling of mucus in the chest, with weakness; difficulty of respiration and anguish. It appears especially adapted to that form of inflammation of the larynx which resembles croup, and where every thing seems to tend upward towards the throat.

DOSE.—One drop of the dilution, or six globules, in half a tumblerful of water, a spoonful to be given every half hour, until amelioration or change.

36*

ſ.—Croup. (*Cynanche Laryngitis. Cynanche Trachietis.*)

Another form of acute laryngitis, which from its dangerous character, is deserving of the most careful and serious attention is croup.

This is usually a disease of childhood, consisting of a high degree of inflammation of the windpipe, with spasm probably of the interior muscles, and an exudation on the inner or mucus surface, with a tendency to the formation of a tough, stringy, membranaceous or viscid substance, which often adheres closely to the interior surface of the windpipe, and at times appears to cover or nearly to cover the tube for considerable length. After this membrane has been allowed to form, the case becomes extremely dangerous. It sometimes terminates fatally in a few hours, though not usually till the third or fifth day.

A predisposition to croup may no doubt be induced by a too highly stimulating diet; the excessive use of candies, mint drops, and aromatic substances, having a smart or biting taste, as pepper, spices, nutmeg, &c.; and this predisposition may no doubt be transmitted from one generation to another, so long as the habit of indulgence continues; all other notions about constitutional taint are simply absurd. What more natural than that a mother, who accustoms herself to the constant use of large quantities of allspice, or of black or cayenne pepper, or cloves, until all the mucus surfaces are burned dry and parched, and compelled to defend themselves against renewed assaults by exuding from their surface an unnatural secretion, with which they cover themselves as with a coat of mail, should transmit to her offspring a disease of those tender and delicate surfaces, upon which the poisons she is accustomed to indulge in are known specifically to act.

An attack of croup usually commences with the symptoms of a common cold; the cough at length becomes shrill or hoarse, with a ringing sound as if the air were passing through a metallic tube; breathing becomes exceedingly difficult, every.inspiration of air being accompanied with a shrill sound, which has by some writers been compared to that made by a chicken when dying with the pip; if there be any expectoration it has a stringy appearance, and is exuded during a fit of coughing; the fever and restlessness are continuous, but may vary in intensity, and the paroxysms are often followed by a profuse clammy sweat, especially of the head and face. So long as the voice is sonorous, there is usually reason to hope; extinction of the sonorous character of the voice is thought to evince the existence of membraneous formations; if the pulse is hard, frequent and intermittent; the inspirations difficult and audible; the features livid or purple; the head thrown back; the cough husky; the voice whispering; the eye glassy and dull, or dilated; the danger is imminent, and recovery if not hopeless, is at least extremely doubtful.

Should the cough at length become more loose and broken, the paroxysms of coughing shorter, the sounds acquire a mucus character, and mucus be discharged to some extent with the cough, gradually becoming less strong and viscid, we have reason to hope for a favorable termination. The remedies most useful in croup have been already described in treating on the subject of laryngitis, but such is the dangerous character of this disease we shall give it a separate consideration.

So far as has yet been ascertained, Aconite, Hepar sulph., Lachesis and Spongia, are here also the most reliable remedies. The other remedies which may become useful or necessary in the course of the treatment, are Antimonium crud., Arsenicum, Belladonna, Bryonia, Cantharis, Iodium, Kali carb., Phosphorus, Tart. emetic, Sambucus.

ACONITE is useful at the outset, to subdue the inflammatory symptoms, and the nervous spasmodic contractions, and should usually be the first remedy resorted to. It is especially indicated by the following additional symptoms: choking, strangling and suffocating symptoms, with a short, dry cough, or with constant attempts to cough, as if from uneasy sensation in the throat; convulsive, hoarse, croaking cough, with suffocative, constrictive spasms; hoarse, croaking voice, or tremulous and stammering, hesitating speech. The modifying effects of this remedy upon the nervous system should never be forgotten.

DOSE.—Two drops of the dilution, or twelve globules, in twelve spoonfuls of water, a spoonful to be given every fifteen minutes, in severe cases, until amelioration or change. In cases less severe, every half hour, every hour, or every two hours. After *Aconite*, give *Spongia* or *Hepar sulph.*

HEPAR SULPH.—After *Aconite*, especially if the skin be moist, or covered with sweat; cough and breathing more loose and free, but still a harsh or hollow cough, with hoarseness; constant rattling of mucus in the throat and chest; ineffectual endeavors to raise something from the throat; or, if the fevers continue, with frequent throwing back the head, grasping at the throat; restlessness; hot skin; rapid and difficult breathing; violent suffocative fits of coughing; husky cough, with soreness; cough, with scraping sensations and itching in the throat, at times increased to vomiting; urine when passed, pale and clear, afterwards turbid, or turbid when passed, or yellow and dark-colored; worse at night; barking cough; breathing anxious; wheezing, with attacks of suffocation, and manifest inability to breathe deeply.

DOSE.—Two drops of the dilution, or twelve globules, in half a tumbler of water, a teaspoonful to be given every two hours, or oftener, in severe cases, until amelioration or change.

LACHESIS is indicated in croup by a dry, short, suffocating and croaking cough, or cough with vomiting; choking cough, or fatiguing, with inability to raise anything; cough after sleeping, or when rising up, or with flow of watery saliva from the mouth, and pains at the pit of the stomach; and if the breathing be short, rattling, croaking or wheezing; spasmodic fits of choking; convulsive spasms; difficulty of swallowing; dread of drinks, especially if there be a general appearance of bloatedness, and much tenacious mucus in the throat; neck and throat sore or sensitive to the touch, or swollen; face swollen, purple or pale, even to a frightful extent; lips swollen and discolored; rapid and feeble and sometimes intermittent pulse; cold sweat; coldness of the feet; asphyxia, with stiffness and swelling of the body; tremulous pulse, and appearance as if dying, or as if already dead.

DOSE.—One drop of the dilution; or six globules, in ten spoonfuls of water, a spoonful every two hours, or oftener, according to the severity of the symptoms, until amelioration or change.

SPONGIA.—Croup is distinguished by rattling of mucus in the lower portions of the windpipe and chest; or if there be expectoration of thick, tenacious mucus with the cough, the skin being moist, and after the more acute inflammation and dry, burning heat have been mitigated by other remedies, such as *Aconite* or *Hepar*, the breathing being still quick, wheezing, anxious and difficult; the cough barking, rough or whistling; the voice husky; or with appearance of fulness; or bloatedness of the chest, throat, face and eyes.

It would also be indicated, if the child place its hand
upon the upper part of the chest, and cry after coughing; or if by any other means it should be ascertained
that there are pains or burnings, or sensations as of
excoriation in the chest accompanying the cough; and
if the windpipe be painful, worse when touched, with
constrictive sensations, or with glandular swellings;
drowsiness; lassitude; out of humor. The urine deposits a greyish white sediment.

DOSE.—One drop of the dilution, or six globules, in ten spoonfuls of
water, a spoonful to be given every two hours, until amelioration or change,
after, or in alternation with *Hepar sulph.*

The above general indications, it is believed will
cover nearly all cases of catarrhal, spasmodic, or simple
inflammatory croup, where the attack comes on suddenly;
and also a large portion of the cases which are truly
membranous, and in cases not too far advanced. If the
remedies above indicated, be wisely and perseveringly
used, a favorable result may be anticipated; and I would
here caution physicians, as well as laymen, who may use
this work, against too hastily leaving our well-tried, and
approved remedies, in difficult and dangerous cases, on
account of the perhaps exaggerated specific virtues of
some newly discovered remedy, the uses of which,
although it may have done good in some given case,
under a certain train of circumstances, or in some
particular locality, are too imperfectly understood, to
afford us indication for exact scientific prescription, as
adapted to other circumstances, and other localities.

The following additional remedies may be consulted.

AMMONIUM CAUST., if the voice be weak; the breathing
labored and rattling; the speech interrupted; the cough
violent; expectoration copious; with fits of suffocation
and spasms.

DOSE.—As for *Belladonna.*

ARSENICUM, in the most desperate cases, and after the use of *Lachesis*, when the cough occurs in paroxysms, with great anguish, weakness, and prostration; coldness of the extremities; cold sweats; attacks of suffocation; stiffness or trembling of the limbs, or of the body; worse in the evening and when lying down. Or croup in persons subject to rash-like, eruptive diseases; or cruptions, with burning itchings; miliary eruptions, and diseases of the skin: scabs, or swellings of the mouth and nose, on taking cold, &c.

BELLADONNA, especially if following a case of scarlatina, in which *Belladonna* has not been used as a leading remedy; or in a case of spasmodic croup, with choking and constriction; inability to swallow; great soreness of the windpipe; and loss of voice. The cough is dry, short, hollow, and barking, excited by the least movement; with paroxysms of sneezing afterwards; worse at night, or in the evening, in bed.

DOSE.—One drop of the dilution, or six globules, in six spoonfuls of water, a spoonful every half hour, or oftener, if the symptoms appear to demand it.

BROMINE.—Hoarse, wheezing, fatiguing cough, having the peculiar sound which characterises croup, attended with sneezing; inability to speak, and violent fits of suffocation; mucus, rattling and wheezing; the breathing being at times slow, deep, and suffocative, at other times rapid and superficial; or labored, oppressed, gasping for air; membranous formations in the windpipe, and suffocative spasms; heat in the face; urine increased; pulse hard and slow; or accelerated.

DOSE.—One drop of the dilution, or six globules, in six spoonfuls of water, a spoonful to be given every half hour, or oftener, according to the symptoms.

NOTE.—The best practitioners give *Bromine* when required for croup, in very low dilutions; about one part to one hundred, or one to one thousand, appears most useful.

CANTHARIS, if there be oppression for breath, with sensation of excessive weakness in the respiratory organs; rattling of mucus in the chest, with cutting pains; especially where there is painful and difficult urination; scanty emission; or urine of a deep red, or of a pale yellow color.

DOSE.—One drop of the dilution, or six globules, in six spoonfuls of water, a spoonful to be given every four hours, usually in alternation with some other remedy.

CHAMOMILLA, for catarrhal croup, attended with great restlessness; tossing about; and alternate chilliness and heat; or with redness and burning heat of the cheeks, or of one cheek; excessive nervous excitability, and fretful humor; and if the cough be dry, spasmodic, convulsive, and especially if it be excited by anger or passion.

DOSE.—Two drops of the dilution, or twelve globules, dissolved in ten spoonfuls of water, a spoonful to be given every half hour, until amelioration or change.

CUPRUM, if there be violent suffocative fits, with cramps and contractions, particularly in the chest, and convulsive efforts; and especially if the cough be dry, with great weakness.

DOSE.—A drop of the dilution, or six globules, to be dissolved in six spoonfuls of water, a spoonful to be given every half hour, until amelioration, or change.

KALI BICHROMICUM or HYDROIDICUM.—If the attack be slow and insidious, symptoms at first slight, becoming very gradually severe, until the sound of the air in breathing becomes shrill and whistling, even quite low down in the windpipe; cough, not frequent, but dry and hoarse, or metallic; throat red and swollen, or covered with something resembling false membrane; head thrown back; offensive breath; diminished temperature; prostration; stupor.

DOSE.—One drop of the dilution, or six globules, in ten spoonfuls of water, a spoonful to be given every half hour, until amelioration or change.

PHOSPHORUS may be given in croup if *Hepar sulph.* and *Spongia* fail of affording relief, and especially if there be a manifest constrictive oppression across the breast; short and difficult breathing with anguish; cough dry, shaking and convulsive, with loss of voice.

DOSE.—One drop of the dilution, or six globules, in six spoonfuls of water, a spoonful to be given every half hour, until amelioration or change.

SAMBUCUS, for catarrhal or true membranous croup, when there is an accumulation of much viscous mucus in the windpipe and throat; the paroxysms of spasmodic suffocating cough are attended with cries, tossing and anguish, and the respiration is quick and wheezing.

DOSE.—One drop of the dilution, or six globules, in six spoonfuls of water, give a spoonful every half hour, until amelioration or change.

TARTAR EMETIC.—In many obstinate cases, especially if there be symptoms of paralysis of the lungs, great difficulty of breathing, face livid and cold, pulse small and rapid, or feeble and slow, great weakness and anxiety, disposition to sleep ; or if there be an excessive accumulation of mucus in the chest, with paroxysms of suffocative cough, and difficult breathing ; especially useful after *Phosphorus.*

DOSE·—One drop of the dilution, or six globules, in ten spoonfuls of water, a spoonful to be given every fifteen minutes, until amelioration or change ; or it may be given every half hour, in alternation with *Belladonna* or *Aconite.*

There are a large number of other remedies which have proved serviceable in croup. A knowledge of their symptomatic indications may be learned from other sources. It is believed that the above will be found sufficient for a work on domestic practice.

10

A disease so nearly resembling croup, as to have been termed by some Spasmodic Croup, by others, Millar's

37

Asthma, or ASTHMA of MILLAR, is deserving of a separate notice in this place.

It is supposed to consist mainly in a spasmodic contraction of the top of the windpipe, there being little or
no evidence of membranous or even of mucus exudation.
The attack commences very suddenly, the breath is drawn
in with difficulty, or with a peculiar crowing or ringing
noise, the face and extremities become purple, the hands
often clenched, the feet and toes drawn up; the attacks
recur frequently at short intervals, whilst the remissions
are usually more perfect and complete, than in ordinary
or true croup; little or no cough, fever, or symptoms of
inflammatory disease, though in the efforts for breath,
the countenance may be flushed and swollen, with an
expression of extreme anxiety and distress.

The remedies usually employed are Aconite, Belladonna, and Sambucus, which may be administered
according to the directions already given under the
article Croup; or where the above symptoms exist, give
first, Belladonna, one drop, or six globules, in six teaspoonfuls of water, a teaspoonful to be administered
every five or ten minutes. If a change do not occur
within one hour, and the danger appear imminent, give
Sambucus in the same manner as Belladonna for one
hour, and then return again to Belladonna, or give
Hyoscyamus, six globules, in six spoonfuls of water, a
spoonful to be administered every ten minutes or oftener,
until a change is effected. After Belladonna or Hyoscyamus, Cuprum, Arsenicum, or Tartar emetic, may be
indicated.

The patient, in a case of croup, should always be kept
of an even temperature, in a room neither too warm nor
too cold, and should be kept in the same room day and

night; the air of the room should be kept perfectly clear and pure, free from all gases, vinegar, camphor and other fumigations, as well as from all odors, and strong-smelling substances. The diet should be mucilaginous, as oat-meal gruel, barley water, toast water, &c., though in some cases, broths made of the lean portions of beef or mutton, or the dark meat of chicken, from which the skin has been carefully taken, may be allowed.

In administering medicines to children, it is not always necessary to give a full spoonful of the medicine. When medicines are administered every five or ten minutes, a few drops of the dilution placed upon the tongue will always proves equally efficacious, and where there is great difficulty in swallowing, and especially if water appear to increase the spasms, a single globule placed upon the tongue at frequent intervals, with occasionally a few drops of the dilution, will be found useful and satisfactory.

Rely implicitly upon the remedies. Never on any occasion resort to fomentations, cataplasms, hot or cold baths, or other old wives' fables, unless specifically called for by some well recognized homœopathic adaptation. Never use warm foot-baths, especially not unless the feet are hot. Let the skin be kept clean and well covered.

In severe cases of croup, physicians of the old school have recourse to tracheotomy, or to opening the windpipe for the removal of the false membrane, and also to caustic applications of the nitrate of silver, but generally with very indifferent success. Much more rational as well as homœopathic, we should think, Dr. C. D. and his son Dr. J. Forsyth Meigs, of Philadelphia, recommend the use of Alum, which in their hands appears to have performed many extraordinary cures, although I am not aware that it has been used in homœopathic practice. Dr. Rush recommends the free use of Calomel, and as high as three hundred grains are said to have been administered to a child in the short space of twenty-four hours. The usual allopathic treatment is by bleeding, blistering, vomiting, and the administration of *Asafœtida* and *Opium*. From such crude and undigested, as well as dangerous and heroic treatment, we turn with pleasure to the simpler and more rational, as well as safer, more efficient, and more successful treatment, which we have indicated above, confident that all persons of truly scientific minds will receive with pleasure the truths which homœopathy alone had the power to unfold and bring to light.

11.—Consumption of the Throat.—Chronic Inflammation of the Larynx. (*Chronic Laryngitis, &c.*)

This disease in its most simple form is only a chronic hoarseness, and has been sufficiently enlarged upon under the article Hoarseness. In its higher grades, however, it becomes one of the most serious and obstinate of diseases. It frequently commences with a slight hoarseness, a little uneasiness in the throat, and perhaps a slight cough, rather a clearing up of the throat or a hawking than a cough. As it progresses, various unpleasant sensations are felt in the throat, such as burning, tickling, itching, dryness and constriction, and sometimes dull, smarting, or acute pain, though in many fatal cases there is little or no pain. The voice is sometimes hoarse, sometimes squeaking, sometimes whispering; the change being more perceptible when speaking loudly, or singing. Cough, if any, usually short and dry at first, and becoming gradually loose, with mucus or purulent expectoration.

- If ulceration takes place, a pricking sensation is not uncommonly felt in the throat, as if from a sharp, pointed body, especially when speaking, and if the disease be in the upper part of the throat, especially in or near the epiglottis, it becomes exceedingly difficult to swallow, and at times whatever is swallowed returns by the nostrils; in other cases there is no difficulty in swallowing; the voice may become hollow, or quite lost, especially if the rim of the glottis is ulcerated, or the vocal ligaments are involved; the discharge becomes purulent or bloody and fetid; patches of lymph detached from the membrane are expectorated; portions of cartilage, ossified and calcareous matter, are sometimes discharged; the symptoms are more generally paroxysmal than continuous; the general health gives way; debility, night sweats, swelling of the limbs, emaciation, loss of appetite, and vomiting or diarrhœa, are premonitions often of a fatal termination.

In this disease there is usually more or less soreness of the windpipe upon pressure. The breathing of cold air, coughing, sneezing, speaking, laughing and swallowing, frequently aggravate or bring on a paroxysm of severe sufferings.

The remedies which have been recommended in this disease, are Argentum, Arsenicum, Belladonna, Carbo veg., Calcarea carb., Hepar sulph., Lachesis, Nitric acid, Phosphorus, Sanguinaria, Spongia, Silicea, Sulphur. Belladonna, Lachesis, Sanguinaria and Sulphur will be found adapted generally in the earlier stages. Arsenicum, Carbo veg., Nitric acid, Phosphorus and Spongia to more advanced forms, and Argentum, Calcarea carb.,

Spongia, Silicea and Sulphur, to the latter stages. As this disease is comparatively of rare occurrence, we shall give but few symptomatic indications.

ARGENTUM is adapted to all cases in which there is a marked sensation of rawness in the throat, or in the throat, mouth and chest; or if there be an appearance of an eruption in the thròat, with sense as if raw; sensation as if some foreign body were sticking to the front part of the larynx, at a small spot, with a feeling of coldness and pressure; frequent inclination to cough, but no relief obtained by coughing; aggravations in the evening; sore throat of public speakers.

DOSE.—Give one drop of the dilution, or six globules, in ten spoonfuls of water ; a spoonful to be taken every four hours, until amelioration or change.

ARSENICUM is indicated if the tongue be of a dark color, dry or cracked, with dryness or burning in the throat, windpipe and chest; frequent stifling sensations, with constrictions; constant desire for drink which affords little or no relief, perhaps aggravates the dryness in the throat; or, if there be ulcerations with burning pains, fetid, bloody and ichorous, or water-colored discharge; or of mucus having a saltish, pungent and bitterish taste; and if there be emaciation, weakness, periodical attacks, shiverings and heats, night-sweats, swelling of the limbs, especially for persons subject to eruptions, nettle-rash, or ulcers with burning pains.

DOSE.—One drop of the dilution, or six globules, in half a tumbler of water; a spoonful to be given every four or six hours, until the symptoms become modified, or some other remedy is indicated.

BELLADONNA, if the voice be weak and squeaking, if the attacks are spasmodic and suffocating, worse at night and in bed; if the least pressure upon the windpipe and throat is attended with choking and suffocation, all the parts being very sensitive to the touch; face pale or flushed; a choking dryness in the mouth; redness of the mouth and tongue, and especially of the throat; or if there be swellings of the glands of the throat and mouth.

DOSE.—One drop of the dilution, or six globules, in half a tumbler of water; a spoonful to be given every six hours for two or four days, then omit medicine four days, or give some other remedy according to the symptoms.

CALCAREA CARBONICA may be given after *Belladonna* to persons of scrofulous habits, with tendencies to ulceration, especially if ulceration in the throat be already established; if the discharge on coughing be thick and yellowish or pus-like, or if blood be mixed with the matter discharged from the throat; especially adapted to persons of a weak, sickly constitution, of a light complexion, blond hair and eyes; or to persons of a lymphatic constitution, with tendencies to corpulency.

DOSE.—One drop of the dilution, or six globules, to be dissolved in six spoonfuls of water; a spoonful to be given night and morning, until some change be observed, after which wait a few days without medicine.

HEPAR SULPHUR also after *Belladonna*, if there be sensation in the throat as of a plug or an internal tumor; stinging in the throat as if from splinters; painful sensibility of the larynx, with weak rough voice; emaciation; hectic fever and sleeplessness; abundant expectoration of mucus with the cough; or swellings, glandular enlargements, &c., and if ulceration be already established; also for persons of unhealthy skin, subject to tubercles, nettle-rash, or to erysipelas.

DOSE.—Give one drop of the dilution, or six globules, dissolved in ten spoonfuls of water; a spoonful to be taken every four hours, until amelioration or change.

LACHESIS, if with a great degree of painful sensibility of the throat there be swellings, burnings and raw sore pains; stiffness and paralysis; soreness affecting only a small spot on the throat, or on the contrary extending

over the whole throat even to the ears; sensation of a
tumor in the throat, or of some foreign body which can
not be detached; difficulty of swallowing, with dread of
drinks; face pale, earthy or yellowish, with redness of
the cheeks, and bloatedness, or wasted and wan; ulcerations even on the palate and throat, with fetid discharge;
gangrenous ulcerations; pulse weak, frequent, intermittent, with cold sweats; after *Belladonna,* and before or
after *Arsenicum.*

DOSE.—One drop of the dilution, or six globules, in six spoonfuls of
water; a spoonful to be given every four hours, until amelioration or
change.

MERCURIUS VIV. or NITRIC ACID, if the disease be
manifestly of syphilitic origin, if there be inflammatory
swellings or ulcerations, involving also the glands of the
mouth and throat; if there be stinging, stitching, excoriating, or cutting pains; discharge of fœtid pus, or of
bloody and corrosive scrum; fœtid or acid night-sweats,
lassitude, emaciation, fever, especially at night; violent
thirst, hoarseness, &c.

DOSE.—One drop of the dilution, or six globules, in ten spoonfuls of
water, a spoonful to be taken every four hours, and continued for two weeks,
or longer; if there be an aggravation of the symptoms, stop all medicine,
or give a much higher dilution of the same remedy; continue the selected
remedy, alternately changing the dilution or omitting all medicine, until a
cure is effected, which will usually take several months. *Nitric acid* frequently produces aggravations in syphilitic affections, preceding a cure.

PHOSPHORUS is useful, if the disease be in consequence
of frequent or long neglected catarrhs, or if it be in consequence of the suppression of some local disease, as
small-pox, itch, measles, scarlatina, &c.; or especially, for
persons of a weak, irritable constitution, the skin being
thin and tender, with disposition to bleed easily from
slight causes; cough, with stinging, and painful sensibility of the throat, loss of voice, hoarseness, and scrap-

ing sensations, as if the parts were raw; cough, dry or moist, or with expectoration of pus, greenish or saltish, or of bloody mucus.

DOSE.—One drop of the dilution, or six globules, in twelve spoonfuls of water, a spoonful to be given every four hours until amelioration of the most acute symptoms; afterwards, every morning and evening, until a cure is effected.

SANGUINARIA has proved efficacious after *Sulphur*, in a case characterised by sensation of swelling, and pain as if the parts were raw, especially during the act of swallowing, the expectoration being whitish mucus, of a saltish taste, with hectic fever.

SILICEA will be found useful, if the cartilages of the throat are involved, and if there be expectoration of pus, or of pus mixed with blood; if the cough be aggravated by cold; pricking in the throat, as if from pins; ulceration of the palate; difficulty in swallowing; frequent sensation as of a hair on the tongue; tongue coated brown, or sore as from excoriation; easy bleeding of the mouth and gums; and especially for persons subject to unhealthy skin, lymphatic tumors and abscesses, obstruction of the glandular system, nervous debility, &c.

DOSE.—One drop of the dilution, or six globules, in six spoonfuls of water, a spoonful to be given every twenty-four hours, for six days; then wait, if possible, without medicine, one week; if improvement set in, give no medicine so long as it continue; afterwards, repeat the medicine, or give some other remedy, according to the symptoms.

SPONGIA is useful in a large number of cases, in scrofulous subjects with dispositions to swellings; with throbbings, and uneasy fulness and bloatedness of the superior parts, and sensations of torpidity or of paralysis of the inferior parts of the body; the voice is weak, husky, and hoarse, the throat is painful to the touch, with sensation of an obstruction; the pains are burning and pressive, or as if raw, the expectoration yellowish. It is useful after *Lachesis*.

DOSE.—One drop of the dilution, or six globules in ten spoonfuls of water, a spoonful to be given every four hours, until amelioration or change.

SULPHUR may be given in nearly all cases, a few doses at the commencement of the treatment, or it may be called for by peculiar symptoms during the progress of the disease, especially if the system fail to respond to the remedy used, if there be a morbid irritability indicative of some concealed psora. The sensations in the throat are tingling, crawling, tickling, itching, with dryness, or there may be hoarseness, roughness, with discharge of mucus or of pus, fœtid or yellowish.

DOSE.—When given as a principal remedy, give one drop of the dilution, or six globules, in ten spoonfuls of water, a spoonful to be given every six hours, until amelioration or change.

12.—Pharyngitis. (*Inflammation of the Pharynx.*)

That part of the throat which lies above and behind the larynx, behind the palate and roots of the tongue, and in immediate contiguity with the œsophagus, (*of which the lower and back part of the pharynx seems to be only an expansion,*) is called the pharynx, being itself a continuation of the same structures as the mouth, windpipe, and throat, and performing similar functions, it will, of course be liable to similar diseases, and to be affected by similar remedies; for it must never be forgotten by those who would prescribe intelligently for the sick, that the nature of a structure, and the function or office performed by any organ, and the kind and degree of exposure to which it may be subject, is of much more importance to the cure, than its locality, or the name of the disease with which it may be affected.

Whilst the larynx, trachea, and bronchia, serve only as a channel for the conveyance of air, and the œsophagus, for the conveyance of food and drink, the pharynx is in some sense a double organ, acting in a two-fold capacity, being itself a kind of expansion, both of the larynx and œsophagus.

In the classification of diseases, the pharynx has usually been considered as a digestive organ, to which class, perhaps, it no less properly belongs, but as its diseases usually connect themselves with the respiratory function, and as some of its diseases manifest themselves by symptoms peculiar to that function, I have concluded that I should make myself more intelligible, and this work more perfect, by treating the pharynx as a respiratory rather than as a digestive organ.

The pharynx as a respiratory organ, presents a large surface, capable of great expansion, proportionate to the rapidity and power with which we draw in and throw out the breath. As an organ of deglutition, it is a capacious reservoir, bag, or sack, the fibres of which, interlacing and intertwining each other, are capable of such an amount of contraction, as to draw the walls of the organ into the closest possible contiguity, forcing out of the pharynx, and down the œsophagus, whatever substance may have been conveyed thither by the action of the mouth and tongue. Diseases affecting its expanded surface, are made sensible in the act of breathing, those affecting its contractive power, in the act of swallowing.

13.—Simple Inflammation of the throat.

Pharangitis simplex is often controlled by a few doses of Aconite, or of Chamomilla. But in other cases, Belladonna, Mercurius viv., Nux vomica, or Sulphur, may be given, according to the directions which follow in the succeeding article, on quinsy sore throat.

" When a spasmodic, almost suffocating constriction

of the gullet takes place," especially manifest in the act of swallowing, "and Belladonna, Mercurius, and Lachesis fail, Calcarea carb. often affords rapid relief."—*Laurie.*

14.—Common Sore Throat. (*Quinsy.*)

This complaint is usually ushered in by a feeling of dryness; heat, and rawness of the throat; with constant soreness, and pain on swallowing; pain often worst in the morning, or after lying down; on examination, the throat will be found to be of a bright red color, perhaps swollen, and in the advanced stages, small, white patches are seen on its surface. After a time, a thick, ropy mucus is secreted, which excites frequent efforts to clear the throat, the discharge being sometimes mingled with blood. If this secretion of mucus is abundant, the red-ness and pain are usually diminished. If there be a frequent disposition to swallow, or to cough, the palate, (or uvula,) will usually be found to be elongated, which at times even produces vomiting. The whole system frequently sympathises with this complaint, and chilliness, heat, loss of appetite, rapid pulse, and headache, occur with symptoms not unlike those of scarlet fever.

After this disease has become established, it frequently goes on to suppuration; the discharge is at times excessive, and even gangrenous. The disease may involve the whole throat, or it may affect only a small portion; or it may be located in the tonsils, palate, or on any of the glands around the throat; be confined to one tonsil, whilst the other is nearly unaffected; or it may be more general. It is most dangerous when it shows a disposi-tion to travel downward, towards the lungs; and chronic inflammation of the larynx, or of the bronchia; and at times, even a rapid and fatal consumption, has been known to follow an attack of this disease.

One attack of this disease always creates or engenders in the system, a predisposition to a second attack, and this predisposition is cumulative, that is, it goes on increasing in proportion to the number and frequency of the attacks; the vital powers fail; the system becomes liable to be disturbed by every change of weather, and other slight causes; and unless arrested by some revulsion of nature, or by the administration of appropriate remedies, if life may hang for a longer or shorter period, it is upon a brittle thread, and its continuance is embittered by a variety of sufferings, the nature and cause of which, many learned and skilful physicians have failed to discover.

The remedies most useful in this complaint are Aconite, Arsenicum, Aurum, Belladonna, Chamomilla, Hepar sulph., Lachesis, Mercurius viv., Nitric acid, Pulsatilla, Rhus tox., Silicea, and Sulphur.

ACONITE may be administered at the commencement of the attack, when the pulse is rapid, the chills and heat frequent or continuous, the inflammation in the throat acute, with dryness, and pricking sensations, aggravated by speaking.

DOSE.—One drop of the dilution, or six globules, in ten spoonfuls of water, a spoonful to be given every two hours, after which give *Belladonna* or *Mercurius viv.*

ARSENICUM is one of the most reliable remedies if the disease assumes a malignant type, or when it prevails as an epidemic, with great prostration of strength, and sinking of the vital powers; nausea and vomiting; inability even to sit upright, without feeling faint; ulcers spread rapidly, take on a livid color, with disposition to slough; or in more advanced stages, after deep, dark sloughs or ulcerations are already estab-

38

lished, having a livid margin; the teeth and lips being covered with a dark sordes; the tongue cracked and tremulous, parched and blackish; pulse small; eyes dull and glassy; acrid discharge from the nostrils; skin hot and dry; excessive thirst, but drinking little at a time; the patient seems rapidly sinking, and a livid colored rash breaks out in blotches here and there.

DOSE.—The same as directed for *Mercurius viv.*

AURUM.—Against a chronic predisposition to malignant sore throat; also if it be a syphilitic or a mercurial complication; the pains seeming to extend even to the loins; fetid smell from the mouth, like strong cheese; ulceration of the palate, or of the tonsils, of a bluish color; and even in caries of the bony structures, with piercing pains, and great sensibility to cold.

DOSE.—One drop, of the dilution, or six globules, in six spoonfuls of water, give a spoonful every four hours, for several days, or until the symptoms are modified.

BELLADONNA, in the most acute cases; the pain in the throat is raw, sore, pressing, burning and shooting, worse when swallowing, and extending into the ears; or there is a sense of spasmodic constriction and contraction, with an uncontrollable desire to swallow; thirst, with dread of drink, or complete inability to swallow liquids; throat swollen, bright red, with accumulation of slimy mucus on the throat and tongue; swelling of the glands of the throat and neck; headache, chiefly in the forehead; stupor or delirium.

DOSE.—One drop of the dilution, or six globules, dissolved in ten spoonfuls of water, give a spoonful every two hours, until amelioration, or change. After *Belladonna* give *Mercurius viv.* or *Lachesis.*

CHAMOMILLA should be given if there is great restlessness, with partial heats, or with partial shudderings and heats, and inability to swallow, especially hot food; the pains are shooting and burning; the glands of the mouth and throat are swollen, red and inflamed; with excessive inquietude, fretfulness, tossing, groaning and weeping.

DOSE.—One drop of the dilution, or six globules, in ten spoonfuls of water, a spoonful to be given every four hours, until amelioration, or change.

HEPAR SULPH. is an important remedy in the earlier stages, when there is a sensation of an internal tumor or plug in the throat; stinging as if from splinters extending to the ears; and dryness, loss of appetite, with bitterish taste, and violent thirst; or in the latter stages, after suppuration begins to be established, to hasten it forward, and to promote a clean and free discharge, it is an almost invaluable remedy.

DOSE.—One drop of the dilution, or six globules, in six spoonfuls of water, give a spoonful every four hours; continue this remedy two or three days, when called for.

LACHESIS, in cases of great prostration, especially if there is great tumefaction, and swelling of the external, as well as of the internal parts; intermittent and periodical sufferings, especially worse after sleeping, and perhaps mitigated while eating. Tumors in the throat, ulcerations, fœtid odor, sharp pains when swallowing food; and before or after *Arsenicum*, with similar symptoms as are mentioned under that remedy; or after *Belladonna*.

DOSE.—One drop of the dilution, or six globules, in six spoonfuls of water; a spoonful to be given every two hours, until amelioration or change.

MERCURIUS VIV. is also one of the most valuable and important remedies, and in a large majority of cases, will prove its claims to notice. Its symptoms are, stinging pains, especially when swallowing, in the throat and tonsils; inflammatory swelling and redness of all the back part of the mouth and throat; constant desire with painful inability to swallow; liquids escape through the nostrils; salivation, profuse and fœtid; tongue moist and white, or dry and brownish, or blackish.

DOSE.—One drop of the dilution, or six globules, in ten spoonfuls of water, a spoonful to be given every two hours, until amelioration or change.

NITRIC ACID, often, and especially if the complaint be syphilitic in its character; the ulcerations are already established, deep, and with stinging pains, as if caused by splinters; there are reddish-brown or copper-colored spots on the skin; the ulcers bleed easily, and the discharge is acrid, and often mixed with bloody serum.

DOSE.—One drop of the dilution, or six globules, in ten spoonfuls of water; give a spoonful every four hours, for two days, afterwards every twelve hours, for two weeks; then wait a few days without medicine.

PULSATILLA, when with swelling, and dark livid redness of the throat and tonsils, there are shootings in the throat when not swallowing, extending at times, into the ears; sensations of enlargement or swelling, with rawness, scraping, and dryness, without thirst; gastric derangement, nausea, bilious vomiting, shivering, and sometimes when there is excessive accumulation of adhesive mucus in the mouth and throat; adapted to females of a mild and phlegmatic temperament.

DOSE.—One drop of the dilution, or six globules, in ten spoonfuls of water, a spoonful to be given every four hours, until amelioration or change.

RHUS TOX. is indicated, if there be fever towards evening, with hot, dry skin; aching, pricking pain when swallowing, lowness of spirits, anxiety, disposition to tears, the pains being low down the throat; and in extreme cases, when there is great muscular weakness, with trembling, sopor, and other typhoid symptoms, it is almost always a reliable remedy.

DOSE.—Dissolve two drops of the dilution, or twelve globules, in ten spoonfuls of water; give a spoonful every twelve hours, four days. Then follow it with some other indicated remedy.

SILICEA, to promote suppuration, and bring forward the ripening abscess and after *Hepar sulph.*, to favor the formation of healthy granulations in the latter stages, is most valuable.

DOSE.—Give a teaspoonful from a solution of six globules, in ten spoonfuls of water, every twelve hours, for two days.

SULPHUR, in obstinate cases, when after the discharge of the abscess the ulcer shows no disposition to heal, may be given with advantage, or may be alternated with *Hepar sulph.* or *Silicea*, until the healing process is established; it will also be found useful for persons of a psoric constitution, either alone, or in alternation with *Rhus tox.*, *Belladonna*, or *Hepar sulph.*, or after *Mercurius viv.*

DOSE.—One drop of the dilution, or six globules, in ten spoonfuls of water, a spoonful to be given every six hours, until amelioration or change.

15.—Chronic Diseases of the Pharynx.—Chronic Sore Throat.

Besides the diseases of the throat to which we have already alluded, and which may acquire a constitutional basis in the system, the throat is liable to take on disease from a variety of other causes, which require a separate consideration.

The complications which may arise from other acute diseases, as scarlatina, &c., will be treated in the chapters which speak of those diseases, respectively. A form of disease of the pharynx, not uncommon in this country, has been described by Dr. Dunglison, in his treatise on the Practice of Medicine, under the head of Folicular Inflammation of the Pharynx, and by Dr. Popkin, as Tubercles of the Pharynx.

It appears on inspection, to consist of small granulations in the external or mucus membrane which lines

38*

the throat, varying in size from the smallest point to that of half a pea, and so thick, that at times, portions of the throat appear to be lined with them. These granulations, especially if they occupy the upper and back part of the pharynx, not unfrequently resemble in appearance, one of the varieties of Acne Rosacæ, on the face, the pimples being slightly elevated, of a reddish purple color, and sometimes patches of adherent mucus of a white color, may cover portions of the throat, between each of the granulations. This disease, like Acne, may also exist a long time, without producing much effect upon the general health; or in persons of irritable, scrofulous, or psoric tendencies, it may result in serious and fatal lesions, either of the throat or of other important organs. It is characterised by uneasy sensations in the upper and back part of the throat, with dryness, and a disposition to clear the throat by hawking. If it affect also the larynx, there will be huskiness of the voice, and frequent cough, generally without fever, or much change in the general health, but with dryness, and sense as of something adhering to the throat. The disease is thought usually to involve the respiratory, rather than the digestive organs, and to affect persons in middle life,—seldom the very young. It is no evidence of the existence of any other chronic tubercular disease. It appears to bear no little resemblance to Acne. Occasionally, these follicles or tumors break, and discharge a small quantity of tough adhesive matter, and at times ulceration succeeds, the ulcers being surrounded by a livid red inflammation.

TREATMENT.—The remedies most useful in this complaint, will be found to be the same as those which are curative of skin diseases and indolent tumors or eruptions.

Arsenicum, Antimonium crud., Bryonia, Calcarea carb., Causticum, Graphites, Hepar sulph., Kali carb., Phosphorus, Rhus tox., Silicea, and Sulphur.

ARSENICUM.—If there be scraping or burning pains; great sensation of dryness, with dryness of the tongue, which may be brownish or cracked; or if there be gangrenous ulcers, or in persons subject to intermittent fevers, or other intermittent diseases; bitter taste in the mouth and throat; expectoration greyish, greenish, saltish or bitter. After *Rhus tox*.

DOSE.—One drop of the dilution, or six globules, in six spoonfuls of water, give a spoonful every six hours, until amelioration or change.

ANTIMONIUM CRUD.—When there is an accumulation of adherent mucus in the throat, with dryness and scraping; when the tubercles are conoid in shape, and of considerable size; for persons subject to degeneration of the skin, or to callous excrescences; and also if there be inflammation and swelling of the upper portion of the epiglottis; tongue coated white.

DOSE.—One drop of the dilution, or six globules, in six spoonfuls of water, give a spoonful every six hours, for two days, then give the same remedy every twenty-four hours, for one week, then wait for the result. If better, repeat the remedy every alternate week, until a cure is effected.

BRYONIA.—Tenacious mucus in the throat, which cannot be expectorated or detached from the throat without effort; sensation of great dryness; sensation as if some hard and pointed substance were in the throat; sensation of dryness and stiffness, particularly behind the palate; tongue dry or dark colored, or wrinkled; shooting sensations, often when turning or moving the throat.

DOSE.—One drop of the dilution, or six globules, in ten spoonfuls of water, a spoonful to be given every four hours, until amelioration or change.

CALCAREA CARB.—If there be excoriating, constricting and shooting pains; the throat being of a deep red color, and covered perhaps with blisters; dryness, and burning pains; hawking up of mucus, with rawness; the expectoration having a taste of iron; and if there be also glandular swellings, sore throat, as if from a plug, and sensation as if the food had lodged in the throat.

DOSE.—One drop of the dilution, or six globules, in ten spoonfuls of water, a spoonful to be given every six hours, until amelioration or change, or give a dry powder, two globules, every morning, each alternate week, in chronic cases. Useful after *Antimonium crud.* or *Bryonia.*

CAUSTICUM.—If there be soreness, roughness, scraping, stinging or burning pains, with hoarseness; sensation as of small tumors; or sticking as from a splinter in the throat, worse on swallowing; or if there be adherent mucus behind the palate, which can at length be expectorated by hawking and straining.

DOSE·—One drop of the dilution, or six globules, in six spoonfuls of water, take a spoonful every twelve hours, night and morning, in acute cases every six hours, until a change is effected. Or alternate with *Hepar sulph.* or *Arsenicum.*

GRAPHITES.—For persons subject to excoriations of the skin, tetters, glandular obstructions, and asthma; and if the sensations in the throat are scraping, roughness and dryness, especially behind the palate, worse in the morning, and relieved by hawking, which causes expectoration of adherent mucus; or, if there be ulcerations with stitches quick and darting; or ulcerative pain with choking, and much mucus; crumbs frequently lodge in the throat.

DOSE.—One drop of the dilution, or six globules, in ten spoonfuls of water, a spoonful to be given every six hours every alternate week, or until some other remedy is demanded.

HEPAR SULPHUR.—For symptoms similar to *Graphites*, especially if there be ulcerations with suct like bases; sensation as of a plug in the throat, with stingings and pressure, extending even to the ears; and difficulty in swallowing.

DOSE.—One drop of the dilution, or six globules, in ten spoonfuls of water; give a spoonful every four hours, until amelioration or change.

KALI CARB.—If there be a copious accumulation of saliva, and at the same time a sensation of dryness, with soreness and blisters on the tongue, mouth or throat; or if there be much mucus on the palate and in the throat; skin dry; respiration obstructed, with itching and burnings.

DOSE.—One drop of the dilution, or six globules, in ten spoonfuls of water; a spoonful every four hours, until amelioration or change.

PHOSPHORUS.—If there be dryness, scraping, smarting, burning, and pressure, with hawking up of mucus, especially in the morning; or if the skin of the palate be shrivelled or covered with purulent vesicles; and frequently with excoriations, or scabby tetters on the lips or angles of the mouth.

DOSE.—One drop of the dilution, or six globules, in ten spoonfuls of water; a spoonful to be given every twelve hours, night and morning for one week, afterwards give some other remedy, according to the symptoms.

RHUS TOX.—In the commencement of the treatment, and for persons of erysipelatous tendencies, if there be dryness, burnings, itchings and crawlings in the throat; worse at night in bed and at rest; much mucus in the mouth and throat, with frequent hawking in the morning; sensation as if something had been torn from the throat.

DOSE.—One drop of the dilution, or six globules, in ten spoonfuls of water; a spoonful to be given every four hours for four days; after which, *Arsenicum, Graphites, Phosphorus, Silicea* or *Sulphur* may be indicated.

SILICEA.—Often after *Phosphorus*, or in the later stages of the treatment in obstinate cases, where there are tendencies to induration, no less than to ulceration; the pains are crawling, itching, smarting, boring and shoot-ing; sensation of a hair on the tongue or in the throat; prickings as from pins, and frequently difficulty of swal-lowing as if the parts were paralysed.

DOSE.—One drop of the dilution, or six globules, in ten spoonfuls of water; a spoonful to be given every twelve hours for four days; after *Silicea*, give *Rhus tox.*, or omit all medicine and wait the result.

SULPHUR, when there are itching burnings, for per-sons of psoric tendencies, and often when other medicines fail to produce their usual effects, may be given to advan-tage; a dose every successive morning for four mornings, either dry on the tongue or in solution, as most conve-nient; to be afterwards repeated or not, according to the symptoms.

16 —Hooping-cough.

This disease is usually epidemic, and is, by many, supposed to be contagious. It is generally confined to children, and persons seldom suffer a second attack. The disease may be very slight, though it is more often distressing, and sometimes fatal. Old school practice, in this disease, no better than old wives' fables, weakened the vital energies, and rendered the little sufferer less able to resist the more acute forms of the malady. Homœopathy, on the contrary, almost always overcomes the more distressing symptoms, and shortens the duration of the disease, without leaving after it any evil conse-quences, calculated to retard the restoration of health.

It is distinguished by a cough, which is spasmodic, and often convulsive, or suffocative, attended, at times, with a peculiar hoop while drawing in the breath, whilst the fits of coughing usually occur while the breath is being thrown outward, from the chest. It is divided into three stages, the febrile, the convulsive, or the nervous stage, and the stage of conva lescence.

The febrile stage is characterised by the symptoms of a severe cold, with cough, and difficulty of breathing.

In the second, or nervous stage, as the fever diminishes, the hooping commences; the cough recurs in paroxysms; the face, perhaps swells and becomes livid; mucus or blood may exude from the mouth or nose; the breathing appears interrupted; but after a deep inspiration, the patient usually quickly recovers, and remains during the intervals, almost perfectly well.

The third stage, is either the period of convalescence, or of prostration, according as the disease has been successfully or unsuccessfully managed from its com-mencement. Unsuccessful cases are liable to assume a chronic form, when emaciation, debility, and sometimes death ensues.

The remedies should be selected for each of the above periods, according to the symptoms attendant upon each, either at their earliest manifestations, or immediately antecedently thereto, and carefully continued, until the disease is found to yield, which will often be in an unex-pectedly short time; and by carefully noting the changes which occur, and adapting the remedies to the remaining symptoms, convalescence will rapidly take place.

For the forming, febrile, or catarrhal stage, the remedies most appropriate, are those given in ordinary catarrh from a cold. They are Aconite, Belladonna, Bryonia, Ipecacuanha, Nux vomica, Phosphorus, Pulsa-tilla, Tartar emetic.

ACONITE.—Dry whistling cough, with fever, and hot dry skin.

DOSE.—One drop of the dilution, or ten globules, in ten spoonfuls of water, give a spoonful every two hours. It should usually be followed with some other remedy, after being continued from twelve to twenty-four hours.

BELLADONNA.—Dry, hollow, barking cough, worse at night; or with sore throat, fever, red flushed face. It is also useful in the more advanced stages, even when the brain appears affected; the child can not endure the light; is impatient of noise, or of movement; headache; more or less delirium; convulsions; and if the paroxysms terminate with sneezing.

DOSE.—One drop of the dilution, or six globules, in six spoonfuls of water, give a spoonful every two or four hours, until amelioration, or change. It is often appropriate before or after *Cuprum*, or after *Helleborus* or *Bryonia*.

BRYONIA is a valuable remedy both in the early and later stages, and is often indicated when there is congestion to the head, and symptoms of an inflammatory condition of the lungs; also when *Belladonna*, and *Helleborus* were insufficient in the later stages, and for similar symptoms.

DOSE.—The same as *Belladonna*.

IPECACUANHA.—Dry cough: with strangulation; great anguish; and when a fresh fit of coughing is excited by the act of breathing, and at almost every breath; coughing fits, with spasmodic stiffness of the body; blueness of the face; anxiety; and with much mucus.

DOSE.—One drop of the dilution, or six globules. in ten spoonfuls of water, give a spoonful every hour for four hours, afterwards every two or four hours, until some other remedy is indicated. It may often be followed by *Nux vomica*.

NUX VOMICA should be given either just before or at the commencement of the second stage, the symptoms being similar to *Ipecacuanha*, and if the paroxysms occur after midnight, or in the morning, and are attended with vomiting. Or it may be given at the earliest stages, if there is acute coryza, with stoppage of the nose; difficulty of breathing; costiveness, and soreness either of the whole abdomen or of the stomach pit.

DOSE.—One drop of the dilution, or six globules, in six spoonfuls of water, a spoonful to be given every four hours, until amelioration or change. Useful after *Ipecacuanha*, and before or after *Belladonna*.

PHOSPHORUS will be found useful in the inflammatory stage, especially if the child complains of a distressing constriction across the chest; if the breathing is short, and the thirst great, with debility; and often after *Aconite* or *Bryonia*, when they appear to be indicated.

DOSE.—As *Nux vomica*.

PULSATILLA.—Loose cough; hoarseness; inclination to vomit; sneezing; weakness of the eyes, with abundant tears; and often with diarrhœa.

DOSE.—The same as *Ipecacuanha*.

TARTAR EMETIC.—For symptoms similar to *Phosphorus*, and especially if there is rattling of mucus in the chest, and retching. This remedy, if given at the commencement of the disease, will often diminish its violence, and at times cut it short.

DOSE.—Same as *Nux vomica*.

For the second or the nervous stage, additional remedies will be found in Carbo veg., Cuprum, Drosera, Opium and Veratrum.

CARBO VEG.—When the first symptoms of hooping appear, worse in the evening, with sore throat; or after the use of *Drosera* or *Veratrum*, to hasten a favorable termination; or if a tendency to vomit still remain in the latter stages. This remedy and *Cuprum* have often been found useful in restoring the tone of the system, so that other remedies which had before appeared to fail, have acted with effect, and completed the cure.

CUPRUM.—When after each paroxysm of cough, there are convulsions and loss of consciousness, which cease when the paroxysms return; also when the paroxysms are very frequent, with rigidity of the body or of the limbs; drowsiness; rattling of mucus in the chest; and congestions to the brain. Before or after *Belladonna*, or in alternation with *Helleborus* or *Bryonia*. It may also be given after *Phosphorus* or *Tartar emetic* in congestions to the lungs or chest, if indicated by its own peculiar symptoms.

DROSERA.—Paroxysms of cough in rapid succession, with a shrill hoop; vomiting; relief on moving about; if there be fever, it is characterised by chilliness, heat and thirst, hot perspiration, especially in the night. Often after *Carbo veg.*

OPIUM.—When there is stupor; anguish; irregular breathing; constipation; and if the indicated remedies do not produce the desired effect.

VERATRUM.—Often, and when there are cold sweats, especially on the forehead; excessive thirst; involuntary urination; vomiting; perhaps fever, with miliary eruptions, or with great weakness; small and quick pulse; apathy and drowsiness; disliking to move or speak. Often useful after *Cuprum.*

The third stage, if the convalescence be favorable, will need no medicine; if unfavorable, the symptoms must be treated as they appear, the cause being properly considered, and the peculiar dyscrasies, or the constitutional condition of the system, taken into the account.

ADMINISTRATION.—In the second stage the remedies may generally be administered as follows: Give *Veratrum* first, either one or two globules on the tongue, or a spoonful of a dilution of one drop, or six globules, in ten spoonfuls of water, immediately after a paroxysm, then wait till the next paroxysm, after which give another dose, and so on after each paroxysm, until from two to four doses are taken, then wait twenty-four hours, and if there be improvement, continue to wait until the improvement ceases, or until the cough becomes worse again. If there be no improvement, select another remedy : or *Drosera* may be administered at the first instead of *Veratrum*, two to four doses ; if there be no improvement in two or three days, select another remedy. *Drosera* is often administered after *Veratrum*. Other remedies may be administered in the same manner.

17.—Bronchitis. Influenza. Grippe.

Inflammation of the Bronchia. Catarrh on the Chest.

This is a disease of the mucus lining of the bronchial tubes, and is divided into acute and chronic. The symptoms of acute bronchitis are chilliness, fever, hoarseness; difficult breathing, or shortness of breath, sometimes threatening suffocation; wheezing, with rattling or whistling, or harsh, rough and broken sounds in the chest; severe cough, frequent and distressing, at first dry and with scanty expectoration, afterwards copious; general weakness; loss of appetite; foul tongue; pale lips, and anxious countenance. If the disease terminate favorably, with a diminution of the fever the breathing becomes easier, and the expectoration thicker less frothy or stringy; if unfavorably, the difficulty of breathing increases, a state of debility or collapse sets in, the body is covered with a cold clammy sweat, the face becomes livid, and mucus accumulates in the chest, which the patient is unable to expectorate; there is usually pain, or a sense of constriction, especially in the upper part of the chest and along the region of the breast bone, which is greatly aggravated by coughing. It is distinguished from influenza by being more confined to the upper part of the chest or thorax, and from lung fever or pneumonia, because in the latter disease the fever, pain, and other sufferings are usually referable to those parts of the chest more distant from the sternum or pit of the stomach ; and by the sputa, which in pneumonia assumes a greyish or rust-colored appearance. A correct diagnosis can however only be made by an experienced physician.

TREATMENT.—The most useful remedies are Aconite, Belladonna, Bryonia and Phosphorus; next to these are Lachesis, Mercurius vivus, Pulsatilla, Nux vomica and Spongia.

ACONITE is almost always required in the earlier stages, when the skin is unusually hot and dry, the pulse strong and rapid, breathing obstructed, cough short and dry, anxiety, restlessness and thirst.

DOSE.—One drop of the dilution, or six globules, in ten spoonfuls of water; give a spoonful every two or four hours, according to the seventy of the attack; after which, give *Belladonna, Bryonia* or *Phosphorus.*

BELLADONNA.—If there be extreme sensitiveness to pain when coughing, either in the chest or head; oppression and constriction as if bound; dry fatiguing cough, worse at night, with short and anxious breathing; and especially for children in insidious cases, coming on suddenly, and threatening suffocation.

DOSE.—One drop of the dilution, or six globules, in ten spoonfuls of water; give a spoonful every three hours, until amelioration or change.

BRYONIA.—Laborious, short and anxious breathing, with constant inclination to take a deep inspiration; dry cough, with burning, pricking pains in the region of the sternum and pit of the throat; dryness of the mouth and lips, with thirst; headache, especially on coughing; shooting pains in the chest and sides.

DOSE.—The same as *Aconite.* After *Bryonia, Phosphorus* is often indicated; or if abundant expectoration follow, *Hepar sulph.* or *Spongia* may be useful.

LACHESIS.—Oppression at the chest, with pressive sensations as if the chest were too full; suffocative breathing, with choking, and sense of swelling and tightness; or with wheezing, and deep, difficult or asthmatic breathing, with anxiety and depression; worse at night after lying down, or after sleeping.

DOSE.—The same as *Belladonna.*

MERCURIUS VIV.—If in addition to the ordinary symptoms there are excessive perspirations; coryza, with acrid discharge; much swelling of the mouth and throat; offensive breath; or dryness in the chest, breathing quick and short, with tickling and fatiguing cough; often after *Belladonna.*

DOSE.—One drop of the dilution, or six globules, in ten spoonfuls of water; give a spoonful every four hours, until amelioration or change.

PHOSPHORUS.—After *Aconite;* respiration oppressive; heat in the chest; constriction, anxiety and oppression; cough dry, with tickling in the throat or chest; aggravated by talking; stringy mucus expectoration, and often with difficulty; and especially if the disease appears to be complicated with pneumonia.

DOSE.—The same as *Mercurius viv.*

PULSATILLA.—After *Aconite,* when the fever is abated, the expectoration thick and abundant; and for persons of mild lymphatic constitution; or for females, when, as not unfrequently happens, bronchitis follows a suppression of the catamenia; and if there be rattling of mucus in the chest; shaking cough, and expectoration of thick and tenacious or yellowish mucus, at times mixed with blood.

DOSE.—One drop of the dilution, or six globules, in ten spoonfuls of water; give a spoonful every four hours, until amelioration, or change.

RHUS TOX. is a remedy which has too frequently been overlooked in affections of the respiratory organs. In addition to the symptoms mentioned under *Bryonia,* its indications are ticklings, crawlings, burnings and shootings, anxiety, and depression, weakness, trembling

39*

and uneasiness; or torpidity, languor and sleepiness;
the cough is short and dry, with weakness and short
breath; tickling low down in the chest, worse in
the evening and at night, or when at rest, and after
waking in the morning, and sometimes attended with
pain in the stomach, or with pressure and squeezing at
the stomach pit.

DOSE.—One drop of the dilution, or six globules, in ten spoonfuls of
water, a spoonful to be given every four hours, until amelioration, or
change.

SPONGIA.—After *Aconite,* when a distinct sonorous
sound, or a mucus, rattling sound, can still be heard
under the sternum or breast bone; the cough being dry
and hollow, and continued through the day, but worse
towards evening; or cough, with scanty expectoration,
viscid and ropy; heat or burning in the chest; respiration
laborious, or inability to breathe, except the head be
thrown backwards.

DOSE.—One drop of the dilution, or six globules, may be dissolved in
ten spoonfuls of water, give a spoonful every three hours, until amelioration,
or change.

18.—Inflammation of the Lungs.   (*Pneumonia.   Lung Fever.*)

When the substance of the lungs takes on inflammation, there are generally rigors, followed by heats, with
great heat of the skin; thirst; restlessness; pulse rapid
and full, or hard and wiry, or quick, weak, and variable;
tongue dry and parched; urine scanty, red, and sometimes scalding; short, distressing, and continuous cough,
aggravated by speaking and breathing; scanty expectoration of viscid, tenacious mucus, which may be at first
nearly transparent, and which appears to arise from low
down in the chest, but soon becomes of a greyish, rusty,
or brick-dust color; interrupted, hesitating speech, with

frequent pauses; and abdominal respiration. Sometimes there is dull pain, and sometimes only a sense of tightness in the chest; the patient lies, either on the affected side, or on his back; his breathing is short, hurried, and difficult; and an unusual degree of heat may commonly be felt in the axilla and region of the ribs. If the disease progress, the face often exhibits patches of redness, and lividity;. the vessels of the neck become swollen and turgid; the pulse weak and irregular, or thready; and the patient may sink, either from exhaustion, or from obstruction of the lungs.

If an abscess form in the lung, a gurgling sound may be heard by applying the ear over that portion of the chest; shiverings usually precede the formation of the ulceration, and a hollow, or cavernous, respiratory sound will follow, after the abscess has been emptied by expectoration and coughing. Abundant expectoration of whitish or yellowish mucus; general sweat; a sudden profuse discharge of urine, with abundant sediment; and sometimes, even diarrhœa, or epistaxis, are regarded as crises, giving promise of a favorable termination.

The most useful remedies are Aconite, Belladonna, Bryonia, Phosphorus, Rhus tox., Tartar emetic, and Sulphur.

ACONITE, in the early or inflammatory stage, can seldom fail to be of use. It should be continued so long as the fever is of a decidedly inflammatory type; the pulse rapid and full; the skin dry; and the thirst excessive.

DOSE.—One drop of the dilution, or six globules, in ten spoonfuls of water, give a spoonful every two hours, until amelioration, or change.

BELLADONNA is indicated by cerebral symptoms;

452   ORGANS OF RESPIRATION,

exanthematous eruptions; flushed face; headache; and other congestive symptoms.

DOSE.—The same as *Aconite.*

These two remedies may often prove sufficient in the milder cases, to subdue an attack.

BRYONIA, especially if the disease be complicated, with pleuritic symptoms, (plueripneumonia,) if there be catching, shooting pains in the region of the pleura, diaphragm, or heart, or in the pectoral muscles; thick coated tongue; constipation, with gastric derangement; or after *Aconite* and *Belladonna* have been given with partial success; and especially if there is an increase of the pains or sufferings, on movement.

DOSE.—The same as *Aconite.*

PHOSPHORUS is regarded as a most invaluable remedy, and by some is relied on in every stage of this disease. It is no doubt most efficient in those advanced and dangerous cases, in which there are muttering delirium, and suffocative paroxysms; laborious respiration; debility; small quick pulse; and threatened paralysis of the lungs; also if there be great prostration; paleness of the face; dimness of the sight; dry cough, especially at night; and great depression of the physical power. Or if there be cold and clammy sweats, with coldness of the breath; tremulous, and scarcely perceptible pulse; sharp, and livid face; frequent cough, with brown, frothy, and rusty colored sputa; dulness of the chest on percussion, so that it seems as if a wall were struck, instead of the chest.

DOSE.—One drop of the dilution, or six globules, may be given in ten spoonfuls of water, every two hours, a spoonful, until amelioration or change.

TARTAR EMETIC.—Extreme oppression, and obstructed respiration, without pain; loose cough, with much rattling in the chest, and expectoration of lumps of mucus without much blood: also, if there be a sensation as if the chest were lined with velvet; a sore pain as if from excoriation, occurring in paroxysms; burning sensations under the sternum, as if the bronchia were inflamed,—that is, the pneumonia being complicated with catarrhal, rather than pleuritic symptoms; respiration, short, oppressed, rendering it necessary for the patient to sit up in bed; intermittent respiration; difficulty of breathing, in paroxysms, especially in the night; oppressed breathing, with difficulty of swallowing; also, if there be much coughing and violent sneezing, with tickling sensations; night cough, or cough after eating, with vomiting the contents of the stomach, and pain in the left side, above the hypochondria.

DOSE.—The same as *Phosphorus*.

RHUS TOX., is an important remedy in the congestive stage, when there is extreme restlessness, anxiety, palpitation of the heart, and redness of the face; also, if the pneumonia has followed severe and long continued exertion, and in cold weather; or been the result of a contusion, fall, blow, or other mechanical injury; also, before or after *Sulphur*, in exanthematous cases.

DOSE.—One drop, or six globules, in six spoonfuls of water, give a spoonful every four hours, until a change is effected, or some other remedy indicated.

SULPHUR.—After *Aconite* and *Belladonna* to complete the cure, when these medicines have acted favorably, and also after *Phosphorus* or *Tartar emetic;* and for persons of scrofulous habits, and when in the advanced stages other remedies fail to produce their accustomed effects; also, in cases of repercussion of some exanthematous disease, and in tuberculous patients, long subject to old chronic coughs; or if there be purulent or serous expectoration; and in case of obstinate constipation,

DOSE.—The same as *Rhus tox.*

REMARKS.—The above are by no means all the remedies which may be found useful in the acute forms of pneumonia, though it is believed they will be found sufficient to cure a large portion even of the most obstinate cases. A number of other remedies, the symptomatic indications for which, we would not have space to describe in a work on domestic practice, will be known and carefully studied, by every intelligent physician. Of these, Arsenicum is adapted to the pneumonia of old persons; also to debilitated, scrofulous, or cachetic constitutions. Aconite is indicated, where there is inflammation or excitement of the arterial system; Belladonna, where there is sensitiveness to movement or to the touch,—also, in cerebral complications; Bryonia, for complications with pleurisy; and Phosphorus and Tartar emetic, where actual congestion of the lungs has taken place. Arnica, to cases from mechanical violence, or if attended with profuse spitting of blood; Mercurius viv., if there are copious night sweats, not alleviated by Bryonia or Phosphorus; Lachesis, Nux vomica, or Opium, in the pneumonia of drunkards, or for persons accustomed to the use of ardent spirits; Pulsatilla, for chlorotic females; and Lachesis, Arsenicum, and China, where there is threatened gangrene of the lungs.

The characteristic rust-colored sputa, usually appears the second or third day; the crisis takes place on the seventh; and the patient often returns to his accustomed avocations on the fourteenth day, if otherwise healthy, and under homœopathic treatment.

19.—Spurious Pneumonia. (*Peripneumonia. Pneumonia Notha.*)

Usually affects the aged, seldom the middle aged or the young. It commences like a common cold, with cough, and alternate heats ,and chills. The cough is generally loose, the sputa white or yellow, slimy and bloody; breathing quick and laborious, with great sense of weight and oppression; pain at a small circumscribed spot, on taking a deep inspiration; aggravated by every thing which causes increased action of the lungs; lying on either side oppressive; patient generally lies on his back; pulse soft and quick; voice low and weak; skin damp, or nocturnal sweats, which afford no relief; symptoms alleviated in the morning.

TREATMENT.—First give Aconite or Mercurius viv., afterwards Belladonna. If this does not complete the cure, return again to Aconite, and after a few doses give Chamomilla.

ARSENICUM is a most important remedy, and will often restore the patient when all other remedies fail, and the case appears hopeless. Especially after *Nux vomica, Ipecacuanha* or *Veratrum.*.

IPECACUANHA, in repeated doses, when *Mercurius viv.* does not afford relief, and attended with anguish or anxiety. Or if the anguish increase, the extremities become cold, and paroxysms of suffocation threaten, give *Veratrum.*

NUX VOMICA is called for when, with a dry cough and difficult expectoration, there is excessive tension, oppression, and sense of fulness, with the sense of weight.

TARTAR EMETIC.—If there be excessive accumulation of mucus in the bronchial tubes. In some cases also *Arnica, Phosphorus, Pulsatilla* or *Sulphur* may be indicated. See also the remedies under Bronchitis, Pneumonia and Pleurisy.

DOSE.—For any one of the above remedies, given in solution, one drop, or six globules, in ten spoonfuls of water, give a spoonful every two to four hours, or if the danger be imminent, every half hour, or oftener, according to the symptoms.

20.—Typhoid or Congestive Pneumonia.

In this disease the accompanying fever is of a low or typhoid character; the pulse slightly changed, or quick and very weak; lassitude; shivering; loss of appetite; skin rather dry and harsh than hot, or having a clammy feel; little or no pain; tongue dry and parched; urine scanty and high-colored; respiration often at first but little affected, but gradually becoming short, quick and laborious; great prostration, and often cerebral symptoms ensue. It sometimes appears to succeed other diseases, as bilious or gastric affections, and is sometimes apparently epidemic. Patients at times survive weeks or months, and at times, at least under old school prescriptions, death takes place in a single day.

REMEDIES.—Arnica, Arsenicum, Opium, Phosphorus, Rhus tox. and Veratrum.

ARNICA has been recommended after Opium, when the disease is clearly defined, the typhoid and cerebral symptoms manifest, and the congested condition of the lungs rendered certain by auscultation and percussion.

DOSE·—One drop of the dilution, or six globules, in ten spoonfuls of water, a spoonful to be given every two hours, until amelioration or change.

ARSENICUM.—Pulse small and weak, or irregular; coldness; rapid failure of strength, and desire to lie down; sleep unrefreshing, uneasy, restless, agitated, with starts and fright; cold and clammy sweats; shiverings or heats, or burnings in the chest; lassitude and oppression, with great prostration; coldness of the body or alternated with burning heat, or with sense of internal heat; irritability or indifference; worse at night, or in bed, and after sleeping.

DOSE.—One drop of the dilution, or six globules, in ten spoonfuls of water, a spoonful to be given every two hours, in desperate cases every half hour, until amelioration, or change.

OPIUM.—Respiration difficult, slow and intermittent, with weak and low voice; obstructed, suffocative, stifling respiration; head bewildered, with dizziness and vertigo; or with heaviness and congestions to the head; violent pulsations and constipation.

DOSE.—The same as *Arnica*.

PHOSPHORUS.—In desperate cases, even with muttering delirium; picking at the bed clothes; suffocative paroxysms; debility and threatened paralysis of the lungs; and when auscultation and percussion reveal a congested or even an indurated condition of portions of the lung.

DOSE.—One drop of the dilution, or six globules, in ten spoonfuls of water, a spoonful every four hours, until amelioration or change.

RHUS TOX. will prove an efficient remedy, as it is clearly indicated by the dry, harsh skin; the scanty urination; dry and parched tongue; short, dry cough, with anxious expression; weakness; sanguineous congestion; prostration; heaviness and pressive fulness; also by its moral symptoms; anxiety; inquietude; stupefaction; delirium.

DOSE.—The same as *Phosphorus*.

VERATRUM is also chiefly indicated when the extremities become cold; the lips and face livid, with clammy sweat on the forehead, and great weakness; sudden prostration; shivering, with slow pulse, almost extinct; delirium, and with desire to run away.

DOSE.—The same as *Arsenicum*.

40

21.—Pleurisy.

The lungs have already been described, as dividing into two large branches, towards the right and left side of the thorax, or upper portion of the chest, above the abdomen, and surrounded by the ribs. Each of these branches is covered with an investiture, sac, or sheath, which serves a two-fold purpose; by its connections with the diaphragm, sternum, spine, and with the walls of the chest, to retain them in position; and also, to protect them from too close contiguity or contact with other organs. This covering, is a reflexion from the membrane or skin of the lungs, and also from the inner walls of the thorax. It is a muscular tissue, its surface being covered with a serous coat, from which is constantly exuded a lubricating fluid, calculated to give ease of motion to the constantly expanding and contracting organs it serves to protect or support. This double sheath, covering, or sac, is called the pleura,—and inflammation of the pleura, is called pleurisy. It partakes more of the nature of a rheumatic affection, than any of the diseases of the respiratory organs we have yet considered, and is characterised by pains of a rheumatic character. These pains are catching, sticking, stitching, cutting, lancinating,—often confined to one spot in the side, arresting the breathing, and greatly aggravated by coughing, or by drawing in the breath. Respiration is difficult and anxious, but with less oppression than in pneumonia; pulse quick and hard; cough short and dry; tongue parched; urine scanty and high colored; patient lies on his back, and if there be effusion in one spot, lying on the opposite side is very difficult. The tendency of inflammation of the serous surfaces, no less than of the mucus surfaces, is to produce effusion; but as the serous surfaces are all shut sacs, that is, have no opening to the external air, this exudation is usually removed by absorption. When, however, the case is neglected, or the absorbent powers weakened by blood-letting, blistering, and other similar expedients, the effused fluid, occupying the space between its own surface and the contiguous organ, gradually dries up, or changes its character, and becomes plastic,—an adhesion ensues, and the neighboring organ becomes closely cemented to the serous coat. In this way, the lungs have been cemented to the pleura, the pleura to the diaphragm and side, this again to the liver, the liver to the stomach, side, and back, laying the foundation either for painful activity, or partial inactivity of these great and important organs.

This, if the pleura be implicated, constitutes one of the forms of chronic pleurisy, which, although it may be alleviated, it is not often possible to cure. Other forms of pleurisy yield readily to medicine.

REMEDIES.—Aconite, Arnica, Arsenicum, Bryonia, Belladonna, Phosphorus, Rhus tox. and Sulphur.

ACONITE will almost always produce a favorable impression within the first twelve hours from its administration, in acute cases; after which, the cure may sometimes be completed with *Sulphur.*

DOSE.—One drop of the dilution, or six globules, dissolved in ten spoonfuls of water, a spoonful to be given every half hour, until amelioration or change.

ARNICA, if from external injury, and after *Aconite* when soreness and pain on movement alone remain; or if pleuritis supervene upon long continued and laborious exertion, and to promote absorption when considerable effusion has taken place.

DOSE.—One drop of the dilution, or six globules, in ten spoonfuls of water, give a spoonful every three hours for twelve hours, then every six hours, until the pains and soreness subside; afterwards give *Sulphur* or *Arsenicum*, if indicated.

ARSENICUM is a remedy on which we place great reliance in extreme cases, where much serous effusion has already taken place; where the respiration is obstructed, and there are asthmatic symptoms, with much prostration of strength.

DOSE and Administration.—The same as *Arnica*.

BRYONIA, génerally after *Aconite*, or often at the commencement, when the shooting, lancinating, burning pains are increased by every inspiration, or by movement; dry cough, or cough with dirty or bloody expectoration, and great aggravation of pain; dry, cracked, brown, or yellow coated tongue; bitter taste, nausea, and perhaps vomiting; aching, painful pressure at the pit of the stomach, and hypochondria; intense thirst; constipation; giddiness, and confusion in the head; aching and shooting pains in the head as if it would burst, especially when coughing; disturbed sleep, with frequent startings; comatose sleep; delirium; burning heat of the skin, or clammy perspiration; aching in the limbs; cough on lying on the side, with impossibility of lying otherwise than on the back.

DOSE.—Two drops of the dilution, or twelve globules, dissolved in ten spoonfuls of water, a spoonful to be given every hour, until amelioration or change.

BELLADONNA, if there is great restlessness or sleeplessness, or comatose sleep with delirium; or if the pains in the side are extreme and unendurable, increased by the slightest touch or movement; pains in the head and eyes; and if the pain and fever return after being alleviated by other remedies.

DOSE.—One drop of the dilution, or six globules, in ten spoonfuls of water, give a spoonful every two hours, until alleviation or change.

PHOSPHORUS, in cases complicated with pneumonia or bronchitis, and in all extreme cases, where the lungs also are implicated, will be found a valuable remedy.

DOSE.—The same as *Belladonna*.

RHUS TOX. is also a valuable remedy in pleurisy, even where adhesions have already taken place, and also if with the shooting, lancinating pains, there is tension, and short breath, with pressure; and in chronic cases relieved by walking and by vigorous exercise, but felt worse when beginning to move, and when at rest. Its symptoms are, shootings, drawings, tension and constriction, with sense of weakness.

DOSE·—The same as *Arnica*.

SULPHUR in almost all cases, may follow *Aconite* or *Bryonia*, or if the fever be not violent, and we suspect effusion already to have taken place, it may be given at the outset, alone, or in alternation with *Aconite, Rhus tox.,* or *Bryonia*, and be continued until the effusion shall disappear; or it may be followed by *Arsenicum*, in cases where that remedy becomes indicated. Also, in cases complicated with pneumonia, to prevent solidification, and favor resolution, it is a most reliable remedy.

DOSE.—One drop of the dilution, or six globules, in six spoonfuls of water, give a spoonful every four or six hours, if in alternation with some other remedy; otherwise every two hours, in severe cases, until amelioration or change.

22 —Asthma,

Is an affection of the lungs and chest, characterised by difficulty of breathing, occurring in paroxysms, attended with suffocation, constrictive sensations, cough, and wheezing. The patient usually sits or stands, his arms elevated so as to lift upward and outward the walls of the chest; often requests the windows and doors to be opened, and makes frequent efforts to expel something

40*

from the air passages by hawking or coughing; the face has an anxious expression; the extremities are generally cold; and there is often cold perspiration on the forehead, face or chest; there is frequently palpitation of the heart or arteries, the pulse is irregular, quick or intermittent, and expectoration does not always afford relief. It has been divided into the dry and the humid asthma; the attacks of the former are much more sudden, violen', and of shorter duration than those of the latter; the cough is slight, and the expectoration scanty; whilst in moist or humid asthma the attacks come on more slowly, and are more protracted, the cough is unusually more severe, expectoration commences early, and when it becomes copious usually affords relief.

The remedies most used by homœopathic practitioners are Aconite, Arsenicum, Belladonna, Bryonia, Cuprum, Ipecacuanha, Lachesis, Moschus, Nux vomica, Pulsatilla, Sambucus, Tartar emetic and Veratrum.

ACONITE.—For persons of a full or plethoric habit; for young persons and children when there is active palpitation of the heart; congestion to the head; vertigo; or when the paroxysm follows some mental excitement.

DOSE.—One drop of the dilution, or six globules, may be infused in ten spoonfuls of water; give a spoonful every half hour, or in extreme cases it may be given every fifteen minutes, or alternated with *Ipecacuanha* or *Belladonna*.

ARSENICUM.—Extreme agitation and moaning; exhaustion and anguish as if at the point of death, with cold perspiration; in confirmed asthmatics, and in old people, when the least exertion brings on a paroxysm; or when paroxysms recur soon after lying down, or with remissions, and continue until after a fit of coughing; a few lumps of viscid mucus filled with vesicles is expectorated; also when paroxysms are liable to be brought on by exposure to cold air, or to changes of temperature; sense of weakness or burning pain.

DOSE.—One drop of the dilution, or six globules, in ten spoonfuls of water; a spoonful to be given every four hours, or oftener, according to the urgency and severity of the symptoms.

BELLADONNA.—For plethoric women, and for children of irritable habits, and if subject to spasms; constriction at the throat, with loss of consciousness, gasping for breath, and constant efforts to dilate the chest; constriction, and feeling as if suffocation would ensue.

DOSE.—The same as *Aconite.*

BRYONIA.—If with the asthmatic symptoms there are pains in the hypochondria, and inability to lie on the right side; or if the patient is constrained to lie on his back; shootings in the chest on breathing deeply, or on coughing, or from movement; difficulty of breath-ing, aggravated by talking or by movement; cough with expectoration, at first frothy, afterwards glutinous, attended at times with vomiting or retching.

DOSE.—One drop of the dilution, or six globules, in ten spoonfuls of water, give a spoonful every hour; in extreme cases, every half hour, until some change is manifested; after which, select some other remedy for the remaining symptoms.

CUPRUM.—For hysterical women after fright or anger, or before or during the menses, when there are spasms, oppression at the chest, with short dry cough, aggravated by talking.

DOSE.—The same as *Belladonna.*

IPECACUANHA.—Spasmodic constriction of the throat in nightly paroxysms, with suffocation and rattling from an accumulation of mucus in the chest; redness and heat, or paleness and coldness, and ghastliness of the face; nausea, and cold perspiration on the forehead; coldness of the feet, anxiety, and dread of suffocation; spasmodic rigidlty; feeling as if dust were being drawn into the lungs.

DOSE.—One drop of the dilution, or six globules, in ten spoonfuls of of water; give a spoonful every half hour, or oftener, for one or two hours, or until four doses are given; afterwards, alternate with *Arsenicum*, or some other indicated remedy.

LACHESIS.—Wheezing respiration after eating, or attacks of suffocation; worse when lying down, or after sleeping, with sensations of fulness or bloatedness; and for women after the change of life.

DOSE.—Same as *Belladonna*.

MOSCHUS.—Asthma of hysterical females, with spasmodic constrictions, and paroxysms of suffocation, commencing with a fit of coughing, followed by distressing oppression, constriction, almost driving the patient to madness and distraction.

DOSE.—The same as *Belladonna*.

NUX VOMICA.—Suffocative tightness at the lower part of the thorax, near the stomach and hypochondria; aching and pressive pains in the region of the liver and stomach, with distension of the abdomen and stomach pit; flatulence; inability to endure the slightest pressure, even from the clothing around the chest or waist; clothing seems to press, even when loose; sufferings worse in the morning, or when walking in the open air, especially if cold; also after exertion; alleviated by lying on the back, or by frequently changing the position; for persons of irritable temperament, and for those addicted to the use of ardent spirits. Before or after *Arsenicum*.

DOSE.—One drop of the dilution, or six globules, in ten spoonfuls of water, a spoonful every half hour during the paroxysm; to be continued afterwards every four hours if necessary; or give *Nux vomica*, a spoonful at three o'clock, in the afternoon, and at bed time, and *Arsenicum* at six and at ten o'clock in the morning, to overcome a predisposition to such attacks, every alternate four days, for one month, then wait till the next attack.

PULSATILLA.—Asthma of females after cessation of the menses; or from suppression by cold; choking, suffocative paroxysms, with death-like anguish, and palpitation of the heart; much mucus expectoration, streaked with blood, which is at times coagulated, sense of fulness and pressure in the chest. Before or after *Lachesis*.

DOSE.—One drop of the dilution, or six globules, in ten spoonfuls of water, a spoonful every two hours until a change is effected. In severe cases alternate with *Lachesis* or *Moschus*. Also after *Aconite*.

SAMBUCUS.—If the respiration be rapid, laborious, wheezing, with anguish, and dread of suffocation; oppression of the chest, as from a weight, and sometimes with swelling and lividity of the face and hands, sometimes general heat, tremor, and inability to speak above a whisper; worse when lying down; also for children, when they wake from sleep in a start, and exhibit many asthmatic symptoms; also if there is much perspiration. Often useful after *Ipecacuanha*.

DOSE.—The same as *Ipecacuanha*.

TARTAR EMETIC.—Oppression at the chest, with excessive secretion of mucus, low down in the bronchia; difficult breathing; suffocative cough; and anxiety at the præcordial region; especially for old persons and children, with paroxysms of retching, choking, and suffocation, especially in the evening.

DOSE.—One drop of the dilution, or six globules, in ten spoonfuls of water, a spoonful to be given every half hour, or oftener, according to the symptoms.

VERATRUM.—In violent attacks of spasmodic asthma, with suffocative symptoms; coldness of the nose, ears, and feet, with cold perspiration especially in females, before the menstrual period; and if aggravated by movement.

DOSE.—The same as *Tartar emetic*.

23.—Determination of Blood to the Chest.

(Congestion of the Chest.)

This condition is distinguished by a sensation of fulness, with weight or pressure, throbbings and palpitation of the heart, attended with anxious expression and short, sighing, and difficult breathing; and sometimes with slight cough. It is most frequent in children and young people, and in persons of consumptive habit. Its exciting causes are undue activity; exposure to heat and cold; stimulants, such as coffee, spices, vinous and alcoholic drinks, or narcotic drugs; repressed eruptions; suppression of accustomed discharges, &c., &c.

REMEDIES. — Aconite, Belladonna, Bryonia, Ipecacuanha, Mercurius viv., Nux vomica, Pulsatilla, and Sulphur.

ACONITE.—For plethoric persons, or with florid complexion; violent oppression, heat and thirst, cough, anxiety, and palpitation of the heart; congestion of females, before, and during the catamenia; followed by *Mercurius* or *Belladonna*, to complete the cure.

DOSE.—One drop of the dilution, or six globules, in ten spoonfuls of water, give a spoonful every half hour, for four hours, afterwards every two hours, until some other remedy be selected, or the more acute symptoms subside.

BELLADONNA.—If, with the oppression, shortness of breath, and palpitation of the heart, there be throbbings in the chest, extending even to the head; cough, mostly at night; internal heat and thirst; also after *Aconite*, unless *Mercurius* be especially indicated.

DOSE.—One drop of the dilution, or six globules, in ten spoonfuls of water, a spoonful every two hours, until amelioration, or change.

BRYONIA.—When with the ordinary symptoms, as anxiety, oppression, palpitation, &c., there are burning heats in the chest, sensation of tightness, and prickings during inspiration.

DOSE.—The same as *Aconite*.

IPECACUANHA.—Often after *Nux vomica*, and for similar symptoms.

MERCURIUS VIV.—After *Aconite*, especially in cases of suppression of customary discharges in females, to complete the cure; and also if there are burnings in the chest, with frequent desire to take a long breath; or expectoration streaked with blood.

DOSE.—The same as *Belladonna*.

NUX VOMICA.—When the affection has arisen from the use of stimulants, or from the suppression of hemorrhoidal discharges; also for females accustomed to profuse menstrual flow, and if the suppression be attended with severe constipation; in irritable, bilious subjects this remedy must always produce favorable results, and will often itself complete the cure. After *Nux vomica*, give *Aconite* or *Sulphur*.

DOSE.—The same as *Aconite*.

PULSATILLA.—When with the constriction, difficulty of breathing, and palpitation, there is ebullition of blood to the chest, with external heat, and aggravation towards evening; also in phlegmatic persons, with hemorrhoidal suppression; and in females with suppression of the menses, especially if they have been suddenly stopped, or if these sufferings appear before menstruation; it may be given after or in alternation with *Aconite* or *Bryonia*, after which give *Sulphur* to complete the cure.

DOSE.—The same as *Belladonna*.

SULPHUR.—After any of the above remedies, and for

similar symptoms, but especially after *Aconite, Nux vomica, Bryonia* and *Pulsatilla.*

DOSE.—One drop of the dilution, or six globules, in ten spoonfuls of water, a spoonful to be given every four hours, four doses, afterwards every morning, to complete the cure.

24.—Spitting of Blood. (*Hæmoptysis.*) Vomiting of Blood.
(*Hæmorrhage from the Lungs.*)

Spitting of blood may be divided into three varieties: First, by effusion from the mucus surfaces.

Second, by congestions, the substance, air vessels, or parenchyma of the lungs, being engorged; throat either in whole or in part, filled with the effused .fluid, which is expectorated by coughing, &c.

Third, by the rupture of a blood vessel in some diseased spot, usually in the body of the lungs, an occurrence not uncommon in tubercular consumption.

The first variety is not at all dangerous, the second but slightly so, and the third is rather an indication of the dangerous condition of the patient, than dangerous in itself. The first variety is perfectly under the control of medicine; the second generally so, and in the third variety, though a patient may die of strangulation, this but seldom happens, and much less frequently from loss of blood.

In such cases do not act too hastily, as haste makes waste, but act calmly, prudently and rightly, and thereby save all the time that is possible. The most dangerous bleedings usually give us the most time, whilst the milder forms more frequently take us by surprise.

TREATMENT.—Place the patient, as quietly as possible, in a half sitting, half lying posture, and let him remain perfectly at rest, without speaking or being spoken to, unless indispensably necessary, and send for a good homœopathic physician. But if no physician or other medicine is at hand, dissolve a spoonful of salt in a tumbler of water, give a teaspoonful of the solution every five, ten, or twenty minutes, until other remedies can be obtained. Or ten drops of Sulphuric acid in a tumbler of water, from which give a teaspoonful as above, until relief is obtained.

REMEDIES.—Aconite, Arnica, Arsenicum, Belladonna, China, Ferrum, Ipecacuanha, Opium, Pulsatilla, Phosphorus and Rhus tox.

ACONITE is indicated for plethoric individuals, or for persons of sanguine temperament, when there is ebullition of blood to the chest; blood gushing up at intervals, with fulness and burning; slight cough; or for the premonitory symptoms, in case of frequent attacks, such as shivering, palpitations, accelerated pulse, anguish, or anxiety, paleness of the face, and aggravations when lying down.

DOSE.—One drop of the dilution, or six globules, in ten spoonfuls of water; give a spoonful every ten or twenty minutes, for two hours; if not relieved give *Ipecacuanha*, or for tuberculous patients, *Phosphorus*.

ARNICA.—In all cases arising from external violence, as from a blow or strain; or for persons who play on wind instruments; and when effusion of blood into the substance (air cells) of the lungs is indicated by constriction and burning low down in the chest, the expectorated blood being warm, sweetish in taste, and with a sensation as if it came from some deep-seated source, or with pain in the region of the shoulders and back; also if there be expectoration of dark colored or coagulated blood, or mixed with mucus, especially if clotted; tickling behind the sternum, with weakness and syncope. Often useful after *Aconite*.

DOSE.—The same as *Aconite*.

41

ARSENICUM, after *Aconite*, if the anxiety, anguish, and palpitation continue, and there be also extreme restless-ness, with dry, burning heat; also, after or in alterna-tion with *Ipecacuanha*, when that remedy has been found insufficient of itself; and after *Nux vomica*, to persons addicted to spirituous liquors, fermented drinks or coffee. If there should be a return of the symptoms after a temporary cessation, give *Sulphur*.

DOSE.—The same as *Belladonna.*

BELLADONNA is useful for women with profuse cata-menia, or at the change of life, and especially if there be cough, with tickling in the throat; sensation of fulness; pressing shooting pains, worse on movement.

DOSE.—One drop of the dilution, or six globules, in ten spoonfuls of water, a spoonful every half hour, until amelioration, or change. Often useful after *Aconite.*

CHINA, if the patient has lost much blood, or is suffer-ing from debility, especially from debilitating discharges; dry, hollow, violent, and painful cough, with taste of blood in the mouth; shivering, with flushes of heat; faintness; cloudiness of sight, and roaring in the head, with sense of lightness and vivacity; short and transient inspirations.

DOSE.—Same as *Belladonna.* After four or six doses, give at longer intervals, or select some other remedy.

FERRUM, after *China*, if this has in severe cases relieved, but there remains great fatigue after talking; slight cough, with expectoration of scanty bright red blood; pain between the shoulder blades, and difficulty of breathing.

DOSE.—The same as *Belladonna.*

IPECACUANHA.—Taste of blood in the mouth; fre-quent short cough; nausea; weakness; expectoration mucus streaked with blood. Useful after *Aconite*, or before *Arsenicum*.

DOSE.—The same as *Belladonna*.

OPIUM.—Cough dry and hollow, with spitting of bloody and frothy mucus; weakness of the voice; drowsiness, with sudden starts; worse after swallowing; difficulty of breathing, with burnings in the region of the heart, and coldness, particularly of the extremities; tremors, especially in the arms. Useful in most difficult cases. For persons addicted to the use of spirituous liquors it may be followed by *Nux vomica*.

DOSE.—The same as *Belladonna*.

NUX VOMICA for persons of irritable temper, when caused by hemorrhoidal suppression, a fit of passion, or exposure to cold; dry cough, with headache; tickling in the chest; worse towards morning. After *Nux vomica*, *Sulphur* is almost always useful.

DOSE.—One drop of the dilution, or six globules, in ten spoonfuls of water, a spoonful every two hours, until amelioration or change. After *Nux vomica*, give *Arsenicum* or *Sulphur*.

PHOSPHORUS, in case of consumption, or ulceration of the lungs; also, after the discharge of blood has ceased to prevent inflammation, or degeneration into consumption, is a most useful remedy.

DOSE.—The same as *Nux vomica*.

PULSATILLA, for females, for suppression of the monthly discharge, or in cases of hemorrhoids; also, if there be expectoration of a dark coagulated blood, with shiverings towards evening, and at night; great anxiety; pain low down in the chest; flaccidity, and weakness at the epigastrium.

DOSE.—One drop of the dilution, or six globules, in ten spoonfuls of water; give a spoonful every two hours. Afterwards give *Sulphur*.

Rhus tox., if there be expectoration of bright red blood, with a sense of constriction, crawling, and short breath; or with pressure at the stomach pit, and desire to take a deep inspiration; weakness, and sensation of trembling; or sensation in the chest, as if something were torn away.

DOSE.—One drop of the dilution, or six globules, in ten spoonfuls of water; a spoonful to be given every hour or two hours, until four doses are taken; after which give *Sulphur* or *Arsenicum.*

SULPHUR, always after treatment with other remedies; also, for persons subject to piles and hemorrhoidal affections; derangement of the menses; or when hœmoptysis arises from suppressed eruptions. To drunkards, it should be given in alternation with *Nux vomica* or *Arsenicum,* and continued some time after the affection ceases, at intervals of three or four days.

DOSE.—The same as *Rhus tox.*

A form of this affection, termed by some Apoplectic Hæmorrhage, in which the patient loses his consciousness, looks as if suffocated, his eyes protruding from their sockets, and bloody mucus issuing from his mouth, is most immediately dangerous, and frequently fatal. The first remedy in this case is *Aconite.* If not better in thirty minutes, *Opium,* and afterwards *Ipecacuanha.* Keep the extremities warm by friction, downwards rather than upwards, and stimulate the circulation by hot bandages, cloths wrung out from hot water, to the head and stomach pit, especially if those parts are hot. Send immediately for a good homœopathic physician.

DOSE, and Administration.—First place a few globules of *Aconite* upon the tongue; then dissolve two drops or twelve globules, in four table-spoonfuls of water, and give a teaspoonful every five or ten minutes. If not better in thirty or forty minutes, give *Opium,* in the same manner, and afterwards *Ipecacuanha.*

25.—Consumption of the Lungs. (*Phthisis Pulmonalis.*)

The symptoms of this disease in its earlier stages, are frequently obscure. When they become manifest the friends and physician too often allow themselves to give up in despair, whilst the patient generally continues to hope on, even to the close of life. In the earlier stages the affection is no doubt often curable. After disorganization of the lungs has taken place, and ulcerations have become established, although something may still be done, a cure is hardly to be expected. In this, as in all other cases, however, the Almighty has reserved the entirely hopeless cases to the moment of death, and no physician is justified in giving up a case to die, whilst the patient still lives.

The earlier symptoms, a short, dry cough, or with a little frothy expectoration, are usually attributed to a cold; but if shortness of breath, with sensation of obstruction, only felt at first after exercise, or after a fit of coughing; fevers, with remissions, especially towards morning, and returning at noon; or remission at about five in the afternoon, and returning before midnight; flushes in the face, heat in the palms of the hands, and soles of the feet, with night sweats supervene, it is time to take the alarm, and seek for aid. These are the unmistakable symptoms of an approaching malady, which may require all the skill and wisdom of a most intelligent physician to meet and cure.

If the above symptoms continue, the emaciation and debility increase; respiration is more difficult; the cough is more severe, and troublesome, especially at night, the fever, if shorter in duration, is followed with more profuse sweats, and the pulse loses tone; the expectoration, at first viscid and frothy, becomes more free, copious

41*

thicker, and less transparent; a circumscribed red patch, often appears on the cheek, or the cheek is faded, and the countenance dejected; these symptoms indicate the commencement of the second stage. In the third stage, there is expectoration, at first, of cheese-like particles, afterwards mixed with pus, mucus, shreds, lymph, and blood, and at times portions of the tissue of the lungs themselves may be expectorated. The bowels which had been costive, are now relaxed; diarrhœas are of frequent occurence, which with colliquative sweats, induce excessive weakness and prostration. The flesh becomes reduced; the face thin; the cheek-bones prominent; the eyes hollow; the hair falls off, the nails curve inwards, and are livid; the feet swell; yet the countenance may be clear, and the eyes have the lustre of health; the mind is often serene and hopeful; the patient seems unconscious of his danger, and often speaks and acts as if he expected a speedy recovery.

In cases which make slow progress, the patient may have a troublesome cough, weakness, and emaciation, chiefly in the winter and spring, whilst he enjoys comparative health in summer, sometimes even for several years. In this case he usually becomes careless of himself, and often loses his life from neglect, or from some sudden attack of inflammation, arising from cold, or other causes.

In other cases the disease makes rapid progress, and terminates in death, often in a few months. This, from the rapidity of its progress, as well as from the severity of its symptoms, has been, not inappropriately, termed galloping consumption. It is most common in young persons, in the periods of development, and in persons of sanguineous temperament, or of sedentary habits.

Tubercular consumption often appears to arise from the transfer of other diseases, such as scrofula, or king's evil, cancer, syphilis, various eruptive diseases, as itch, tetters, and eruptive fevers, as erysipelas, small-pox, scarlet fever, &c., to the lungs and chest. When these causes can be certainly detected, the disease might properly receive the name of scrofulous consumption, cancerous consumption, syphilitic consumption, &c., but these distinctions have not been sufficiently studied, to enable us to form an acurate diagnosis, and it is, no doubt, often from not understanding the cause, that physicians of every school have failed in curing consumptive diseases.

TREATMENT.—In the treatment of consumption it may emphatically be said, consult causes, and if the disease or dyscrasia which has produced the consumptive cough, or tubercles, or ulcerations, could be cured if it affected other organs or tissues, a cure should never be despaired of, because the lungs are the seat of the disease. The lungs often recover from the most severe forms of inflammation and congestion. Why should they not then, recover from other kinds of irritation? The interior surface or lining of the lungs, is a mucus surface, having a very close analogy to the interior surface of the mouth and throat, as well as to the skin. Why should not remedies, which given on the tongue, will cure ulcerations of the mouth and throat, and of the extremities, even of the fingers and toes, also cure the same kinds of ulcerations, if they exist on similar surfaces, in the lungs and chest? Evidently they may do so, and the reason why consumption is yet reckoned among the incurable diseases, is because its cure has never been attempted in faith, by any true student of nature, in obedience to her law of cure; but looking upon consumption as a disease in itself, of some peculiar concealed, and fatal character, the physician has discharged his arrows in the dark, at a masked image, whilst the disease has been left to pursue its course, until the fountains of life have been broken, and death has secured another victim. I shall be excused, therefore, in this place, for repeating, in the treatment of consumption, consult causes; and with a wise reference to these causes, prescribe your remedies, as if any other organ, having similar tissues, were similarly affected; continue your treatment, after it is wisely determined on, perseveringly, obstinately. You will often have success, where it is least expected.

Again, it is not to be admitted, because allopathic physicians, relying upon external applications mainly in the cure of skin diseases, ulcerations and tumefactions, when they occur upon the external parts, have always been at fault when the same diseases occur upon any of the internal organs, and where direct application to the diseased surface is impossible, that therefore homœopathy, which almost always succeeds in curing these external diseases by internal remedies, should imagine herself also unable to cure the same diseases, when they occur internally, and upon similar tissues.

Every true homœopathist then should assume "consumption can be cured," and should enter upon a systematic course of observations, trials and expedients, until he discovers the nature of the disease, and all the circumstances upon which a cure may be dependant.

TREATMENT.—If consumption be a disease sui generis, to which the lungs and the internal organism are alone exposed, it is probable that the remedies necessary in its treatment are but few, and their application simple. But if consumption be only a term indicative of a variety of morbid influences, any one of which, acting upon the complex and susceptible tissues of which the lungs and internal organs are composed, may produce degeneration and death, then the number of remedies applicable in the treatment will no doubt be increased, and more skill, knowledge and judgment will be necessary in their application. I shall in this treatise adopt the latter view, and in that view will remark that nearly all the remedies useful in coughs and other affections of the respiratory organs, nearly all the medicines adapted to ulcerations, tubercles, cancerous and syphilitic affections, are likely to be called for in some of the forms of disease called consumption. We have room in this place to give the indications for but a few of these remedies, and must refer the reader to the chapters which treat on those diseases in other portions of this work, or to the pathogenesis of the medicines, for further information. The remedies I have selected from a great number which may be found useful, are Aconite, Arsenicum, Belladonna, Calcarea carb., China, Kali carb., Lycopodium, Phosphorus, Pulsatilla, Sepia, Stannum, Sulphur, and I doubt not there are forms of consumption to which Aurum mur., Bryonia, Nux vomica, Mercurius viv., Manganum, Nitric acid, Rhus tox., Sambucus, Tartar emetic, Silicea, and various other remedies are adapted.

I shall give the symptomatic indications for Aconite, Belladonna, Calcarea carb., Lycopodium, Phosphorus, Sepia, Stannum, Sulphur.

ACONITE is most frequently called for in the congestive variety, attended with considerable active inflamma-

tions, in persons of sanguineous temperament, and naturally of a full habit, in the so-called galloping consumption, to be given in alternation with *Sulphur*, when that
remedy appears indicated ; also at times with *Pulsatilla*,
or *Sepia*, to females affected with chlorotic symptoms;
also, often in those protracted cases, worse in winter;
and when there is a repercussion of some exanthemata.

BELLADONNA is applicable to persons subject to erysipelatous inflammations, phlegmonous ulcerations, glandular swellings, &c.; also to cases following scarlatina,
angina tonsilaris, and many other forms of glandular
disease. It is thought to have cured a few cases, but
in common with *Aconite*, is as yet known more as an
adjuvant or a palliative to certain acute symptoms, and
is usually administered in alternation with some other
remedy.

DOSE.—Give either of the above remedies, one drop, or six globules,
in ten spoonfuls of water, a spoonful every four hours, until amelioration
or change.

CALCAREA CARB.—Cough, with irritation, as if produced by feather dust; cough with mucus low down
the throat; cough dry, violent, evening and night, with
pulsations; cough dry, exhausting, with pain in the
chest; cough day and night; rattling in the lower part
of the windpipe, near the throat pit; expectoration
offensive, brown and mixed with pus; violent cough by
day, with rattling, sputa being lumpy, purulent, greenish or yellowish, at times attended with vomiting;
stitches in the chest and sides of the chest on coughing,
breathing deeply, moving about, and bending towards
the painful side; burning in the chest; chill with thirst;
evening fever every third day, first heat in the face,
then chills, night sweats; debilitating local perspiration
on the chest at night; unquenchable thirst; diarrhœa,

with cutting pains; alternation of diarrhœa with constipation; disposition to hemorrhage; menstruation profuse every three weeks; disposition to weep; emaciation; want of strength; great exhaustion after exercise.

DOSE.—One drop, or six globules, in two spoonfuls of water, a spoonful to be given every twelve hours, until amelioration, or change.

LYCOPODIUM.—Cough dry and violent at night, with expectoration by day, or day and night, or in the morning; purulent expectoration, with rattling on the chest, or expectoration of blood and pus, or of greenish, musty, rancid, greasy sputa, with putrid taste; the pains are stitching, burning, gnawing, with pressure; oppression, and difficult breathing; cannot lie on the left side; feeble pulse; chills towards evening, with flashes of heat; lingering fever and night-sweats; clammy sweat, constipation, or purulent diarrhœa; discharges of blood, inward debility, loss of strength, emaciation; mental exhaustion, with apprehensions for the future; sadness, wilfulness, irritability and depression of spirits; the pains often extend through the chest from the front to the back.

DOSE.—The same as for *Calcarea*.

PHOSPHORUS.—Cough, with tickling in the chest and throat; roughness; hoarseness; dryness; every word causes a short hacking cough; night cough, with stitches disturbing sleep; dry cough, or with bloody expectoration, or of pus and blood; yellowish, purulent, saltish, or greenish expectoration; or whitish, or of white mucus.

Stitches in the chest, in the windpipe, about the pit of the throat, especially in the left side, a spot in the side being sensitive to the touch; sore pains, or burning pains in the chest, or pain under the left chest when lying on it, cannot lie well on the back, and not at all on either side; burnings, stingings, and soreness in the chest and side difficulty of breathing, with oppression; lancinating, constricting, or oppressive pains, sense of pressure. Evening chills, with flashes of heat, or with dry heat, especially in the palms of the hands; circumscribed redness of the cheeks; morning sweats; night sweats; clammy sweats; irritability, fretfulness, anxiety.

Certainly useful when there is a great amount of congestion, as if from chronic pneumonia, and in the inflammatory variety, and probably when consumption arises from repercussion of some exanthematous disease, as scarlatina, measles, &c. In purulent tubercular consumption it will aid in overcoming the congested condition of those portions of the lung in immediate proximity to the tubercles, and in developing a more healthful action.

DOSE.—The same as *Belladonna.*

SEPIA.—Hoarseness; agitation and painful soreness in the chest, with pains on motion; oppression, stitches in the left side when coughing or breathing; morning and evening cough, with saltish, tenacious sputa raised with difficulty; purulent sputa; night sweats; sour sweat in the morning; useful for females long subject to leucorrhœa or to menstrual affections, also for some forms of eruptive disease.

DOSE.—The same as *Belladonna.*

STANNUM.—For mucus consumption, with tickling, scratching sensations in the throat, and when the cough is excited by talking, laughing, singing, &c.; constant tendency to cough, with sensation of mucus in the chest, especially along the windpipe; cough night and morning; violent fatiguing, shaking cough, at one time dry, at another moist; at one time tenacious, at another loose; cough day and nights, with copious mucus expectoration, at times in lumps, yellow, offensive, or greenish, nauseous, and sweetish, at times watery and thin; chest raw and sore; pains all over the chest, pressure as from a weight and tension; feeling of faintness as if numb, with weakness, or sensation of weakness; rattling breathing; oppression, dislikes to speak; difficulty of breathing when moving, and at night; tightness, want of air, and sense of suffocation; chills frequent over the back, with heat of the hands, or burning of the hands and feet; dryness of the mouth; seething of the blood; night and morning sweats; flashes of heat; small and quick pulse; weakness of the limbs; emaciation.

DOSE.—The same as *Belladonna.*

SULPHUR.—Cough at any time of the day or night, short, barking, frequent, either dry or with expectoration; either of mucus or pus; thick, yellowish, or greenish, or bloody, or when whole lumps are coughed up; the sensations are oppressive, especially on drawing the arms together, feels as if the chest would split when coughing; gnawing burning sensations in the left side; difficult breathing, with tightness, or with burning, whistling and rattling in the chest; pressure under the breast bone; chills and sour night-sweats; can sleep only on the back; pains in the sacrum; weakness and languor, especially after exercise.

DOSE.—Give a powder in the morning every four days.

For DIET and REGIMEN.—See Chronic Cough, page 399 and 400.

42

CHAPTER X.

DISEASES OF THE CIRCULATORY APPARATUS.

1.—Angina Pectoris.

THIS affection is usually confined to persons who have passed the meridian of life, who are of a rheumatic or gouty diathesis, or of a corpulent habit, exposed to much mental uneasiness, or addicted to intemperance. The following are the more common symptoms. Sudden paroxysms of agitation in the chest, felt more on the left side, near the lower portion of the sternum or breast-bone; a sudden feeling of constriction and suffocation, so that if walking, the patient is obliged to stop; at first only brought on by extra exertion, but afterwards by the most trivial excitement, or mental effort, error in diet, or indigestible food; and finally coming on suddenly, and unexpectedly, without any assignable cause, even in bed, or when asleep. The pain is usually severe and ex-cruciating, at first confined to the chest, but afterwards extending to the left shoulder, the deltoid muscle, and frequently the entire length of both extremities. Parox-ysms may terminate in a few minutes, or continue for hours, or the patient may never be free from agonizing, constricting pains. In severe cases the countenance becomes pale, haggard, and contracted, with an expres-sion of extreme anguish, the eyes sunken, the body cold, and perhaps cold, clammy sweats, respiration difficult and rapid, palpitation, and perhaps intermittent pulsations of the heart, anxiety, and a feeling as of approaching death; the pulse is usually slow, feeble, oppressed, and intermittent; it may, however, be quick, strong, and irregular, when the skin is usually warm, and face flushed. The digestive functions also are often deranged. An attack may terminate as suddenly as it came on; or soreness may remain about the chest for considerable time.

REMEDIES.—Aconite, Arnica, Arsenicum, Belladonna, Bryonia, Digitalis, Ipecacuanha, Lachesis, Phosphoric acid, Sulphur, and Veratrum.

ACONITE.—For recent cases, and for plethoric persons; or when paroxysms are attended with a full throbbing pulse, heat of the skin, flushed face, and rapid pulsations of the heart; and generally in the commencement of the treatment, will be found of service.

DOSE.—One drop of the dilution, or six globules, in ten spoonfuls of water, a spoonful to be given every fifteen minutes, in some acute cases, otherwise every half hour, or every two hours, until amelioration, or change.

ARNICA. — When the pains are constrictive and burning, as well as drawing and tearing; with anguish almost insupportable, extending to the back, and under the shoulder blade, also along the side, and down the left arm; with stiffness of the nape of the neck, and drawing towards the left side; numbness and prickings of the fingers, as if from a blow at the point of the elbow; accompanied with a smothering sensation at the heart, as if it had ceased to beat, relieved at times by pressure over the heart; especially in arthritic subjects, with tendencies to ossifications; and for persons subject to long continued and protracted labor in a sitting posture, with intermittent palpitations and pulsations.

DOSE.—The same as *Arsenicum.*

484   DISEASES OF THE

ARSENICUM has been administered often, and with the best success, where there was excessive difficulty of breathing from the slightest movement, as from getting into bed, or from turning in bed; palpitations, with anguish, and feeling of approaching death; face pale and haggard; great debility; feeble, irregular, and intermittent pulse. If relief be not obtained, give *Veratrum* or *Ipecacuanha.*

DOSE.—One drop of the dilution, or six globules, in ten spoonfuls of water, give a spoonful every half hour, for two hours, afterwards give a spoonful every four hours, until amelioration or change.

BELLADONNA.—After *Aconite,* if the paroxysms return, and if there be a pain, with soreness, and sensitiveness to the touch, rather than a constrictive pain, in the region of the heart; other symptoms being similar to *Aconite.*

DOSE.—The same as *Aconite.*

DIGITALIS. — For more advanced cases, when the attacks recur more frequently, and suddenly, without assignable cause, the pulse being intermittent and slow, palpitations violent, with shudderings; contractive and tearing pain; paralytic pullings and tearings in the arms and fingers, with numbness of the hands; drawing pains in the bones, and stiffness and tension in the muscles, and nape of the neck.

DOSE.—The same as *Arsenicum.*

Various other remedies have been recommended in this affection, and there are others which by their pathogenesis, would frequently seem to be indicated.

Thus Hydrocyanic acid, or Kali Hydrocyanicum, when Arsenicum has failed to relieve. Veratrum if there is coldness of the extremities, cold sweats, and slow, depressed intermittent pulse. Lachesis to prevent returns, and for symptoms similar to Veratrum, especially if the patient be worse after sleeping. Nux vomica and Sulphur, if the digestive functions are deranged, and if the attacks are attended or succeeded by flatulence. Also China, Ferrum, Nux vomica, Phosphoric acid, and Sulphur, if there are local congestions, combined with debility. Arsenicum, Aurum, Cannabis, Colchicum, Ignatia, Lactuca virosa, Natrum mur., Sepia, and Spigelia, are also remedies which may at times exert a beneficial influence; as may also Calcarea carb., and Lycopodium, and perhaps Phosphorus.

2.—Acute Pericarditis. (*Inflammation of the investing membrane of the heart.*)

The pericardium encloses the heart and roots of the large vessels issuing from it, somewhat as the pleura encloses the lungs; and the interior surface next the heart, like the interior surface of the pleura, is a serous surface, constantly pouring forth a serous exudation. If the pericardium takes on inflammation it is called pericarditis; and it is manifest, that as inflammation may arise from various causes, so pericarditis may assume various forms, each form constituting a distinct variety of disease. The symptoms at times set in with marked severity, at other times they are so insidious and deceptive as to produce considerable disorganization before attracting attention. Indeed, disorganizations have been found, on dissection, to have existed to a great extent, which have entirely escaped attention.

The symptoms usually manifest are sharp, burning, pricking, darting pains in the region of the heart, with acute fever. The pains shoot to the left shoulder and shoulder blade, and frequently extend down the arm; are aggravated by deep inspirations, by pressure in the

42*

spaces between the ribs, and in the region of the heart, or on the stomach pit. The patient cannot lie on the left side, but lies easiest on the back; breathing is rapid, irregular and laborious, especially on movement; a feeling of contraction, restlessness, anxiety, and frequent syncope. The pulse is accelerated, at times hard, full and vibratory, at other times feeble, irregular and intermittent, whilst if the ear be applied to the region of the heart, its action may be found to be tumultuous and violent. This inequality is thought to be of great importance, as it will often enable us to decide in doubtful cases by comparing the strength of the action of the heart with that of the pulse. Again, when copious effusion has taken place, the practised ear will discover that the sounds of the heart appear distant, muffled and disguised, whilst they are heard, with their usual distinctness and intensity, near the upper part of the breast bone, in the carotid and subclavian arteries. This effusion, as in all inflammations of serous surfaces, consists of an increased secretion, which from the nature of the inflammation becomes a kind of plastic lymph, and ultimately creates adhesions, or it forms water, and lays a foundation for dropsy on the chest, or hydrothorax. The extremities not unfrequently become œdematous, or enlarged. The affection resembles pleuritis, both in its nature and duration, though differing in the name of the affection, and the organ implicated.

REMEDIES.—Aconite, Arnica, Arsenicum, Belladonna, Bryonia, Cannabis, Lachesis, Spigelia and Sulphur.

ACONITE should be given in frequently repeated doses in the acute inflammatory stage, and even if the case be implicated with previous disease of the heart, effusion may be prevented, and a cure speedily effected. For plethoric, sanguineous, lymphatic patients, give *Belladonna* in alternation with *Aconite*. If the action of the heart continues tumultuous, with oppression, anxiety and constriction, give *Cannabis* also, if symptoms of effusion are manifest. *Bryonia*, instead of *Cannabis*, if there are sharp, pricking pains about the heart, increased by breathing, and by movement; also for slight effusions. *Spigelia* in the earlier stages, when there are severe lancinations in the cardiac region, or pain as if the heart were compressed or squeezed, distressing oppression on movement or speaking, and when complicated with endocarditis.

ADMINISTRATION.—Any of the above remedies may be given, one drop of the dilution, or six globules, in ten spoonfuls of water, a spoonful every three hours, until amelioration or change. After the above treatment, if the disease appears to be overcome, give *Sulphur*, a dose every twelve hours, for four days.

Other remedies are Arnica, Arsenicum, Lachesis and Veratrum.

ARNICA.—If the disease arise from external injury, from long protracted labors, especially in a sitting posture, with the head bent downwards, in arthritic subjects, and with liability to calcareous deposits; and if the patient complain of pains as from a bruise, painful prickings, or compression in the heart, with giddiness in the head.

DOSE.—One drop of the dilution, or six globules, in ten spoonfuls of water, a spoonful to be given every two hours, for twelve hours, afterwards every four hours, until amelioration or change

ARSENICUM.—After *Aconite*, when there are strong palpitations, with rapid pulse, intense thirst, burning pains, anxiety, fainting, restlessness; or in a more advanced stage, when the respiration is hurried and laborious; worse when moving; inability to lie on the left side; pulse feeble and irregular.

DOSE.—The same as *Arnica*.

LACHESIS may be given, if anxiety or vexation appear to have hastened the disease; if there is great oppression for breath, with fulness and pressure, or as if the chest were too full; palpitations with anxiety, and with cramp-like pains; and cough with choking sensations, or with stitches, fainting fits, and cold sweat; also if there are pulsations extending into the 'ears; worse after lying down or after sleeping.

DOSE.—The same as *Arsenicum*.

VERATRUM, if the extremities become cold, or a cold sweat covers the forehead or other parts; pulse slow and intermittent; nose sharp, and the features sunken and contracted.

DOSE.—The same as *Arsenicum*, which it may follow in these all but hopeless cases.

Pericarditis is most frequently met with, in connection with Acute Rheumatism. We should therefore, always examine the region of the heart in such cases, that the disease may not attain an incurable height before it is detected. When acute pericarditis is not complicated with previous organic disease of the heart, by the proper application of remedies, a cure may always be expected.

Chronic Pericarditis, often exhibits nearly the same symptoms as the acute variety, differing only in duration, and perhaps in intensity, and liable to be frequently reincited by colds and other causes. If, in the progress of acute pericarditis, adhesions have formed between the apex of the heart and the pericardium, other serious organic lesions, as hypertrophy, and dilatation, are likely to follow. The signs by which these adhesions are detected, are not always distinctly marked. But when the pericardium is also adherent to the walls of the chest, and the adhesions are close and rigid, the heart will always be found pulsating in close contact with the ribs; its pulsations will be seen and felt more plainly than usual, drawing in the spaces between the ribs at each pulsation; and if enlargement of the heart, upwards and downwards ensue, a projection will be strikingly observable about the ends and the cartilages of the middle ribs.

TREATMENT.—When the effused lymph has become organised, the adhesions being extensive, may so materially interfere with the motions of the heart, as to be only susceptible of alleviations by medicine; but previous to such organization, whilst the exudation is still partly of a serous character, even in chronic cases, a cure may sometimes be effected. The remedies usually applicable, are the same as in the acute variety, and perhaps, also, Aurum muriat., Calcarea carb. or Phosphorus, Lycopodium, Silicea, Colchicum, Ledum, and others. Arnica, Bryonia, and Sulphur, should never be forgotten. Remedies should be exhibited less frequently. Calcarea, Silicea, and Sulphur, only once in twenty-four hours; other remedies may be given every four hours, or as directed in acute pericarditis, for a few days; then omit medicine for a few days, then give again as before.

3.—Inflammation of the Lining Membrane of the Heart.
(Endocarditis.)

The symptoms observable in this disease, are still more uncertain and obscure, except to a physician, than those of pericarditis.

Tumultuous, irregular action of the heart from oppression; anxiety, faintness, some pain often referred to the sternum or epigastrium, are more commonly noticed. To a practised ear, the sounds of the heart are at first louder, the impulse greater, often attended with a vibration or tremor, but not always more frequent than in health. Afterwards, the sound seems double, prolonged, rough, and finally blowing or grating, as if the blood were flowing back through the defectively closed valves. The exact location of the various abnormal sounds of the heart, is of little consequence, in domestic practice, and the limits of this work will not allow me to enter upon the description. When the above symptoms are present, we are justified in supposing the inflammation to be in the tissues or substance of the heart; and although it is better to apply immediately to a physician, the following remedies will generally be of service: Aconite, Arsenicum, Belladonna, Digitalis, Nux vomica, Pulsatilla, Spigelia, and Veratrum.

ACONITE is useful in acute cases, the pulse being hard, full, and vibratory; sharp, pricking pain in the region of the heart; and in alternation with *Belladonna*, if the brain also, is affected, causing delirium, and sometimes stupor; also, *Aconite* for pressing together in the region of the heart; palpitations, with anxiety; oppression of the chest, and relaxation of the limbs; slow throbs, near or in the heart; pain in the left side of the thorax; disproportion between the heart-beats and pulse-beats; pulse beats three times to the heart's once; enlargement or hypertrophy of the heart.

DOSE.—Give one drop of the dilution, or six globules, in ten spoonfuls of water; a spoonful every hour, in very acute cases every half hour, until amelioration or change.

ARSENICUM.—Anxiety in the region of the heart; violent and irregular pulsations of the heart, with feebleness of the pulse; indistinctness or roughness of the sounds of the heart, heard loudest at the end of the third rib, near the left side of the sternum; frightful palpitations, especially at night; irregular and violent; loss of contractile powers; pinching, burning, and soreness around the heart.

DOSE.—The same as *Nux vomica.*

BELLADONNA.—Pains, aching or sore, or throbbing, in the left chest, or shooting and cutting, as from knives; also, around the heart; irregular, unequal contractions of the heart, with occasionally intermitting pulse; clucking, or trembling of the heart, with palpitation on ascending, as in going up stairs; throbbing pain under the sternum, near the epigastrium; violent and persistent throbbings and palpitations, with jarring even of the head and neck; adapted to congestions of the chest, to prevent and modify inflammations, rather than to subdue actual affections of the heart itself; but often controlling those exacerbations, which frequently light up the irritation anew.

DOSE.—The same as *Aconite.*

DIGITALIS.—Increased activity of the heart, with slowness of the pulse; palpitations which rouse one from sleep; commotion of the blood with great anxiety, forcing one to get out of bed, and quickness of the pulse; congestions to the head; noise and roaring in the ears; beatings of the heart scarcely perceptible, very soft and weak; unequal intervals between the pulsations; very irregular pulsations; homœopathic to dilatation, with thinning of the walls of the heart when the palpitations are feeble, oppressed, more or less distressing, frequent and prolonged, the pulse soft and feeble, and if the debility of the heart be great.

DOSE.—The same as *Nux vomica.*

NUX VOM.—Palpitation in frequent short paroxysms; pulsating throbs; great anxiety· long continued spas-

modic contraction, with difficult respiration and extinction of the pulse; the face livid, the eyes protruded, and
the hands clasped over the heart; exactly the opposite of
Digitalis, it is homœopathic to hypertrophy, and contraction with thickening. ˙

DOSE.—One drop of the dilution, or six globules, in ten spoonfuls of
water; give a spoonful every two hours, until amelioration or change;
should usually be given in the afternoon, and if adapted, *Arsenicum* may
be given in the morning.

PULSATILLA.—Passive congestions, with venous distension, and tedious affections of the heart; hypertrophy,
with dilitation of the right side of the heart; excessive
accumulation and activity of the venous blood; useful
when the right side of the heart is implicated; usually
for females, and for persons of a quiet phlegmatic temperament.

DOSE.—The same as *Aconite.*

SPIGELIA.—Increased impulse of the beats of the heart,
elevating the walls of the chest; want of harmony between
the beats of the heart and pulse; point or apex of the
heart beats too near the nipple, and sometimes even outside the nipple; valvular murmurs at different points;
oppression and palpitation; violent and audible beatings
felt through the clothing, with anxious oppression, especially in the morning; wave-like, vibratory, or undulatory
motion of the heart.

DOSE.—Same as *Nux vomica.*

VERATRUM.—Affections of the heart, complicated with
derangement of the stomach; nervous palpitations, worse
after meals; the apex of the heart beats out of its usual
place; bulging of the ribs over the heart; visible and
violent action of the heart; sounds loud and clear, or
with abnormal murmurs; intermittent pulse; nervous
irritability.

DOSE.—One drop of the dilution, or six globules, in ten spoonfuls of of water, a spoonful to be given every half hour in extreme cases; in other cases, every two or four hours, until amelioration or change.

A great number of other remedies are also homœo-pathic to different forms of heart disease. In the earlier stages of endocarditis, *Aconite* and *Belladonna* will gene-rally be found of service. *Arsenicum* in complicated cases of long continuance, and when organic changes have taken place. Also, Bismuth, Calc. carb., Carb. veg., Colchicum, Croton, Digitalis, Graphites, Lachesis, Natrum mur., Nux vomica, Phosphorus, Rhus tox., and Sepia, will be care-fully studied by the physician, of which the limits of this work will not allow a more extended notice.

Diseases of the heart are much more common than is generally supposed. They are not always immediately dangerous. They are thought most frequently to arise as a complication in the course of rheumatic and arthritic diseases, but may be incited by a variety of other causes.

4.—Carditis. (*Inflammation of the substance of the Heart.*)

This is usually complicated with peri and endocarditis. If a large portion of the heart suffer severe acute inflamma-tion for a considerable period of time, a fatal result must no doubt be expected; but in a great number of cases, having the most acute symptoms, something may still be done. The symptoms and the indications for reme-dies are however the same as in pericarditis, and in endocarditis.

These inflammations may produce hypertrophy, that is, thickening or enlargement of the substance of the heart, in which case there will be difficulty of breathing, and whilst the impulse of the heart's action will be increased, the natural sounds will be diminished, pulse full and strong, but vibratory.

43

Remedies most useful in this condition, are Arsenicum, Bismuth, Nux vomica, Pulsatilla, Phosphorus, and Graphites.

Dilatation, or enlargement of the capacity of one or both cavities of the heart, the symptoms of which are palpitation and difficulty of breathing on any sudden emotion; impulse of the heart's action diminished; natural sounds increased, with soft, feeble, undulating pulse.

REMEDIES.—Arsenicum, Aconite, Arnica, Belladonna, Digitalis, Lachesis, Pulsatilla and Spigelia.

Disease of the valves of the heart, which may be inferred if by placing the hand over the region of the heart, a purring tremor, or inquietude, is felt under the fingers, or if by the ear a bellows sound or a rasping sound can be distinguished; palpitations and difficulty of breathing, aggravated by exercise, or by mental exertions; swelling of the feet towards evening, and at length discoloration of the face, and of the extremities; dropsy of the feet and legs, and of the cavities of the body.

REMEDIES.—Asafœtida, Arsenicum, Belladonna, Croton, Digitalis, Graphites, Lachesis, Phosphorus, Pulsatilla, Rhus and Spigelia.

Heart diseases, excited by the frequent use of Mercurius, also in syphilitic patients, require Aurum mur., China, Hepar sulph., Lachesis and Nitric acid.

In gouty subjects, Arnica, Colchicum, Calcarea carb., Lycopodium, Nux vomica, Rhus tox., Silicea and Sulphur.

For rheumatic cases, Aconite, Arnica, Arsenicum, Bryonia, Belladonna, Colchicum, Lachesis, Nux vomica, Pulsatilla, Spigelia and Sulphur.

For controlling attacks of congestion, Aconite, Aurum, Arsenicum, Belladonna, Cocculus, Coffea, Digitalis,

Lachesis, Lycopodium, Nux vomica, Opium, Phosphorus, Plumbum, Pulsatilla and Sulphur.

Anuerism of the aorta, or enlargement (dilatation) of
the great artery which conveys the blood from the heart,
known by a loud wheezing or rustling at the upper
part of the sternum or breast bone, perceived by placing
the hand over the part; rattling at the throat; oppression of the chest; pulse unlike at the wrists; if the
anuerism is large, the pulsation will be single, and the
sound dull under the sternum; whilst in a healthy state,
the pulsation will be double, and the sound clear; or
the pulsation may be single, the impulse increased, and
the sound louder than when in health. The symptoms
differ according to the situation, size and form of the
anuerism; if it press against the gullet, it may impede
deglutition, or occasion a constant guggling, clucking
sound. If it press upon the spine, it may cause pains
in the back, and various nervous phenomena, with
debility. It may press upon one of the bronchial tubes,
or involve a portion of the lung, and occasion cough, &c.

REMEDIES.—Arsenicum, Arnica, Belladonna, Croton,
Digitalis, Lachesis, Rhus tox., Zincum.

Aneurism, or dilatation of an artery, is distinguished
by the appearance of a tumor which pulsates, and which
disappears on pressure, but returns as soon as the pressure is removed.

TREATMENT.—Apply gentle pressure to the part, and
treat with internal remedies, such as Arsenicum, Arnica,
Carbo veg., Causticum, Digitalis, Lachesis, Rhus tox.,
Spigelia and Zincum.

At times a number of small arteries and veins become
enlarged and united together, forming a Pulsating Tumor of considerable size, in the treatment of which in

addition to the above remedies, Pulsatilla, Silicea and Thuja may be of service; also Hamamelis virg.

Inflammation of the Arteries if in consequence of a wound, requires Rhus tox. If there be also contusion, Arsenicum; and if the inflammation extend towards the heart, Aconite. In advanced stages, Pulsatilla, or Arsenicum may be required.

Inflammation of the veins, when after external injury, burning pains are felt, deep in the right hypochondria, extending downward and backward, and towards the left side, or in the left side, near and below the kidneys, or in the abdomen, extending towards the stomach and liver; with distension of the right side; bitter taste; whitish, brown, or yellow tongue; vomiting; yellowness of the eyes, and of the face; give Nux vomica; or give Pulsatilla, Arsenicum, or Lachesis; and afterwards give Sulphur.

In chronic inflammation of the veins, give Arnica, Carbo veg., Calcarea carb., Lycopodium, Plumbum.

Swelling of the veins, (Varices or Varicose veins,) distinguished by chronic enlargement, dark blue or purple color of the veins, of the leg and other parts; often appearing in knots, or swollen spots, of large and uncertain size, in women during pregnancy, and at the change of life, and often in men of hœmorrhoidal, venous, congestive habits, and terminating at times, in extensive œdema of the limbs, indolent or sloughing ulcers, with bleeding, and attended with burning, shooting, and stinging pains, is a very common affection, which may be greatly relieved, and oftentimes entirely cured, by the use of such remedies as Arnica, Arsenicum, Causticum, Lachesis, Lycopodium, Hamamelis vir., Nux vomica, Pulsatilla, Silicea, Sulphur, and Thuja; also, Apis mel., Millefolium, Carbo veg., and Zincum.—See Ulcers.

For general inflammation of the veins, Tartar emetic
For burning in the veins, Bryonia, Arsenicum: and
if with stinging, Silicea.

Pulsation of the veins, Belladonna, Graphites, Sepia,
Pulsatilla.

Any of the remedies above enumerated may be administered in water, for each of the above conditions,
according to the directions given for pericarditis and
endocarditis; administering medicines more frequently
if the sufferings are acute, or the pains severe.

CHAPTER XI.

DISEASES OF THE NERVOUS SYSTEM, INCLUDING THE BRAIN AND SPINAL CORD.

1.—Rush of Blood to the Head. (*Congestio ad Caput.*)

MANY individuals who lead a sedentary life, are
subject to what is termed rushes of blood to the head.

CAUSES.—Intense mental application, habitual use of
wine and other stimulants, may be recorded among the
exciting causes, particularly with those who inherit a
predisposition to the disorder.

SYMPTOMS.—A sense of fulness of the head and neck,
and also a conscious cognizance of the beating of the
arteries throughout the body; heat, redness, and turgidity,
or pallor and puffiness of the face; anxious expression
of the countenance; frequent attacks of giddiness, particularly after sleeping, or sitting in a warm room, or on

43*

exposure to the sun when out in the open air, headache generally above the eyes in the forehead, aggravated by coughing or stooping; dimness of vision; buzzing in the ears; tightness around the throat; oppressed breathing; furred, red-pointed, or enlarged and very red looking tongue; dyspepsia and constipation; drowsiness by day, and restlessness at night.

The principal remedies, are Aconite, Arnica, Belladonna, Coffea, Chamomilla, Ignatia, Mercurius viv., Nux vomica, Opium, Pulsatilla.

ACONITE is the principal remedy to begin with in all new cases, or such as have very recently happened, and it generally proves the only remedy required, either for children or adults.

DOSE.—Dissolve one drop, or six globules, in half a tumbler of water, and give a spoonful every three hours, until amelioration or change. Use *Belladonna*, if necessary, as directed.

BELLADONNA is useful after *Aconite*, when required. It is one of the most important remedies in the treatment of congestion of the head. It is indicated when there is great distension of the vessels of the head, attended with severe, pricking, burning pains in one-half of the head, aggravated by the slightest movement or the least noise; fiery redness of the face and eyes, and bloated; sparks before the eyes; dimness of vision; dark spots; buzzing in the ears; redness of the throat; attacks of fainting; and great inclination to sleep.

DOSE.—Dissolve one drop, or six globules, in six teaspoonfuls of water, and give a teaspoonful every three hours, until amelioration or change.

ARNICA is more particularly indicated, when the rush of blood is occasioned by external violence; severe falls or bruises, followed by stupefaction; vertigo; sensation of pressure or coldness, over a small circumscribed space; disposition to close the eyes,—to be frightened,

—and to vomit. This remedy is otherwise indicated, when there is heat in the head, with coldness of other parts of the body; sensation of obtuse pressure on the brain; painful burning or throbbing in the cranium; humming in the ears; vertigo, with confused vision, especially on assuming the erect posture after being for sometime seated.

DOSE.—When the difficulty has been occasioned by a fall or blow, &c. Dissolve one drop, or six globules, in six teaspoonfuls of water, and give a teaspoonful every three hours. At the same time prepare a lotion for external use, by adding five drops to half a tumbler of water, and bathe the head and back. When for other cases, dissolve as before, and give a teaspoonful every two hours until amelioration or change.

COFFEA may be used when the difficulty arises from excessive joy; when there is excessive liveliness, almost uncontrollable; great heaviness of the head; or aggravation of the sensation when speaking; sleeplessness.

DOSE.—The same as for *Arnica*.

CHAMOMILLA is called for, when the rush of blood is brought on by a fit of passion,—particularly in children.

DOSE.—The same as *Coffea*.

IGNATIA, when the difficulty has been brought on by stifled grief or vexation.

DOSE.—One drop, or four globules, to be given in a teaspoonful of water every night for a week, or until the patient is quite recovered.

MERCURIUS VIV. is indicated, when there is congestion with sense of fulness, or as if the head was compressed by a band; aggravation at night, with darting, piercing, tearing, or burning pains, and a proneness to perspiration.

DOSE.—In all respects as directed for *Arnica*.

NUX VOMICA is very efficacious, when the difficulty arises from sedentary habits, intense study, or excessive indulgence in spirituous or vinous liquors, &c. It is accordingly, one of the best remedies for rush of blood to the head, induced by such causes. It is also of service in irritable persons, when the same arises from a fit of passion. It is especially indicated, when there is distension of the veins, with violent pulsation in the head; heat and redness, or paleness, or sickly hue of the face; attacks of giddiness; violent headache, particularly in the forehead and over the eyes, aggravated by intense thought, or any attempts at mental application; also by stooping and coughing; disturbed sleep; nervous excitability, and disposition to be angry at trifles; constipation.

DOSE.—Dissolve one drop, or six globules, in half a tumbler of water, and give a spoonful every four hours during the attacks, but to prevent a recurrence of them, or to obviate a predisposition to them, give a spoonful at night, half an hour before retiring to rest.

OPIUM is of great service, in congestion arising from fright, and one of the best remedies in serious congestions arising from other causes, such as from drinking iced water when heated, &c. It is indicated by vertigo, heaviness of the head, humming in the ears, dulness of hearing, *stupor*, or when the attack is occasioned by *debauch*, with pressure in the forehead, from within outwards, with redness and bloatedness of the face, great depression, fugitive heat, violent thirst, dryness of the mouth, nausea or vomiting.

DOSE.—Dissolve one drop, or six globules, in half a tumbler of water, and give a teaspoonful every four hours, until manifest improvement or change.

PULSATILLA is more particularly indicated, when congestion takes place in young girls at the critical age, or in all cases occurring in cold lymphatic temperaments, with the following symptoms: distressing pains in one side of the head, of a pressive character, or if the pain commence in the occiput and extends to the root of the nose, and *vice versâ;* sense of weight in the head, aggravated when sitting; vertigo; inclination to weep; face pale, or red and bloated; coldness or shivering.

DOSE.—Dissolve one drop or six globules, in four tablespoonfuls of water, and give a spoonful every four hours, until relieved.

Several other remedies are useful in this difficulty, answering to the causes that give rise to it; as,

DULCAMARA, when brought on by getting the feet wet.

LYCOPODIUM, when dependent on habitual constipation.

CHINA, when brought on by debilitating losses.

SULPHUR, should for the most part follow *China*, four days after, and *Calcarea* after *Sulphur*.

DOSE.—Of the selected remedy, one drop, or six globules, in a spoonful of water, twice a day, until amelioration or change.

DIET.—This should be strictly in accordance with the diet table of the first chapter. No stimulants whatever should be used.

2.—Inflammation of the Brain and its Tissues.—Brain Fever.
(*Phrenitis. Encephalitis.*)

The characteristics of this disease are exceedingly various, as the symptoms are more or less modified by extent and duration of the disease, by age and sex, and by constitution and temperament; but the general symptoms are, coma, or inclination to sleep; delirium, with signs of determination of blood to the head.

When the tissues of the brain are involved, the pain is more violent, than when inflammation attacks the substance of the brain. But paralysis more frequently accompanies the latter form.

Much assistance can be derived, in ascertaining whether the brain is the seat of the affection or not, by examining the eyes and general expression of the countenance. In the first stages, the pupils are observed to be more or less contracted, but as the disease advances, they often become dilated.

Occasionally, there are premonitory symptoms, such as rush of blood to the head; sense of weight or pressure, and sometimes shooting or darting pains in the head; and also, feverish symptoms, ringing in the ears for the space of a week preceding the attack.

There are also, giddiness and sense of weight on the crown of the head; pulse rather quick, and the heat of the skin somewhat increased at night, attended with restlessness and tossing about; and moreover the patient is observed to be irritable and annoyed at trifles; anomalies in the mental powers, may then be observed, such as stupefaction, drowsiness, and slight delirium, or great excitability, in which the patient is affected with the slightest noise, and there is a brilliant and animated expression of the eyes, which are blood-shot, with fiery redness of the face, and violent delirium.

The accompanying fever is more or less according to the seat of the inflammation or the constitution and temperament of the patient; the pulse varies much in the course of the day; sometimes regular, at others intermitting; sometimes quick and weak, at others strong and slow; either a slow or rapid pulse indicates danger; the patient often complains of heat in the head when the extremities are cold; the eyes look heavy and void of expression when there is stupor or a tendency in this direction; sometimes there is uncontrollable vomiting, the stupor becomes more apparent, convulsions appear, and death sooner or later takes place.

From the fact that children possess a more delicate structure of the brain and its membranes, they are more liable to inflammation of the organ, and it is well to observe critically the symptoms that sometimes affect them, such as heaviness and a tendency of the head to gravitate backwards, attended with pain, which can only be ascertained in young children by manifest inclination to raise their hands to the head; intolerance of light; poroxysms of temper, sometimes followed by vomiting and tendency to costiveness; drowsiness, wakefulness or starting during sleep.

And again, when a child is observed to be continually boring its head against the pillow, or thrown into a fit of screaming from the slightest ray of light or noise, or is prone to a heavy sleep, having great heat in the head, swelling and redness of the face, throbbing of the blood-vessels of the head and neck, great agitation and continual tossing about, particularly at night, or when the eyes are red and sparkling, convulsed or fixed, dilated pupils, which appear not to move, there is reason to fear that the brain has become involved in some febrile difficulty.

CAUSES.—Inflammation of the brain may be the consequence of any thing tending to irritate it,—it may arise from the extremes of temperature,—from the abuse of ardent spirits, external injuries of the head, concussion or falls, intense mental emotions, and excesses of all kinds; overtasking the faculties of children is a fruitful source of the disease, repressed eruptions, contagious diseases or rushes of blood to the head, and sometimes a transfer of inflammation to the brain from the stomach or lungs.

The remedies most to be relied upon in this affection are Aconite, Belladonna, Bryonia, Cuprum met., Hyoscyamus, Opium, Stramonium and Zincum.

ACONITE should be immediately called into requisition at the commencement of the attack, when the skin is hot and dry, rapid pulse, and the usual indications of inflammatory fever.

DOSE.—Dissolve one drop, or six globules, in half a tumbler of water, and give a teaspoonful every three hours, until there is a diminution of the pulse, perspiration or moisture appears on the skin; after which the intervals may be extended to six hours, and continued until general and progressive improvement takes place, unless some other remedy seems to be indicated; in such an event select another remedy.

BELLADONNA is one of the most important remedies in this affection. It is indicated when there is great heat in the head; redness and swelling of the face, with violent pulsation of the arteries of the neck; boring the head into the pillow, and increase of suffering from the slightest noise, and extreme sensitiveness to light; violent shooting and burning pains in the head; eyes red and sparkling, and protruded, with wild expression; contraction or dilation of the pupils; violent and furious delirium; loss of consciousness; sometimes low muttering, convulsions, vomiting, and involuntary evacuations of fæces and urine.

DOSE.—Of a solution of one drop, or six globules, in half a tumbler of water, give a teaspoonful every three hours, until amelioration or change; if the first dose, or even the second or third, &c., appears to aggravate, discontinue until reaction takes place; but if improvement supervenes, repeat the medicine only once in six or eight hours, and so on until permanent relief or change. Should repeated doses of this remedy fail of the desired result, proceed with the remedy which next follows.

BRYONIA will frequently be found of great efficacy in children, when *Aconite* and *Belladonna* have produced but trivial improvement, and the symptoms indicate a tendency to dropsy of the brain.

DOSE.—Dissolve one drop, or six globules, in half a tumbler of water, and give a teaspoonful every three hours, until amelioration or change; but if only partial relief should be obtained after giving four doses of *Bryonia*, wait three hours, and proceed with *Hyoscyamus*.

CUPRUM METALLICUM.—Under the head of *Scarlatina* we mentioned the good effects of this remedy, when the eruption becomes repressed, and the brain becomes to a considerable extent involved in the difficulty, presenting certain characteristic symptoms. It is also called for in a peculiarly sensitive, rather than an irritable or inflammatory condition of the brain, which not unfrequently appears in children during the course of difficult dentition, or during other acute sufferings. The following symptoms will indicate its use, viz.: crossness and fretfulness, or apathy and indifference, restless and disturbed sleep. As the disease progresses, drowsiness and inability to sleep; not able to hold the head erect; a flushed face; dryness of the mouth, without thirst; disgust for food; nausea and vomiting; torpor of the bowels, except in some very rare cases of diarrhœa; shudderings, followed by heat, and occasionally burning; occasional perspiration; variable pulse, generally rapid, but not always full; augmenting of the fever towards evening and at night; twistings of the muscles, and grinding of the teeth during the aggravations.

DOSE.—Dissolve one drop, or six globules, in half a tumbler of water, and give a teaspoonful every four hours, until the immediate symptoms yield; then at intervals of six hours, until general improvement or change ensues.

HYOSCYAMUS is indicated when there is drowsiness; loss of consciousness; delirium about ones own affairs; unable to articulate; tongue coated white; frothy mucus about the lips; pupils distended; eyes fixed; dry and parched skin; redness of the face, and picking of the bed-clothes.

DOSE.—Dissolve one drop, or six globules, in half a tumbler of water, and give a teaspoonful every three hours, until amelioration or change.

OPIUM is indicated when there is lethargic sleep; half open eyes, and confusion and giddiness after waking; congestion of the brain; complete apathy and absence of all complaint.

44

DOSE.—Dissolve one drop, or six globules, in half a tumbler of water, and give a teaspoonful (or otherwise three globules, dry, upon the tongue,) every two hours, until amelioration or change.

STRAMONIUM is indicated when there is starting or jerking in the limbs when asleep; almost natural sleep, followed by absence of mind after waking, but sometimes attended with moaning and tossing about; eyes fixed; apprehension of some dreadful event; utters cries; redness of the face; feverish heat, with moisture of the skin. In many of the symptoms this remedy bears a close resemblance to *Belladonna*, with the exception of being indicated by the more prominent existence of spasms, and less acuteness of pain in the head.

DOSE.—Dissolve one drop, or six globules, in half a tumbler of water, and give a teaspoonful (or otherwise three globules, dry, upon the tongue,) every three hours, until amelioration or change.

ZINCUM.—This remedy may be employed after *Bella₄ donna*, or in alternation with it, in case that remedy produces only partial relief. In those deep-seated affections of the brain, threatening paralysis of the organ, indicated by loss of consciousness, half-closed eyes, dilated pupils, and insensible to light, icy coldness of the extremeties, and perhaps of the entire body, blueness of the hands and feet, interrupted respiration, diminution and weakness of the pulse, this remedy has been found unusually efficacious.

DOSE.—Dissolve one drop, or six globules, in three tablespoonfuls of water, and give a teaspoonful every hour, until amelioration, and afterwards every four hours. Three globules, dry, may be used at the same intervals.

For those cases of inflammation arising from repercussed exanthemata, *Rhus tox.* has been found serviceable. This remedy, with *Belladonna, Lachesis* and *Mercurius*, will afford the principal remedial means to be employed in such cases.

DOSE.—Of the selected remedy, the same in all cases as directed for *Cuprum metallicum.*

3.—Apoplexy. (*Apoplexia.*)

Apoplexy is a sudden loss of consciousness and motion during which the patient to all appearance is dead, the heart and lungs however continue in motion, though somewhat disturbed. There are many forms of apoplexy, and yet there can be no classification entirely void of objections. It is no easy matter to discriminate between the different kinds of apoplexy, for the external symptoms are not always such as tally with the internal injury. Thus, serous apoplexy may resemble sanguineous so perfectly in the appearance of the symptoms that it is utterly impossible to tell the difference. The same remark is true about congestion or effusion, it is impossible to tell the difference from the symptoms. It is therefore requisite that we should treat the malady in accordance with the symptoms that manifest themselves. *And as successful treatment must be had, if at all, (in many cases,) when the premonitory symptoms manifest themselves, they are as follows:* great inclination to sleep; general feeling of dulness or heaviness; dimness before the eyes; buzzing in the ears; hardness of hearing; heavy, profound sleep, and snoring respiration; frequent yawning, and fatigue after the least exertion; acute pains in the head; vertigo or giddiness; fainting, irritability of temper; loss of memory; forgetfulness of words or things; double or acute vision; difficulty of swallowing; numbness, torpor, or pricking sensation in the extremities; rush of blood to the head, with beating of the temporal arteries; red face; quick pulse, hard and tense.

TREATMENT.—The principal remedies employed in the treatment of this distressing disease, are Aconite, Belladonna, Ignatia, Lachesis, Nux vomica and Pulsatilla.

ACONITE is indicated in all cases in which there is congestion of the head, with full, quick pulse; red face; throbbing of the arteries of the temples, neck, &c. `

DOSE.—One drop, or four globules, morning and evening.

BELLADONNA is indicated when the symptoms of congestion do not yield to *Aconite*, or in the event of there having been only a partial amelioration effected by the remedy, or further, if the following symptoms present themselves: redness or bloatedness of the face; injection of the conjunctiva; violent beating of the carotid and temporal arteries; noises in the ears; darting pains in the head; violent pressure in the forehead, aggravated by movement, by the least noise, or bright light; double vision, and almost all the symptoms relative to the eyes, mentioned in the premonitory symptoms of the disease; dryness of the nose, with unpleasant smell, and bleeding at the nose; difficulty in swallowing; slight attacks of paralysis of the face; and heaviness and paralytic weakness in the limbs.

DOSE.—Of a solution of one drop, or six globules, in half a tumbler of water, give a teaspoonful (or two globules, dry upon the tongue,) every six hours, until amelioration, or change. If there appears the slightest aggravation of symptoms, whether medicinal or not, the medicine should be discontinued, and *Aconite* substituted in its place.

IGNATIA is indicated when the premonitory symptoms are brought on by sudden grief, or from suppressed continual excitement, especially when there is moaning and sighing.

DOSE.—One drop, or six globules, may be dissolved in six teaspoonfuls of water, and a teaspoonful may be given every four hours, or else, three globules, dry upon the tongue, at the same intervals, until amelioration, or change.

LACHESIS is indicated by vertigo confusion and humming in the ears; nausea, and inclination to vomit.

It is especially suited to those who are accustomed to sedentary habits, and indulgence in wine and the pleasures of the table; particularly when there is frequent abstraction of mind; vertigo, with congestive pains deep in the brain, or severe, aching pains at the left side of the head, and lowness of spirits; face pale and puffy, or turgid and somewhat livid, pulse weak and slow.

DOSE.—Dissolve one drop, or six globules, in half a tumbler of water, and give a teaspoonful every half hour, or two globules, dry on the tongue, every half hour, until the threatening symptoms pass away, and then, only every two hours, until a general amendment, or change results.

NUX VOMICA is particularly indicated against threatened apoplexy in sedentary subjects, addicted to the use of ardent spirits, or too great indulgence in the pleasures of the table; or to those who have long been affected with dyspepsia, either bilious or nervous, and have consequently more or less of rheumatic or gouty disposition; and also when the following symptoms are present: deep-seated headache, at the right side, with vertigo; confusion and humming in the ears; nausea, and inclination to vomit; turgescence of the capillaries of the face, or redness only of one cheek; drowsiness; feeling of languor, with great disinclination to exertion, either mental or bodily; cramps in the limbs, especially at night; weakness of the joints; constipation; retention of urine; irritability of temper; aggravation of the symptoms in the morning, or after a meal, and also in the open air; bilious, sanguine, or nervous temperament.

DOSE.—Dissolve one drop, or six globules, in half a tumbler of water, and give a teaspoonful every six hours. If only a partial improvement is effected, within six hours after the fourth dose, follow with *Lachesis*.

PULSATILLA is better adapted to *complete apoplexy*, than to remove the *premonitory symptoms*. Its use is

44*

indicated by lethargy; loss of consciousness; the patient lies speechless; bloatedness, and bluish red hue of the face, occurring after a full meal, which has been hurriedly swallowed; or sudden loss of the power of movement; palpitation of the heart; pulse almost entirely suppressed; snoring respiration. This remedy is best suited to the lymphatic, or phlegmatic temperament.

DOSE.—Dissolve one drop, or six globules, in half a tumbler of water, and give a tablespoonful (or otherwise three globules, dry,) every half hour, until the pulse improves, and afterwards every two hours, until general amendment or change. If, after three doses of the remedy, the pulse exhibits no improvement, proceed with the use of *Ipecacuanha.*

IPECACUANHA is indicated when the attack has arisen from a full or hurried meal, and may be employed after or in alternation with *Pulsatilla.*

DOSE.—In every respect as directed for *Pulsatilla.*

OPIUM, in real Apoplexy, when the disease has attained considerable height, is regarded one of the most important remedies to commence with, when the attack has arisen from hard drinking, especially when the following symptoms are present: slow, stentorious, or snoring breathing; red and bloated face; heat of the face and head, which are covered with sweat; pupils dilated and insensible to light; stupor; tetanic rigidity of the entire frame, or convulsive movement and trembling in the extremities; foaming at the mouth. In elderly persons this remedy is of primary importance.

DOSE.—Dissolve one drop, or six globules, in four tablespoonfuls of water, and give a teaspoonful (or three globules, dry, on the tongue,) every fifteen minutes, until the more alarming symptoms disappear, and afterwards every two hours, until prominent amendment or change results.

ARNICA is indicated in Apoplexy, when it comes on after a hearty meal, with loss of consciousness, drowsiness or stupor; snoring respiration, moaning or inarticulate muttering; involuntary evacuations; paralysis of the extremities, or of the left side; strong and full pulse.

DOSE.—Dissolve one drop, or six globules,'in three tablespoonfuls of water, and give a teaspoonful (or otherwise three globules, dry, upon the tongue,) every twenty minutes.

BELLADONNA for apoplexy, is indicated when there is deep sleep and loss of consciousness; speechless; mouth drawn on one side; convulsive movement of the limbs, or muscles of the face; paralysis of the right side; dilated and stationary pupils; face red and bloated.

DOSE.—Dissolve one drop, or six globules,·in three tablespsoonfuls of water, and give a teaspoonful (or otherwise three globules, dry, on the tongue,) every twenty minutes, until there is a change in the more alarming symptoms, of the pulse in particular, and then every two hours, until the patient exhibits signs of returning consciousness. But if the paralysis of the right side remains, repeat the remedy every six hours, until some further signs of improvement.

During the attack of apoplexy, the patient ought to be placed in a cool room, with the head raised, or put in such a position as will least favor determination of blood to the head; the clothes ought to be loosened, especially about the neck, and the feet and legs allowed to hang down. It may also be well to apply friction to increase the force of the circulation in the feet and legs. In some cases perhaps it would be well to put the feet in a warm bath, stimulated with mustard.

4.—Acute Inflammation of the Spinal cord and its Membranes.
(*Myelitis. Meningitis. Spinalis.*)

The entire length of the spine is liable to inflammation, and it is indicated by pain more or less severe, either in the small of the back, or in the upper portion of the back and neck. The slightest movement aggravates the pain, and there is a marked increase of the sensibility of the skin in various parts, as may be inferred from the dread the patient manifests at the slightest touch. There is also sharp pain in the region above the stomach, sometimes spreading over the whole region of the bowels, that becomes augmented on pressure; palpitation of the heart; sensation of constriction and weight in the forepart of the chest, with oppressed respiration; small, quick, hard pulse.

If only a part of the cord is affected, the symptoms vary according to the locality of the inflammation. Thus when the inflammation is seated in the cervical portion of the cord, there is squinting, spasm of the pharynx, lock-jaw, loss of voice, spasm or other abnormal conditions of the muscles of the neck, chest and superior extremities, with general clonic convulsions.

When the dorsal portion is implicated, there is a tendency of the body to bend backwards; there is also labored respiration, and sometimes great difficulty in breathing.

When the lumbar region is the seat of the inflammation, there is retention of urine, or paralytic or spasmodic affections of the pelvic viscera.

It matters not which portion of the spinal cord is implicated, the extremities are either convulsed or paralysed.

When the membranes that invest the cord are the seat of the inflammation, the sensitiveness of the surface is very much augmented, and the spasms more frequently general and of a tonic character.

When confined to the cord there is less sensibility, but the muscles of the extremities are affected with clonic spasms or paralysis, and only those of the back in a tonic state of contraction.

When the membranes only are implicated, the bowels

are constipated; when the cord is the seat of inflammation, the bowels are subject to diarrhœa. The symptoms produced from inflammation of the (anterior) front part of the cord, and the (posterior) back part, are essentially different. One abnormally alters the power of *motion*, and the other of *sensibility*.

CAUSES.—Exposure to cold, damp atmosphere, and external injuries, appear to form the leading exciting causes of this inflammation.

5.—Chronic Inflammation of the Spinal Cord and its Coverings.

This difficulty is generally accompanied with a trivial degree of local pains, and its prominent features chiefly consist, in derangement of the functions of the viscera, deprivation or diminution of the sense of feeling, cramp, palsy, and emaciation. The chronic form is not only more tedious, but more dangerous, than the acute form of the disease. It may terminate when confined to the substance of the cord, in softening, induration, suppuration, gangrene, in effusion of serum, pus, or blood; or when the membranes have been the seat of inflammation in the thickening of their structure.

TREATMENT.—In the treatment of the acute form, Aconite, Belladonna, Bryonia, Hyoscyamus, Stramonium, and Sulphur, are the chief remedies.

ACONITE is indicated, in all cases where the accompanying fever is present, and must be given in repeated doses.

DOSE.—Of a solution of one drop or six globules, in two tablespoonfuls of water, give a teaspoonful every two hours, until the fever subsides. If, after three doses, the fever is not allayed, discontinue for four hours, and commence again, and so on, until the fever subsides.

BELLADONNA is indicated, when the cervical portion

ɔf the cord is implicated; if from the delirium there is apprehension of the inflammation extending to the brain.

DOSE.—Dissolve one drop or six globules, in half a tumbler of water, and give a teaspoonful every hour, until the more violent symptoms of inflammation subside; (two globules dry, upon the tongue, may be administered in the same way,) after which, give a teaspoonful every four hours, and continue until decided amendment or change.

BRYONIA is often of service, when there is delirium, anxiety for the future, the mind running on very anxious thoughts, and in a severe despondency; when there is severe dry heat of the whole body, the eyes being glassy, and apparently suffused with tears, are dull and turbid; the face burning and red, and the lips dry, cracked, and swollen; the tongue dry, or when there are convulsive movements in the arms, and painful stiffness of the knees; hot, dark colored, and scanty stools; short, interrupted, and oppressed breathing, with violent pulsation of the heart; this medicine being of service more particularly, when the upper portion of the cord is implicated.

DOSE.—Dissolve one drop or six globules, in half a tumbler of water, and give a teaspoonful every two hours, until a degree of improvement becomes apparent, and subsequently, if yet indicated, every six hours, until decided amendment or change.

HYOSCYAMUS is also required, when the inflammation is high up on the cord, and when there is violent jerking attended with cries; or when there is an unmeaning smile, quick pulse, and swollen turgid veins; redness of the tongue; spasmodic clenching of the eyelids, with dilated pupils; or red, immovable and convulsed eyes; difficulty in swallowing drinks; frothy saliva about 'the mouth; extreme sensitiveness of the stomach to the touch; and involuntary discharge of excrement and urine. The remedy is also indicated, when there is inflammation of the whole cord, that produces protracted spasms, and also, in cases where inflammation has been caused by external injuries.

DOSE.—One drop, or six globules, may be dissolved in two tablespoon-fuls of water, and a teaspoonful, (or otherwise, three globules dry upon the tongue,) may be given every half hour, until amelioration of the spasmodic symptoms, and otherwise as directed for *Belladonna.*

STRAMONIUM is particularly indicated, when the dorsal or cervical portion of the cord is implicated; when there are violent and frantic fits of delirium, the face being deep red, puffed and bloated, and the expression pecu-liarly vacant; grinding of the teeth, or great distortion of the features; suppression of the urine, and alvine discharges; trembling of the hands and feet, and con-vulsive jerking or spasmodic attacks, affecting the arms in particular, but sometimes also the legs; bending back-wards of the body, in the form of an arch; imperfect articulation, or total loss of speech; eyes sparkling and fixed, pupils dilated, insensible to light, no attention being paid to objects passed before the eyes.

DOSE.—Dissolve one drop, or six globules, in half a tumbler of water, and give a spoonful, (or otherwise, three globules dry, on the tongue,) every twenty or thirty minutes, until the more urgent symptoms subside, or gene-ral change ensues; and subsequently. if still indicated, give a teaspoonful every three hours, until there is a decided amendment or change.

SULPHUR very frequently proves of service, either as an intermediate remedy, when some other remedy that appears to be indicated, seems to have little effect, or does not promptly moderate the symptoms; and also, when severe or general exhaustion appears to supervene, after severe attacks of inflammation of the upper or lower portion of the cord, or more particularly, when, notwithstanding the previously directed treatment, gene-ral convulsions take place, attended with clenching of the teeth; or when the patient sinks into complete lethargy; or when delirium of a low moaning kind, succeeds to more violent frenzy, the eyes half open, the respiration snoring and difficult, and the body motionless and lying upon the back, except as it is slightly shaken by feeble jerkings of the limbs; incoherent attempts to communicate the wants and wishes; extreme sensitiveness, or entire insensibility of the eyes to light; no motion of the pupils, which are dilated; trembling of the eyelids; dry and cracked tongue; putrid and frothy evacuations; involuntary passing of urine.

DOSE.—Dissolve one drop, or eight globules, in half a tumbler of water, and give a teaspoonful, (or otherwise, two globules, dry upon the tongue,) every twenty or thirty minutes, until a degree of improvement becomes apparent, or there is necessity for returning to one or more of the preceding remedies, if indicated by the symptoms; in which case discontinue the *Sulphur*, or otherwise continue its use, by giving a teaspoonful every three hours, until amelioration becomes decidedly manifest, or change.

6.—Palsy. (*Paralysis.*)

Paralysis consists in being deprived of the power of motion, through the agency of the will. It for the most part comes on suddenly, but in some instances it is preceded by numbness, coldness, paleness, and slight convulsive jerking, or twitching in the parts affected. The treatment must be regulated according to the originating cause. When this difficulty arises from apoplexy, for its treatment see the article apoplexy.

TREATMENT.—The chief remedies employed in the treatment of paralysis, are Arnica, Bryonia, and Sulphur.

ARNICA.—When the weakness affects the joints generally, or the hip, and knee, in particular.

DOSE.—Three globules, in a teaspoonful of water, or one drop in the same quantity of water, may be given night and morning, for a week, or until change, then pause for six days, and then repeat again, if there is not decided convalescence resulting from the first course; if from the second course there is not decided improvement, proceed with the use of *Sulphur.*

BRYONIA is decidedly indicated when the paralysis affects the lower limbs, to greater degree than other parts of the body.

DOSE.—In every respect as directed for *Arnica*, follow with *Sulphur*, if necessary, as there directed.

RHUS TOX. is the most preferable if the arms, hands, and fingers, are the chief seat of the paralytic affection, or if both upper and lower extremities are involved in the difficulty.

DOSE.—The same as directed for *Arnica*, and follow with *Sulphur*, as there directed, if necessary.

SULPHUR.—In all obstinate and protracted cases of paralysis, *Sulphur* is of paramount importance, and may be employed as directed, after each of the foregoing medicines, or in alternation with either of them, and particularly after remedies that appear to have been indicated, and yet seem to have had little effect.

DOSE.—If this remedy is to be given after one that has previously been indicated, give one drop, or three globules, four days after the last dose of the former remedy, and then for three successive mornings give the same dose, and then discontinue for a whole week, and if necessary after this recur to the use of the remedy first indicated, or continue with the *Sulphur*, another course, and so on, until amelioration or change.

This difficulty has sometimes been relieved, if not cured by *electricity* or *galvanism*, but to be of service, it must be moderately applied. There can be no harm in resorting to its use, when frequent painful jerkings take place in the affected parts.

7.—Tetanus. Spasm.

This disease is characterised by general spasmodic rigidity of the muscles. There are four varieties noted by pathologists, viz.:

TRISMUS. *Lockjaw.*

OPISTHOTONOS. *When the body is bent backwards.* A

45

common affection that results from the spasmodic contraction of the muscles, sometimes to such a degree that the back of the head touches the heels.

EMPROSTHOTONAS, *means when the body is·bent in an opposite direction, or forwards;* this a rare form of the disease.

PLEUROSTHOTONAS, *means when the body is bent one side.* This is a still more rare affection or variety.

Tetanus in either form is chiefly occasioned by exposure to cold, or else by irritation, resulting from some injury done to a tendon or nerve. When it results from cold, it is termed *idiopathic* tetanus; when from irritation from a local injury, it is termed *traumatic* tetanus. It is of much more frequent occurrence in warm than cold climates. In this and other climates the amputation of a limb, or the twitching of a nerve by a ligature, are not unfrequently the sources of the disease. When it occurs from an external cause, it sets in about the eighth day, sometimes later; but when it supervenes on exposure to cold, it usually declares itself much earlier. In some cases the attack comes on suddenly and with great violence; but it more generally comes on by degrees, only a slight stiffness being experienced at first in the back part of the neck, together with an uneasy sensation at the root of the tongue, difficulty of swallowing, and oppressive tightness of the chest, and a pain at the lower extremity of the breast-bone, extending to the back; impeded respiration, pale countenance, small pulse, high colored urine, and constipation of the bowels; a stiffness also takes place in the lower jaw, which after awhile increases so much that the jaws are compressed together so tightly that it is almost impossible to allow the smallest opening between them, and this is what is called lockjaw. In some cases the spasmodic contractions extend no farther, in others they return with great frequency and augmented severity, extending to the arms, back, abdominal muscles and lower extremities, so as to bend the body in either the one or the other directions described.

Ultimately the tetanus becomes general, the eyes become fixed and immovable, the whole countenance frightfully distorted, and expressive of great anguish; irrregular pulse; severe exhaustion, and a fatal termination of the sufferings generally about the fourth day, if the case be acute, at which time it consists of one concentrated spasm. In some cases the fatal termination is protracted considerably beyond the stated period.

The spasmodic action does not continue without remission; sometimes the muscular contractions appear to have some abatement, but are immediately renewed when the patient attempts to drink, speak or move.

TREATMENT.—The remedies for this severe malady are Arnica, Belladonna, Hyoscyamus, Lachesis, &c.

ARNICA is indicated when the disease has been produced from irritation, arising from local injury, which is by far the most dangerous form of the disease. It should be used internally and externally.

DOSE.—For internal use, dissolve one drop, or six globules, in three tablespoonfuls of water, and give a teaspoonful every two hours, or three pellets dry on the tongue at the same intervals, until manifest improvement or change; but if no apparent benefit be effected in the course of twenty-four hours, pause six hours after the last dose, and proceed with some other remedy.

BELLADONNA is one of the most useful remedies, in this distressing complaint, and particularly for that form brought on by a cold, or in lockjaw. It has also proved useful after *Arnica*, when the disease has been brought on by local irritation. The indicating symptoms are, sensation of constriction in the throat, with tightness at the chest; grinding of the teeth; spasmodic clenching of the jaws; distortion of the mouth; foaming, interrupted swallowing, and a renewal or aggravation of the paroxysms on attempting to drink.

DOSE.—Dissolve one drop, or six globules, in three tablespoonfuls of water, and give a teaspoonful, if it is possible to introduce it into the mouth, every four hours, until a degree of relaxation becomes apparent, and afterwards, morning and evening, until some manifest change for the better or worse. The medicine, if more practicable, may be administered, by putting three globules at a time into the mouth or inside the lips, or if impossible to introduce into the mouth at all, the lips and nostrils may be moistened with the solution.

HYOSCYAMUS is a remedy that may be used in connection with *Belladonna*, in *trismus* or lockjaw, and other forms of tetanus.

DOSE.—The same as directed for *Belladonna*, not to be used for four hours after the last dose of *Belladonna*.

LACHESIS is indicated, when the muscles of the back are contracted, so as to draw the head backwards towards the heel. *Stramonium, Opium,* and *Rhus tox.*, are severally remedies to be called in requisition for the treatment of the same symptoms.

DOSE.—Of either, in all respects as directed for *Belladonna* or *Arnica*.

MERCURIUS VIV., has been called into requisition, as an effectual remedy in trismus, of an inflammatory character, with swelling of the angle of the lower jaw, and tension of the muscles of the throat and neck from cold.

DOSE.—One drop, or six globules, may be dissolved in four teaspoonfuls of water, and a teaspoonful, (or otherwise, three globules dry, upon the tongue,) may be given every half hour, until a degree of relaxation takes place, and afterwards every two hours, until a change.

NOTE.—When it is absolutely impossible, from the clenching of the jaws, to administer medicine by the mouth, the effect of olfaction or smelling must be tried, or the lips must be bathed with the solution, or it may be administered in the form of an *enema*, a few drops to a half pint of water; in this way, it has been found very efficacious.

8.—Delirium Tremens.—Potatorum. (*Mania é potu.*)

This is a disease brought on by persistent inebriation, and consists of an affection of the brain, and is peculiar to drunkards and opium eaters, and very rarely occurs except from these causes, although it is said, excessive bleedings or losses, may bring on an exhaustion that. may prove the source of the disease; the intemperate use of ardent spirits, however, either vinous, malt, or distilled liquors, more frequently prove the exciting cause than any thing else. The disease generally comes on in drunkards, during the state of prostration which ensues, when they have in a great measure given up, or been suddenly deprived of their accustomed stimulus.

The symptoms of delirium tremens, are extreme irritability of temper; weakness of memory, but constant activity of mind; anxiety, and uncontrollable restlessness, with increased muscular motion.

The appetite is generally good, though often impaired from the previous habits, and the tongue is sometimes foul but moist. Soon after these premonitory signs, wakefulness sets in, and not much sleep can be obtained afterwards; and what is obtained, seems unrefreshing and disturbed by frightful dreams, imaginary visions and sounds; fixed ideas then take possession of the patient's mind, .such as the supposition that some one is bent on accomplishing his downfall, by depriving him of liberty, or of doing him some other injury, &c.; yet he generally dreads being alone; the speech is generally stuttering and inarticulate; the countenance quick, wild, and exceedingly variable, according to the prevailing impression of the mind; the face is generally pale and sallow; the eye rolling, restless, expressive; the skin damp, or covered with perspiration, and very rarely above the natural temperature; there is commonly, a tremulous motion of the hands and muscles.

As the disease advances, sleep is completely banished; great disposition to talk; constantly occupied; and when the disease is fully developed, delirium supervenes; the pulse soft and compressible, seldom quick. The corporeal activity in some respects, corresponds to the restlessness of the mind, and it is difficult to confine the patient to his bed, or keep him in his room. At the same time, exhaustion is liable to come on very rapidly, and the patient is prone to lie down from fatigue. Convulsions sometimes take place, somewhat serious, but seldom fatal. The disease seems to be entirely confined to the nervous system, and the above symptoms will enable us to discriminate between this disorder and inflammation of the brain, or its meninges.

TREATMENT.—The principal remedies employed, are Aconite, Belladonna, Calcarea, Nux vomica, Opium, Hyosyamus, Lachesis, and Sulphur.

ACONITE may be employed when there is any indication of fever, or heat in the head, as may *Belladonna*, when there is, before the delirium sets in, severe pain in the head; when the eyes appear red, and the face flushed.

DOSE.—Dissolve of either, one drop, or six globules, in three table-spoonfuls of water, and give a teaspoonful every three hours, until amelioration or change.

CALCAREA.—After *Sulphur* has been employed in cases of long standing; this remedy may be given four days after the last dose of *Sulphur*, if the patient be of a full habit of body; or if the lymphatic constitution be a characteristic of the patient. Or this remedy may be used after any of the other remedies employed in the treatment of the disorder, if it be inveterate, and of long standing.

DOSE.—Dissolve one drop, or six globules, in half a tumbler of water, and give a tablespoonful four days after the last dose of the preceding remedy, and repeat every twelve hours, for two days, then discontinue for two days, and repeat, or recur to the former remedy, if still indicated.

NUX VOMICA is one of the most important remedies in the commencement of the disease, and may be the means of arresting its further progress, when administered at this period.

DOSE.—One drop, or four globules, in a tablespoonful of water, may be given, and repeated in twelve hours, and afterwards every twenty-four hours, (at bed time,) until the premonitory symptoms subside, or there is a change that calls for some other remedy.

OPIUM is indicated when the disease becomes fairly established, and the patient is affected with delirium or convulsions, and we find an aggravated degree of all the symptoms observed at the commencement of the attack. *Nux vomica* may also be used in connection with *Opium*, when the digestive function is deranged. The remedies in such a case may be used alternately.

DOSE.—OF OPIUM SINGLY. Dissolve one drop, or six globules, in three tablespoonfuls of water, and give a teaspoonful, and repeat in half an hour, and in one hour repeat again, and then every three hours, until amelioration, or change. Or in alternation with *Nux vomica* every four hours, until decided amelioration, or change.

HYOSCYAMUS AND LACHESIS are both useful in the treatment of the disorder, in the stage when the delirium appears.

DOSE.—The same as directed for *Nux vomica.*

SULPHUR, in some cases of long standing, and of an obstinate and untractable character, may be employed additionally, or in regular rotation with *Nux vomica* and *Opium.*

DOSE.—The same as directed for *Nux vomica.*

It sometimes happens that *Nux vomica* or some other

remedy is indicated, and when administered according to directions, appears to produce but little effect; under such circumstances, *Sulphur* or *Calcarea* may be employed as *intermediary* remedies; of either, give one drop, or four globules, in a spoonful of water, twelve hours after the last dose of the remedy that precedes, and then repeat in twelve hours; pause twenty-four hours, and recur to the remedy indicated as before.

9.—Epilepsy.—Fits. (*Epilepsia. Morbus sacer.*)

The characteristics of this disease are convulsions, with loss of consciousness and voluntary motion, and generally by foaming at the mouth.

It usually comes on in sudden attacks, or fits; sometimes, however, it is preceded by pain in the head; dimness of vision; flashes or sparks of fire; (linitus aurium) palpitations; flatulency and languor, or by a peculiar feeling, partaking partly of pain, and partly of a sense of cold, beginning in some remote part of the body, as in the toes, abdomen or fingers, and proceeding gradually upwards towards the heart or head; generally during the fit the muscles of one-half of the body are more severely agitated than those of the other, and those connected with respiration are always more or less implicated; the eyes are frightfully convulsed, and turned in various directions; at length they become fixed, so that the whites of them alone are seen; the fingers are firmly clenched, and the muscles of the jaw are often the seat of spasms, which often lacerate the tongue when it becomes thrust out, immediately before the violent or sudden closing together of the teeth. The mouth is frequently filled with phlegm, which requires considerable force to expel it; it generally becomes frothy by the effort.

The face during the fit is of a livid color, dark-red, or pale, or alternately red and pale, or pale on one side and red on the other; the fæces and urine are sometimes passed involuntarily. On the abatement of the spasms, the patient gradually recovers. Sometimes vomiting will terminate the attack.

The memory and judgment are often temporarily impaired for some little time after the fit, and a sensation of languor, or exhaustion, or uncomfortable feeling about the head, and weight, are sometimes complained of.

But few patients die of a fit, yet it sometimes happens that they will occur in succession, or with increasing intensity, until a comatose state ensues, and the patient sinks.

Idiocy often is the result of this disease.

The disease is curable without much difficulty when it occurs before the age of puberty, and also when it is purely sympathetic, by the administration of homœopathic remedies.

When it occurs after the age of puberty, and is constitutional or hereditary, and has been of long duration, it is not easy to bring about a cure. It is, however, in the most inveterate cases, possible to lengthen the intervals between the attack, and also to bring about some mitigation of their violence, by persevering in judicious homœopathic treatment.

TREATMENT.—This disease must not be treated *haphazard*, for much depends upon a correct course, and this has to be regulated by the character and causes, as well as by the symptoms of the malady; the latter merely guides us in selecting one from a class of remedies.

The remedies employed for the most part are Bella-

donna, Cuprum, Hyoscyamus, Ignatia, Lachesis, Nux
vom., Opium and Stramonium. -

BELLADONNA may be employed at the commencement
of the attack, when there is a crawling and torpor in the
upper extremities; jerking of the limbs, especially of the
arms; convulsive movement of the face, eyes and mouth;
rush of blood to the head, with vertigo; bloatedess and
redness of the face; or on the other hand, paleness and
coldness of the face, with shivering and dread of light,
with fixed or convulsed eyes, dilated pupils; obstruction
of the throat, rendering the patient unable to swallow;
cramps of larynx and throat, and danger of suffocation;
foam at the mouth; involuntary discharges from the
bowels, and of urine; oppression of the chest and anxious
respiration; renewal of the fits on the slightest contact or
the least contradiction; loss of consciousness; unable to
sleep after the fit is over; constant agitation and tossing,
or deep lethargic sleep, with grimaces and smiles, and
waking with starts and cries.

DOSE.—Dissolve one drop, or six globules, in six teaspoonfuls of water,
and give a teaspoonful (or otherwise four globules dry upon the tongue),
immediately after the attack, and as a preventive of return; repeat the dose
night and morning for a week, until there is decided amendment or change.

CUPRUM.—When the commencement of the fit is in
the fingers and toes, or in the arms, or retraction of the
thumbs; this remedy is indicated, and especially when
there is loss of consciousness and speech; salivation,
sometimes of a frothy character; eyes and face red;
recurrence of the fits about every moon, and especially
at the menstrual period.

DOSE.—Dissolve one drop, or six globules, in six teaspoonfuls of water,
and give a teaspoonful (or otherwise three globules dry upon the tongue),
immediately after the attack, and give the same every night and morning
for a week, before the anticipated attack begins again, take the medi-cine
night and morning.

HYOSCYAMUS.—This remedy is indicated when the face is bloated, and when there is bluish color of the lips; foam at the mouth; prominent eyes; convulsive movements of certain limbs, or of the whole body; violent tossing about; retraction of the limbs; renewal of the fits on attempting to swallow the least portion of liquid; cries; grinding of the teeth; loss of consciousness; unnoticed emission of urine, cerebral congestion; deep and lethargic sleep, with stertorious breathing.

DOSE.—As directed for *Belladonna.*

IGNATIA is indicated when the attack is brought on by grief, and when there are convulsive movements of the limbs, eyes, muscles of the face and lips; throwing back of the head; retraction of the thumbs; bluish or red face, or red on one cheek and paleness on the other; or redness and paleness alternately; frothing at the mouth; spasms in the throat and larynx, with threatening suffocation and difficult deglutition; loss of consciousness; frequent yawning or drowsy sleep; great anxiety and deep sighs between or before the attacks; paroxysms or fits every day.

DOSE.—Dissolve one drop, or six globules, in four teaspoonfuls of water, and give a teaspoonful every six hours, or otherwise three globules dry upon the tongue.

LACHESIS.—The indicating symptoms are loud cries; falling and want of consciousness; foaming at the mouth; cold feet; belchings from the stomach; pale face; dizziness or vertigo; heaviness in the head, and sometimes pain; palpitation of the heart; distended abdomen; half sleep, or deep sleep; nausea, &c.

DOSE.—Dissolve one drop, or six globules, in four teaspoonfuls of water, and give one immediately after the attack, and repeat night and morning after, unless more urgent symptoms should call for more frequent repetition; or if it suits better, four globules may be given dry upon the tongue, after an attack, and repeated every six hours, until amelioration or change.

Nux vomica.—This remedy is indicated when there is shrieks, throwing back of the head, trembling or convulsive jerks of the limbs or muscles; renewal of the fits after disappointments or contradictions, or from anger; unobserved passing of fæces and urine; sensation of numbness of the limbs; vomiting; profuse perspiration; costiveness; full of ill-humor between the attacks.

DOSE.—Give one drop, or four globules, after a fit, and repeat the dose twelve hours after; then, as a preventive, give a drop, or four globules, every evening for a week.

Opium is the remedy when the fits occur at night or in the evening; throwing back of the head, or violent movement of the limbs, particularly the arms; loss of consciousness; closed fists; deep somnolency after the fits.

DOSE.—One drop, or four globules, in a spoonful of water, may be given every four hours, until four doses have been taken, and then every twelve hours for four days, and so on after each attack, until a change

Stramonium is more particularly serviceable when there is throwing back the head or convulsive motion of the limbs, and especially the upper part of the body and the abdomen; haggard and pale face; stupid expression; bloated; red face; unconscious, insensible, and sometimes cries, &c.; the fits come on by being touched, or by the sight of any brilliant objects.

DOSE.—Precisely as directed for *Opium*.

Arsenicum may be called into use when the fits are attended with burning in the stomach, vertebra and abdomen.

DOSE.—Dissolve one drop, or eight globules, in four teaspoonfuls of water, and give a teaspoonful (or otherwise three globules, dry, on the tongue,) every three hours, until amelioration or change.

For Chronic Epilepsy, Sulphur, Calcarea, Silicea, Stannum, Cicuta, Cocculus, Mercurius and Veratrum may be called into requisition.

Sulphur is indicated when the attack is preceded

by a sensation as if a mouse were crawling over the muscles.

CALCAREA, when the fits occur at night.

SILICEA is indicated in Chronic Epilepsy after *Calcarea*.

STANNUM, for tossing about the limbs; retraction of the thumbs; paleness of the face; backward traction of the head; loss of consciousness, and the fits come on in the evening and at night.

DOSE.—For either of the above remedies in Chronic Epilepsy, dissolve one drop, or eight globules, in half a tumbler of water, and give a tablespoonful night and morning, for a week, and then discontinue for a week, provided there is no recurrence of the fits, after which the course may be repeated, and so on until there is a permanent amelioration or change.

During a fit the patient should be placed in a horizontal position, and such precautions should be taken as will obviate any injury which may be sustained by the violence of the convulsive movements; something should be inserted in the mouth to prevent any violence being done to the tongue; the cravat should be loosened or removed, and so should stays; cold water should be sprinkled over the face, especially when the breathing is much affected by a spasm of the muscles concerned in breathing. When the fit occurs in plethoric subjects, give a dose of *Aconite* and follow with *Belladonna*, if relief is not speedily brought about.

DIET AND REGIMEN.—Persons subject to fits ought to live on a plain diet, easy of digestion, and in.great moderation. When there is plethora with a tendency to congestion, stimulants should be entirely avoided. Persons very much the opposite, require a more generous diet, but care should be taken not to overload the stomach; excessive exertion of any kind must be abstained from.

46

10.—Neuralgia. (*Nerve pain. Face ache. Tic doloreux.*

The meaning of the term neuralgia is pain in the nerve, and it is usually of an excruciating character; it is experienced with great acuteness under the eye, before the ear, shooting half over the face, into the eye, and into the brain. The paroxysms generally continue for shorter or longer periods, sometimes days, sometimes weeks, and even longer. It is not always confined to the face. As the nerves extend throughout the body there may be pain in the nerve in almost any part. The disease is obstinate, and sometimes baffles all attempts at cure.

The principal remedies used in curing this distressing malady, are Arsenicum, Belladonna, China, Colocynth, Lycopodium, Platina, Spigelia, &c.

ARSENICUM is indicated when there is a tendency to periodicity in the attacks, and the pains are of a burning, pricking and rending character, and are experienced around the eyes, and occasionally in the temples; aggravated by cold, and temporarily relieved by heat.

DOSE.—Dissolve one drop, or six globules, in four spoonfuls of water, and give a spoonful every three hours, until during the interum, beginning immediately after the paroxysm. Should the paroxysm not return so soon, or should it return earlier, discontinue the medicine for two days, and then commence again, if necessary.

BELLADONNA is indicated in facial neuralgia, when there are darting pains in the cheek-bones, nose, jaws, or temples, or in the neck, and clenching of the jaws; twitches of the eyelids, and excruciating pain in the ball of the eye; for almost every form of face-ache, or *tic doloreux*, this remedy is a polycrest.

DOSE.—Dissolve one drop, or ten globules, in half a tumbler of water, and give a teaspoonful every four hours, for two days, unless there should be an earlier amelioration, in which case give a teaspoonful every twelve hours, or if it suits better, three globules dry on the tongue, every twelve hours, until complete amelioration or change.

CHINA is indicated in the same way as *Arsenicum*, when there is an apparent tendency to periodicity in the attacks, and when the pains are excessive, and there is extreme sensibility and soreness of the skin.

DOSE.—Dissolve one drop, or ten globules, in half a tumbler of water, and give a tablespoonful three times a day, during the intermissions, if the paroxysms should be retarded, or they should come earlier than expected, discontinue after three days' trial, for a week, and then, if necessary, begin again.

COLOCYNTH. is particularly indicated, when there is violent rending and darting pains, which chiefly occupy the left side of the face, aggravated by the slightest touch, and extend to the head and temples.

LYCOPODIUM is particularly useful when the symptoms are much the same as described under the preceding remedy, with the exception of the torpor and creeping, and particularly when the right side of the face seems to be the part affected.

DOSE.—One drop, or ten globules, may be dissolved in half a tumbler of water, a tablespoonful may be given every evening for four days, or intil a change, then pause two days, after which, proceed again, if necessary, until there is permanent relief.

PULSATILLA is a useful remedy for facial neuralgia, when there is a feeling of coldness and torpor in the affected side of the face, with severe spasmodic pain in the cheek bone, with a sensation of crawling and aggravation, or renewal of the suffering in the evening, and when in a state of rest; lachrymation; redness of the face, &c.

DOSE.—In all respects as directed for *Belladonna*.

Neuralgia is often attendant on other difficulties, such as *Prolapsus uteri*, in such cases, *Sepia*, *Aurum*, if produced from taking the blue pill, *China*, if from miscarriage, &c.

DOSE.—Of either, one drop, or four globules twice a day.

SPIGELIA is also a useful remedy when the pain extends into the head, and is excruciating; aggravated by the slightest touch.

DOSE.—One drop, or four globules, in a spoonful of water, every four hours, until a change.

11.—Chorea. *St. Vitus's Dance.*

This disease is characterised by regular and uncontrollable movements of portions of the body, and sometimes, though rarely, of the whole body; sometimes one entire side, and it has been observed that the left more frequently suffers than the right; at other times the affection is limited to certain parts, as the face, lower jaw, one arm or single muscles. The motions are most strange and fantastic, occasioning grimaces of the face, when limited to this region, and singular movements of the extremities, when they are particularly affected, &c.

TREATMENT.—The remedies suited to other irritations of the *nervous centres*, are for the most part useful in this difficulty. The principal are Belladonna, Pulsatilla, Stramonium, Hyoscyamus, Nux vomica and Sulphur.

BELLADONNA, if the face is implicated; *Hyoscyamus*, if the tongue or lower jaw; and also *Stramonium*, for the affection of any of the muscles about the head and neck. *Pulsatilla, Nux vomica* and *Sulphur*, if the extremities are affected.

DOSE.—One drop, or six globules, of the selected remedy, may be dissolved in a spoonful of water, and given every morning.

12.—Stammering.

This difficulty is a form of chorea, affecting the muscular organs of speech. The remedies found most useful are Belladonna, Hyoscyamus, Sulphur, Causticum and Calcarea.

DOSE.—Of the selected remedy, dissolve one drop, or six globules, in four spoonfuls of water, and give a spoonful every morning.

To produce a useful effect in the treatment of this difficulty, it is necessary that the patient when taking remedies should subject the voice to exercise, observing to prolong the sound of the voice, and to speak often very slowly and distinctly, and persevere until amelioration or change.

13.—Headache. (*Cephalagia. Hemicranea.*)

Headache is seldom a disease by itself, it is more a symptom of some constitutional difficulty, or of general disease, and under such circumstances has to be treated according to the other symptoms in connection. As for instance, when it arises from indigestion; derangement of the stomach; cold in the head; mental emotions; fulness of the blood vessels of the head; or from any other disorders. The remedies most appropriate to the treatment of these different disorders, will be the best suited to remove the headache.

We may, however, subjoin a few remedies for headache in general, whether dependant on some other disease or not.

BELLADONNA is indicated, when there is pain in the head that is nearly constant, increased by motion either of the head or body, and especially on stooping, or moving the eyes; or when a bright light or the most trivial noise tends to aggravate the pain, which consists of a dull pressure of the top of the head, or merely on one side; sometimes very violent, almost depriving the patient of consciousness, depriving him of rest, &c.

DOSE.—Dissolve one drop or six globules, in four tablespoonfuls of water, and give a tablespoonful every six hours, until amelioration, or change.

46*

BRYONIA is more particularly indicated, when there is aching, piercing, tearing pain, at a fixed spot, daily after a meal, or after sleep, or pain coming on in the morning and disappearing in the afternoon, and returning again in the evening with undue violence, with a sensation as if the head were pressed together, particularly at the temples; burning tearing pain over the entire head, and shootings in one side of the head, and all the pains are increased by motion, attended with chilliness or shivering; they are sometimes relieved or made to disappear by a fit of vomiting. If the remedy proves inefficient, follow with *Nux vomica* or *Rhus tox.*

DOSE.—One drop, or four globules, in a tablespoonful of water, may be given every four hours, until amelioration or change. In chronic cases, give a similar dose night and morning for several days. If no favorable change ensues, select another remedy.

RHUS TOX. is indicated, when there are rending and shooting pains, extending to the root of the nose; headache after a meal, with desire to lie down; burning or pulsating pains; fulness and weight in the head, or when the headache is renewed on going into the open air; undulation of the brain when walking, at every step; sensation of motion in the head, as from water, or as if the contents of the cranium were in a loosened state; sensation as if something were crawling in the head.

DOSE.—Three globules, in a teaspoonful of water, every four hours, in acute cases, or one drop in four spoonfuls of water, and give a spoonful every four hours. In chronic cases, only once in twelve hours; in either case, until amelioration or change.

NUX VOMICA is indicated, when the headache arises from cold; intense shooting pains; piercing, rending, or stunning pain, confined to a small space, or single spot, which is sensitive to the touch; and for most of the symptoms arising from indigestion or cold, or from stimulating drinks.

DOSE.—Dissolve one drop, or six globules, in four tablespoonfuls of water, and give a teaspoonful every three hours, in acute cases, but every twelve hours in chronic cases, until amendment or change.

PULSATILLA, for headache attendant upon the menstrual period, characterised by rending pains, with heaviness of the head, and for uncomplicated headache in persons of mild dispositions or lymphatic temperaments.

DOSE.—Dissolve one drop, or six globules, in six teaspoonfuls of water, and give a teaspoonful every three hours, for one day, and afterwards at intervals of twelve hours, until decided change.

SEPIA is indicated, for periodical headache, that comes on in paroxysms. It is better suited for persons of mild temperaments and females, and especially those subject to hysteria, and when the following symptoms are present; viz., pain in the vertex and occiput, that disposes the patient to assume the recumbent posture; hemicranea, or pain in one side of the head; sharp, shooting pains through the temples; worse in the afternoon or evening, or early in the morning; sometimes producing nausea; sense of fulness, giddiness or vertigo, on rising, accompanied with coldness of the hands and feet.

DOSE.—Dissolve one drop, or eight globules, in four tablespoonfuls of water, give a spoonful immediately after the paroxysm, and repeat night and morning for three days, and recur again to the remedy, at the first indication of a succeeding paroxysm, and so on, until amelioration or change.

CHAMOMILLA is indicated, for headaches that occur in impatient individuals, who become exasperated by the slightest pain, or who exhibit symptoms or expressions of suffering, apparently from the most trivial causes, and seemingly uncalled for; and also, for semilateral headaches, of a rending or shooting character, sometimes extending into the upper and lower jaw; and also, when the head perspires during the continuance of the pain.

DOSE.—Dissolve one drop, or eight globules, in four tablespoonfuls of water, and give a teaspoonful every four hours, (*in acute cases*,) until decided amelioration or change. In *chronic* cases, give a similar dose, at intervals of twelve hours, until decided relief or change.

SULPHUR is a useful remedy, in chronic headache, occurring daily, or every eight days; worse in the morning or at night; attended with heaviness and confusion of the head; incapability of mental exertion; pain as if the head would split, especially on moving about in the open air; great tenderness of the scalp and falling off of the hair.

DOSE.—One drop or four globules, may be dissolved in a spoonful of water, and given every morning and evening, until improvement or change; then discontinue for a week; if in the meantime, the improvement has been going on, there is reason for longer discontinuance; but if the improvement be only partial, which takes place during the first course, and remains stationary afterwards, recur again to the remedy as before.

CALCAREA is indicated, in chronic headache attended with a sensation of extreme coldness, either internally or on the scalp, when the pains affect the entire head, or merely the forehead, one side of the head, or the crown, and are of a stunning, aching, throbbing, or hammering description, compelling the patient to lie down, &c.

DOSE.—The same in all respects as for *Sulphur*.

ARSENICUM, for periodical headaches, of an excruciating and unbearable character, almost driving the patient to despair; aggravated by taking food, extending to the gums; tenderness of the scalp, temporarily relieved by cold applications to the head.

DOSE.—In acute cases, give one drop or four globules, in a teaspoonful of water, every four hours, until decided amelioration or change. In *chronic cases*, this remedy may be used consecutively with *Veratrum*, at intervals of twelve hours, until decided amelioration or change.

AURUM is indicated, for headaches in hysterical patients, attended with buzzing, or noises in the head, or pain as if the head had been bruised, especially on rising in the morning, or during mental occupation.

DOSE.—As directed for *Chamomilla,* or *Nux vomica.*

CHINA, LACHESIS, MERCURIUS, and VERATRUM, are remedies that may be consulted with reference to headaches, according to indications.

DOSE.—Of the selected remedy, the same as directed for *Arsenicum,* in both the acute and chronic form.

In the treatment of headaches, much advantage is to be derived from a knowledge of the causes which produce them; we will therefore state concisely:

1. Headache from determination of blood to the head, Aconite, Belladonna, Pulsatilla, &c.

2. Headache from cold in the head or catarrh, Aconite, Arsenicum, China.

3. Headache from rheumatism, Bryonia, Chamomilla, Nux vomica, Pulsatilla, &c.

4. Headache from disordered bowels, Ignatia, Ipecacuanha, Nux vomica, Veratrum.

5. Headache from constipation, Bryonia, Lycopodium, Nux vomica, Opium, &c.

6. Headache arising from affection of the nerves, (*Nervous Headache,*) Aconite, Bryonia, Coffea, Nux vomica, Pulsatilla, Sepia, Sulphur, &c.

7. Headache caused by suppression of eruptions, Belladonna, Calcarea, and Sulphur.

DOSE.—Of the selected remedy, one drop, or six globules, may be dissolved in half a tumbler of water, and a teaspoonful may be given every two, three, four, or six hours, according to the severity of the disease, until amelioration or change.

14.—Sick Headache.

This affection must be treated in accordance with the habit, temperament, and constitution of the patient, together with the accompanying symptoms.

The most important remedies are Arsenicum, Belladonna, Nux vomica, Sepia, Veratrum, and Colocynth. (See dyspepsia.)

The disease is often dependent upon other affections, such as disturbance of the uterine function, torpidity of the liver, and nervous irritability. Remedies suited to these different complaints, will be the most effective in affording relief.

15.—Giddiness.—Vertigo.

This difficulty arises from various causes, and is often connected with foul stomach, profuse evacuations, and the abuse of stimulants and narcotics. (See Dyspepsia, &c.)

When persons are subject to giddiness, which is not attendant upon constitutional derangement, Aconite, Arnica, Chamomilla, Nux vomica, Pulsatilla, &c., may be employed as indicated.

DOSE.—The same as directed for headaches.

16.—Weakness or Loss of Memory.

This difficulty may occur from several causes, and should be treated with reference to the particular one producing the difficulty.

1. If produced from weakness or losses, China.
2. If from blows on the head, Arnica.
3. If from intoxication, Nux vomica.
4. If from grief, Ignatia, &c.

DOSE.—Of the selected remedy, the same as directed under headaches.

CHAPTER XII.

DISEASES INVOLVING VARIOUS ORGANS AND REGIONS.

In the chapter on fevers, we treated of gout, rheumatism, &c., inasmuch as these diseases are uniformly dependent upon a peculiar febrile difficulty. We will now proceed to consider other difficulties, not yet considered.

1.—Inflammation of the Psoas Muscle. (*Psoitis.*)

The indications of the presence of this disease, are pain in the region of the kidneys, hip, and downwards to the leg; the limb can neither be stretched out, or drawn upwards without pain; in walking there is hobbling in the gait, with the body inclined forward; turning in bed, or lifting aggravates the pain. Sometimes there is external swelling. A psoas abscess is not usually dangerous, unless it discharges itself into the cavity of the abdomen, or produces caries. More frequently the abscess discharges in the groin, through the anus, perinæum, or thighs.

TREATMENT.—The remedies employed the most successfully, are Aconite, Belladonna, Colocynth, Hepar sulph., Silicea, and Staphysagria.

ACONITE is indicated when there is considerable degree of fever present in the commencement of the difficulty. This remedy should be followed by *Belladonna.*

DOSE and Administration.—Dissolve one drop, or six globules, in half a tumbler of water, of either remedy, and give a teaspoonful every three hours. If, after using the *Aconite* two days, and there is no amelioration, commence with the use of *Belladonna* in the same way, until it becomes necessary to resort to another remedy, or change.

COLOCYNTH. is indicated when there is a sense of contraction in the psoas muscles when walking, and the disease is more of a chronic nature.

DOSE.—One drop, or four globules, dissolved in a spoonful of water, repeated every six hours until amelioration, or change.

HEPAR SULPH. is indicated when there are rigors, followed by throbbing and increase of pain in the affected part, and we are led to believe that suppuration is about taking place.   It is well to precede the use of this remedy with a dose or two of *Staphysagria*.

DOSE.—Dissolve, of *Staphysagria*, one drop, or six globules, in half a tumbler of water, and give a teaspoonful every six hours, for three days, and then *Hepar sulph.* in the same way, until suppuration takes place.

SILICEA is indicated when the bones become affected from the abscess, or when an abscess has arisen from diseased vertebræ.

DOSE.—One drop, or six globules, every night and morning. *Staphysagria* may follow this remedy when an offensive sanies is discharged.

Hip Disease.

Under the head of *sciatic rheumatism*, when treating of *rheumatic fevers*, we gave some of the characteristics of hip affections.   There are, however, two other difficulties which sometimes affect the hip, more malignant and painful than *sciatica*, which we regard worthy of attentive consideration under the head of *hip disease*.

2.—Pain in the Hip. Hip-gout. Rheumatism of the Hip.
(*Coxalgia-coxagra.*)

The symptoms of this disease are pain in the hip-joint, dependent upon a true gouty inflammation, almost universally of an acute description; the pain is extremely violent, and extends from the hip-joint to the neighboring parts, and renders motion exceedingly painful, either in walking, rising, sitting down, or turning in bed.

Hip-gout usually assumes the irritable character, runs its course quickly, and forms an active local inflammation, which speedily suppurates when unchecked.

When suppuration takes place the pain becomes obtuse, pressing and throbbing; the inflammatory fever becomes suppurative in its character, which is evinced by shivering and shuddering, alternately with heat, to which a number of other sufferings become adjoined, such as pain the knee, swelling, and spontaneous luxation.

TREATMENT.—Aconite, Arsenicum, Belladonna, Chamomilla, Colocynth., Hepar sulphur, Pulsatilla and Rhus tox.

ACONITE is useful when the affection is attended with considerable degree of fever, or inflammation of the joint itself exists from the first.

DOSE.—Dissolve one drop, or six globules, in three tablespoonfuls of water, and give a teaspoonful every four hours, until amelioration or change.

ARSENICUM is one of the most useful remedies when the pain shoots along the interior of the thigh, like a stream of hot fluid, which augments on the slightest motion or change of temperature; great prostration of strength, which is not so much during the intervals between the paroxysms; paleness of the face; oppression at the chest; attacks of faintness from trifling exertion.

DOSE.—In all respects as for *Aconite*.

BELLADONNA is particularly called for during the inflammatory stage, when the patient suffers much from pain. It may be alternated with *Mercurius*, if the symptoms are such as to call for their use in this way.

DOSE.—Dissolve one drop, or six globules, in six teaspoonfuls of water, and give a teaspoonful every four hours. If used in alternation with *Mer-*

47

curius, give of the one remedy a teaspoonful, and four hours after one of the other, and so on every four hours, until amelioration or change.

CHAMOMILLA is of great efficacy in recent cases, where there is marked increase of pain at night in the bed.

DOSE.—One drop, or four globules, every three hours.

COLOCYNTH.—In chronic cases, where the fever and pain are less severe, though constant, and the pain is of a squeezing description, as if the entire joint were pain-fully bound, and also when the attacks are brought on by violent emotion or anger.

DOSE.—The same as directed for *Belladonna.*˜

HEPAR SULPHUR is called for in case of exudation, and may follow *Mercurius*.

DOSE.—One drop, or four globules, every six hours, until better or change.

MERCURIUS is indicated when the disease is attended with halting in the gait, and sharp burning pains, worse at night and at every movement, attended with sweats at night; it is also useful when exudation is about to take place, or has taken place.

DOSE.—The same as *Aconite* and *Belladonna*.

PULSATILLA is of great service in mild cases of hip disease, that partake merely of a rheumatic character, when the patient has wrenching pains in the *hip-joint*, aggravated towards night, and even when in a state of rest.

DOSE.—One drop, or six globules, morning and evening.

RHUS TOX. is particularly called for when there are darting, tearing or dragging pains in the hip-joint, attended with tightness and stiffness in the muscles, aggravated or chiefly felt during rest; also great pain felt in the joint when rising from the seat.

DOSE.—The same as *Mercurius*.

Chronic inflammation of the hip-joint is what is most commonly called "*hip disease.*" It is seated in the bones that form the joint, and particularly in the socket. When the disease is about making its appearance, the pain may be felt in the knee, hip-joint, or a slight weakness of the part affected, attended with limping; afterwards, emaciation and elongation of the limb itself takes place, and as the complaint progresses a severe pain is felt behind the head of the thigh bone, which becomes increased by pressing the bone towards the socket; the pain extends down to the knee, ankle and foot, accompanied by fevers, restlessness, and flattening of that part of the *nates* which is generally fullest and roundest, depression of the crest of the ilium, and distortion of the spine.

The disease is most commonly found among children, but no age, sex, or station in life, is exempt from its attacks. It is peculiarly insidious in its approach, the pain in the knee being the first symptom denoting its presence, hence it is sometimes mistaken for disease of the knee-joint, but this would be an unfortunate mistake, for it is the only symptom of the incipient stage of the disease, that may direct to a timely treatment, that may obviate the formation of matter in the socket, and the luxation of the joint.

CAUSES.—Constitutional taint, such as scrofula, undoubtedly is the frequent source of the disease; but it is more frequently attributed to mechanical injury, or exposures, &c.

TREATMENT.—The principal remedies employed, are Belladonna, Colocynth., Rhus tox., and Sulphur.

BELLADONNA is more especially called for in the inflammatory stage, when the patient suffers considerable pain. It may be well to alternate this remedy with *Mercurius* in the early stage of the disease.

DOSE.—One drop, or four globules, may be given three times a day, in a spoonful of water.

COLOCYNTH. has been found of much value in this disorder, either after *Belladonna* and *Mercurius*, or in preference from the first. Its use is indicated by a feeling in the hip-joint, as if tightly bound by an iron clasp, and pain extending down the limb, and stiffness in the hip-joint.

DOSE.—One drop, or four globules, every six hours, until amelioration or change.

RHUS TOX. is particularly useful in the first stage of the disorder, when there is dragging or tearing pains in the hip-joint, aggravated by pressing the head of the femur into the socket, attended with stiffness of the muscles, most painful when in a state of rest, and severe pain on arising from a sitting posture.

DOSE.—The same as for *Colocynth.*

SULPHUR, CALCAREA, and SILICEA, are required for the most part in chronic cases. *Sulphur*, if the disease arises from scrofula, or psoric metastasis. *Calcarea* is particularly useful after the first stage has passed off. *Silicea*, when there is abscess or caries. There are other remedies that may be considered, as *Hepar sulph.*, *Phosphoric acid*, *Phosphorus*, and *Lachesis*.

DOSE.—Of the selected remedy, one drop, or four globules, every morning and evening. If, after two days, no improvement takes place, proceed with some one of the other remedies named, and so on in the same manner with others.

3.—Affections of the Knee.

When the knee-joint is affected, particularly when the disease begins in the synovial membrane, Silicea forms one of the best remedies, and in addition, Aurum, Calcarea, Lycopodium, Nitric acid, and Phosphoric acid.

Calcarea and Sulphur may be used when the inflammation exists in consequence of the effects of mercury; and Bryonia, China, Nux vomica, Rhus tox., or Sulphur, when it results from gout or rheumatism; Sulphur and Calcarea are thought applicable to scrofulous enlargement of the knee. When there is suppuration, Mercurius and Hepar sulph., when serous infiltration, Silicea and Sulphur. In white, glossy, doughy swellings of the knee, Pulsatilla is an excellent remedy, whether the swelling be painful or otherwise. In persons of scrofulous habit, Iodine may be used in connection with Pulsatilla, a dose of one in the morning and the other in the evening.

DOSE.—Of any of the remedies mentioned, when indicated, one drop, or six globules, in a spoonful of water, every twelve hours.

DIET AND REGIMEN.—In acute inflammatory difficulties of the hip-joint, the diet should be the same as in acute fevers, but in the *chronic* form, the diet should be light and nutritious, avoiding all stimulants.

4.—Affection of the Organs of the Senses.—Diseases of the Eyes.

In the treatment of diseases of the eye, great care should be exercised, to avoid all injurious applications. There is no salve or ointment, eye-water, or lotion, that is to be recommended for the eyes, for all of these preparations are deleterious, and should be avoided, and internal remedies should be relied upon. Cold water may be used freely, externally, unless the eyes are affected with erysipelas, which is known by the redness that usually surrounds them. It does good in common inflammations from a cold.

Luke-warm water may also prove a source of relief
47*

under circumstances where there is considerable heat in the eyes, and discharge of acid tears.

INFLAMMATION AND SWELLING OF THE LIDS.—Sometimes the lids are swollen and red, when the eyeballs are not affected.

TREATMENT.—The remedies are, Aconite, Chamomilla, China, Euphrasia, Hepar sulph., Nux vomica, Mercurius, and Rhus tox.

ACONITE is indicated, for red, hard swelling, with burning heat and dryness; shining as if transparent; burning, with tension and copious secretion in the eyes and nose.

DOSE.—Dissolve one drop, or six globules, in six teaspoonfuls of water, and give a teaspoonful every three hours, until change. *Hepar sulph.* if necessary, may be given after *Aconite,* to effect a cure.

BELLADONNA is the remedy to be employed, if the lids are paralyzed, or the lids stick together, and are red and swollen.

DOSE.—The same as for *Aconite.*

CHAMOMILLA is indicated, when the upper lids feel heavy as lead.

DOSE.—The same as *Aconite.*

CHINA is indicated, when there is sense of crawling inside of the lid, increased in the evening, with running tears.

DOSE.—The same as for *Aconite.*

HEPAR SULPH. is a remedy that may be used after several of the other remedies, as *Aurum, China, Belladonna,* &c., and is indicated when pressing pain remains, or the lids feel sore.

DOSE.—One drop or four globules, to be given twelve hours after the last dose of the preceding remedy, and repeated every morning until a cure is effected.

EUPHRASIA.—This remedy is very useful in chronic inflammation of the eyelids, that is characterised by itching in the day time, and by their sticking together in the night; red, and somewhat swollen, with the edges ulcerated, wet and purulent, with dread of light, constant catarrh, attended with headache and heat of the head.

DOSE—The same as for *Aconite*.

RHUS TOX. is particularly useful for inflammation of the inner surface of the lid, and when the eyes are contracted as if by spasm, or when pus is discharged from under the lids.

DOSE.—The same as for *Aconite*.

NUX VOMICA is particularly indicated when the edges of the lids burn, itch, and feel very sore when touched, and stick together towards morning.

DOSE.—Dissolve one drop, or six globules, in half a tumbler of water, and give a teaspoonful every three hours, until amelioration or change. This remedy may be used with advantage after *Euphrasia*.

MERCURIUS VIV. should be employed when the lids turn outwards, and there is pricking, burning and itching, or when there is no pain.

DOSE.—The same as directed for *Nux vomica*.

Stye.—Hordeolum.

This is a little hard tumor, much like a dark red boil, generally in the corner of the eye, and although small, is sometimes attended with severe inflammation and fever, causing more or less pain and suffering. It is slow in suppurating, and seldom bursts spontaneously.

TREATMENT.—The remedies are Pulsatilla, Staphysagria and Sepia.

PULSATILLA is to be employed on the first appearance of the stye, and in most cases no other remedy will be required to remove it.

DOSE.—One drop, or six globules, may be given every morning, until amelioration or change. If *Pulsatilla* is only partial in its effects, *Staphysagria* is the best remedy to proceed with.

STAPHYSAGRIA is particularly indicated when the swelling degenerates into a hard, white tumor, after the use of *Pulsatilla.*

DOSE.—In all respects as directed for *Pulsatilla.*

SEPIA is particularly applicable in scrofulous subjects, and in obstinate cases.

DOSE.—The same as directed for *Pulsatilla.*

Inflammation of the Eye.—Iritis.

This affection affects both the eye-balls and lids in some instances, and at others only the eyes.

TREATMENT.—The remedies employed are Aconite, Belladonna, Chamomilla, Euphrasia, Ignatia, Nux vomica, Pulsatilla, Rhus tox. and Veratrum.

ACONITE is the best remedy for inflammation of the eyes, when the disease comes on suddenly, and increases rapidly, when the whole eye is red, or full of red veins, runs much and is quite painful, and also when the eyes are sore from cold, which is accompanied with catarrh, sore throat, &c.

DOSE.—Dissolve one drop, or six globules, in half a tumbler of water, and give a teaspoonful every three hours, until amelioration or change.

BELLADONNA is indicated when the white of the eyes is quite red, or large red veins, discharge of acid tears, sensitiveness to the light, deep-seated spasmodic pains, with catarrh and excoriations of the nose.

DOSE.—The same as for *Aconite.*

CHAMOMILLA is adapted to children when there is pricking, pressing and burning in the eyes, as if they gave out heat, lids swollen and closed in the morning, or very dry.

DOSE.— In all respects the same as for *Aconite.*

EUPHRASIA is of great service when there is pressure in the eyes, increased secretion of acrid tears, contractions of the lids, the eyes very red, and attended with headache and catarrh in the evening.

DOSE.—Dissolve one drop, or six globules, in half a tumbler of water, and give a teaspoonful every three hours, until amelioration or change.

IGNATIA is indicated when the white of the eye is affected and the pain is very severe; profuse discharge of tears; dread of light, attended with catarrh.

DOSE.—One drop, or four globules, may be given in a spoonful of water, every twelve hours, until amelioration or change.

Rheumatism affecting the Eyes.

NUX VOMICA is indicated when the corners of the lids are exceedingly red, more so than the eyes, and the balls are blood-shot, and smart as if salt or sand were in them, and there is increased secretion of tears; the patient cannot bear the light, particularly in the morning; fever usually attends this condition of the eyes, and is worse in the morning and evening.

DOSE.—Dissolve and take as directed for *Euphrasia.*

PULSATILLA is very useful after the first inflammation has been removed by *Aconite*, when severe pains still remain of a piercing, boring and cutting character; cannot bear the light; pains worse in the afternoon and evening.

DOSE.—In all respects as for *Euphrasia.*

RHUS TOX. and BRYONIA may be employed after *Pulsatilla* has removed the pain, when there is redness remaining, burning, or sensation as from sand under the lids; worse in the evening and at night; the lids so swollen that opening the eyes give pain in the head.

DOSE.—The same as for *Euphrasia*, for either remedy.

VERATRUM is particularly indicated when there is tearing pain interrupting sleep at night; intolerable headache; much heat in the eyes, and a sensation of dryness.

DOSE.—As for *Euphrasia.*

For simple, uncomplicated sore eyes, when small watery blisters are on the eyes, and the light becomes offensive, Euphrasia, Bryonia and Rhus tox. When the light becomes less offensive, and the pain more violent, so that. every vein can be seen, Nux vomica, Chamomilla and Ignatia.

For scrofulous difficulties, see "scrofulous sore eyes."

Gout affecting the Eyes.

When gout attacks the eyes, the remedies found of the greatest service are Aconite, Antimonium crud., Belladonna, Cocculus and Colocynthis.

ACONITE is useful as the first remedy, especially when there is heat and burning in the eyes, with pressive and darting pains, particularly on moving the eyes; redness and inflammation, with intolerable suffering; excessive flow of tears; sparks before the eyes; dread of light; weight and fulness in the forehead; strokes and beatings in the head.

DOSE.—Dissolve one drop, or six globules, in four tablespoonfuls of water, and give a teaspoonful every three hours, until amelioration or change.

ANTIMONIUM CRUD.—Cocculus or Sulphur may be advantageously employed after *Aconite*, when there is nausea or vomiting; redness and inflammation of the lids, or canthi, with itching and sticking together of the lids at night.

DOSE.—Of either, the same as directed for *Aconite.*

BELLADONNA is of great service when the pain is very oppressive all around the eye, above it or alongside of it; pricking pain about it, sensation as if the eye were being torn out or pressed in; when the pain is intermittent; flashing before the eyes; appearance of fog or mist before the eyes; and when the symptoms are accompanied with giddiness and headache so severely as to be deprived of consciousness.

DOSE.—The same in all respects as directed for *Aconite*.

COLOCYNTHIS is particularly indicated when the eyes are sore and inflamed, attended with severe cutting pains, which extend into the head, pressing particularly into the forehead or on one side of the brain, drawing pains extending into the nose, causing great agitation and restlessness.

DOSE.—The same in all respects as directed for *Aconite*. The remedy may be used in alternation with *Belladonna*.

Scrofulous Sore Eyes.—Scrofulous Opthalmia.

In scrofulous subjects, the disease often manifests itself in the eyes. It is met with in children who suffer from this complaint, or in grown persons who have had the taint of the disease in them from childhood. When the eyes have once become weakened from the disease, they are liable to subsequent attacks of the same disorder; from cold and other causes, the disease may be so excited as to affect the sight and produce ulcers on the ball of the eye.

TREATMENT.—The remedies found most useful are, Arsenicum, Belladonna, Calcarea, China, Dulcamara, Hepar sulph., Mercurius, and Sulphur.

ARSENICUM is usually indicated, when the pains are of a burning character, as if produced by burning coals, and when spots are seen in the eye.

DOSE.—One drop, or four globules, may be given twice a day.

BELLADONNA is of service, when there is a sensation of pressure in the eyes, which is worse when they are turned upward, and when red veins, ulcers, or pustules, can be seen on the eye-ball.

DOSE.—One drop, or four globules, three times a day.

HEPAR SULPH. is useful after *Belladonna*, and espe-cially for children who have been dosed with calomel; when the lids are red and sore, and painful to the touch, as if bruised; and also, when from touch, they close convulsively, and can scarcely be moved; unable to bear light in the evening; dulness of the eyes, or other-wise, brilliant appearance of the eyes; spots on the ball; sensation as if the eyes were pressing from their sockets.

DOSE.—One drop, or six globules, every morning for several days.

CALCAREA is indicated, when there are ulcers on the eyeball, attended with itching; burning when reading in the evening.

DOSE.—In all respects as for *Hepar sulph.*

CHINA should be given, when there is considerable pain in the eyes, in the evening; sensation as if sand were in them; and also, when there is a dull or hazy appearance of the eye on inspection.

DOSE.—One drop or four globules, every morning.

DULCAMARA is indicated, in scrofulous sore eyes, when cold is the exciting cause, and when there appears to be thick fog before the eyes, and flashes of light from them, attended with pain over the eyes, aggravated when at rest, and worse when the patient is quiet.

DOSE.—One drop, or four globules, morning and evening.

MERCURIUS VIV. is well suited to the affections in children, who have taken no Mercury; when the pains are cutting, especially in straining the eyes; worse in the evening, and in a warm bed; the eyes full of tears; sen-sitive to light; burning in the open air; sight clouded;

small pustules on the ball of the eye, that occur at every fresh cold. This remedy is especially useful after *Bella-donna.* '

DOSE.—In all respects as directed for *Dulcamara.*

SULPHUR, is a remedy that will prove of service after the use of *Mercurius* or *Belladonna,* but not after *Hepar,* although it may take the place of this latter remedy. It is particularly indicated, when the lids are contracted in the morning, and the light of the sun is dreaded by the patient, on the account of its destroying the sight, and when there appears to be a mist before the eyes, dimness of the cornea, or when the white of the eye appears very red, bloodshot, and little spots upon it; when the flow of tears is increased; severe pressure in the eyeball.

DOSE.—One drop, or four globules, may be given every evening for a week, and then discontinue for the same length of time. If the patient is better, continue the intermission.

Catarrhal Inflammation of the Eyes.

This difficulty may arise from a common cold and obstruction of the tear passages, and may be cured by the use of Chamomilla, Lycopodium and Hepar sulph.

DOSE.—Of either, dissolve one drop, or six globules, in half a tumbler of water, and give a tablespoonful morning and evening, until amelioration or change.

Syphilitic Sore Eyes.

This affection may be cured by Mercurius, if the patient has not been previously treated with mercury in the allopathic form; under other circumstances Nitric acid, Aurum, Sulphur, &c.

DOSE.—Of either, dissolve one drop, or six globules, in four table-spoonfuls of water, and give one morning and evening; if after four days there is no decided improvement, proceed with the next remedy.

Gonorrhœal Inflammation of the Eyes

This difficulty can be eradicated generally by the use of Pulsatilla, Arnica and Sulphur.

48

DOSE.—One drop, or six globules, of either, dissolved in a spoonful of of water, twice a day.

Fungus cancer of the eyes (fungus hæmatodes,) will require Thuja, Carbo animalis and Phosphorus, one dose of either, every day, until change.

Cataract.

The remedies that have proved the most successful in this difficulty are Conium, Phosphorus, Cannabis, Sulphur, &c.

DOSE.—One drop, of either, or six globules, every twenty-four hours, dissolved in a spoonful of water. After the use of *Conium* for *ten days*, discontinue for about the same length of time, in order to allow the remedy sufficient time to act, and then if there has been little or no change, proceed with the use of *Phosphorus* or *Sulphur*.

Specks on the Cornea. Opacity of the Cornea.

These specks, sometimes left on the cornea from preceding inflammation, may be removed by Belladonna, Euphrasia, Sulphur and Calcarea

Squinting. Strabismus.

The cure for squinting is seldom found among remedial agents, to be taken internally, still some remedies may afford material aid to the ordinary mechanical means resorted to in effecting a cure, and some cases have been radically cured by the administration of Hyoscyamus or Belladonna, when the affection had been of recent standing.

DOSE.—Dissolve one drop, or six globules of the remedy employed, in six teaspoonfuls of water, and give a teaspoonful every three hours, for two days, and then discontinue the same length of time, and then proceed with the use of another remedy, if necessary.

Weeping or Watery Eye.

This difficulty consists in the continual flow of tears from either one or both of the eyes. It may proceed from an obstruction of the tear duct, or the cause may merely be a relaxed condition of the glandular aparatus of the eye. If from an obstruction there is no remedy better adapted to effect a cure than Petroleum, but if this should not prove effectual, resort may be had to Stramonium, Calcarea, Pulsatilla, Sulphur, Lachesis, &c. But if the difficulty occurs from merely a relaxed condition of the glandular apparatus, the most suitable remedies are Spigelia, Euphrasia, Pulsatilla, &c.

DOSE.—The selected remedy may be given twice a day in doses of a drop, or four globules, until amelioration or change. The remedies may be tried in the order laid down above, each for two or three days, to be succeeded by at least an interval of two days before another remedy is proceeded with.

Bloodshot Eyes.

This derangement may arise from several causes, such as blows, falls, retching, straining, vomiting, coughing, crying, &c., and it usually disappears of itself. But in some rare instances it proves obstinate and requires remedial aid. In such an event, the external use of Arnica may facilitate a cure. In other cases, though rare, Belladonna, Chamomilla, Nux vomica, &c., may be required.

DOSE.—One drop, or four globules, every six hours, but if no relief is obtained by the time the fifth dose is taken, proceed with the next remedy For external use, twelve drops may be dissolved in half a tumbler of water.

Short or Near-sightedness. Myopia.

This difficulty though dependent in a measure upon the peculiar structure of the lens, has been partially, and in some rare instances, completely removed by medicines, Pulsatilla, Sulphur, Carbo veg., Phosphoric acid, Petroleum. Of these, Pulsatilla and Sulphur.

DOSE.—Dissolve one drop, or six globules, in a half tumbler of water, and give a tablespoonful every morning. If after using one remedy three mornings no improvement is produced, after two days proceed with another remedy.

Attacks of Blindness.

This ephemeral difficulty may be produced from evo-
lutions taking place in the system; it may come on
suddenly or gradually towards evening. Aconite for
sudden attacks, Belladonna or Veratrum for that which
comes on towards evening.

DOSE.—One drop, or four globules, of *Aconite*, every three hours, and
of *Belladonna* every six hours. If after two days there is no improvement,
resort to other remedies. *Hyoscyamus* is a remedy that proves of great
service under particular circumstances, when the patient sees spots or
objects before the eyes.

5.—Inflammation of the Ear. (*Earache. Otitis. Otalgia.*)

Inflammation of the ear is characterised by violent
pain in the ear, with sensibility to noises, attended with
more or less fever. Earache may also arise from toothache, or be a purely neuralgic affection. When the pain
is excessive, it may communicate with the whole head,
and may bring on delirium, or even inflammation of the
brain.

OTITIS.—The remedies employed in this difficulty are
Belladonna and Pulsatilla, and protective means.

PULSATILLA is regarded an effective remedy, and one
drop, or six globules, may be given every three hours;
at the same time cover the ear with cotton, so as to
protect it from noise and the air, if the seat of the
inflammation be internal.

BELLADONNA will be required if the pain penetrates
into the brain, attended with great agitation, vomiting,
coldness of the extremities, and other dangerous
symptoms.

DOSE.—Of a solution of one drop, or six globules, in half a tumbler
of water, give a teaspoonful every three hours, until amelioration or change.
Should there be an aggravation after the first three doses, discontinue
until a natural reaction takes place.

OTALGIA, when there is no inflammatory symptoms, but simply neuralgic pains in the ear. The remedies may be Arnica, Calcarea, China, Mercurius, Nux vomica, &c.

ARNICA is adapted to very sensitive persons, who experience a return of pain from every exposure, with oppression and stitches behind the ears; also tearing, heat, and irritability at any loud noise.

DOSE.—Dissolve one drop, or six globules, in half a tumbler of water, and give a teaspoonful every three hours, until amelioration or change.

CALCAREA CARB. is useful when the pains are confined to one side, deep in the ear, so violent and painful as to drive the patient to distraction; especially when the pain is on the right side, or worse after midnight, or in the forenoon.

DOSE.—One drop, or four globules, in a spoonful of water, every morning and evening, until amelioration, or change.

CHINA is suitable when the patient has more pain in the external ear, with redness, pricking, and tingling inside.

DOSE.—The same as for *Calcarea*.

MERCURIUS VIV. is indicated if the patient perspires without being relieved; tearing pain, extending to the cheeks; burning externally, and feels cold internally.

DOSE.—The same as for *Arnica*.

NUX VOMICA is particularly indicated when violent earache occurs from a fit of passion, or in irritable angry persons.

DOSE.—The same as for *Arnica*.

Other remedies, such as Chamomilla, Dulcamara, Hepar sulph., Phosphoric acid, Pulsatilla, Platinum, and Sulphur, may be resorted to in particular cases.

GENERAL TREATMENT.—Resort to no external appli-

48*

cations. Oil introduced into the ear, may become injurious, heating vapors may weaken the organs of sense of hearing.

Warm water applied on a sponge or soft linen cloth, may sometimes relieve the pain, without doing injury; avoid cramming cotton into the ear.

Running of the Ears.   Otorrhœa.

This complaint results from a variety of causes, and in some instances, proves very obstinate and difficult to cure. It is better not to suppress the discharge, for this may produce serious consequences. The use of the syringe should be discarded, and oil is certainly of little avail, any article that becomes hard, is still worse; but the ear may be cleansed with luke-warm water, a little fine wool may be put into the ear, in winter, to protect it from cold, and during the summer, as a protection from flies, which sometimes deposit their eggs in them; but even this resort should be with great caution, when the discharge smells offensively.

TREATMENT.—Belladonna, Calcarea, Mercurius, Pulsatilla, and Sulphur, are among the principal remedies.

BELLADONNA is one of the remedies for running from the ears, after *scarlet fever*. It may be used in alternation with *Mercurius.* '

DOSE·—Dissolve one drop, or six globules of *Belladonna*, in six teaspoonfuls of water, and give a teaspoonful every six hours, for three days; and then dissolve of *Mercurius*, in the same way, and give a teaspoonful every six hours, for three days, and of *Belladonna* again, &c., but if these remedies prove insufficient, resort to *Hepar sulph.*

MERCURIUS is useful, in running from the ears, either after *scarlet fever* or *small-pox*, when the discharge is bloody, attended with pricking pain, and offensive.

DOSE.—The same as directed for *Belladonna*, but if the patient has taken much Calomel, *Hepar* may be substituted for the *Mercurius*.

CALCAREA is indicated, for purulent and tedious discharge, and one drop, or four globules, may be dissolved in a spoonful of water, and given once every week. *Mercurius* may be administered first, and in six days after *Calcarea*.

SULPHUR is also indicated, in these purulent tedious discharges, to be administered in the same manner as directed for *Calcarea*, one week after *Mercurius* has been given, and continued as long as the case requires, or its usefulness is apparent.

LACHESIS, PULSATILLA, SILICEA, DULCAMARA, and other remedies, may prove useful in chronic otorrhœa, but they should be duly affiliated in accordance with the symptoms.

DOSE.—The same as directed for *Calcarea* and *Sulphur*.

Suppression of the Discharge.

PULSATILLA, MERCURIUS, and BELLADONNA, when the neck becomes hard and swollen, after the suppression of the discharge.

DOSE.—Of either, one drop, or four globules, daily, in the morning.

BELLADONNA, BRYONIA, DULCAMARA, and MERCURIUS, if severe headache occur after the suppression.

DOSE.—The same as for *Pulsatilla, Mercurius,* &c., until the running becomes established.

If the irritation which keeps up the running should not be removed, it is by far the best, that the running should remain; or otherwise, the disease may spend its force upon the brain, and produce violent inflammation and death.

Deafness. Hardness of Hearing. Dysecoia.

This difficulty is usually connected with diseases that must be cured in order for the deafness to cease. It is frequently caused by some obstruction of the ear.

TREATMENT.—The most useful remedies to remove hardness of hearing, are Calcarea, Mercurius, Nitric acid, Phosphoric acid, Phosphorus, Pulsatilla, and Sulphur.

DOSE.—One drop, or six globules, every morning for a week; if this does not produce the effect, proceed with the next remedy.

FOR DEAFNESS ARISING FROM CONGESTION, Belladonna, Hyoscyamus, Phosphorus, Sulphur.

DOSE.—In all respects as directed for *deafness*.

NERVOUS Deafness, may be relieved by Causticum, and Phosphoric acid.

DOSE.—The same as for *deafness*.

RHEUMATIC or CATARRHAL Deafness, may be removed by Arsenicum, Calcarea, Mercurius, Nitric acid, Pulsatilla, Arsenicum, &c.

DOSE.—The same as for *deafness*.

DEAFNESS FROM SUPPRESSED ERUPTIONS, may be relieved by Causticum, Graphites, Sulphur, &c.

DOSE.—One drop, or six globules, may be taken morning and evening for a week; if without the desired result, proceed with the next remedy.

When Deafness occurs from Measles, Carbo veg., and Pulsatilla. When from Scarlet Fever, Belladonna, and Hepar sulph. When from Small-pox, Mercurius viv., and Sulphur. When from the abuse of mercury, Aurum, Nitric acid. When from the Enlargement of the Tonsils, Aurum, Mercurius, Nitric acid. When it is the sequel of Fevers, and other disorders, Phosphorus, Phosphoric acid, Veratrum. When it occurs from suddenly checked discharge from either the nose or ears, Hepar sulph., Lachesis, Pulsatilla, &c.

DOSE.—The same as for *deafness from suppressed discharges*.

Buzzing or Noises in the Ears.

This affection is generally connected with the incipient stages of deafness, and running from the ears, or it may be produced by cold. The remedies are Nux vomica, if from cold; Pulsatilla, when worse in the evening. Mercurius, when attended with perspiration. Sulphur, when the noises become annoying, and difficult of endurance, &c.

DOSE.—The same as directed for *deafness from suppressed discharges.*

6.—Bleeding at the Nose. *Epistaxis.*

This affection often occurs during the course of many diseases, and frequently is a source of benefit to the patient. In a general way, it is better not to interrupt the bleeding, unless too violent and too long.

The efforts usually made, to arrest bleeding at the nose, with cold water, sponge, vinegar, &c., often prove a source of injury instead of relief, and great caution should be exercised in the use of such agents. Extending the arm and hand upwards over the head, will often arrest the bleeding of the nostril on the same side of the arm that is raised, whether right or left.

TREATMENT.—The principal remedies are, Aconite, Arnica, Belladonna, Bryonia, Cina, China, Nux vomica, Pulsatilla, Rhus tox., and Sulphur.

ARNICA is a suitable remedy, when the bleeding of the nose is occasioned by a blow, fall, or any external injury, and also, when the nose feels hot, or itches, and the blood is of a light red color.

DOSE.—One drop, or four globules, in a spoonful of water, may be given and repeated in the course of a day, if necessary.

ACONITE.—When the difficulty occurs in consequence of being overheated, or by reason of determination of blood to the head, or by drinking wine; it is well suited to persons of full or plethoric habit, when affected with fever, flushed face, throbbing of the temporal arteries, &c.

DOSE.—Dissolve one drop, or six globules, in half a tumbler of water, and give a desert-spoonful every three hours, until amelioration or change.

562 DISEASES INVOLVING

BELLADONNA may be indicated as an alternating remedy with either of the two remedies above named, (*Aconite* and *Arnica*,) when the bleeding takes place at night, or comes on again in the morning, or arises either from being overheated or drinking wine.

DOSE.—The same in all respects as for *Aconite*, when used by itself, or every three hours, alternately when used with another remedy, until amelioration or change.

BRYONIA is indicated when the bleeding is prolonged in a warm room, or in warm weather, or from drinking wine; and also when the patient is of an irritable disposition, and the bleeding occurs more frequently at night, awaking the patient out of sleep.

DOSE.—In all respects as for *Aconite*.

CINA is indicated when the bleeding of the nose occurs in children subject to worms.

DOSE.—The same as for *Aconite*.

CHINA is especially indicated for persons of weak, debilitated constitutions, when the bleeding is prolonged, and when there is marked paleness of the face, coldness of the extremities, fainting, &c.

DOSE.—The same as for *Aconite*.

NUX VOMICA is indicated for bleeding that usually returns in the morning, and particularly when the difficulty is brought on by drinking wine, or being overheated, or in habitual inebriation.

DOSE.—The same in all respects as directed for *Aconite*.

PULSATILLA is best suited for females of mild, quiet disposition, or such as have scanty menstrual discharge; also for that bleeding of the nose which takes place during a cold, or stoppage of the nostrils.

DOSE.—The same as for *Aconite*.

RHUS TOX. is indicated when the difficulty is brought on by great exertion, such as by lifting or straining, and is worse every time the patient stoops.

DOSE.—The same as directed for *Aconite.*

SULPHUR, taken once or twice a week, will be found of great service in correcting that condition of the system which favors frequent recurrence of the difficulty.

DOSE.—One drop, or six globules, in a tablespsoonful of water.

DIET AND REGIMEN.—The diet in all cases should be simple, and the patient should be kept cool and quiet.

Swelling of the Nose

This affection springs from various causes, sometimes from contusions, at others from certain diseased conditions of the body.

TREATMENT.—The remedies that in general are found to be the most useful, are Arnica, Belladonna, Bryonia, Hepar sulph., Mercurius viv., Sulphur, &c.

ARNICA is indicated when the nose is swelled in consequence of having received a blow, or when the swelling occurs without any apparent cause, attended with itching pain in the upper part of the bone of the nose, as from a blow.

DOSE.—Dissolve one drop, or six globules, in three tablespoonfuls of water, and give a teaspoonful every two hours, until amelioration or change.

BELLADONNA is indicated when the swelling arises from catarrh. *Hepar sulphur* when the nostril is red, swollen and sore. *Mercurius* when there is watery running from the nose, making it sore, red, shining and swollen. *Bryonia* in painful tedious swelling. *Sulphur* in swelling with black spots on the nose. *Phos. acid* in chronic swelling, with red spots on the nose. *Causticum* for warts on the nose. *Rhus tox.* when the point of the nose is red. *Arsenicum* when it presents a coppery red ness, accompanied with a craving for spirituous liquors.

DOSE.—For each remedy the same as directed for *Arnica*, with the exception of *Sulphur*, *Causticum* and *Arsenicum*, which should be administered in the same dose twice a day, until better or change.

HEPAR SULPHUR is useful when the nose has been made sore by *calomel;* a dose three times a day.

Against swelling of the interior of the nose, *Sepia, Aurum, Silicea, Hepar sulph., Causticum* and *Nitric acid,* are the remedies.

DOSE.—Of the selected remedy, one drop, or six globules, in a spoonful of water, night and morning; if after three days no improvement takes place, proceed with the next remedy.

CARIES.—When the bones of the nose appear to be affected, (caries) whether from scrofula or the abuse of mercury, *Aurum* is the remedy; when from other causes, *Mercurius viv., Hepar sulph., Lachesis, &c.*

DOSE.—One drop, or six globules, of the selected remedy, in a spoonful of water, morning and evening.

OZÆNA.—This disorder consists of an ulcer in the nose, from which a fetid purulent matter is discharged.

SYMPTOMS.—Slight inflammation and swelling of the sides of the nose, attended with sneezing, flow of mucus obstructing the nostril, sometimes producing slight hemorrhage, or sometimes as the inflammation and ulceration extends, the mucus assumes the character of pus.

TREATMENT.—Pulsatilla, Sulphur, Calcarea, Lycopodium and Natrum muriaticum, are the chief remedies for the first stage.

DOSE.—One drop, or six globules, may be given every morning, of the remedy selected; if not relieved in four days, proceed with the next remedy.

In the second stage, when there is discharge of pus, Aurum and Mercurius are the remedies. The former if the disease arises from the abuse of mercury, and the latter when it arises from other causes, such as syphilis or scrofula.

DOSE.—One drop, or six globules, in a spoonful of water, every morning and evening, until amelioration, or change. *Conium* or *Thuja* may be found requisite, in the same dose, to complete a cure.

CANCER OF THE NOSE.—This disease has been combatted by the use of Arsenicum, Aurum, Carbo veg., Sepia, Silicea, and Sulphur.

DOSE.—The same as directed for *Ozæna*, or ulceration in the nose.

POLYPUS OF THE NOSE is a pear-shaped tumor springing from the lining membrane of the nose, having only a small attachment at its root, and expanded below. Sometimes it is hard and fleshy, and at other times, soft and tender. The common kinds resemble an oyster.

TREATMENT. — The remedies that have proved the most successful, are Calcarea, Sanguinaria, Sepia, and Staphysagria.

DOSE.—The same as directed for *Ozæna* or *Cancer*,

Baldness or Loss of Hair.

The most useful treatment for this misfortune, in numerous instances, is the judicious use of cold water and the brush; but in some cases remedies are useful, as for instance,

1. When the hair falls out from debilitating causes, China and Ferrum.

2. If the hair falls out in consequence of perspiration, Mercurius.

3. If after the use of quinine, Belladonna.

4. If after the abuse of mercury, Carbo vegetabilis.

5. If after much grief or trouble, Phosphoric acid and Staphysagria.

6. If after inflammatory diseases and nervous fevers, Calcarea, Hepar sulph., Silicea, &c.

49

7. For recent baldness, and that which appears in early life, Tincture of Cantharis, in the proportion of one drop, to two ounces of lard, mixed up together faithfully, and applied externally, while the same remedy may be administered internally.

DOSE.—Of the selected remedy, in either case, dissolve one drop, or six globules, in half a tumbler of water, and give a teaspoonful every six hours, until a change.

Dandruff.

This squamous difficulty may often be overcome by the use of Lycopodium, especially when there is headache, or when it is attended with itching.

DOSE.—One drop, or six globules, in the morning.

7.—Offensive Breath.

This unpleasant affection is sometimes dependent upon other derangements of the system, which must be cured in order to relieve it. But at other times it results from a want of cleanliness, in allowing tartar to accumulate on the teeth, or from sore mouth, or leaving particles of food; simply washing the mouth, two or three times a day.

In other cases when there is no perceptible cause, Chamomilla, Nux vomica, Pulsatilla, or Sulphur may be employed.

DOSE.—Of the selected remedy. One drop, or six globules, dissolved in a spoonful of water, may be given every morning, until the difficutly is removed.

AURUM, PULSATILLA and SULPHUR are the remedies suited to remove the difficulty in young girls at the age of puberty.

DOSE.—One drop, or four globules, every morning.

When the difficulty appears to be the result of

previous salivation, with mercury or calomel, Carbo veg., Hepar sulph., Nitric acid, &c.

DOSE.—One drop, or six globules, of the selected remedy, in a spoonful of water, every morning. If no relief takes place for a week, proceed with the the next remedy.

8.—Cramps in the Legs.

VERATRUM is recommended to remove the tendency to the difficulty, and *Colocynth.* and *Sulphur*, if necessary to effect a cure.

RHUS TOX. when the difficulty occurs when sitting.

SEPIA, NITRIC ACID, and LYCOPODIUM when the difficulty is experienced in walking.

NUX VOMICA and RHUS TOX. when the attacks occur at night.

CALCAREA, when it occurs on stretching out the limb.

DOSE.—Of the selected remedy. One drop, or six globules, in a spoonful of water, night and morning, for a week. If without salutary effect, select another remedy.

9.—Goitre. (*Bronchocele. · Derbyshire neck.*)

The main feature of this difficulty consists in disfigurement of the neck, arising from the swelling of the thyroid gland; as this gland enlarges, considerable obstruction to free inspiration arises from the pressure which it exerts against the windpipe. Women especially of mountainous districts, are the most subject to the affection; they are more prone to it than men, particularly those women who have suffered from severe labors. Something inherent in the constitution, without doubt, is a frequent source of the difficulty.

TREATMENT.—In recent cases, Iodine and Spongia. In long standing cases, Calcarea, Carbo veg., and Sepia.

DOSE.—One drop, or six globules, every morning, for a week, then discontinue for a week, and proceed again in the same manner.

SEPIA AND THUJA are useful when the superficial veins of the swelling are in a varicose and painful state.

DOSE.—One drop, or six globules, every morning and evening.

BELLADONNA is indicated when the difficulty is acute, and arises from a cold. *Aconite*, if the accompanying fever runs high, and the skin over the region of the swelling is red.

DOSE.—Dissolve one drop, or six globules, in half a tumbler of water, and give a tablespoonful three times a day.

MERCURIUS is indicated when there is no discoloration of the skin, and also when symptoms of suppuration have set in.

DOSE.—Dissolve one drop, or six globules, in four tablespoonfuls of water, and give a teaspoonful every four hours, until the abscess bursts. If *Mercurius* does not produce the desired result so speedily, resort to *Silicea*, and give one drop, or four globules, morning and evening.

Sweating Feet.

The fact that some individuals are troubled with a disagreeable clammy sweating of the feet, to such an extent as to require a change of stockings twice or three times a day, would seem to argue that some diseased condition of the system was the source. The difficulty not only annoys the patient, but others, from the fact that the utmost attention to cleanliness is insufficient to remedy the complaint.

TREATMENT. — Silicea and Rhus tox. are foremost among the homœopathic remedies. The latter may be given one drop, or six globules, every morning, for a week, and if improvement sets in then or soon after, a few days may elapse, and then the same remedy may be given every other day for a week, but should no amelioration result, resort to the other remedy. The use of these two remedies alternately, three days apart, may also prove useful, not only in curing the difficulty, but in obviating the ill effects of its sudden suppression.

10.—Sleeplessness. (*Vigilance. Agrypnia.*)

In the article on Sleep, in Chapter I., may be found some practical remarks, useful to consider, with reference to normal amount of sleep required to promote health; whenever anything interrupts the natural state of health, or interferes with what the economy requires, either too much or too little sleep may be the consequence. It will be seen, therefore, that sleeplessness is but symptomatic of some other disturbance, and can only be remedied by the removal of the diseased condition, as for instance,

NUX VOMICA is indicated when sleeplessness has been produced by intense mental application, continued up to the period of retiring to rest; or by sedentary habits, or the habitual use of coffee and other stimulants. .

DOSE.—One drop, or six globules, night and morning, and a discontinuance of the practices that produced the difficulty.

PULSATILLA is indicated for sleeplessness produced by overloading the stomach.

DOSE.—The same as for *Nux vomica*, and a discontinuance of the habit that produced the disturbance.

COFFEA is a useful remedy when the difficulty originates from excessive joy. *Ignatia*, when the affection arises from grief, vexation, &c. *Opium*, when it arises from fear or fright. *Belladonna*, when it arises from the same or similar difficulties. *Aconite*, when anxiety or agitating events disturb sleep or produce wakefulness. *Hyoscyamus*, when it arises from nervous excitement in sensitive or irritable subjects.

DOSE.—One drop, or six globules of the selected remedy, in a spoonful of water, every evening at bed-time, until the difficulty is overcome.

PHOSPHORIC ACID and SEPIA are useful remedies when sleeplessness occurs in hysterical or hypochondriacal persons.

DOSE.—The same as for *Coffea* or *Ignatia.* .

49*

Nux vomica, Sulphur and Lycopodium are indicated when sleeplessness is occasioned by cold feet. It is necessary at the same time to resort to friction for the purpose of promoting active circulation, as well as frequent bathing the feet in cold water.

DOSE.—Of either remedy, one drop, or six globules, in a spoonful of water, at bed-time, until amelioration or change. If the one selected produce no improvement, proceed with the next remedy.

Lachesis, Stannum, Pulsatilla and Secale are indicated when the sleep is prevented by burning heat, in the feet, and *Nitric acid*, *Silicea* or *Calcarea*, when the same occurs from a harsh, dry condition of the skin.

DOSE.—One drop, or six globules of the selected remedy, in a spoonful of water, night and morning, until amelioration or change, *Graphites* and *Sepia* are sometimes useful, used in the same way.

Nightmare. Incubus.

This disagreeable affection is dependent upon certain diseased conditions of the system, which can be remedied by homœopathic remedies.

Aconite is useful, when there is considerable fever, quickness of the pulse; thirst; palpitation of the heart; oppression of the chest; anxiety and agitation.

DOSE.—One drop or six globules, dissolved in two spoonfuls of water; one spoonful may be given to remedy the immediate symptoms, but when indicated by the general condition of the patient, the same dose may be given night and morning, until amelioration or change.

Nux vomica, is the remedy, when night-mare results from sedentary habits, or indulgence in wine or other stimulants.

DOSE.—Six globules, or one drop, may be dissolved in three teaspoonfuls of water, and a teaspoonful given every night at bedtime, for a week, or until decided amelioration or change.

Pulsatilla, when the difficulty arises from derangement of the digestive functions, in consequence of gross living, late suppers, &c.

DOSE.—In all respects as directed for *Nux vomica.*

OPIUM may be employed in all severe cases, when there is labored or snoring respiration, the eyes only half closed, the mouth open, the countenance expressive of great anguish, and moist with cold perspiration, and twitching of the muscles.

DOSE.—Dissolve one drop, or six globules, in three teaspoonfuls of water, and give a teaspoonful night and morning, for a week ; then discontinue for a week, and recur again to the remedy if necessary, until amelioration or change.

SULPHUR, or SILICEA, may be employed, when any of the foregoing remedies do not suffice to effect a cure.

DOSE.—One drop, or four globules, may be given every night at bedtime, and the exciting cause of the attacks must be removed.

DIET AND REGIMEN.—The diet should be simple, when under treatment, and there should be daily exercise in the open air. A shower-bath may sometimes be resorted to, or sponging with cold water every evening.

11.—Rupture. (*Hernia.*)

By Hernia, is meant the protrusion of any of the abdominal viscera from the cavity of the abdomen. It is a common affection, and consists of several varieties, according to situation.

1. *Inguinal Hernia*, which takes place near the groin.

2. *Umbilical Hernia*, which has its position near the navel.

3. *Scrotal Hernia*, which makes its appearance near the scrotum.

CAUSES.—It may be produced by any severe exercise, by straining to lift heavy weights, riding on horseback, vomiting, parturition, jumping, &c.

TREATMENT.—In recent cases, the treatment may consist entirely of internal remedies, and they will be found sufficient to effect a cure; but in other cases, well-adapted trusses may be requisite.

Strangulated Hernia.

This difficulty is brought about, by not wearing a suit-able truss, and by too much exertion; the protrusion becomes incarcerated or strangulated, and requires to be reduced, and it is of importance to know how it should be accomplished.

1st. The patient should lie on his back, with a pillow under his hips, so that the ruptured part should be higher than the rest of the abdomen; he should then incline a little to the ruptured side, so that the abdominal muscles may be relaxed as much as possible, and then another person, or the patient himself, can generally reduce the hernia.

2d. The reduction is accomplished, by gentle pressure upon the protrusion with one hand, while with the fingers of the other hand, the tumor is grasped so as to direct it backwards, through the aperture from whence it protrudes. The efforts should be continued gently and patiently, a sufficient length of time to gradually effect the reduction. When the tumor is so sensitive as to forbid pressure without occasioning severe pain, appro-priate remedies must first be used.

ACONITE and NUX VOMICA, may be used alternately, every six hours, for one or two days, in *doses* of one drop, or four globules, after which it frequently returns itself; or if any aid is required, a rag dipped in warm water, gently placed upon the tumor, may be all that will be required to effect the reduction.

ACONITE may be given, when there is violent burning in the abdomen, as from hot coals; the least touch, giving pain and sickness at the stomach, bitter or bilious vomitings, nervousness, and cold perspiration.

DOSE.—Dissolve one drop, or six globules, in half a tumbler of water, and give a spoonful, and repeat every time the pain occurs.

VERATRUM is useful after *Aconite*, when the latter remedy produces only temporary relief, without any other good effect.

DOSE.—The same as for *Aconite*, and give a teaspoonful every two hours, for six or eight hours. If after this, efforts should fail to reduce the hernia, *Sulphur* may be employed ; give one dose and wait awhile ; if the patient falls asleep, do not disturb him.

NUX VOMICA is indicated, when the pain is less violent, and the vomiting not so much, but the breathing difficult, occasioned by taking cold or being overheated, or from vexation or improper diet.

DOSE.—In all respects as for *Veratrum*.

OPIUM is indicated, when the patient becomes red in the face, and the abdomen becomes distended, or when there is offensive eructations and vomiting.

DOSE.—Dissolve one drop, or six globules, in half a tumbler of water, and give a teaspoonful every fifteen minutes, until there is a change. If the vomiting is accompanied by cold sweat, or the extremities become cold, give *Veratrum* in the same manner, and afterwards *Belladonna*, if the *Veratrum* after one or two doses produces no relief. But if the abdomen becomes sensitive to the touch, give *Aconite* and *Sulphur*, as before directed.

ARSENICUM and LACHESIS are indicated when the symptoms are very alarming.

DOSE.—Give one drop, or six globules of *Lachesis*, in a spoonful of water, and follow in two hours with *Arsenicum*, if there be no relief, and repeat this latter remedy every four hours, until amelioration or change.

In all cases of Strangulated Hernia, the services of a well-educated and experienced physician should be had if possible. But in nearly all cases of recent standing, when there is no strangulation, *Aconite* and *Sulphur* will prove effectual, administered as above.

DIET.—In obstinate and painful forms of hernia, the diet should be simple and easy of digestion.

12.—Fainting. (*Syncope. Swooning.*)

Fainting may be caused by sudden transitions from cold to heat; great fatigue; intense pain; loss of blood; protracted abstinence from food; grief, and other severe emotions of the mind.

Whenever the difficulty occurs, the patient should be placed in a situation to be favored with a current of pure fresh air, and freed from tight clothing about the neck, chest and abdomen, and placed on his back in a horizontal position. Cold water may also be sprinkled in the face and neck, if necessary, to aid in effecting restoration; sometimes spirits of camphor may be applied to the nose, should the before-mentioned remedies fail to produce the desired benefit.

TREATMENT.—The following group of remedies will be found useful in the treament of this difficulty; Aconite, Coffea, Hepar sulph., Lachesis, Nux vomica and Veratrum.

ACONITE is indicated when there is rush of blood to the head, accompanying palpitation of the heart; or when the attack comes on at the time of assuming the erect posture, attended with shivering and flushing of the face, followed by death-like paleness.

DOSE.—Dissolve one drop, or six globules, in half a tumbler of water, and give a teaspoonful when there appears the first indication of the attack, and repeat if necessary in one hour, and again in four or six hours. If the attacks occur frequently after the first, have recourse to the succeeding remedies.

COFFEA, after *Aconite*, in highly excitable subjects, and particularly when the fainting has arisen from fright.

DOSE.—As directed for *Aconite*.

HEPAR SULPH. is indicated when fainting generally comes on towards evening.

DOSE.—One drop, or six globules, in a spoonful of water, every morning, (fasting,) for a week. Then after a few days' suspension, if the difficulty is not overcome, recur to the remedy again, and so on until amelioration or change.

LACHESIS is of service when asthmatic symptoms either precede or accompany the fainting, and also vertigo, paleness of thé face, bleeding at the nose, and cold perspiration.

DOSE.—The same as for *Hepar sulph.*

NUX VOMICA is serviceable when the fainting occurs after a meal, or after taking exercise, or there is nausea, with paleness of the face, and when the patient immediately after recovery complains of pain in the stomach, sparks before the eyes, dimness of the sight, anxiety and trembling, or oppression at the chest.

DOSE.—Dissolve one drop, or six globules, in half a tumbler of water, and give a teaspoonful night and morning for a week, or until amelioration. Then discontinue for a week, and proceed again if necessary, until amelioration or change.

VERATRUM may be employed when the fainting is excited by fatigue, or when they are preceded by a feeling of extreme anguish, or dejection and despair, attended with convulsive closing of the mouth, or moving of the eyes and lids.

DOSE.—The same as directed for *Nux vomica.*

Some additional remedies have also been found useful after any of the above remedies, when little benefit has been received. *Phosphoric acid* is useful after *Nux vomica; Moschus* for fainting fits occurring in the open air, attended with spasms in the chest, or followed by headache.

DOSE.—In all respects as directed for *Lachesis.*

13.—Pains in the Loins. (*Notalgia.*)

This affection is more commonly symptomatic, being produced by other difficulties, such as piles, whites, &c., the removal of which, depends very much upon the the successful treatment of the difficulties which give rise to it. But when it occurs under other circumstances, it must be treated with reference to the cause and the symptoms.

TREATMENT.—The remedies employed, are for the most part Calcarea, Nux vomica, Rhus tox., and Sulphur.

NUX VOMICA is indicated when the difficulty has been produced by habitual indulgence in spirituous liquors, in conjunction with late hours, and sedentary habits.

DOSE.—Dissolve one drop, or six globules, in four spoonfuls of water, and give a spoonful every twelve hours, for two days, and then wait a few days, and proceed again if necessary, and so on until relieved, or change.

RHUS TOX. may be employed when the difficulty has been caused by a strain, from heavy lifting, or sudden turning of the body, or any other violent exercise.

DOSE.—Same in all respects as for *Nux vomica.*

SULPHUR and CALCAREA are both useful remedies, and may be employed after *Nux vomica* or *Rhus tox.,* when the pain is continued after the use of these latter remedies.

DOSE.—The same in all respects as for *Nux vomica.*

14.—Dropsy. (*Hydrops.*)

Dropsy is a preternatural swelling of the whole body, or parts of it, occasioned by a collection of watery fluid. It is distinguished by different names, according to the part affected, viz:

1. Anasarca, or dropsy of the cellular membrane.
2. Ascites, dropsy of the abdomen.
3. Hydrothorax, dropsy of the chest.
4. Hydrocephalus, dropsy of the brain.
5. Hydrocele, dropsy of the testicle.
6. Hydrometra, dropsy of the womb.

Anasarca.

This form of dropsy consists in an unnatural accumu. lation of water under the skin, in the cellular membrane. Sometimes the skin is rendered inflamed and swollen by the accumulation of the fluid, and not unfrequently appears of an erysipelatous character. In most cases this affection is but the consequence of some other disease, often met with in combination with general dropsy. It sometimes, however, constitutes the primary disease, arising from an excitable condition of the part involved. The acute form of the disease for the most part affects those who are in the prime of life.

It makes its appearance suddenly, from exposure to cold, when the body is heated; drinking cold water when in the same condition.

SYMPTOMS. — Oppression at the chest, attended occasionally with cough and pain, are among the first indications of the system being invaded by the disease, especially on drawing a full breath; in the course of a few hours the patient begins to swell, first in the face, and then from the face it spreads downwards, to the trunk and lower limbs; the urine is scanty, and high-colored; in some cases the pulse remains normal, at others it becomes accelerated, and is attended with heat and dryness of the skin, and then in some cases it is weak and feeble. If the disease is not checked the swelling will go on, until the functional processes are all performed with great difficulty, especially that of respiration, so that the patient cannot lie down. The *sthenic* or primary form of the disease may terminate fatally in a few days.

That form of the disease which is dependent upon an exhaustion of strength, comes on slowly; it afflicts those

obliged to dwell in damp or dark apartments, not sufficiently ventilated, and those fed upon an unwholesome
diet. It may also be superinduced by sedentary habits,
depressing emotions, excessive depletion, diarrhœa, or
dysentery; it is generally attended with thirst and scanty
secretion of urine; the feet are observed to swell first,
and the swelling gradually ascends higher, until it pervades the entire body; the pulse varies; sometimes there
is fever and dry skin; sometimes the bowels are costive,
at other times loose.

This form of dropsy sometimes is superinduced after
scarlatina and other acute exanthemata in children. It is
apparently of an inflammatory character, connected with
imperfect cutaneous transpiration, or obstructed secretions and execretions; exposure to wet or cold favors its
occurrence.

TREATMENT.—Arsenicum, Bryonia, China, Helleborus;
Mercurius and Phosphorus, are among the principal remedies employed.

HELLEBORUS is particularly called for where there are
febrile symptoms, with constriction in the chest, and
lancinating pains in the extremities, and almost entire
suppression of the urine; or when there is a sort of
half sleep with great debility and looseness of the bowels;
shivering, rapid respiration, and much thirst. *Arsenicum*
is often advantageously employed after *Helleborus*.

DOSE.—One drop, or ten globules, in a half-tumbler of water; give a
teaspoonful every four hours, until four doses have been given, and then
every six hours, until amelioration or change.

BRYONIA is of great service when the disease arises
from an exhausted condition of the system, if there is
oppression of the chest, with acute pricking pain during
a full inspiration, or when the swelling increases by day

and diminishes by night, attended with constipation, *China* is a good remedy to follow up the treatment with, and so is *Lycopodium* when there is obstinate constipation. .

DOSE.—The same in all respects as for *Helleborus*.

PHOSPHORUS is indicated when Anasarca is attended with inflammation of the lungs.

DOSE—Of a solution of one drop, or ten globules, in four tablespoon-fuls of water; give a teaspoonful every two hours, until three doses have been given, and afterwards every six hours, until decided amelioration or change.

MERCURIUS VIV. is useful either in acute or chronic Anasarca, accompanied with oppression at the chest; constant, short, dry cough, with disordered liver; general heat; thirst; great weakness.

DOSE.—Dissolve one drop, or ten globules, in half a tumbler of water, and give a teaspoonful every half hour, when the symptoms are acute, until there is a decided amelioration or change; and afterwards, the intervals may be extended to two or three hours; and in chronic cases, give the medicine only twice in a day, morning and evening, and continue for a week, and then omit a week and commence again, and so on until the patient is relieved or another remedy is called for.

ARSENICUM is indicated when there is much debility, or when disorder occurs in combination with gastritis, or affections of the heart, or other viscera; constriction of the chest, and oppression, and a sense of suffocation on lying down, particularly upon the back; dry, hard skin; extremely pale; tongue red and parched; intense thirst; rending pains in the trunk and limbs; extreme weakness and prostration; feeble and irregular pulse; coldness of the extremities. This remedy may be alternated with *Helleborus*.

DOSE.—The same as directed for *Mercurius viv.*

CHINA is indicated when the difficulty is combined with affections of the liver and spleen, or when occasioned by loss of blood, diarrhœa or dysentery. Many of the other remedies may be employed after the use of *China*, if indicated.

DOSE.—The same as for *Mercurius viv*.

Dropsy of the Abdomen.   Ascites.

This form of dropsy may be complicated with ana-sarca and other local dropsical complaints.   It is a watery effusion in the cavity of the *peritoneum*, which causes much swelling of the abdomen.   In most cases there is swelling of the lower extremities, or other parts of the body.   Sometimes the disease comes on so gradu-ally as to lead to the belief that it is mere corpulency, and at others it makes its appearance so suddenly as to mark it at once as a difficulty of this kind.

The premonitory symptoms often make their appear-ance in the form of fever, restless nights, thirst, disor-dered digestion, foul tongue, nausea or vomiting, cos-tiveness, scanty flow of urine, high-colored; pain in the small of the back and region of the liver.

The collection of the water is often sufficient to render the abdomen tense, and dull sound on percussion; and when the affection is considerable, the swelling gravi-tates to the side towards which the patient inclines; and a sense of fluctuation may be felt by placing the hand on one side of the abdomen and striking the oppo-site side sharply with the other.

When ascites succeeds any worn-out condition of the system, exhausted from chronic disease, whether in adults or children, the termination will very likely be unfavorable.   When the disorder sets in as a consequence of Scarlet Fever, &c., although a serious malady, it may not necessarily be considered in the light of a fatal dis-order.

TREATMENT.—Helleborus, Arsenicum and China, are the principal remedies.

HELLEBORUS is equally useful in the treatment of this disease and Anasarca, particularly when it is brought on by excitability.

DOSE.—The same as for the same remedy under *Anasarca.*

ARSENICUM is mainly useful in the treatment of this affection, when there is great debility and extreme prostration, and has arisen from the depressing effects of other diseases. In acute cases the remedy is speedily efficacious, in the chronic form it is valuable, and also in cases complicated with organic derangement of some important viscus.

DOSE.—Dissolve one drop, or ten globules, in half a tumbler of water, and give a teaspoonful every half hour for the acute symptoms, until some mitigation becomes apparent, and then every two hours; four hours, and even six or twelve hours may intervene between the doses, according to the urgency of the case. In chronic cases, the same dose may be given every night and morning for a week, and then omit for a week, and commence again if necessary, and so on, until decided amelioration or change.

CHINA is indicated when the Ascites has resulted from debilitating losses, and also in the chronic form when it arises from organic disease of the liver or spleen. It is further indicated by short, dry cough, either with or without expectoration; extreme paleness of the skin; general chilliness; small, feeble, slow pulse; frequent inclinations to urinate, followed by scanty discharge. This remedy may be associated with *Arsenicum* and *Ferrum.*

DOSE.—Dissolve one drop, or ten globules, in half a tumbler of water, and give a teaspoonful every four hours, until a decided change, or otherwise resort to the associate remedies.

ZINCUM METALICUM is indicated in dropsical affections, especially when pain and disagreeable sensations are experienced in the region of the kidneys.

DOSE.—The same as for *China.*

50*

Dropsy of the Chest. (Hydrothorax.)

This form of dropsy may exist either in complication with Ascites or Anasarca, or without it. One or both sides of the chest may suffer from a collection of the fluid. Sometimes the exudation is lodged in the cellular texture of the lungs, as well as in the sacs of the pleura.

SYMPTOMS.—The commencement of the disease may be indicated by a sense of uneasiness at the lower portion of the breast bone, attended with some difficulty of breathing, which is greatly increased by exertion or by lying down; a troublesome dry cough at first, but afterwards accompanied with expectoration of thin mucus; swelling of the feet towards evening. Aside from these symptoms, we meet those common in all forms of dropsy, such as pale skin, thirst, scanty urine, &c. The patient may be able to detect the disease himself by the fluctuation of the fluid, on particular movements of the body.

The physician may detect the presense of the fluid by percussion or auscultation. The former yields a dull sound, and by the application of the ear to the chest the respiratory murmur will not appear distinct, if at all. Sometimes one side, and at other times, both sides of the chest appear swollen, and the intermediate spaces between the ribs become more apparent.

As the disease advances, the breathing becomes more difficult, particularly at night, when it often excites a dread of suffocation; the extremeties become more swollen, and the patient has fits of anxiety and palpitation of the heart; sometimes there is numbness, in one or both arms, and inability to lie down. The final termination of the disease, is in the suffocation of the patient, and he dies from asphyxia, unless arrested in its progress before it has advanced so far that remedies can exert no control.

Inflammation of any of the serous membranes in the cavity of the chest, may give rise to the difficulty, as well as organic lesions of the heart and lungs, and their chief vessels, and also disease of some of the viscera of the abdomen, as induration of the liver, &c.

TREATMENT.—The group of remedies found the most useful are, Apis Mellifica, Arsenicum, Colchicum, Dulcamara.

APIS MELLIFICA, is indicated in Hydrothorax, when there is sensation of heat •throughout the chest, accompanied by a kind of suffocating feeling impeding the respiration, and when there is a feeble intermittent pulse, and inability to lie down.

DOSE.—Dissolve one drop, or six globules, in half a tumbler of water, and give a teaspoonful every three hours, until amelioration or change.

ARSENICUM is particularly indicated, when there is distressingly impeded respiration after going up stairs, constant thirst, and inclined to drink but little at a time, great difficulty of breathing on getting into bed, however gently the act may be performed, attended with palpitation of the heart, and excessive anguish and apprehension; impeded respiration from lying down, or from turning in bed during the night; coldness and swelling of the feet; pale and greenish hue of the skin; pains in the back and loins.

DOSE.—In all respects as directed for *Arsenicum*, in *Ascites*. It may be associated with *Carbo veg.*, *China*, *Ferrum*, used in a similar manner.

COLCHICUM, SPIGELIA, and DULCAMARA, will each exert a palliative effect, when the disease is complicated with organic lesions of the heart and great vessels. *Aconite* may be employed, when there is febrile symptoms. *Dulcamara,* when the suffering is worse in cold, damp, and foggy weather.

DOSE.—Of either, the same as directed for *Apis mellifica.*

Dropsy of the Brain.—Hydrocephalus.

This disease, commonly reckoned among the diseases of infancy, and often termed, *Water in the Head,* or *Dropsy in the Head,* is not exclusively confined to children in the early period of life; we may therefore consider the disease here.

SYMPTOMS.—Headache, particularly in the front part of the head; nausea; vomiting; dilatation of the pupils; stupor; very slow pulse; and convulsions.

CAUSES.—Inflammation of the meninges of the brain. It is liable to occur in scrofulous children of large heads, in whom the fontanels remain for a long time unclosed. The disease comes on sometimes so insidiously, as to betray but very few, if any symptoms. Teething, in young children, may be the exciting cause, or some derangement of the stomach. In other cases, the symptoms are apparent, as follows: hot skin, quick pulse, chiefly at night, but often variable; the child becomes peevish, when raised from a horizontal position, and sometimes, is seized with fits of screaming, grinding the teeth, redness of the face and eyes, *strabismus,* or squinting, convulsions, and stupor.

Dropsy of the brain exhibits nearly the same symptoms as are produced by worms, or extreme exhaustion, and may be confounded with these affections. But the history of the case, and close scrutiny, may be able to determine the distinction.

Acute Dropsy of the Brain.

The first indication of acute dropsy of the brain, of the low or insidious form, is great languor and tendency to fatigue from the slightest exertion; the child totters in its walk, or is averse to movement altogether; very fretful; does not like to be moved; complains of pain in the back of the head and neck, in the limbs and stomach, which is irritable; vomiting being induced whenever the patient sits upright, or is placed in an erect posture. The head is hot; the eye looks inflamed, or the pupil is contracted, and the countenance wears a bold expression; obstinate constipation of the bowels; scanty urine, &c.

As the disease progresses, the child loses all sense of pain; lies quiet, unless disturbed; drowsiness, or stupor gradually comes on, the head sinks upon the pillow, the eyes half closed, the pupils dilated or immovable; or attended with impaired or double vision, or squinting; a partial, or else a complete cessation of sickness; sometimes combined with a slight return of appetite, takes place at this stage; but emaciation progresses rapidly. The child moans and sighs, and frequently lifts its hands to its head; with a tremulous motion.

Following these symptoms, convulsions of greater or less intensity becomes apparent; constant moaning and raving, and complete loss of consciousness; the eyes are dim, glazed, and turn upwards; uniform quick pulse throughout the entire disease; or having become slow and feeble at the close of the first stage; it may be aroused or accelerated for a short period, and then decline; the upper and lower extremities become relaxed; the abdomen drawn up, and the breathing very irregular; and the scene may terminate in a severe convulsion.

The disease of the *acute* and *inflammatory* form sets in very suddenly, with fever and violent convulsions, causing the death of the child in three or four days. In other cases the child is seized with severe headache; the face is red; the head is hot, and full; throbbing in the temples; and the child starts at the slightest noise; the eye is more brilliant than usual, and sensitive to light; the pulse is full and quick, at first, and the breathing hurried and difficult; the stomach is exceedingly irritable; the tongue white and furred, and often enlarged; and severe constipation or unnatural discharges of green color from the bowels; scanty urine, or altogether suppressed; an expression of terror and pain; the hand frequently raised to the head; extremely frightful, particularly when taken up from the bed, and occasionally wild, piercing, and frantic screams; as the disease advances, the pulse becomes slow, feeble, and irregular, easily accelerated, however, by any movement. The sequel and termination of the inflammatory form does not differ from the insidious and low form.

Chronic Dropsy of the Brain.

This form of the disease generally sets in insidiously, without any previous acute stage, although in some instancss it is the sequel of the acute form. The head gradually enlarges, while the face retains its natural size, and sometimes in very young children the bones of the head separate to a considerable extent, and a sense of fluctuation can be detected on pressure.

Languor, lassitude, and emaciation are the first general symptoms observed, and frequently one or more of the senses are impaired, or entirely destroyed as the disease advances. In some cases the intellect is preserved for a considerable time. Sometimes the head acquires an enormous size, so that it cannot be kept erect on the account of the feeble frame that supports it. Sometimes general convulsions occur, causing a permanent rigidity of the limbs, at other times the convulsions are partial, affecting only certain sets of muscles, as of the face, or one of the limbs. When there is an attempt to keep the head erect, it is attended with giddiness, and sometimes heat and pain in the head; · vomiting and fever during the night, and moving of the head from side to side, or burying the head in the pillow; working of the tongue and lips, or lower jaw; and frequently squinting, or cross-eyed.

It has been remarked that the more acute the inflammation, the greater is the prospect of cure, in general cases of dropsy of the brain.

When a copious perspiration breaks out, and the accelerated condition of the pulse passes away, together with the oppression of breathing, and the urine flows more freely, it is regarded a good indication.

When, on the other hand, the disease comes on gradually and insidiously in the wake of some other malady, and especially in children of scrofulous habits, the prospect of recovery is very obscure, though in some instances cures may be accomplished.

Continued slowness, and weakness of the pulse, or its sudden fall, attended with dilated and fixed pupils, and irregular and laborious respiration, are unfavorable indications.

When the chronic form follows the acute, or when, during its progress there is delirium, convulsions, and stupor, it generally proves fatal. But when the chronic form becomes regularly confirmed, the child may, in some instances, live on for years, and come to its death from some other disease.

The fatal termination is generally preceded by drowsiness, convulsions, and relaxation of the limbs. But the immediate cause may be found in some other disease, such as inflammatory affections of the chest, pulmonary consumption, or ulceration of the bowels.

Water on the brain occurs very frequently during the course of other diseases, such as Scarlet fever, Measles, Summer complaint, difficult Dentition, Hooping cough, &c., being insidiously transferred to the brain. It is, therefore, particularly incumbent to guard against the invasion of the brain, by any of these diseases. The premonitory symptoms, however, of the disease taking this course, are often absent, and stupor, convulsions, or paralysis may be the first indications of the brain or its membranes becoming thus secondarily affected.

TREATMENT.—Remedies should be employed in the earliest period of the disease to have a salutary effect. Those found the most useful, are Aconite, Belladonna, Bryonia, Hoyoscyamus, Helleborus, Mercurius vivus, Opium, Stramonium, Sulphur and Zincum metallicum.

ACONITE is indicated at the commencement, when the skin is hot and dry, the pulse quick, and particularly if the patient exhibit the appearance of a full habit of body, and the face has the color of robust health.

DOSE.—Dissolve one drop, or six globules, in six teaspoonfuls of water and give a teaspoonful every morning for a week, unless decided change occurs at an earlier period, then omit the medicine for a week, and then proceed with the remedy again, and so on as before, until some distinct manifestation of improvement or change.

BELLADONNA is particularly indicated when there is great heat in the head; face bloated and red, with strong pulsation of the arteries of the neck; severe pain in the head, and inclination to bury it in the pillow; or moving the head from side to side; sufferings aggravated by the least noise; extreme sensitiveness to the light; frequent flushes of heat; violent shooting and burning pains in the head; eyes red and sparkling; unusually brilliant, and protruding with wild expression; contraction or dilatation of the pupils; sickness at the stomach; violent delirium; drowsiness and stupor; loss of consciousness; frantic dreams; occasionally low mutterings; grinding of the teeth; convulsions and vomiting, and even involuntary discharges from the bladder and bowels.

DOSE.—The same as directed for *Aconite.*

HYOSCYAMUS is especially indicated when there are violent convulsions, loss of consciousness, or inarticulate speech; redness of the face; wild fixed look; white coat upon the tongue, with frothy phlegm about the lips; dilatation of the pupils; dry and parched skin; thirst; diarrhœa; and picking at the bed clothes with the fingers.

DOSE.—As directed for *Aconite* or *Belladonna.*

MERCURIUS is useful after *Belladonna,* when this latter remedy has only produced partial good effects, and when the bowels are much relaxed.

DOSE.—The same as for *Aconite, Belladonna,* &c.

BRYONIA is indicated at the commencement when there is heat in the head with great thirst; dark redness of the face; convulsive movement of the eyes; delirium; sudden starts, with cries and constant inclination to sleep; continual movement of the jaws as if chewing; yellow coat upon the tongue; distended abdomen; pain on passing urine, or else suppression; hot dry skin; hurrried respiration and constipation.

DOSE.—As directed for *Aconite,* or in severe cases, a teaspoonful, or a globule, dry upon the tongue, may be given every three hours, until amelioration or change.

HELLEBORUS NIGER is useful after *Bryonia* has produced temporary benefit, and may be employed in all

51

severe cases from the commencement. When the danger is not removed by this remedy in a few hours, it may be followed by *Sulphur*, and also if spasms are present.

DOSE.—One drop, or six globules, dissolved in three teaspoonfuls of water, and a teaspoonful every four hours, or two globules dry upon the tongue at the same intervals, until improvement appears to be manifest; and every six hours, until decided amelioration or change.

STRAMONIUM will be found useful in some instances, when the symptoms are analogous to those for which *Belladonna* or *Hyoscyamus* are indicated, and especially when the pain in the head is less acute, and more frequent convulsive movements, &c., the skin being hot and moist.

DOSE.—Of a solution of one drop, or six globules, in six teaspoonfuls of water; give a teaspoonful every four hours, until amelioration or change.

OPIUM is indicated particularly when there is lethargic sleep, with snoring respiration, half open eyes, and giddiness or confusion after waking, and complete apathy and absence of complaint.

DOSE.—The same as for *Helleborus*.

SULPHUR is more particularly serviceable, to be used occasionally during the time another remedy is employed. When this other remedy has produced a limited good effect a single dose of sulphur may be given, and in three hours after the indicated remedy may be proceeded with. It is also of great service in completing a cure after an attack of the acute inflammatory form.

DOSE.—If as an intermediary remedy, give two globules in a teaspoonful of water; and then in three hours, or six or twelve hours, if possible to wait as long, resume the treatment with the previous remedy, if appropriately employed. If used to complete a cure, one drop, or four globules, in a spoonful of water, may be given every morning until the cure is effected.

ZINCUM METALLICUM is indicated in the last stage against symptoms of incipient paralysis of the brain.

DOSE.—The same as directed for *Helleborus niger*, until the warmth returns and the pulse grows stronger, then recur to the other remedies as indicated.

LACHESIS, DIGITALIS and ARSENICUM are remedies that may be employed. *Lachesis* in the last stage of a low form of the disease, if any hope remains. *Digitalis*, when the pulse is slow, weak, and irregular. *Rhus tox.* may also be employed in the low, protracted variety, and *Arsenicum* when the face is pale, and great debility and emaciation, with quick, weak, and irregular pulse.

DOSE.—Of either as directed for *Helleborus*.

DIET AND REGIMEN.—The diet should be exceedingly simple, for those children weaned from the breast, while the nurse's diet, should be simple and easy of digestion, in order to afford proper nourishment to those who have not been weaned; or if children when afflicted with water upon the brain, cannot move, the food should be prepared for them, with reference to the irritable condition of the stomach, and in no case should it be stronger than the secretion of the breast.

Dropsy of the Testicle. Hydrocele.

For the description and treatment of this affection, see Diseases of the Urinary and Genital Organs.

Dropsy of the Womb. Hydrometra.

For the treatment of this affection see Diseases of Women.

CHAPTER XIII.

CAUSUALITIES

Concussions. Wounds. Dislocations. Bruises. Sprains. Fractures, &c.

1. BY CONCUSSION OF THE BRAIN is understood, the effect produced by violent shaking, or a blow upon the head. The symptoms vary according to the degree of injury which the brain has sustained. When the concussion is very severe, there is a sudden suspension of sense and power of motion, which generally results in death. When slight, a mere stunning or confusion, with more or less headache, is produced, succeeded by acceleration of the pulse, vertigo, and sickness.

Then again, when the violence done is more severe, yet not so much so, as to cause fatal termination, the patient may be rendered insensible, and incapable of movement; his limbs become cold; the pulse slow, weak, and intermittent; and laborious and snoring respiration. This has been termed the *first stage of concussion.*

The *second stage* is that which follows, as the patient begins to recover, the pulse and respiration improve, and warmth begins to be felt in the extremities. The sensibility to touch then returns, and the patient vomits, but still remains in a dull, confused state, and almost unconscious of external impressions.

The *third stage* takes place after the gradual subsidence of the first effects of the concussion, and the patient become enabled to respond to questions spoken in a loud tone, when active inflammation of the brain sets in, or begins to develope itself with all its characteristic symptoms, (See Inflammation of the Brain, &c.,) and unless checked, the result will be unfavorable.

TREATMENT.—To remove the immediate effects of concussion of the brain, when not very severe, Arnica is sufficient.

DOSE.—Dissolve one drop, or six globules, in three tablespoonfuls of water, and give a teaspoonful every three hours, until amelioration, or change. If there be an external wound, the injured part may be bathed with a lotion made of ten drops of the tincture, to an ounce of water, twice a day.

When, however, the concussion results in inflammation of the brain, or hydrocephalus, which will be indicated by the characteristic symptoms, the same treatment must be pursued, as that described under the head of these diseases.

DIET AND REGIMEN.—After any serious injury to the head, the patient should not be allowed any stimulating liquids for several weeks, he ought also to be kept quiet, and free from excitement of any kind.

2. CONCUSSION OR CONTUSION OF THE CHEST.—When this injury is inflicted, and soreness, or a sensation as if from incipient suppuration, with heat and throbbing is experienced in some particular spot, and there is chilliness, fever, restlessness, cough, and spitting of blood; and when sneezing, coughing, or a full inspiration aggravates the pain, &c., Aconite and Arnica, may be given in alternation.

DOSE.—Of each, dissolve one drop, or six globules, in separate tumblers, in four tablespoonfuls of water, and give a teaspoonful alternately, every four hours, until decided amelioration or change.

PULSATILLA is indicated, when a concussion of the chest is attended by a sensation as if there were an internal excoriation or wound.

51*

DOSE.—Of a solution of one drop, or six globules, in four tablespoonfuls of water, give a teaspoonful every six hours, until the patient is better or change.

MERCURIUS is indicated, when there is a continuance or increase of the cough, with expectoration of thick yellow mucus, occasionally streaked with blood.

DOSE.—The same as for *Pulsatilla.*

NUX VOMICA is indicated, when the expectoration has a sweetish taste, and is accompanied with difficulty in breathing.

DOSE.—The same as for *Pulsatilla.*

CHINA is useful, when a degree of delicacy of the chest remains behind after the use of any of the preceding remedies, and when there is a tendency to suffer from shortness of breath, and dry cough and paleness of the face, impaired appetite, restless, and unrefreshing sleep.

DOSE.—The same as for *Pulsatilla.*

BRYONIA is of service, when there is the manifest effects of a shock to the nervous system, with pains in the limbs, &c., produced by making a false step or stumbling.

OPIUM is indicated, when the accident has been accompanied with fright.

ACONITE, when accompanied with fainting.

CHAMOMILLA, when from extreme pain, convulsions ensue.

DOSE.—Of either of the above remedies, the same as directed for *Pulsatilla.*

Sprains.

This class of troublesome injuries, are best treated with *Arnica,* at the commencement, both as an internal remedy, and externally as a lotion.

DOSE.—One drop, or six globules, in a spoonful of water, may be taken daily, and a lotion of ten drops to a half tumbler of water, may be applied externally, three times a day.

RHUS TOX. may also be regarded a useful remedy ; to be used in the same manner as prescribed for *Arnica*.

BRYONIA, PULSATILLA, and RUTA, are remedies that may be used internally, in the same manner as directed for Arnica, when there is continuance of the pain, attended with heat and aggravation on movement.

Strains

Strains are generally the effects of over exertion, either of lifting, or of some powerful and sudden exercise.

BRYONIA is indicated, when there are pricking pains experienced in the back, aggravated from the slightest movement of the arms and trunk. If only partial relief is obtained, *Sulphur* may be employed to effect or complete a cure.

RHUS TOX. is indicated when headache results from a similar source, or when the pains are confined to the extremities. If this should fail of obtaining complete relief, *Calcarea* may follow.

VERATRUM is of service when sickness and great pain in the abdomen are produced by the effects of a strain.

DOSE.—One drop, or six globules of *Bryonia*, in a teaspoonful of water, may be given night and morning, until four doses have been taken, then pause four days, and begin with *Sulphur* in the same manner. *Rhus tox.* when indicated may be used the same as *Bryonia*, and then followed in the same way with *Calcarea* as prescribed for *Sulphur*. *Veratrum* when indicated may be given in the same dose, night and morning, until amelioration or change.

Wounds

There are six varieties of wounds subject to homœopathic treatment:

1. *Incised wounds*, such as are produced by a sharp sword or knife, and not accompanied by any contusion or laceration, easily healed.

2. *Lacerated wounds*, are those in which the muscular fibres are torn asunder, instead of being divided by a sharp knife; and the edges, instead of being even and regular, are jagged and unequal, and rarely healed without suppuration, and frequently succeded by violent inflammation.

3. *Contused* or *bruised wounds*, are those occasioned by some blunt instrument being brought in violent collision with a part of the body. These wounds are sometimes severe and dangerous, being prone to terminate in mortification and sloughing.

4. *Punctured wounds*, are those caused by a pointed instrument.

5. *Gun-shot wounds*, produced from the shot from a gun, partake both of the character of lacerated and contused wounds.

6: *Poisoned wounds*, are such as are produced by the bite of venomous and rabid animals.

TREATMENT.—The first object to be attained in the treatment of all wounds, is to arrest the hemorrhage. This is to be done by various means, as, by the *tourniquet*, compression, ligature, application of *cold water* or *ice*, and *astringents*.

APPLICATION.—Cold water or ice may be applied by saturating several folds of linen rags, or lint pads, and applying them to the wound, remoistening and reapplying as fast as they become hot, until the local pain and inflammation subsides.

Wounds of the arteries are generally the most serious, and may be distinguished by the bright color of the blood, which issues very rapidly in jets, while that which flows from the veins has a dark purple hue, flows smooth and uninterrupted.

When wounds only implicate vessels of a small size, they cease to bleed spontaneously or as soon as the wound is dressed; but when larger vessels are implicated, the tourniquet or compression should immediately be resorted to.

ARNICA and CALENDULA are employed to arrest hemorrhage from the mouth, and from fungous tumors and other diseased surfaces; and they may be employed both externally and internally.

DOSE.—One part of the tincture of *Arnica*, or *Calendula*, to sixteen parts of water, will form a lotion with which to saturate linen rags, which may be placed over the wound after the sides of which are drawn together, and secured by wrapping a strip of linen around the injured limb.

When considerable hemorrhage takes place after the extraction of a tooth, the best way of suppressing it is by a compress of lint pushed into the socket from whence the tooth has been dislodged. A solution of salt or alum may also have the desired effect.

CHINA is indicated when from loss of blood there are severe fainting fits, with deadly paleness of the face, or when the countenance assumes a livid appearance and when there are other signs of great exhaustion from the same cause.

DOSE.—One drop, or six globules, in half a tumbler of water; give a teaspoonful every hour; if this proves insufficient to arouse the patient, give a little wine and water, and subsequently *Arnica*, and *China* again if necessary.

It is further necessary in the treatment of wounds of every description after the bleeding is arrested, to remove all extraneous matter of whatever description, such as sand, splinters, shot, rags, &c., then place the lips of the wound together accurately by bandages, plasters, &c.

Deep-seated wounds may suppurate; and under such circumstances it is necessary that they should be dressed with strips of plaster, with sufficient space between the strips to allow the matter to escape.

TREATMENT.—The constitutional treatment of wounds of all kinds requires in the commencement the adminis tration of a few doses of *Arnica*. The patient at the same time should be kept as cool and as free from inquietude and anxiety as possible; he should live moderately, avoid- ing stimulants of every description. If the subject be robust and strong, and the sympathetic fever runs high, a *dose* of four globules, or one drop of *Aconite*, in a spoon- ful of water, should be given; and in three hours follow- ed with *Arnica*, and so on alternately until amelioration ensues. The only local application to relieve pain should be lint dipped in cold water, often moistened.

Lacerated Wounds.

Wounds of this description should be carefully cleansed; as far as possible the gaping parts should be brought together, and secured by plasters, and the limb, or body should be placed in the most suitable condition for insuring union, by first intention. The wound may be dressed with lint dipped in cold water, and frequently renewed, if it becomes inflamed and painful. If, on the other hand, the wound suppurates, and becomes intensely painful, cold water must not be used.

CHAMOMILLA followed by *Hepar sulph.*, should be administered for the purpose of producing a healing action. Should these fail, *Silicea* and *Sulphur* used in alternation, may produce the desired result. (See Ulcers.)

DOSE.—Of the selected remedy, dissolve one drop, or six globules, in three teaspoonfuls of water, and give a teaspoonful morning and evening, for . three days; if, however, the second dose has not succeeded in effecting material improvement, proceed with the next remedy.

Contused Wounds. Bruises.

In the treatment of wounds of this description, *Arnica* must be given internally, and cold water must be applied as above. When there is considerable extravasation of blood, ten drops of the *Tincture of Arnica*, in half a tumbler of water, should be applied as a lotion, to promote absorption, and otherwise forward the cure.

RHUS TOX has been particularly recommended, when the joints, synovial membranes, or tendons become bruised. *Ruta* is recommended if the membrane surrounding the bone becomes injured. If there is blood collected beneath the membrane, it is better to make an incision into the membrane to let it out; or even if there is matter there, causing severe suffering. After which the treatment to be pursued is the same as directed for open abscesses.

ARNICA may be prescribed internally, when the contusion has jammed or squeezed the limb nearly flat, or otherwise disfigured it.

CHINA is indicated when gangrene threatens, and the skin has assumed a livid and black appearance.

LACHESIS and ARSENICUM are also remedies to be used under similar circumstances. But under such circumstances, amputation becomes imperative in most cases, and the aid of a competent surgeon becomes necessary. When this operation of amputation has been performed, the stump should be dressed with lint, and dipped in cold water, *Arnica* should be given internally; and afterwards *Aconite* may be employed on the accession of the fever, and the ensuing stages may require *Calendula, Hepar, Silicea, &c.*

DOSE.—One drop, or six globules, of the selected remedy in a tablespoonful of water, every three hours. If no improvement takes place within twenty-four hours, proceed with the next remedy.

Punctured Wounds.

The treatment to be pursued in wounds of this description, is the same as for wounds in general. Punctured wounds of the abdomen require the internal administration of *Aconite* in order to prevent active inflammation, which so frequently follows in such cases. *Belladonna* is required after *Aconite*, when symptoms of peritonitis have already made their appearance.

DOSE.—One drop or six globules, in a spoonful of water, every three hours.

Cure by the first intention must not be attempted, unless compression by means of adhesive plaster, or a bandage, can be effected throughout the entire extent of the puncture.

When suppuration ensues, Mercurius, followed by Hepar, may be prescribed. Belladonna, Chamomilla, and Rhus tox. may be found serviceable in the event of excessive local inflammation.

CICUTA will be indicated if there are spasmodic twitchings.

BELLADONNA and RHUS TOX., if the inflammations partake of an erysipelatous character.

ACONITE is indicated when the constitutional disturbance is severe.

ARNICA, however, will be found sufficient to subdue most of the symptoms, when administered in time.

DOSE.—Of the selected remedy, one drop, or four globules, in a spoonful of water, every three hours, until amelioration, or change.

If lock-jaw or tetanus supervene upon a punctured wound, Arnica must be employed, and followed, if required, by other remedies suited to this complaint. (See Tetanus.)

Gunshot Wounds.

The treatment of this kind of wounds, is much the same as directed for *lacerated wounds*. A weak solution of Arnica, may be used in preference to cold water, in some instances, at the commencement. When a bullet, or splinters of bone, are lodged in the wound, or any other incongruous substance, they should be removed with as little irritation as possible, if they press on some important viscera, or vital part; but if otherwise, it will for the most part, be better to allow them to remain, especially when deeply seated, or difficult to be found, until loosened by suppuration, which process may be accelerated by the administration of Hepar sulph., Silicea, and Sulphur.

DOSE.—Of the selected remedy, one drop, or six globules, in a spoonful of water, every night and morning, until suppuration takes place.

In the event of fever, gangrene, and other difficulties attending gunshot wounds, see what is said of the treatment of contused wounds.

AMPUTATIONS.—When a joint is greatly injured, or much of the soft parts, together with the important vessels and nerves are carried away by a gunshot wound, leaving the bone entirely bare; also, in case of destruction of both the soft parts and the bone, or when the bone is shattered and the important vessels lacerated, or when a limb is torn off, or any other serious injury done that renders the prospect of saving the limb hopeless, amputation should be performed.

ACONITE, according to Dr. Wurzler, is of important service, after any operation of the kind, in removing the pain, and for preventing the fever pertaining to wounds, from making its appearance.

DOSE.—One drop, or six globules, in a spoonful of water, every three hours.

Poisoned Wounds.

These wounds are generally produced by the bites of venomous serpents, mad dogs, &c.

TREATMENT.—The usual domestic remedy is radiating heat; the manner of applying it, is by means of a red-hot coal or iron, placed as near the wound as possible without burning the skin, or causing too sharp pain, and the heat should be kept up by a succession of instruments heated for the purpose. Care should be taken to limit the action of the heat to the wound, and to continue it till the affections produced by the venom are observed to diminish.

" In the case of a *bite of a serpent*, it will be advisable to take from time to time, a gulp of salt and water, or a pinch of kitchen salt, or of gunpowder, or else.pieces of garlic." (Laurie.)

If bad effects arise, notwithstanding this, give a wine-glassful of brandy, every five minutes, until the sufferings are relieved, and repeat again, should the sufferings recur.

ARSENICUM should be given, if the shooting pains are aggravated, and proceed from the wound towards the heart, and if the wound becomes bluish, marbled or swollen, and is attended with vomiting, vertigo, and fainting.

DOSE.—One drop, or six globules, in a spoonful of water, and give every half hour, until there is an amelioration, and then cease until a reappearance of suffering.

BELLADONNA is useful after *Arsenicum*, when this latter remedy has had no influence.

DOSE.—The same as directed for *Arsenicum*.

PHOSPHORIC ACID, or MERCURIUS, will generally prove beneficial in chronic affections arising from the bite of a serpent.

DOSE.—One drop, or six globules, in a spoonful of water, every night.

SENEGA or ARSENICUM may prove of service if morbid affections or ulcerations exhibit themselves in consequence of a bite from a *rabid man* or animal; *Hydrophobin* is also a remedy regarded of some service.

DOSE.—One drop, or six globules, every three hours.

ARSENICUM is useful in the treatment of wounds poisoned by the introduction of animal substance in a state of putrefaction, which are frequently inflicted during dissection of diseased bodies.

DOSE.—One drop, or six globules, every six hours, in a spoonful of water.

Preventives against bad effects from poisoned wounds,— application of dry burning heat as soon as the wounds are inflicted.

Dislocations. Luxations.

Violent pain attends these difficulties. There is swelling, distortion of the joints, loss of motion, with an alteration in the shape, length and direction of the limb.

TREATMENT.—The first thing necessary is to reduce the dislocation, and this should be done by the surgeon as soon as possible after the injury has been received.

MEDICAL TREATMENT.—*Arnica* and *Aconite* should be given in alternation if there is excessive pain and inflammation; at the same time a weak solution of the tincture of *Arnica* should be applied to the affected joint, whether before or after the dislocation is reduced.

DOSE.—The same as directed for *lacerated wounds*.

Fractures.

The way to determine whether there is a fracture or not, is by the symptoms; if there is pain, swelling, deformity, and sometimes shortening of the limb, loss of power, and crepitation or rubbing of the broken surfaces of bone together on bending the limbs. There are several varieties of fractures, all requiring nearly the same *medical treatment.*

1. *Transverse*, or immediately across the bone.

2. *Oblique*, or running from side to side in an oblique direction.

3. *Longitudinal*, or running lengthwise of the bone.

4. *A simple fracture*, is one in which the bone is broken without there being at the same time a wound of the soft parts.

5. *A compound fracture* consists not only of the simple fracture, but in addition an external wound, caused by the protrusion of the bone through the integuments.

6. *A complicated fracture* involves that of the bone. attended with a wound of a large artery, extensive laceration of the soft parts, or with the dislocation of a joint.

7. *A comminuted fracture* is that in which the bone is broken into several pieces.

TREATMENT.—Whenever it is discovered that a limb is fractured, the patient ought to be placed on a litter of any kind at hand, whether a bed or a board, and removed to the nearest place of shelter; or if not far distant, to his own home. The greatest care should be exercised in lifting or removing the patient from one place to another, or else a simple fracture may be converted into a compound one, or into a complicated variety from a laceration of the soft parts, &c. In the case of simple fractures the reduction should be effected immediately. One drop, or four globules of *Arnica*, should be given as soon as the fracture is reduced for the purpose of preventing the invasion of undue inflammation, and of promoting the re-union of the fracture. *Ruta* has likewise been recommended as useful in some cases, used the same as the *Arnica.*

Burns and Scalds. (*Ambustiones.*)

The amount of danger arising from burns depends upon several conditions. An extensive scald or burn frequently proves fatal in a short time. The degree of danger to be apprehended from either is to be determined by its depth and extent, its particular seat, the age, temperament and habit of body.

TREATMENT.—When the burn or scald is so slight as only to affect the skin, the injured part held for a couple of minutes to the fire, will effect a cure.

ARNICA is of great service, in superficial burns.

CARBO VEG. often relieves, when the pain is excruciating.

COFFEA, when the pain is severe, causing great restlessness.

DOSE, and Application.—One drop, or six globules, in three spoonfuls of water, and give a teaspoonful every three hours, until amelioration or change. Ten drops of *Tincture of Arnica*, in two tablespoonfuls of water, may be employed as a lotion, to bathe the injured part, ten minutes after the accident.

In severer injuries from burns and scalds, the affected parts may be bathed in heated alcohol, or oil of turpentine; observing to keep the surface moist, and protected from the air.

The application of raw cotton is of great service, when the burn extends over a large surface. If there are any blisters, it is well to puncture them, and bathe the affected part with tepid water, and then apply the carded cotton in several layers, (three or four); when suppuration takes place, remove the upper layer only, and substitute fresh.

. HEPAR SULPH. is of the greatest service, at the same time.

DOSE.—One drop, or one grain, may be dissolved in half a tumbler of water, and a dessertspoonful may be given every twelve hours.

52*

CHINA will sometimes be found useful after *Hepar sulph.*, when the discharge has been excessive.

DOSE.—One drop, or six globules, in a spoonful of water, three times a day.

SOAP is extremely useful in burns, where not only the cuticle, but the true skin has been destroyed; pure white soap is the best for this purpose, but castile or other kinds of soap may suffice.

APPLICATION.—Place a cake of the soap in the bottom of a mug, and fill the mug with hot water, and immediately pour off all the water with the exception of about a tablespoonful; with a common shaving-brush make a thick lather, and spread it upon linen in the form of a plaster; apply it to the injured part, and secure by a bandage. It is well to puncture carefully any blisters, and all loose skin should be removed before the soap is applied. The whole surface of the sore should be covered with soap, and the air carefully excluded; at first, the soap will cause an aggravation of sufferings, but very soon it will afford relief. The plasters may be renewed every day, until the injury is completely healed.

URTICA URENS OINTMENT.—An emollient salve or ointment, having the medicinal properties of the nettle, may be used with great advantage.

APPLICATION.—Prepare the sore by puncturing the blisters, and removing any folds of dead skin, and then spread the salve on fine linen, and cover the entire surface of the sore, excluding the air as before; renew every day, as with the soap.

ACONITE is essentially serviceable for extensive inflammation, with considerable fever, or when the system has received a severe shock from fright at the time of the injury. *Opium* is also of use, in case of fright producing any shock at the time.

DOSE.—One drop, or six globules, every four hours, until better or change.

The TINCTURE OF URTICA URENS, may be used precisely the same as *Arnica.* So may *Creosote-water, Crocus sativus*, &c.

ARSENICUM, and NITRIC ACID, are useful after the first stage has passed away.

DOSE.—One drop, or four globules, morning and evening.

DIET AND REGIMEN.—During the febrile stage of a burn, the diet should be simple. After the fever has passed off, and the burn begins to heal, a more substantial diet, free from condiments, &c., may be employed.

Exposure to Heat. (*Overheating.*)

Sometimes in hot weather, over-exertion may cause heat in the head, and flushed face; under such circumstances it is unsafe to drink cold water, until sufficient time has elapsed for the body to cool off.

ACONITE will generally afford speedy relief in such cases, and generally prevents the occurrence of other troublesome consequences.

BELLADONNA will be indicated when there is violent headache, with congestion, fever, vomiting, sleeplessness, great anguish, or despair, and a sense of weight at the forehead on bending forward, or on stooping, as if the forehead would burst.

BRYONIA will be indicated when there is ill humor, and apprehension of some future misfortune; and also when there is headache with loss of appetite; a degree of fever, with thirst, or diarrhœa; results from exposure to the sun, or other heat, during exertion.

SILICEA will be indicated if nausea is the principle symptom that results from exposure to heat.

CARBO VEG. may be employed against headache from overheating, with weight over the orbits, and pain in the ball of the eye, in looking at any object intently.

DOSE.—Of any of the remedies. Dissolve one drop, or six globules, in half a tumbler of water, and give a teaspoonful every two hours, until amelioration or change.

Stings of Insects

The. stings of insects, such as bees and wasps, frequently produce febrile irritations, and it is found that the smell of the spirits of camphor will speedily alleviate them.

ACONITE should be administered when there is considerable inflammation, with swelling supervening.

ARNICA should also be employed both internally and externally, as directed for wounds. Should the tongue be the part where the sting is inflicted, as may be the case, the mouth may be rinsed with a solution of a teaspoonful of Tincture of Arnica, in half a tumbler of water.

BELLADONNA and MERCURIUS VIV. may also be employed, if found necessary.

DOSE.—For internal administration. One drop, or ten globules, of either, dissolved in half a tumbler of water, give a teaspoonful every three hours, until amelioration, or change.

LEMON JUICE, as well as ARNICA LOTION, may be employed to relieve the pain and itching caused by the bites or stings of gnats. *Arnica lotion* may also be employed to relieve the effects, where persons have been severely stung by nettles.

Fatigue.

Over-exertion will sometimes result in a sensation or feeling as if all the limbs were bruised, the joints being painful; under such circumstances consult the following remedies:

ARNICA when there is excessive fatigue, and sore feeling and pain on moving about.

DOSE.—One drop, or four globules, in a spoonful of water, repeated every twenty-four hours, until relieved.

RHUS TOX. when there are pains in the joints, &c., arising from lifting, or violent physical exertion of any kind.

DOSE.—The same as directed for *Arnica.*

CHINA will frequently assist in restoring the strength, when there has been profuse perspiration.

DOSE.—One drop, or six globules, in a spoonful of water, every six hours, until better, or a change.

VERATRUM is indicated when there is a tendency to fainting from the effects of excessive fatigue.

DOSE.—The same as for *China.*

COFFEA will be found useful when exhaustion has been the result of violent exercise combined with abstinence from food.

DOSE.—One drop, or four globules, every four hours, until better or change.

COCCULUS is a useful remedy when fatigue occurs after the most trivial exertion, either of body or mind; *Veratrum* and *Calcarea* may also be resorted to when *Cocculus* proves insufficient.

DOSE.—The same as for *Coffea.*

When running produces palpitation of the heart, pain in the side and aching in the extremities, *Aconite* may be employed, or else *Bryonia*, should the *Aconite* fail of affording relief. *Arnica* will remove a stitch in the side brought on by running.

DOSE.—One drop, or six globules of the selected remedy, in a spoonful of water every six hours, observing to change if no relief is obtained in twenty-four hours.

Apparent Death. (*Asphyxia.*)

It is known that individuals sometimes, to all appearances, suddenly expire, when in fact there is but a mere suspension of animation; and inasmuch as absolute and sudden death frequently occurs when it might be mistaken for a suspension of the kind, it is well in all cases where there is the least uncertainty to exercise the greatest care,—to do nothing that may cause death, and not to permit an interment until certain signs of putrefaction become manifest.

Apparent death may result,—1st, from hunger; 2d, from a fall; 3d, from suffocation; 4th, from lightning; 5th, from drowning; 6th, from cold or being frozen; 7th, from noxious vapors.

From hunger.—When an individual has been long without food, and animation has merely become suspended in consequence, warm milk may be given repeatedly, the smallest possible quantity at a time; it may be given drop after drop at first, and gradually increased to a teaspoonful; after a short interval, a small quantity of beef tea and a few drops of wine; after animation has been restored, and the patient has had a sound sleep, a small meal may be given; but it is better that the patient should be fed little at a time, and often, that he may gradually return to his natural mode of living; any deviation from this rule will prove in the highest degree dangerous.

From a fall.—When animation becomes suspended from a fall, the patient should be carefully placed upon a bed in a quiet place, with his head high, and then four globules of *Arnica* placed on his tongue, and the services of a medical man should be had that he may ascertain whether there is any fracture or signs of life; *Arnica* may be repeated, and also administered in injec. tions.

INJECTION.—To half a tumbler of water add a teaspoonful of *Tincture of Arnica.*

From suffocation, hanging or choking.—If there is a mere suspension of animation from these causes, the same may be restored by removing all tight clothing and placing the patient in a proper position, the head and neck rather high, quite easy and not bent forward; gentle friction may then be employed, and an injection of ten globules, or one drop of *Opium*, in half a tumbler of water, may be administered very slowly, and repeated every fifteen minutes while gentle friction is applied to the ribs; examine the eyes and see if they contract, or hold a mirror to the mouth to see if the breath dims it; surround the patient with warm clothes, place heated bricks to the feet and about the person, if no change is produced in an hour, pound a *bitter almond* fine, and mix it in a pint of water, and give it in injections, putting a few drops into the mouth or nose.

From lightning.—When animation is suspended from lightning, the patient should be placed in a current of fresh air, and cold water should be showered upon the face, neck and breast; warm friction should be applied if the body is cold, and the lungs should be inflated. *Nux vomica*, four globules, may be placed upon the tongue, and the neck may be rubbed with a solution of one drop of the tincture in a half pint of water.

From drowning.—To restore animation that has become suspended from drowning. The body should be stripped and rubbed, and wrapped in blankets and placed in a warm bed. The throat, mouth and nostrils should be wiped and cleansed, and then if no reaction takes place, put a few globules of *Lachesis* upon the tongue, keeping up the rubbing.

Should these efforts fail, or should the *Lachesis* not be at hand, the body may be surrounded with warm applications. A warming pan filled with live coals may be passed up and down the spine; bottles or bladders filled with hot water may be placed about the body; hot bricks may be placed at the pit of the stomach, and at the soles of the feet; use friction, with hot flannels, flour of mustard and other stimulants, or in the absence of other means, rub the body briskly with the hand.

To restore breathing, close the mouth and one nostril, and introduce the pipe of a common bellows into the other, at the same time carefully drawing down and pushing back the upper part of the windpipe, in order to allow a more free admission of the air; blow the bellows gently in order to inflate the lungs, till the chest be a little raised; the mouth and nostrils should then be set free and the chest should be moderately pressed by the hand. Continue this process until there are manifest signs of life. Electricity or galvanism may be of service if obtainable, by passing a current through the chest. These means may be persevered in until the signs of death are unmistakeable.

When the patient shows signs of life, a drop of spirits of camphor may be placed upon the tongue, or spirits of hartshorn may be applied to the nostrils, and when he can swollow, small quantities of warm stimulating drink may be given, but till then nothing of the kind should be attempted.

And finally, let it be well understood, that no time should be lost in the treatment of such cases as the above; avoid all rough usages; never hold up the body by the feet, roll it on casks, nor rub it with salts or spirits, or adopt any other violent measures. .

From cold, or being frozen.—When animation becomes suspended in consequence of exposure to cold, the patient should be gently removed to a place of shelter, or cool room, as a moderate degree of heat might prove an obstacle to restoration, and he should not be exposed to a draught of air.

He may then be well covered with snow, the mouth and nostrils being left free, and be placed in such a position that the melted snow may readily run off, when it must be again renewed. If ·there is no snow, a bath of very cold water or cold salt water may be substituted, the body being immersed therein for a short time: After which the body should be covered with cloths taken out of cold water, and the whole covered tightly with dry blankets. When every part of the body has lost its rigidity the patient should be properly cared for, and as the parts become pliable they may be rubbed with snow, if it is to be had, until they begin to have a healthy appearance; after which they should be wiped perfectly dry, and rubbed with the naked hand, until vitality appears to be perfectly restored.

These measures should be persevered in for several hours, or until it becomes manifest that restoration is impossible.

When restoration is effected the pain usually experienced may be alleviated by *Carbo veg.* or *Arsenicum.*

53

DOSE.—Of a solution of one drop, or six globules, in half a tumbler of water, give a teaspoonful every half hour, until a mitigation of the sufferings or change.

The patient must not be exposed to heat of any kind for considerable length of time after animation has been restored, otherwise serious consequences may be the result.

From noxious vapors.—When animation is suspended from such causes, remove the body into a fresh current of air, and dash cold water on the neck, face and breast, observing to keep up external warmth by such means as have been recommended for persons drowned, and also to inflate the lungs. Opium and Aconite must be employed after restoration has been effected.

DOSE.—One drop, or six globules, of *Opium* in a spoonful of water, every two hours. If three doses produce little or no effect, proceed with the use of *Aconite* in the same way.

Hydrophobia.

This disease, which literally signifies a fear or dread of water, arises in consequence of the bite of a rabid animal, or it may be a symptom arising from some diseases of the nervous system.

SYMPTOMS.—When it arises from the bite of a rabid animal, the first indications are generally anxiety, uneasiness and disturbed sleep. The eyes are glassy, inflamed, and sensitive to light; also ringing in the ears; giddiness and paleness of the countenance; frequent paroxysms of chilliness; oppressed respiration; rapid, irregular, small, contracted pulse; a loss of appetite. These symptoms generally occur after the elapse of an indefinite period, and sometimes after the bitten part seems quite well.

In the *second stage,* the wound, which may have already become completely healed, begins to assume somewhat of an inflammatory appearance, and a slight pain and heat, at times attended with itching, is felt in it. At this stage, it breaks out afresh, and an ulcer, with elevated margins of proud flesh, secreting an offensive, dark-colored discharge is afterwards formed, and wandering, drawing, and shooting pains, from the affected part upwards towards the throat, present themselves; these symptoms increase daily; the patient complains of a state of confusion in the head, or giddiness, with sparks before the eyes; is afflicted with sudden startings, spasms, sighing, and is fond of solitude; the pulse is small, irregular, and intermittent; the breathing laborious and uneasy; the skin cold and dry, and chilliness generally, though more particularly in the extremities, is complained of; then hiccough, colic, and palpitation succeed; the patient looks wild; the eyes have a fixed, glassy, and *shining* appearance; the swallowing is obstructed by a sense of pressure in the gullet, which occasionally renders every attempt to swallow liquids ineffectual; convulsions take place in the muscles of the face or neck. In this stage, however, the swallowing of solids is performed with tolerable ease. In ordinary cases, the patient remains affected in the above manner for a few days, after which the disease passes into the *hydrophobic* stage, in which it is utterly impossible for him to swallow the smallest drop of liquid; and the moment that any fluid, especially water, is brought in contact with the lips, it causes the patient to start back with horror and dread, although he may be suffering from the most excessive thirst; even anything that tends to remind him of water, produces indescribable anxiety, uneasiness, convulsions, and furious paroxysms of madness; he dreads even to swallow his own saliva, which he constantly spits from his mouth.

Vomiting of bilious matter soon comes on, succeded by intense fever, great thirst, dryness and roughness of the tongue, hoarseness, and fits of delirium, or madness, with disposition to bite and tear everything within reach, followed at intervals by convulsive spasms.

These attacks usually last from fifteen to thirty minutes, and when over, the patient is restored to reason, but remains in a state of great despondency, and finally, the paroxysms return more frequently, and in some instances, a fit of furious delirium closes the frightful scene; in others, nature sinks exhausted, after a severe attack of convulsions. The disease may be communicated to the human subject, from the bites of dogs, cats, or other animals of the canine race, which which have been previously innoculated with the virus.

It is said by the most reliable authors upon the subject, that the human species are the least susceptible of contagion from the hydrophobic virus. Scarcely one out of thirty, of those actually bitten by a rabid animal, suffer from the effects; yet it is necessary to exercise every precaution against the danger.

When the bite of a rabid animal occasions no abrasion of *the skin, there is not the slightest danger.*

In the homœopathic treatment of this disease, and its prevention, the following remedies may be employed, viz: *dry or radiating heat,* Belladonna, Cantharides, Hyoscyamus, Lachesis, and Stramonium.

BELLADONNA.—This remedy, according to Hahnemann, given every three or four days, is the most certain preventive against hydrophobia; still, it is well after having been bitten, to apply *radiating heat.* This should be done by the readiest means at hand; a red-hot iron, or live coal, placed as near the wound as possible, without burning the skin, or causing too sharp pain, and the heat should be continued for an hour, or until the patient begins to shiver, and stretch himself.

DOSE.—Of *Belladonna*, one or two globules, dry upon the tongue, every three days, as a preventive; during the time, the patient should be allowed to pursue his regular employment, and his mind should be kept from dwelling upon his misfortune, as much as possible.

CANTHARIDES is also useful as a preventive, as well as a curative remedy. Its use is indicated by great dryness, and burning in the mouth and throat, much aggravated on attempting to swallow; paroxysms of fury, alternating with convulsions, which are renewed by any pressure on the throat or abdomen, and also by the sight of water; fiery redness and sparkling of the eyes, which become prominent and frightfully convulsed; spasms in the throat, excited by the pain produced by the act of swallowing, especially fluids; continually burning, tittilation, and other irritating sensations, in the lower part of the abdomen.

DOSE.—Three globules, placed upon the tongue, or one drop of the dilution, at every threatening of a return of the convulsions, until benefit ensues.

BELLADONNA as a curative, is indicated when there is drowsiness, with ineffectual efforts to sleep, in consequence of excessive anguish and great agitation; sense of burning; great burning in the throat, with accumulation of frothy mucus in the throat or mouth; frequent desire for drinks, which are spurned on being presented, or a suffocating or constrictive sensation in the throat on attempting to swallow; inability to swallow; with glowing redness, and bloated appearance of the face; pupils immoveable, and generally dilated; great dread; occasional desire to strike, spit at, or bite or tear everything; inclination to run away; continual tossing about; great

53*

physical activity, with twitching in various muscles, especially those of the face; ungovernable fury; foaming at the mouth; and tetanic spasms.

DOSE.—The same as for *Cantharides.*

HYOSCYAMUS is indicated either before or after *Bella-donna,* where the convulsions are severe, and of long duration, and when there is less inclination to spit or bite, but a desire to injure those near in some manner or other; dread of liquids, on account of the pain of swallowing; spitting out the saliva for the same reason; excessive convulsions, with loss of consciousness, occuring soon after an attempt to swallow; and in other respects for similar symptoms, as detailed under *Belladonna.*

DOSE.—The same as for *Belladonna.*

STRAMONIUM is chiefly indicated when strong convul-sions result from fixing the eye on brilliant objects, or whatever reminds the patient of water; fits of laughter and singing; convulsions severe, attended with un-governable fury; and in other respects, for symptoms similar to those under *Belladonna* and *Hyoscyamus.*

DOSE.—The same as *Cantharides*

LECHESIS may be employed as soon as the convulsions take place.

DOSE.—Two or three globules, or one drop, every time the convulsions return, until better, or decided symptoms of medical action make their appearance. Should no benefit result, have recourse to the other remedies.

Mental Emotions.

As many affections arise in consequence of the control which mental emotions exercise over the human organ-ism, such as fright, anger and grief, we will briefly point out the treatment.

OPIUM is indicated for any affections which have been

brought on by sudden fright, with terror, horror, or fear. It may be used in alternation with *Aconite* or *Ignatia*, when necessary.

DOSE.—One drop, or six globules, of the selected remedy, may be dis. solved in half a tumbler of water, and a teaspoonful may be given every three hours; if in alternation, give one three hours after the other, in rotation.

ACONITE is indicated when the system is laboring under the joint influence of fright and passion, and particularly if there is fever, heat in the head, and headache.

DOSE.—One drop, or six globules, every four hours.

PULSATILLA in cases of fright, fever, and timidity, when the effect is upon the stomach and bowels; cold feet; suitable for sensitive persons.

DOSE.—Dissolve one drop, or six globules, in three teaspoonfuls of water, and give a teaspoonful every two hours, until better, or change.

BELLADONNA, when there is particular liability to be startled by trifles, or extreme nervous excitement after a fright, &c.

DOSE.—Two globules, repeated if necessary, in four hours.

IGNATIA for affections caused by grief, or suppressed emotions.

DOSE.—One drop, or six globules, repeated every six hours, until amelioration or change.

CHAMOMILLA, when the sufferings arise from vexation, or a disposition to irritability, or attended with great anguish and mental depression.

DOSE.—The same as directed for *Ignatia.*

NUX VOMICA for affections arising from sudden fits of passion or rage.

STAPHYSAGRIA for anger and vexation arising from just cause.

DOSE.—Of either, three globules, repeated every six hours, if necessary.

620   CASUALTIES.

ARSENICUM is indicated for great weakness and prostration, arising from a fit of passion.

DOSE.—Dissolve one drop, or six globules, in two tablespoonfuls of water, and give a teaspoonful every four hours, until better or change.

BRYONIA is indicated for coldness and shivering over the whole body; loss of appetite; nausea; vomiting, &c., brought on by a fit of passion.

DOSE.—The same as for *Nux vomica*.

COFFEA against the ill effects of excessive joy.

HYOSCYAMUS against the injurious consequences of jealousy, or disappointed love.

IGNATIA and PHOSPHORIC ACID for sufferings from unrequited affections.

PULSATILLA, BELLADONNA and PLATINA against the effects of mortification.

SAMBUCUS, when the effects of fear or fright, such as snoring respiration, has failed of being relieved by *Opium*.

DOSE.—Of either. Three globules in a teaspoonful of water, every three hours, until decided amelioration or change.

DIET AND REGIMEN.—When there is feverish excitement, let the diet be the same as directed for fevers. If derangement of the digestive organs, (see Indigestion.)

CHAPTER XIV.

WOMEN AND THEIR DISEASES; OR, DISEASES OF WOMEN.

Menstruation.

MENSTRUATION is a healthy function, and should be unattended with sufferings of any kind; but with the present enervating habits, and the various deleterious influences which prevail, it usually demands the careful attention of the physician. Even in females, otherwise apparently healthy, it may be delayed, or it may be preceded or followed by various sufferings, as spasms, cramps, hysteria, and other complaints. In temperate climates, this secretion usually makes its appearance from the thirteenth to the sixteenth year. In warmer climates, it may appear as early as the ninth, and in colder ones, not earlier than the twentieth. Its healthy continuance is not more than four or five days, though it may continue eight or nine days, or even longer; or it may only show itself for a few hours, at each returning period. It should return regularly every twenty-eight days, and finally cease at about the age of forty-five years, though it may cease earlier, or continue later. This period of cessation is called the change of life, and from the general disturbance of health it is apt to create, it has been sometimes called the dodging period.

Menstruation Obstructed.—Delay of the first Menses.

When the menses do not make their appearance so early in life as is usually expected, if the girl be bright, cheerful and active, if her health appear good, and no derangement is observable, medical interference is unnecessary and unjustifiable. In such a condition of affairs, the work should be left to nature.

But if there are congestions to the head; flushed face; constriction of the chest; palpitations; dulness; sleepiness; if her appearance is melancholic, or stupid, or sad; her countenance pale; if she is slender and feeble, and weak; or bloated, swollen and sluggish; a little attention at this period may save much suffering and expense in after life.

The remedies most useful, or most frequently required in these circumstances, are Pulsatilla and Bryonia.

PULSATILLA, if she is of slender make; feeble habit; pale countenance; mild disposition; inclined rather to weep than to be angry or fretful; and is always better when in the open air.

BRYONIA, if the face is flushed; the head feels full; the nose bleeds frequently; inclined to be costive; and if there be symptoms of congestion to the head and chest, with constriction and palpitation of the heart.

ADMINISTRATION.—Give either of the above remedies, according to their indications, a dose, either in powder or in solution, every morning, for one week; if the symptoms abate, wait a week without medicine, and afterwards give *Sulphur*, a powder every morning, one .week; if not better, apply to a physician, or see the article Chlorosis, which follows, for other medicines and their indications.

REGIMEN.—Fresh air, moderate exercise and a simple diet, are of the utmost importance to persons in this condition. Bathing when rising in the morning or re-

tiring at night, avoiding exposures to night air, dampness, cold or wet feet, and strictly observing the homœopathic regulations as to diet, &c., will greatly facilitate
the recovery.

Chlorosis.—(*Green Sickness. Emancio Mensium.*)

When in addition to the delay of the first menses, and
the symptoms above enumerated, such as weariness,
languor and debility, the patient becomes emaciated,
face pale, lips blanched, or with flushes of heat and redness, depraved appetite, with longing for such innutritious substances as chalk, &c., and the appearance is as
of one going into a decline; the condition has received
the name of Green Sickness, or Chlorosis. In this affection there is sometimes cough, which may be harsh and
dry, or with expectoration, bloody or in clots. Bowels
irregular, confined or relaxed; abdomen distended, and
with borborygmus or flatulence, especially after eating,
and in the evening; limbs frequently swollen and cold;
headache, short breath and palpitation of the heart.

REMEDIES.—Bryonia, Calcarea carb., Ferrum, Natrum
muriaticum, Plumbum, Pulsatilla, Sepia and Sulphur.

BRYONIA, for congestions to the head or chest; harsh,
dry cough; coldness and shiverings, or dry, burning
heat; constipation or colic; pressure in the stomach, as
from a stone; bitter taste; yellow, coated tongue; and
with bleeding at the nose.

DOSE.—One drop, or six globules, in a spoonful of water, morning
and evening.

CALCAREA CARB., in the worst cases, and after the failure of other remedies, when the limbs are swollen and
the difficulty of breathing great; afterwards *Ferrum*, to
prevent a relapse; especially if after *Calcarea* the pale

and sickly lôok continue; or give *Calcarea* and *Sulphur*, in alternation, in case of tuberculous diathesis, with cough.

DOSE.—Of either, the same as for *Bryonia*.

FERRUM, if after *Calcarea* the pale and blanched appearance of the countenance continue; with debility, want of appetite, nausea.

DOSE.—One drop, or six globules, in a spoonful of water, morning and evening.

LYCOPODIUM, along with or after *Calcarea*, when there is obstinate constipation; extreme languor; also if there is a tubercular tendency, with cough.

DOSE.—The same as for *Ferrum*.

NATRUM MURIATICUM, in obstinate cases, with habitual constipation; and if the sufferings appear periodically.

PLUMBUM, in obstinate cases, with swelling of the limbs or of the abdomen; and when there is no organic disease.

DOSE.—Of either, the same as for *Ferrum*.

PULSATILLA, when chlorosis is accompanied with derangement of the stomach, and frequent semilateral headaches; shooting pains to the head and teeth; shifting from side to side; aching in the forehead, with pressure at the crown of the head; difficulty of breathing, with suffocative sensations, palpitations, or sudden heats; diarrhœa and leucorrhœa; pains in the loins, with sense of weight; spasms in the stomach; nausea or vomiting; hunger, with dislike to food, or want of appetite; periodical expectoration of dark coagulated blood; swelling of the feet and ankles; with fatigue, especially in the legs; cold hands and feet, or with alternate heats.

DOSE.—One drop, or six globules, morning and evening, in a spoonful of water, until amelioration or change.

SEPIA, after *Pulsatilla*, or if there be disposition to hysteria; sallow complexion; dark or yellowish spots on the face; colic and pains in the limbs as if bruised

DOSE.—The same as for *Pulsatilla*.

SULPHUR, pressive and tensive pains in the back of the head and nape of the neck, or pulsative pains with determination of blood to the head; humming in the head; pimples on the forehead; voracious appetite; sour and burning eructations; pressive fulness and heaviness; bowels irregular; pain in the loins; fainting; excessive fatigue in the limbs; difficulty of breathing; great depression, especially after talking; emaciation, irritability, sadness, melancholy, weeping; tendency to take cold; enlargements of the abdomen occurring at this period have been cured by *Lachesis*, and also by *Apis mel.*

DOSE.—One drop, or six globules, may be dissolved in a spoonful of water, and taken every twenty-four hours, until a change.

The diet and regimen to be observed in chlorosis is the same as for menstruation obstructed which see.

Tardy Menstruation.

After menstruation has become established it may show itself less frequently than the usual periods, or be delayed considerably beyond the twenty-eight days. In such cases avoid all stimulating beverages, all highly seasoned dishes, all malt or other liquors, and all quack medicines. Strengthen the system by exercise, keep the feet dry and warm, and the head cool, the mind cheerful and happy, pay every proper attention to cleanliness, diet, &c., and take one of the following remedies: Arsenicum, Bryonia, Belladonna, Cocculus, Cuprum, Lachesis, Lycopodium, Phosphorus, Pulsatilla, Sulph. acid., Sepia and Veratrum.

ARSENICUM is suitable for cases attended with weakness, swellings, paleness, and sensations of heat or burnings, and if the sufferings are intermittent.

DOSE.—Dissolve one drop, or six globules, in half a tumbler of water and give a teaspoonful morning and evening, until amelioration or change

BELLADONNA, if whilst the menses are frequently delayed, they are copious when they do occur; determination of blood to the head; redness of the eyes; intolerance of light; giddiness; full bounding pulse; bleeding at the nose.

DOSE.—The same as for *Arsenicum.*

BRYONIA.—Bleeding at the nose instead of the menses; or with congestions of the head or chest; constipation.

DOSE.—The same as for *Arsenicum,* except repeat three times a day.

COCCULUS, given every alternate four days, when there are nervous symptoms; contracting, pinching pains in the pelvic region; oppressed respiration; scanty discharge, black or very dark; weakness, agitation, sighing, groaning, scarcely able to speak.

DOSE.—Dissolve one drop, or six globules, in ten spoonfuls of water, and give a spoonful every six hours, for four days, and then wait four days, without medicine.

CUPRUM for spasms, or if they are threatening; nausea; vomiting; cramps in the calves, with screaming; also, for convulsions.

DOSE.—The same as for *Bryonia.*

LACHESIS, when there is bloatedness; fulness; coldness of the extremities; worse after sleeping, and after *Pulsatilla.*

DOSE.—Dissolve one drop, or six globules, and administer the same as directed for *Arsenicum.*

LYCOPODIUM for costiveness, in tuberculous cases; and when *Bryonia, Lachesis,* or *Pulsatilla* fail, after these remedies.

DOSE.—The same as for *Arsenicum.*

PHOSPHORUS for females of light and delicate form, with weak chest, lively disposition, and predisposed to coughs and lung diseases; or if, instead of the menses, there be expectoration of blood.

DOSE.—The same as for *Arsenicum.*

PULSATILLA.—Pains low down in the abdomen, and across the small of the back; giddiness; fulness about the head; headache, with nausea; paleness, with flushes of heat; coldness of the hands and feet, or general coldness; roaring in the ears; partial deafness; sour taste after eating; nausea and vomiting; loss of appetite; desire for acids; palpitations; soreness of the breast; crying and laughter; sadness and melancholy; and disinclination for active exercise.

DOSE.—One drop, or six globules, in half a tumbler of water, give a teaspoonful every four hours, until amelioration or change.

SEPIA, after *Pulsatilla* or *Arsenicum,* and in similar cases; also, when there are eruptions or tetters; or if the patient is subject to a yellowish leucorrhœa.

DOSE.—The same as for *Pulsatilla.*

SULPHUR at the close of the treatment; or if there be heat in the head; giddiness; palpitation of the heart; shortness of breath; loss of appetite; nausea after eating; sleepiness; emaciation; or mental depression.

DOSE.—One drop, or six globules, in a spoonful of water, every morning each alternate week.

Suppression of the Menses. (*Amenorrhea.*

Usually caused by some sudden exposure; wetting the feet; strong mental emotions,—as fright; or it may occur in diseases of the lungs, liver, uterus, &c.; in which case, it is only symptomatic, and will subside with the original affection. Suppression from sudden incidental causes, will generally be relieved by Aconite and Pulsatilla, four or six doses of each, taken at intervals of twenty-four hours. If not Aconite, Belladonna, Bryonia, China, Graphites, Kali carbonicum, Sepia, Sulphur, and Veratrum, should be consulted.

ACONITE, if the suppression arise from fright; congestion to the head or chest; redness of the face; throbbing or acute pains in the head; at times, delirium or stupor; sick stomach and fainting. If Aconite does not afford relief, or the relief be partial, give *Opium*. If there be nausea, give *Veratrum;* and if long continued constipation, *Lycopodium*.

DOSE.—Dissolve one drop, or six globules, in four tablespoonfuls of water, and give a teaspoonful every six hours, until amelioration or change.

BRYONIA, if there be swimming in the head; heaviness with pressure towards the forehead; aggravated by stooping; pains in the chest; dry cough; bitter or sour eructations; pain in the pit of the stomach after eating; rising of food; pains in the small of the back; and also, pains in the lower part of the abdomen, of a drawing character; constipation.

DOSE.—In all respects as for *Aconite.*

BELLADONNA after *Aconite,* if there are congestions to the head; bleeding at the nose; and when *Aconite* is not sufficient.

DOSE and Administration.—The same as for *Aconite.*

CHINA may be useful in chronic cases, and for debilitated subjects.

DOSE.—One drop, or six globules, morning and evening, in a spoonful of water.

GRAPHITES, for persons subject to eruptive diseases, and with pain in the ovarian region.

DOSE.—One drop, or six globules, every twenty-four hours, in a spoonful of water.

KALI CARBONICA.—Paleness of the face, alternating with redness; palpitation of the heart; difficulty of breathing; and if there is a tendency to erysipelatous eruptions.

DOSE.—The same as for *China.*

PULSATILLA will usually afford relief, especially if the suppression result from a chill; or if there be headache confined to one side; pains shooting to the face, ears, and teeth; palpitation of the heart; flushes of heat; nausea; vomiting; pressure in the lower part of the abdomen; frequent desire to pass water; leucorrhœa; with inclination to melancholy or tears.

DOSE.—The same as for *Aconite,* after which it is often suitable.

SEPIA, for women of delicate constitution; sallow complexion, or with yellowish spots on the skin; nervous headache, worse in the morning; toothache; giddiness; melancholy and sadness; pain in the limbs, as if beaten; frequent colic; pain in the loins; nervous debility; delicacy, and tenderness of the skin; or with tendency to herpetic congestions; pains in the head with nausea and vomiting.

DOSE.—The same as for *China.*

SULPHUR, if there be pressive headache, chiefly in the occiput, extending to the nape of the neck; or one-sided headache; or pain over the eyes, with heat and throbbing; heaviness; confusion; giddiness; dimness of sight; bluish circle around the eyes; pimples in the face; disposition to hemorrhoids; constipation, with ineffectual efforts at stool; or loose, slimy evacuations; spasms in the abdomen; numbness in the limbs; pains in the loins; fatigue and weakness; irritability, or disposition to melancholy. (See also Tardy Menstruation.)

DOSE.—One drop, or six globules, in a spoonful of water, every twenty-four hours.

54*

DIET AND REGIMEN.—For each of the above enumerated conditions of the menses, the hygienic treatment
should be essentially the same. All sources of physical
or mental depression should be carefully avoided, and all
undue excitation, either of the physical or mental
powers; late hours; loss of sleep; night air, and exposure
to dampness, or wet feet; also sleeping too long,
especially too late in the morning; lying upon feather
beds, especially with the head covered during sleep, or
in too close apartments; breathing impure air; hot and
crowded rooms; exciting or depressing passions or
emotions; and all stimulating drinks, all highly seasoned
food, all spices, perfumery, and strong aromatic substances, must always be highly injurious.

The patient should have a reasonable supply of good
and wholesome food, and it should always be taken at
regular intervals. The stomach should never be overloaded, and the food should not be in too great a variety.
Coarse bread, (or Graham bread,) wheat and Indian bread,
or bread made of oatmeal; potatoes, tomatoes, ripe fruit,
if they agree, either raw or cooked, and taken in
moderation; milk and cream, soft boiled eggs, with a
little butter and salt, will form the principal articles of
diet. A small piece of beef or mutton, once each day,
at dinner, may be allowed. The drink should be water,
black tea, cocoa, or chocolate, homœopathically prepared;
but on no account should green tea, coffee, beer, or
mineral water, or any of the stimulating or effervessing
drinks be permitted.

Menstruation too soon or too frequent.

If the menses appear too early, that is, too frequently, say every two or three weeks, the irregularity may arise from a variety of causes, and the treatment should generally be commenced with one of the following remedies.

Belladonna, Calcarea carb., Ipecacuanha, Natrum mur., Nux vomica, Platina, and Sulphur.

BELLADONNA, if there be pains in the head, with heat; flushed face, and cold feet; profuse menses, with bearing-down pains; and pressure outward; and especially if there be dryness of the throat.

DOSE.—One drop of the dilution, or six globules, in ten spoonfuls of water, give a spoonful every two hours, four doses, afterwards every six hours, until alleviation or change.

CALCAREA CARB., for persons of relaxed muscular fibre; weak, cachectic, or plethoric; subject to menorrhagias, diarrhœas, or blenorrhœas, with pain in the abdomen; and also in scrofulous subjects. It should never be given to persons of strong, nervous fibres, and when the menses are deficient.

DOSE.—One drop of the dilution, or six globules, in a spoonful of water, every morning for four days, then wait four days. Useful after *Belladonna.*

IPECACUANHA, for passive hemorrhages, where feebleness, dulness, nausea, and coagulated discharges prevail.

DOSE.—The same as *Belladonna.*

NUX VOMICA, when the menses are too early, whether too scanty or too profuse; and when there are spasms, colic, nausea, faintness, dragging sensations; or sensations of weight, or pressure at the epigastrium; fulness, or bloatedness, or sensations of soreness or pain, as from a bruise; with drawing sensations, extending to the thighs, and pressure outward.

DOSE.—One drop of the dilution, or six globules, in four spoonfuls of water, a spoonful every two hours through the afternoon; giving at the same time, a dose of *Calcarea carb.*, or of *Sulphur*, in the morning when the above symytoms are present, will always effect a cure.

NATRUM MUR., for symptoms similar to *Nux vomica*; and also if there be shiverings, or sensations of paralysis, with intermittent sufferings; headache; moroseness; sadness; cramps; and drawing, cutting, and contractive pains.

DOSE.—One drop of the dilution, or six globules, in four spoonfuls of water, may be given every six hours, a spoonful two days;after or in alternation with *Ipecacuanha* or *Nux vomica;* or it may be given in chronic cases, a drop in a spoonful of water, every morning, for four days, then omit four days, and repeat again so long as may be necessary to complete the cure.

Menstruation too Profuse.

When menstruation is excessive or continuous, longer than usual, attended with pains in the back, loins and abdomen, resembling labor pains, the medicines most suitable are Calcarea carb., China, Chamomilla, Crocus, Ignatia, Ipecacuanha, Nux vomica, Platina, Sabina and Sulphur.

CHINA, for too copious or long-continued discharge, and after the use of other remedies; debility.

DOSE.—One drop of the dilution, or six globules, in four spoonfuls of water. Give a spoonful every two hours, or for the subsequent debility, every six hours until amelioration, or change.

CHAMOMILLA, when the discharge is dark colored and clotted, with griping pains, extending from the small of the back towards the abdomen; thirst; coldness of extremities and fainting; also after *Nux vomica.*

DOSE.—One drop of the dilution, or six globules, in four spoonfuls of water, a spoonful to be given every two hours, for twelve hours, six doses; if no change within the next twelve hours select some other remedy.

CROCUS, when the discharge is dark colored, clotted or viscid; very copious, and returning too early.

DOSE.—The same as *Chamomilla.*

IGNATIA, when it continues too long, attended by yawning and hysterical symptoms.

DOSE.—One drop, or six globules, in ten spoonfuls of water; give a spoonful every four hours, until a change is effected, or some other remedy selected.

IPECACUANHA, flooding of bright red blood after labor, repeated every three, six or twelve hours; also in all severe cases it may be the first remedy administered, unless there are strong reasons to the contrary.

DOSE.—One drop, or six globules, in a spoonful of water, should be given every two hours in extreme cases, in those less urgent every six or twelve hours, until a change is effected. After *Ipecacuanha*, *Nux vomica* or *Arsenicum*, may frequently be found useful.

NUX VOMICA, when too copious and early, continuing too long, stopping and returning frequently; for those making use of coffee and other stimulants; spasms in the abdomen; pains in the limbs; nausea; fainting; restlessness, and angry mood.

DOSE.—One drop, or six globules, in ten spoonfuls of water; give a spoonful every four hours, from three o'clock in the afternoon, four doses, after *Ipecacuanha*, and to be followed by *Chamomilla*, if relief be not obtained.

PLATINA, when too profuse, and consisting of thick, dark colored blood; attended with bearing down pains; venereal and general excitability.

DOSE.—The same as *Ignatia*.

SABINA, for plethoric, robust persons, liable to miscarry; discharge profuse, bright red color, with rheumatic pains in head and limbs; pain in the loins and weakness.

DOSE.—The same as *Chamomilla*.

SULPHUR and CALCAREA, after the failure of other remedies, and given two or three times during the intervals, (allowing ten or twelve days to elapse between the doses,) may be found successful.

Rest in a horizontal posture is in most severe cases imperative.

Menstruation painful.—Menstrual Colic.—(*Dysme iorrhœa.*)

This may occur either with scanty or profuse menstruation, or the function may appear otherwise healthy, and be attended with severe pains.

The most useful remedies are Belladonna, Chamomilla, Pulsatilla, Nux vomica, Lachesis, Coffea, Cocculus, Causticum and Veratrum.

BELLADONNA.—Pain in the back and lower abdomen, as if the parts would fall out; congestion of blood to the head; confusion of sight; frightful visions; disposition to bite; screams; redness and puffiness of the face; ineffectual efforts for stool, with much straining; and especially in profuse menstruation.

DOSE.—One drop of the dilution, in ten spoonfuls of water, (or six globules;) give a spoonful every quarter hour, for two hours. If not better, select another remedy.

CHAMOMILLA.—Pains like labor pains; pressure from the small of the back downwards and forwards; colic, with sensitiveness to the touch, and discharge of blood, dark colored and coagulated.

DOSE.—The same as *Belladonna*.

COFFEA.—Colic, with sense of fulness and pressure; violent spasms; grinding of the teeth; wringing of the hands, screaming and groaning; nervous excitement; delirium; coldness, numbness and stiffness; difficulty of breathing, and groaning.

DOSE.—The same as *Belladonna*.

COCCULUS. — Spasms; cramps; flatulency; nausea; faintness, and pressive colic.

DOSE.—One drop of the dilution, or six globules, in four spoonfuls of water; give a spoonful every half hour.

CAUSTICUM.—Cutting pains in the small of the back; spasms; hysterical symptoms; with yellow complexion.

DOSE.—The same as *Cocculus*.

LACHESIS.—If there be diarrhœa, ·with violent tenes. mus, usually commencing before and continuing after the menses.

DOSE.—Give a drop of the dilution, or six globules, in a spoonful of water, after every discharge of diarrhœa.

NUX VOMICA.—Writhing pains in the abdomen, with nausea; pains in the back and loins as if dislocated; sense as if bruised even in the bones; spasms and pricking pains, or paroxysms of pressing and drawing pain; sensation of distension as if the abdomen would burst; frequent desire to pass water; most useful in menorrhagia

DOSE, and Administration.—One drop of the dilution, or six globules, in ten spoonfuls of water; a spoonful to be given every half hour, commencing at two o'clock in the afternoon, after giving *Chamomilla* or *Belladonna* in the morning. .

PULSATILLA.—Feeling of heaviness as if from a stone in the lower abdomen, with violent pressure even in the small of the back, and a sensation of drawing and numbness extending down the thighs, especially when in a sitting posture; pressure in the rectum, ineffectual efforts for stool; inclination to pass water; useful in amenorrhœa and scanty menses; and if the symptoms change frequently, or the pain move from place to place.

VERATRUM.—Menstrual colic with nervous headache; nausea and vomiting; coldness of the extremities; weakness, faintness, or fainting fits, and diarrhœa.

DOSE.—Of *Pulsatilla* or *Veratrum*, one drop, or six globules, in six spoonfuls of water; give a spoonful every fifteen minutes, four doses if no change takes place in four hours, select some other remedy.

Cessation of the Menses.   Change of Life.   Menstrual Climacteræ.   (*Menoposia.*)

Whilst this change is in progress there is usually more or less disturbance of the general health, such as vertigo; headache; flushes of heat; paleness and debility; nervousness; irregularity in the urinary discharges; pains in the back and loins, extending down the thighs, with creeping sensations; heat in the lower part of the abdomen, and occasional swelling of the extremities; piles, and violent itchings of the private parts.

Usually this change approaches gradually; the menses at first become irregular, either at longer or shorter intervals, the quantity discharged also being either greater or less than formerly. The fluid may be mixed with mucus, or the flow may come on suddenly, continue for a short period, and then stop as suddenly. It may even be so profuse as to amount to a hemorrhage. Occasionally it gradually ceases without being attended with any unpleasant symptoms, and after it entirely ceases the health may become better than it had ever been before.

The most important remedies are Pulsatilla and Lachesis.

Administration. —First give *Pulsatilla,* one drop, or six globules, in four spoonfuls of water; a spoonful each evening four days, then omit all medicine four days, then give *Lachesis* in the same manner. If the symptoms abate, wait whilst the improvement continues; if not, repeat the medicines as before.

Other remedies are Aconite, Apis mellifica, Arsenicum, Bryonia, Cocculus, Ipecacuanha, Ignatia, Sepia and Sulphur, which should be administered the same as Pulsatilla and Lachesis. Proper attention should be paid to diet, clothing, exercise, &c. All stimulants should be avoided; exercise in the open air and bathing will be found advantageous. The clothing should be warm and comfortable, and all sudden changes avoided.

ACONITE if there is vascular excitability; humming in the ears, or beatings, with roarings and whistlings; quick pulse; nervous excitability, and weeping; or fretful, desponding ideas about herself; or vacilation of spirits and feelings.

DOSE.—One drop of the dilution, or six globules, dissolved in six spoonfuls of water, may be given, every four hours a spoonful, two days, or until the vascular excitement ceases; after which select another remedy.

APIS MELLIFICA, if dropsical symptoms supervene, or if there be swelling or bloatedness, and congestions, with derangements of the urinary secretions.

DOSE.—The same as *Lachesis*.

ARSENICUM, when the change is succeeded by metorrhagia; when dropsy is also threatened; or if congestions of the liver and spleen, asthmatic symptoms, general debility, and nervous prostration, accompany the change.

DOSE.—One drop of the dilution, or six globules, in ten spoonfuls of water; give a spoonful every six hours. After *Ipecacuanha* or *Bryonia*, should those medicines have been previously indicated.

BRYONIA, if there is congestion of the lungs or chest, with pleuritic symptoms, or dyspepsia, distension of the abdomen, pains and soreness in the region of the spleen, and if there is a tendency to dropsical effusion.

DOSE.—The same as *Aconite*, and repeat at intervals of one or two weeks.

COCCULUS, for spasms in the hypogastrium, with bilious nausea and vomiting; rumbling, as of wind in the abdomen; eructations; cramps; convulsions; paralysis; numbness, especially if it be transient or partial; and if there be a sense of emptiness, or vacuity, with want of vital energy, after which give *Sulphur*, or *Arsenicum*.

DOSE.—One drop of the dilution, or six globules, in ten spoonfuls of water, give a spoonful every half hour, during a severe attack, or every six hours in milder cases, two days, to be repeated after four or eight days, if necessary.

Hysterics. (*Hysteria.*)

Unmarried ladies between the ages of fifteen and thirty-five, are most subject to attacks of hysteria. They usually occur about the menstrual period.

The symptoms are, anxiety, depression, and weeping; difficulty of breathing; palpitations, and nausea; generally pain in the left side, passing upward to the throat, with sensation of a ball in the throat; suffocation; stupor; insensibility; spasmodic clenching the teeth; the body twisted about or becoming rigid; and the limbs stiff or convulsed. There are fits of laughing, crying, or screaming, incoherent talking, and foaming at the mouth, and hiccough. Or an attack may commence with violent spasmodic pain in the back, extending to the sternum, or becoming fixed at the stomach pit; with clammy perspiration; pale, death-like countenance; coldness of the extremities; and weak, almost imperceptible pulse. The attack usually passes off with eructations, sighing, and sobbing, followed by a sense of soreness of the whole body. It is frequently excited by sudden emotions; a predisposition to it may be stimulated by an inactive life, the frequent use of stimulants or cathartics, depressing conditions of mind, &c.

REMEDIES.—Coffea, Cocculus, Cuprum, Ignatia, Lachesis, Platina, Pulsatilla.

COFFEA.—Spasms, with jerking, agitation, screaming, or crying, cold perspiration, &c.

DOSE.—Give a teaspoonful in water, every fifteen minutes, until relief is afforded.

COCCULUS or CUPRUM, for general spasms, with clenching of the jaws, foaming at the mouth, &c. If relief be not obtained, give *Veratrum*. .

IGNATIA, for hysteria attended with nausea and

fainting; chilliness; paleness of the face; dimness of sight; intolerance of light and noise; shrieking for help, and suffocative constriction of the throat; difficulty of swallowing; heat of the body; distension of the abdomen, with hardness; twisting drawing, and pressing pains; yawning and stretching; the fit terminating with a deep sigh; scanty and difficult menses.

DOSE.—Of *Cocculus, Cuprum,* or *Ignatia.* One drop of the dilution, or six globules, in six spoonfuls of water, give a spoonful every ten or fifteen minutes during the spasms, afterwards every two or four hours, to prevent their recurrence, for a few days.

PULSATILLA, for persons excessively chilly, or inclined to tears, or to alternate tears and laughter; silent melancholy; very sensitive, with nervous paroxysms; and if there is suppression of the menstrual flow.

DOSE.—One drop of the dilution, or six globules, in ten spoonfuls of water, give a spoonful every half hour, four doses; afterwards every two to four hours, until perfect relief is afforded.

Other remedies which may be indicated, are

ASAFŒTIDA, especially if the fits proceed from some morbid irritation in the abdomen, affecting the uterus; if there be bloatedness, fulness, and tension; and if the globus hystericus be a prominent characteristic of the fit, the unpleasant sensations appearing to arise from within; involuntary twitchings and jerkings; irregular and intermittent affections; sensations of numbness, and heaviness, in different parts of the body; or spasmodic distress for breath, as if from asthma; with fulness, bloatedness, and choking sensations.

DOSE.—One drop of the dilution, or six globules, in ten spoonfuls of water, a spoonful every fifteen minutes, for four doses; afterwards every two hours, until the above symptoms are controlled.

AURUM. — Hysterical spasms; alternate tears and laughter; morbid sensibility; religious melancholy; despair; oppression at the chest, almost to suffocation; with a fine eruption around the lips, face, and forehead.

DOSE—One drop of the dilution, or six globules, in ten spoonfuls of water, a spoonful to be given every half hour; after the fit every four or six hours, to prevent a recurrence.

BELLADONNA may be given, if, during the fit, the face is red and tinged, the veins of the neck swollen, and symptoms of determination of blood to the head.

DOSE.—The same as *Aurum.*

CONIUM.—Hysteric fits, if accompanied with chilliness; menstrual suppression; acrid leucorrhœa, with colic; induration of the os uteri; spasms, with trembling of the limbs; excessive irritability, with weakness; pulsations in the carotids, globus hystericus, anxiety and tears.

DOSE.—The same as *Aurum.*

MOSCHUS.—Syncope, or fainting fits, with but little excitement of the muscles, or of the arterial system; or if there are spasms and convulsions, especially at the pit of the stomach, and in the thorax; indefinite pains; general sensation of coldness; great desire for brandy, or for beer; nymphomania.

DOSE.—The same as of *Asafœtida.*

NUX MOSCHATA.—Muscular spasms, alternated with debility; sudden changes; hysteric laughter; vertigo; rigidity and insensibility; distension of the stomach and abdomen after eating; menses retarded, with headache, pain in the back, languor, pain at the stomach pit, water-brash; menses thick and dark, or with vicarious leucorrhœa.

DOSE.—The same as *Asafœtida.*

SECALE.—Convulsions, with frequent changes of the mind and body; alternate laughing and crying; depression of spirits and despondency, with thoughts of self-destruction; spasms of the bladder; retention of urine, with frequent and violent efforts; menses profuse.

DOSE.—One drop of the dilution, or six globules may be given in four spoonfuls of water, every half hour a spoonful, until four spoonfuls are taken; afterwards every six or twelve hours, according to the symptoms.

VERATRUM, for hysterical spasms from fear, rage or fright; spasmodic clenching of the jaws; coldness of the extremities; convulsive jerkings, with numbness or stiff- ness; syncope or fainting from the least movement; cold perspiration on the forehead, or coldness and heat in different parts; grinding of the teeth.

DOSE.—The same as of *Asafœtida*.

Hysteria is a very frequent attendant upon such dis- orders as Chlorosis, Amenorrhœa, Menorrhagia, &c., for the treatment of which see those articles. See also *Tetanus* and *Lockjaw of Infants*.

If violent spasmodic hiccough prevails, give Bella- donna or Nux vomica, a dose every fifteen minutes in water, four doses, or give those remedies in alternation.

TREATMENT.—During the fit, place the patient in an easy posture, with a free access of cool air; remove every thing tight from around the body, especially from the waist and throat, and sprinkle the face with cold water.

A predisposition to hysteric fits may generally be overcome by the administration of some of the foregoing remedies, or by remedies adapted to some morbid condi- tion upon which hysteria is nearly always dependent. For further information consult a physician.

Leucorrhœa. Whites. (*Whitish discharge from the Vagina.*)

This discharge is at first usually slight, and unattended by any unpleasant sensation; but if neglected it com- mouly increases in quantity, till it becomes excessive and

55*

very troublesome;) the general health suffers, the appetite fails, the pulse becomes weak; pains in the back and loins, lowness of spirits and debility ensue. At times the sight is affected, the eyes become dull and heavy, or surrounded with a livid or yellowish circle, or the face pale and bloated.

The discharge also at times becomes greenish, yellow- ish, dark brown, or almost black, or like dirty water, and is attended by painful excoriations and ulcers in the parts. The exciting causes are numerous. Inatten- tion to cleanliness, strains, the frequent use of debilitating or stimulating medicines, falling of the womb, excessive sexual indulgence, and the use of pessaries, &c., are among the principal. It is frequently at first a catarrhal affection, and like all other catarrhs is liable to become chronic. In scrofulous, psoric or syphilitic patients, it is most obstinate and troublesome.

REMEDIES.—Calcarea carb., Causticum, Cocculus, Na- trum mur., Pulsatilla, Sepia and Sulphur.

CALCAREA CARB., for lymphatic females of light com- plexion, who have too copious and too frequent men- struation; the leucorrhœa is of a milky appearance, worse immediately before the menses, and often attended with itching and burning, or with pains shooting through the parts, and with falling of the womb.

DOSE.—Of *Calcarea*, one drop or six globules, in a spoonful of water, every morning, one week, after which omit all medicine one week.

CAUSTICUM.—Profuse leucorrhœa, having the odor of the menses, flowing mostly at night, with pain in the back and loins, and excoriation.

DOSE.—The same as *Calcarea*.

COCCULUS.—Leucorrhœal discharge during pregnancy, mixed with blood, or like water in which meat had been washed; colic and flatulency, or leucorrhœa, immedi-ately before and after menstruation.

DOSE.—One drop, or six globules, in four spoonfuls of water, a spoon-ful every six hours, four days, after which wait four days, or select another remedy.

NATRUM MURIATICUM.—Discharge copious, transparent, whitish and thick; mild or acrid; yellow complexion; with headache; diarrhœa, with slimy evacuations; colic, and intermittent sufferings.

DOSE.—One drop, or six globules, in a spoonful of water, every morning.

PULSATILLA, in a majority of cases, especially if the discharge is thick, like cream; or corrosive, with itchings, taking place either before, during, or after menstruation; or if caused by fright; or in young girls, who have not menstruated.

DOSE.—One drop, or six globules, in four spoonfuls of water, a spoon-ful every six hours, four days, afterwards, every night at bed time two weeks; if no alleviation, give *Sulphur*, and repeat the remedy.

SEPIA.—Discharge yellow, or greenish, or fœtid, and sometimes with excoriations; bearing down pains; fre-quent desire to pass water; swelling of the abdomen; and yellow color of the skin.

DOSE.—The same as *Pulsatilla*.

SULPHUR, for inveterate cases, the discharge corrosive and burning; or preceded by colic; also, when it follows suppressed eruptions or ulcerations.

DOSE.—One drop, or six globules, in a spoonful of water, may be given in the morning, for one week; after which, wait one week, then select a remedy for the remaining symptoms.

Falling of the Womb. (*Prolapsus Uteri.*)

SYMPTOMS.—Bearing down, dragging sensations, in the lower part of the abdomen; drawing from the small of the back, and around the loins and hips; pressure low down, towards the private parts; weakness, soreness, and faintness, often at the pit of the stomach; numbness of the lower limbs; frequent desire to pass water; nervousness, &c.; all these symptoms aggravated to a great degree by a long walk, by severe exercise or labor, by lifting, or by carrying any weight. Of the exciting causes, getting up too soon after confinement, and engaging in too laborious employments at that time, is one of the most common; next to this, perhaps, the weakening effects of cathartics and other drugs; tight lacing; the injudicious application of the bandage, by ignorant midwives; injuries from overlifting, strains, &c., are also frequent causes, and also large doses of ergot, and other allopathic drugs.

The remedies are, Aurum, Belladonna, Calcarea carb., Nux vomica, and Sepia.

ADMINISTRATION.—Give a dose of *Nux vomica*, at three o'clock, and another at bedtime, daily, for four days; if not better, give *Aurum*, in the same manner, and then return again to *Nux vomica*. If better, wait four days without medicine and afterwards give *Calcarea*. Or, if it be attended with a yellowish leucorrhœa, give *Sepia*, one powder each day four days. Continue this alternation four weeks, and afterwards give *Calcarea carbonica*.

The following pathogenic indications will generally be found useful.

ARNICA should always be given if the prolapsus be the result of a contusion, or blow, or kick; also *Arnica* or *Rhus tox.* if from a strain or wrench, as in lifting; and if there be a discharge of blood from the uterus; spasmodic retention or involuntary emission of urine; abdomen hard and swollen, with flatulence, colic, and ischuria.

DOSE.—One drop of the dilution, or six globules, in four spoonfuls of water; give a spoonful every six hours, or oftener, for one or two days, until the above symptoms are modified.

AURUM.—Prolapsus, with induration of the womb; dejection of spirits; melancholy; sensitiveness to pain;

heaviness or weight in the abdomen; hands and feet cold like ice, and dyspeptic symptoms.

DOSE.—One drop of the dilution, or six globules, in four spoonfuls of water, a spoonful every six hours, two days; afterwards, give a drop, or six globules, every morning for one week, if necessary, follow with *Nux vom.* and return in a few weeks, or after the next monthly period to *Aurum,* in the same manner.

BELLADONNA.—Pressure as from a heavy load in the hypogastrium, or as if all the contents of the abdomen would fall out, especially if usual early in the morning, or if worse in the morning; distension of the abdomen; heaviness even in the thighs, with weakness; drawing pains all about the pelvis, or lower part part of the abdomen; cramp-like pain low down at the extremity of the spinal column; leucorrhœa and menorrhagia; excessive sensibility and irritability, especially if aggravated by the slightest touch; tenesmus of the rectum; spasms, and even convulsions.

DOSE.—One drop, or six globules, in four spoonfuls of water; give a spoonful every two hours in acute cases; in less severe cases, every six or twelve hours, until a change is effected, or another remedy selected.

CALCAREA CARB.—Often after *Belladonna,* especially if there be relaxation of the system in scrofulous subjects; weariness; desire to urinate when walking, with inability or difficulty in retaining the urine or fæces; too profuse and too frequent menstruation; and weakness of the muscular system, whether in the delicate and spare, or in the plethoric and full.

DOSE.—One drop, or six globules, in a spoonful of water, every morning, four days between each menstrual period, until a change is observed.

NUX VOMICA.—If a varicose condition of the vessels of the uterus be the cause of the descent, and the vagina, or the parts below the womb are also implicated; when there is a relaxed condition of the muscles; pressure towards the genitals, especially when walking, or after walking;

dragging, aching pain in the back, also from the abdomen to the thighs. It is also adapted to the dyspeptic symptoms which frequently accompany this complaint, as sense of weight at the stomach-pit, flatulence, constipa tion, oppression, and desire to lie down; to the nervous irritation and prostration, as well as to the spasmodic and periodical symptoms frequently accompanying severe cases. *Nux vomica* and *Calcarea* are most useful when the menses are too profuse.

DOSE.—One drop of the dilution, or six globules, in six spoonfuls of water; give a spoonful every two hours in acute cases, in other cases, daily at three o'clock in the afternoon.

SECALE CORNUTUM is indicated in prolonged bearing down and forcing pains, urging towards the genital organs, with profuse menstruation; depression; lowness of spirits, and thoughts of suicide.

DOSE.—One drop of the dilution, or six globules, in ten spoonfuls of water; give a spoonful every four or six hours in extreme cases; continue it afterwards daily for some weeks, unless its primary symptoms should appear, when all medication may be suspended.

SEPIA.—Menses variable, or occurring before the time, the flow being interrupted; with loss of appetite; nausea; constipation; and heat in the womb; pains in the back and abdomen, slight, but much increased by exercise; constant desire to pass water; pressure as if the contents of the stomach would fall out, the patient crossing the legs frequently as if to prevent it; applicable to women of feeble and delicate frame, sensitive skin, nervous habits, and weak but not relaxed muscular fibres, easily strained; also if there is a yellowish leucorrhœa, with itchings and eruptions.

DOSE.—The same as *Aurum.*

There are many other remedies applicable to cases of prolapsus, as Kreosote, Mercurius, Platina, Conium, Stannum, &c., for the indications of which see their patho. genesis, or consult a homœopathic physician. Much advantage may at times be derived from a properly adjusted supporter, provided it be not worn too long, or too constantly; whilst the injudicious application is always productive of injury, often of serious magnitude. There are also many cases of prolapsus in which rest in a recumbent posture, generally on the back, with the limbs flexed upward towards the abdomen, and the hips elevated, should be positively enjoined; yet, in many chronic cases, such a requirement, often insisted on by a certain class of practitioners, would be absolutely inju. rious, and retard the cure. Of circumstances of this nature, it requires skill and wisdom to form a correct judgment, and a thoroughly educated physician should always be consulted.

Swelling or Enlargement of the Womb. — Tympanites of the Womb. (*Physometra.*)

The cavity of the womb is occasionally distended with air, in which case, a manifest enlargement may be perceived at the lower portion of the abdomen, with sensations of fulness or bloatedness, and often attended with hysteria. If the air is secreted from the vessels of the womb itself, it may escape with a noise perceptible to the patient; if it arise from the decomposition of some substance within the womb, as from portions of the placenta, or the menstrual fluid being retained within the cavity, or from similar causes, it will only subside when the exciting cause shall have been removed, either by resolution, or by a discharge of the offensive substance.

The remedies which have been used, are Lycopodium, and Phosphoric acid. Some have also recommended injections into the womb of pure luke-warm water. The expediency of such applications, may well be doubted. If resorted to, it should be by the directions of an experienced physician, and after due consideration.

The above remedies may be used alone, or in alternation.

DOSE.—One drop, or six globules, in four spoonfuls of water, a spoonful to be given every six hours, until the symptoms subside; afterwards every twenty-four hours, until recovery.

Dropsy of the Womb. (*Hydrometra.*)

In simple dropsy of the womb, there are usually present, such symptoms as indigestion, nausea, vomiting, flatulence, weight or tension in the abdomen, especially in the lower portion, frequently costiveness, slow fever, and painfulness. There may be a constant dropping, or oozing of a serous fluid through the vagina, or it may escape in gushes, or if the mouth of the womb be closed by any cause, as adhesive inflammation, or hardened mucus, the fluid may be retained within the cavity of the womb, giving rise to great distension of its walls, and of the abdomen. It is often difficult to distinguish from pregnancy, many of the symptoms of which, it frequently simulates, and during the period of which, it may also occur. If, on a careful examination, however, it be certain that pregnancy does not exist, and if the suffused fluid be retained within the cavity of the uterus, it may be easily drawn off with a catheter, after which, the administration of the proper remedies will generally be found to perfect a cure.

If it occur during pregnancy, the abdomen will be found to enlarge much faster than usual, or to attain an undue size; other parts of the body, as the lower limbs and even the face and hands may become œdematous;

inconveniencies naturally resulting from enlargement of the abdomen, such as difficulty of walking, and sense of oppression, even causing the patient to pass her nights in a chair, may be experienced; the patient suffers from unusual debility; there may be cough and constipation; excessive vomitings; even uterine contractions and watery discharges from the vagina before labor. The prognosis is much more favorable to the mother than to the life of the infant. If it survive in such cases it is mostly pale and feeble.

Another form of serous exudation from the womb, sometimes occurs after delivery. There is, in place of the lochia, a discharge, at first like dirty water, after a day or two becoming more clear, and soaking through all the clothing if it be profuse. It more commonly occurs in patients who are languid, relaxed, of lymphatic constitution, and feeble.

The above forms of dropsy are efficaciously treated by homœopathy. All errors in diet must be corrected, and the constitutional condition of the patient must be carefully considered.

Remedies will be found in Aconite, Apis mel., Arsenicum, Bryonia, China, Calcarea, Ignatia, Nux vomica, Pulsatilla, Secale, Sepia and sulphur.

ACONITE in the commencement may often be useful, or in alternation with *Calcarea, Pulsatilla,* or *Sulphur,* when these remedies are indicated.

DOSE.—One drop of the dilution, or six globules, in six spoonfuls of water, a spoonful every four hours, or every eight hours, will often be sufficient to modify the case, and promote a favorable change.

APIS MEL., if there be suppression of the customary urinary discharges; pale watery urine; or profuse urination with œdema, either general or local, whether of the

56

abdomen face or extremities, will be found a useful and reliable remedy.

DOSE.—It may be given the same as *Aconite*, and should be continued for four or eight days, unless a change should sooner be observed, when it may be followed by *Arsenicum*, if necessary.

ARSENICUM, for symptoms similar to *Apis mel.*, accompanied with weakness; desire and inability to lie down; sense of suffocation; scanty and thick urine; also frequently after *Nux vomica* and *Pulsatilla*, when those remedies have been indicated.

DOSE.—The same as for *Apis mel.*

BRYONIA is adapted to cases in which there is difficulty of breathing, or shortness of breath; vomitings; cough, with oppression; pain in the hypochondria; enlargement of the liver or spleen; constipation; for plethoric persons with dark hair and eyes, or for meagre, hypochondriacal, nervous persons, of dark complexion, with chronic hepatic complaints.

DOSE.—The same as *Apis mel.*

CALCAREA CARB.—For weak, cachectic, exhausted subjects, with tendency to scrofulosis, and for persons of lymphatic constitutions, with loose, flabby muscles, and copious mucus or menstrual discharges, subject even when in health to leucorrhœa, or blenorrhœa, *Calcarea* is especially adapted, to restore the general health, and incite a healthy action; and after the more prominent symptoms have been subdued by other remedies.

DOSE.—One drop of the dilution, or six globules, in a spoonful of water, may be given every morning four days, afterwards leaving its action undisturbed two weeks, when the condition of the patient should be considered anew, and other remedies may be selected. It may often follow *Pulsatilla*.

CHINA.—When the effusion has been the result of debility, or loss of fluids, hæmorrhages, or mucus discharges; or has occurred after severe acute diseases, in which *China* or *Quinia* has not been given as a medicine, (in which case give *Bryonia* or *Arsenicum ;*) or if it is the effect of want of nourishment, or the result of indigestion, dyspepsia, &c., the skin being of a yellow color, or loose and flabby.　•

DOSE.—One drop of the dilution, or six globules, in ten spoonfuls of water, give a spoonful every four hours two days, afterwards every night and morning four days, then wait its effects.

IGNATIA.—If it has been produced by grief, or by concealed anxiety, for sensitive, nervous persons, subject to melancholy, hysteria, dysmenorrhœa, chlorosis, or dyspepsia, with scanty menstruation, and weakness of the sexual organization.

DOSE.—The same as *China.*

NUX VOMICA.—When hepatic affections have been the producing cause, may be given after or in alternation with *Bryonia;* also if there is constipation; frequent or difficult urination, or frequent urgent desire; difficulty of digestion, or gastric affections, with vomitings after eating; adapted to sanguineous, choleric temperaments, as *Ignatia* is also to dry, nervous, melancholic, hysterical subjects.

DOSE.—One drop of the dilution, or six globules, in four spoonfuls of water, give a spoonful every three hours, commencing at three o'clock in the afternoon. If in alternation, *Bryonia* may be given in the morning, *Nux vomica* in the afternoon.

PULSATILLA is a valuable remedy in all the different forms of dropsy, being adapted to mild and easy temperaments, to persons of amiable, inoffensive dispositions, who often weep, but are seldom angry, and who are subject to leucorrhœa, and if the bowels are not costive, but generally relaxed, *Calcarea carb.* should often follow *Pulsatilla.*

DOSE.—The same as *Apis mel.*

SECALE is adapted rather to the physiological and pathological conditions upon which hydrometra is dependent, than to the serous exudations or the dropsical condition of the womb itself. It is adapted to lymphatic, relaxed, languid subjects, where excessive tendencies to hæmorrhage exist ; where there is want of contractile muscular power ; abdomen excessively inflated and distended ; frequent, loose, perhaps slimy or involuntary evacuations, or having a putrid smell ; urine suppressed or scanty, hot and burning, or clear like water ; with burning and shooting pains in the abdomen, epigastrium and limbs.

DOSE.—One drop of the dilution, or six globules, in ten spoonfuls of water, give a spoonful every four hours two days. It is suitable after *Apis mel.*, *Bryonia* or *Nux vomica*, and should often be followed by *Calcarea carb.*

SEPIA may be useful after *Pulsatilla*, for persons of weak constitution, tender and delicate skin ; subject to herpetic eruptions, with burning itchings ; or to brownish or liver-colored spots ; or to lassitude, or paroxysms of weakness, with distention of the abdomen as if it would burst ; urine turbid or dark, or fetid, with white sediment. The pains are generally shooting, pricking or burning, with jerkings and paralysis.

DOSE.—The same as *Secale.*

SULPHUR may be given at the close of the treatment, or during the progress of the disease, especially to persons of psoric tendencies, long subject to itchings, or eruptive diseases of the skin ; waterbrash, or dyspeptic conditions, with indigestion and gripings, aggravated by eating and drinking, but mitigated by bending forwards ; and especially when *Nux vomica* or *Bryonia* have been indicated and afforded partial relief.

DOSE·—One drop of the dilution, or six globules, in a spoonful of water, every morning.

For removing the effused fluid, the remedies most appropriate are generally Apis mel., Arsenicum, Bryonia, Pulsatilla. For the early treatment, Aconite and Sulphur, and sometimes Secale; for the constitutional dyscrasias, Calcarea, Nux vomica, Sepia and Sulphur.

REGIMEN.—See Dropsy, page 576.

Inflammation of the Ovaries. (*Ovaritis.*)

This is not an uncommon affection, and may result from a variety of causes. It is no doubt, one of the fruitful sources of dysmenorrhea. It may be generally recognised by pain more or less acute, on one or both sides, along the groins, or in front of the hips. The pain may be shooting, burning, aching, or throbbing. If the inflammation be attended with tumefaction, a circumscribed swelling may often be perceived by examination through the walls of the abdomen; or at other times, if a careful examination be made through the walls of the vagina, or the rectum, a small, hard tumor or gland is detected with the finger, moving easily within the pelvis.

In connection with the above symptoms, there are sometimes itchings or burnings in the private parts, gastric affections, headache, constipation, diminished urinary secretions, fever, and often derangement of the whole nervous system. It is frequently subacute or chronic, coming on insidiously, and accompanied by various derangements of the general health.

REMEDIES.—The most useful remedies are, Apis mellifica, Antimonium crud., Arsenicum, Belladonna, Cantharis, Cannabis, Cocculus, Conium, Graphites, Hepar sulph., Iodium, Kali carbonica, Lachesis, Nux vomica, Phosphorus, Pulsatilla, Sepia, and Sulphur.

56*·

APIS MELLIFICA is indicated, if the pains are stinging and burning, the urinary secretion much affected, and especially in dropsy of the ovaries, the tumefaction being excessive, and urination scanty.

DOSE.—One drop of the dilution, or six globules, in four spoonfuls of water; give a spoonful every four hours two days, afterwards, every night and morning.

ARSENICUM also, in ovarian dropsy, or in ovaritis with burning pains, and in patients subject to chronic eruptions, if there be sensations of weakness and faintness, either with profuse menses, or with almost entire suppression.

DOSE.—The same as for *Apis mellifica.*

CANTHARIS more especially, for the most severe, burning pains in the ovarian region, extending into the thighs, with cutting pains when passing water, or after *Arsenicum,* when that remedy has only alleviated the symptoms.

DOSE.—A drop of the dilution, or six globules, in four spoonfuls of water, give a spoonful every four hours, four doses; afterwards, give a dose every morning four days, or until another remedy be selected.

GRAPHITES.—Tensive or drawing pains in the region of the ovaries; swelling of the ovaries; sensation as if everything were forced downwards towards the private parts; menses slow, scanty, pale, or suppressed; during the menses, violent, cutting pains, headache, nausea, weakness, and swelling of the cheeks; immoderate expulsion of fetid wind, with pinchings, and cramp-like pains. Also if there are flushes of heat in the face; livid circle around the eyes; eruptions on the face, as if the skin were raw; and especially if the dryness and burnings, the diminution of sexual desires, &c., indicate induration, with loss of function, *Graphites* will often be found a valuable remedy.

DOSE.—One drop of the dilution, or six globules, in six spoonfuls of water, give a spoonful every four hours. In chronic cases, give a drop of the dilution, or six globules, in a spoonful of water, once a day, for one week, then omit one week, and return again to *Graphites.*

HEPAR SULPHUR, when with the pains in the ovarian region, there is profuse menstruation, with disposition to herpetic eruptions, and to suppurations. Also, for similar symptoms, *Lycopodium*, and especially if there be obstinate constipation, and much rumbling of wind in the abdomen, tympanites, &c.

DOSE.—Of either of the above remedies, the same as for *Graphites*.

IODIUM, also, for dropsical ovaritis; and when there is extensive tumefaction; in scrofulous subjects; and if the menses be profuse.

DOSE—One drop, or six globules, in four spoonfuls of water, give a spoonful every four hours, for one month ; if no change, give *Arsenicum* or *Apis mellifica*, and afterwards return again to *Iodium*, if necessary.

KALI CARB. — Also when accompanied by gastric affections; the menses being too feeble and too frequent; corrosive, with itching, gnawing, and burning sensations.

DOSE.—The same as *Graphites*.

KREOSOTUM, when at each monthly period, burning pains are felt, most severe in the thighs, but also, in one or both ovaries; with constipation.

DOSE.—The same as *Arsenicum*.

LACHESIS ought to be found useful in ovaritis, and is indicated by tumefactions, with pressive pains; hysterical affections, especially the globus hysteria; menses feeble, tardy, and of short duration; pains from the ovary to the uterus; spasms, colic, cuttings, &c., before and during the menses; pains in the small of the back, and a sensation in the hips, as if broken; pains like labor pains; pressure in the stomach; nausea and eructations; more especially if the affection be of a phlegmonous character, affecting the interior coatings of the ovaries, and fallopian tubes; and if all the sufferings are worse after sleep.

DOSE.—The same as for *Apis mel.*

Dropsy of the Ovaries.   (*Hydrops Ovaries.*)

Ovarian dropsy usually commences with an uneasy sensation in one side of the abdomen, near the hip, or the groin; there may be a sense of pressure or weight; numbness; irregularity of the menses, irritation in the region of the bladder; scanty secretion of urine; or frequent urgent desire to urinate; nausea and fainting. There is also irregular enlargement of the abdomen; constipation and hemorrhoids are common; and frequently sympathetic pain or distension of the breast; swelling of the feet, or one foot, and Hysteria, are attendant symptoms.

In general, if the above symptoms prevail, and if there is a sense of numbness in the thigh, on the affected side, we will be safe to conclude that the ovary is affected, although no tumor can yet be felt in the abdomen; but if while the above symptoms are present, we can plainly distinguish a circumscribed tumor in the lower portion of the abdomen, generally near the hip, moveable, the size and general appearance of which, is not affected by a change of position, there is left no reasonable doubt of the existence of an ovarian tumor, the nature of which must be learned from the general condition of the patient, and would require a kind of knowledge not attainable from a work on domestic practice.

The remedies are the same as those given for hydrometra. (See page 648.) The pathogenic indications also are nearly the same. (See also Ovaritis, page 653.)

Inflammation of the Labia and Vagina.

Inflammation of the labia is attended with a painful, burning, hard, dry, and red swelling of the labia; very sensitive to the touch. It is at times caused by the rupture of the hymen; at times it is the result of difficult labor; or it may arise from cold, and similar causes. If from mechanical cause, give Arnica, one drop of the dilution, or six globules, in ten spoonfuls of water, a spoonful every four hours, and apply a lotion of ten parts of the tincture in one hundred parts of pure water, with which bathe the parts night and morning freely, and the inflammation will speedily subside.

If the inflammation be the result of a cold, to patients subject to phlegmonous or other erysipelatous affections give *Rhus tox.* as directed for *Arnica*, omiting the lotion; and for scrofulous subjects, with glandular affections, if it does not speedily yield to *Rhus tox.* give *Mercurius* in the same manner; or *Belladonna* instead of *Rhus tox.*, may at times be most efficient, when a pressing, bearing down pain is complained of, with fulness and sense of weight.

DOSE.—Of *Rhus tox.* or *Belladonna*, the same as *Arnica*, omiting the lotion in case of *Belladonna*.

Pregnancy.

This may truly be said to be the most interesting, as well as the most responsible period in the life of woman. At this moment commences a connection between herself and her offspring, a connection so close, so intimate, and so inseparable, that her health becomes its health, her life its life, and her happiness its happiness. Even its mind, its disposition, its habits, its loves and its hates, are now being formed by her own, so that it may be said to reflect her image, to be modeled after her likeness, or to be cast in the mould which her hand has made. It is not her actions merely, her feelings, her impulses, her emotions, form into beauty or stamp with deformity, not the mind alone but also the body, the physical conformation of her future offspring.

It is the duty of the mother, therefore, at this period, to pay all proper attention to herself, and a duty which has always been due to herself alone, is now rendered every way imperative by her obligations to her children, to her husband, and to the world.

These duties are naturally divided into two classes, physical and mental.

The physical duties or obligations embrace the subjects of diet, exercise, dress, and care of health, each of which will be considered in order.

The diet should be simple, purely nutritious, generous but not excessive, and all stimulants should be perfectly discarded. Nothing can be more detrimental to life than the use of poisonous drugs during this interesting period. Coffee, wine, pepper, spices, spiced meat, sausages, &c., &c., cannot but exert their baneful influence at such a period when all the newly formed and delicate organs are most susceptible to impressions. But the diet should be generous, good meats daily, (once a day is sufficient,) bread, milk and vegetables, with ripe and rich fruits, will always be found sufficient for persons whose taste has not already become depraved, and for those who have, it is not possible for books to place any limit to their depravity. If some ladies indulge in deleterious drugs, spices, &c., others will no doubt indulge in wines, brandy, ardent spirits, opium, &c.; and others again in other forms of excitement, the names of which would fill a volume, and the deleterious influences of which can never be numbered or computed.

Exercise.

This is absolutely necessary during the period of pregnancy to the enjoyment of health. Passive exercise, such as riding in a carriage, is not alone sufficient. It is a mistake also to suppose that laborious avocations are inconsistent with the healthy development of the child or the condition of the mother. It is only necessary first that the labor should not be irksome; second, that it should not be too long continued after it becomes fatiguing; and third, that it should not expose to sudden strains, as in lifting or reaching, or to jars or falls, as in jumping, &c. A person in this condition falls much more frequently or from slighter cause than at other times, and a fall is attended with manifold greater danger. In addition however to the usual exercise of accustomed labors, exercise should be taken regularly in the open air for amusement and enjoyment. Exercise then should be of two kinds, first for labor, and second for enjoyment; but the one is not sufficient without the other; riding on horseback would be to most women inadmissible; in a carriage would more frequently be admissible, but walking for pleasure in the open air is peculiarly healthful, especially in the morning.

Dress.

This should be free and open. No part of the dress should be tight, or girt about the body. The limbs should also be free, and every thing that invests them sufficiently loose to give free action to the blood. Even small shoes which pinch the feet should not be worn, and the garter should not be drawn too tightly. Artificial supports should be avoided, and the muscles generally allowed full play. Strings drawn too tightly around the waist may induce club feet and other deformities in the child, and perhaps prolapsus uteri, or other displacements, or lingering and protracted labors on the part of the mother.

The dress should always be adapted to the season, and care should be taken to avoid catching cold.

Care of Health.

Every proper attention should now be given to this important particular, the preservation of health.

The mother should not allow herself to be sick. The various ailments she will be told by other women are inseparable from her condition, she should be taught to regard as contrary to nature, and demanding immediate relief. She should early consult some experienced and well educated physician, and listen implicitly to his councils, avoiding all old wives' fables, and especially should she never take any doses of any kind of drugs, any opening laxative or cathartic medicines. Magnesia, oil, senna, salts, paregoric, camphor, &c., &c., including every article brought from the apothecary should always be absolutely prohibited. They weaken the natural powers of the mother, excite undue irritations, and often materially affect the health, and even the life of her offspring, and may be the source of many of the so called hereditary diseases.

Of the Mental Habits.

It has already been remarked, that the habits of mind, the impulses and emotions of the mother, at this period, will influence her offspring. This is true to the highest possible degree. It will mould the features, and give form and symmetry to the body, as well as convey its impress to the mind, and stamp the character.

It is the duty of the mother then, to cultivate proper intellectual habits. Her own mind should have previously received its education, its training, that she may have sources from which to draw images of beauty, and scenes of delight; and she should endeavor to keep it not crammed, but properly supplied with such beautiful images, combined as they are in nature, with useful objects. The mind should not now be severely taxed. It should rather be unbent, and in some degree relaxed. Yet it should be employed, usefully, actively, happily; and this employment will contribute to the intellectual, as well as physical conformation of her offspring. A state of indolence and imbecility, either of mind or body, is never to be admitted.

Unsightly and unpleasant objects, should not be seen, or if seen, the mind should not be permitted to dwell upon them. Brooding over unpleasant impressions can scarcely fail of being both physically and mentally injurious.

Not only intellectually, but morally and socially, the habits and condition of the mind of the mother, are important to the character of her child. If the beautiful and the true should engage her attention, the pure and the good should enliven and enkindle her heart. She should be and feel, during this interesting period, just as she would wish her son or her daughter to be and feel. By the unalterable decree of the Divinity, impressions indulged by the mother during this period, as they are received by her own highly impressible and delicate organization, are conveyed from each of those organs, to the corresponding organs of the child she bears, and she is thus forming, for good or for evil, for virtue or for vice, one who is hereafter to be her happiness or misery, her honor or her repoach. Enough has been said upon this delicate subject. Let her feelings be good and pure, as

57

her thoughts are beautiful and true. Her sons shall sit among nobles, and her daughters among princesses.

The mind should also be guarded against despondency, uneasiness about the future, or depression of spirits. Some females, whose spirits are generally good, suffer much from depression during this period, or while nursing. If, notwithstanding good resolutions, and proper mental efforts, the feeling becomes irresistible, one of the following remedies will generally be found useful.

ACONITE, for despondency, preceded by excitement, the skin being hot, and the pulse frequent, with presentiment of approaching death.

BRYONIA, if the inequietude and fear of the future, be attended with irrascibility and gastric derangement.

CALCAREA CARBONICA.—Excessive dejection, great lassitude; also, when there is suppression of the secretions, obesity and plethora; and in persons predisposed to consumption.

NATRUM MURIATICUM.—Melancholy, with weeping; uneasiness about the future; and for obstinate cases, not yielding to *Nux vomica.*

NUX VOMICA.—Morning sickness and melancholy; great uneasiness; impaired appetite; constipation; fretfulness.

CHINA.—Lowness of spirits during the nursing period, when the energies of the mother appear to be too severely taxed; or when nursing is continued too long; or from rearing twins; also, *Aurum, Lachesis,* or *Pulsatilla,* may at times be found useful.

DOSE and Administration.—Any of the above remedies may be given, one drop of the dilution, or six globules, in a spoonful of water, every night and morning, until alleviation or change.

The practice of bleeding, so prevalent for a long time, and among some of the less enlightened of old school physicians even to the present time, for plethora, sensations of fulness, and tendency to congestions, which usually attend pregnancy, is in all cases to be avoided. It is always positively injurious. It diminishes the patient's strength, renders her more liable to miscarriages, floodings, convulsions, and nervous affections, and is besides, not unfrequently an injury to the child. It saps the fountains from whence it draws its support, changes the natural healthy current of life, diverting it into other channels; and increases the liability to irritation afterwards both with the mother and child.

Continued Menstruation

When menstruation continues during pregnancy, certainly if beyond the first month, it is to be regarded as a deviation from nature's law, and should receive medical aid. Remedies may usually be found by consulting the article Menorrhagia, or if a sanguineous mucus discharge be attended with severe spasmodic pains low down in the abdomen, give Cocculus, or if there be a copious dark viscid discharge, give Crocus.

PLATINA, for profuse discharge, with severe bearing down pains.

PHOSPHORUS.—Cutting pains in the back, with occasional vomiting, attended with discharge of blood.

ADMINISTRATION.—Administer the remedies in water during the periods of suffering, one drop of the dilution, or six globules, in ten spoonfuls of water; give a spoonful every half hour, until the severe symptoms are alleviated, afterwards every four hours, until the alleviation becomes perfect; afterwards give two powders of *Sulphur*, and wait till the next monthly period.

Vertigo and Headache

Another derangement not uncommon to this period is vertigo or giddiness, with sense of fulness and pain in the head, frequently accompanied by dulness, lightness, and a disinclination to employment; sleepiness, or at times sleeplessness ; dimness of sight; sparks before the eyes ; disposition to fall forwards, often when stooping; headache, with a feeling of weight on the top of the head or back of the neck; palpitations, nervous tremblings, &c. These symptoms are usually worse in the morning. They often commence as early as the fourth week.

REMEDIES.—Aconite, Belladonna, Nux vomica, Opium, Platina, Pulsatilla and Sulphur.

ACONITE, for plethoric persons, of florid complexion, and nervous temperament; if there be giddiness, as if intoxicated on rising from a seat, or faintness and dim-ness of sight on rising from the bed; pressure in the forehead; stupifying pains; eyes red and sparkling; intolerance of light; black spots before the eyes.

BELLADONNA.—Congestion to the head, with stagger-ing and trembling; buzzing in the ears, cannot bear a noise : heavy pressive pains on the top of the head, and in the forehead over the eyes ; expansive pains; violent throbbings; redness and soreness of the face and eyes; sparks before the eyes ; double vision; worse in the morning.

DOSE.—One drop of the dilution of either of the above remedies, or six globules, in ten spoonfuls of water, a spoonful to be given every four hours, until amelioration or change.

NUX VOMICA.—For females of a hasty temper, or of sedentary habits; or for those who use wine or coffee; giddiness or confusion in the head, with cloudiness of sight, and buzzing in the ears; tearing, drawing or jerking pains, or periodical pains; worse in the morn. ing, and better in the open air; constipation; insipid, or acid, bitter, or putrid taste.

DOSE.—One drop of the dilution, or six globules, in ten spoonfuls of water, a spoonful every two hours, each afternoon, for four days; give a powder of *Sulphur* in the morning afterwards; if no relief be afforded, select some other remedy.

OPIUM.—Giddiness, with stupidity; drowsiness; imperfect sleep; puffed face, and thick, heavy breathing; illusions of the senses.

DOSE.—The same as *Belladonna.*

PLATINA.—Gradually increasing headache, until becoming violent it diminishes as gradually; headache produced by vertigo or by passion; constant disposition to spit, with tasteless or sweetish saliva; for nervous or hysterical females; symptoms worse during rest, relieved by movement.

DOSE.—The same as *Belladonna.*

PULSATILLA.—Giddiness, worse after stooping, with transient blindness, and staggering; throbbing, shooting pains; one-sided headache, worse every other day, often attended with numbness of the limbs; worse afternoon, and evening, better in the morning.

DOSE.—The same as *Nux vomica.*

SULPHUR.—Congestion of blood, pulsative pains, and sensation of heat in the head; vertigo when seated, and after a meal, also with nausea at times, and fainting; weakness and bleeding at the nose; confusion in the head; difficulty of thinking, worse morning and evening. One-sided headache, or occupying the top or the back of the head, or the forehead over the eyes, with dimness of sight; aggravated by movement, walking in the open air, and by meditation; periodical or inter-·

mittent headaches, worse morning or evening, or at night.

DOSE.—One drop of the dilution, or six globules, in ten spoonfuls of water, a spoonful every four hours, for two days, then every twelve hours for the succeeding two days, or until some other remedy shall be chosen.

Morning Sickness.

Nausea, vomiting, heartburn, and other gastric disturbances, are the most common, and the most troublesome acccompaniments of pregnancy. They commence about five or six weeks after conception, and continue until the sixteenth week, when they usually cease. In some cases, however, they continue with slight modifications, to the end of gestation. They usually occur on rising in the morning, and are often troublesome, for two or three hours, sometimes they return in the evening.

The remedies are Arsenicum, Ipecacuanha, Natrum mur., Nux vomica, Phosphorus, and Pulsatilla.

ARSENICUM will be useful for vomiting after eating or drinking, with fainting, emaciation and weakness.

IPECACUANHA.— Also if there is great uneasiness about the stomach; vomiting of drink, and undigested food, or of bile, bowels loose or relaxed.

NARTUM MUR.—Obstinate cases with loss of appetite; waterbrash; pain and soreness at the pit of the stomach.

NUX VOMICA.—Especially if the nausea occur while eating, or immediately afterwards; acid and bitter risings; hiccough; sense of weight at the pit of the stomach; constipation; irritability.

PHOSPHORUS and MAGNESIA, if *Arsenicum* fail in cases where it is indicated.

PULSATILLA, for symptoms similar to *Nux vomica*, especially when there is craving for acids, wine, &c.,

with whitish coated tongue, and instead of constipation, diarrhœa, or alternations of each.

ADMINISTRATION.—Give of the selected remedy, morning and evening, for three days. If not better select some other remedy.

Where diarrhœa accompanies morning sickness, give first Ipecacuanha; if not relieved, or if the cure be partial, follow it with Arsenicum, and afterwards give Natrum mur., or Phosphorus, if necessary.

If constipation accompany, give first Nux vomica, to be followed, after four days, by Sulphur, and if the cure be not perfect, by Natrum mur., or Magnesia. To ladies who have always been subject to scanty menstruation, give Pulsatilla.

Constipation.

When this affection cannot be relieved by exercise; by drinking a full draught of cold water on retiring at night, and on rising in the morning; by eating fruit, or similar means, take a dose of Nux vomica at three o'clock in the afternoon, and another at bed time, every other day, for one week; if relief is obtained give Sulphur, one dose in the morning, four successsive ·days, and await the result. If not relieved, give Lycopodium, four doses each day, for four days, say night and morning, ten o'clock, and four o'clock; or give Bryonia, Ignatia, or Opium, the same as Lycopodium. (See Constipation, page 212.)

Diarrhœa

Occurs less frequently during pregnancy than constipation, and is more dangerous. If allowed to continue, the health must suffer, and serious consequences may follow.

REMEDIES.—If the tongue is coated white, and the evacuations are watery, the stomach also being affected, Antimonium crud., or Tartar emetic, will often be sufficient. Mercurius, if the discharge is greenish, with straining and tenesmus. Phosphorus often in extreme cases, and after Antimonium. Pulsatilla, Sepia, and Sulphur, will also be found useful. (See Diarrhœa, page 219.)

DOSE.—Give one drop, or six globules, of the selected remedy in a spoonful of water, every four hours, until a change is manifest, or another remedy is indicated.

Itchings. (*Pruritis.*)

Women are not unfrequently annoyed during this period by a troublesome itching of the private parts. It may be occasioned by a vitiated condition of the secretions, or by an eruption resembling the thrush of infants; or the parts may assume a dark, red color, with excoriations, and oozing of a thin, watery secretion, attended with intolerable itchings. It is not confined to the period of pregnancy.

TREATMENT.—The parts should be frequently cleansed by ablution in water. A solution of borax in water, is also often of service. A cloth wet with cold water, and applied to the parts on going to bed at night, the whole being closely covered with canton flannel, or some other warm covering, will frequently be useful. Mercurius, Rhus tox. and Sulphur, are the principal remedies.

ADMINISTRATION.—Give *Rhus tox.*, one drop, or six globules, in ten spoonfuls of water, a spoonful every four hours, and on the following morning give *Sulphur*, one dose.

If the case be of the apthous variety, this treatment may be followed by *Mercurius*.

DOSE and Administration.—The same as *Rhus tox.*, and afterwards give *Sulphur*.

If this course does not relieve, consult Pruritus, page 355.

Fainting and Hysteric Fits

Are not uncommon, nor are they particularly dangerous if properly attended to. Attention to diet, exercise, and air, will often prevent them; if not, trace the cause if possible, and remove it. Tight lacing, the use of stimulants, warm rooms, &c., would be sufficient cause. If called suddenly to a case, admit fresh air freely, sprinkle the face with cold water, and give a powder of Belladonna. Afterwards, administer the remedies as indicated in other parts of this work, (see Hysteria,) or give Aconite if there be full pulse, plethoric habits, and sanguineous congestion to the head or chest; and Belladonna, especially to females who have been troubled with profuse menses, and if there is fulness about the head, with flushed face.

COFFEA, for nervous females, with agitation, abdominal spasms, difficult breathing, and cold sweats.

CHINA, when there has been loss of blood, hemorrhage, weakness, &c.

CHAMOMILLA, if caused by anger.

IGNATIA, for severe headache, as if a nail were driven into the head, with melancholy and frequent sighing; and if caused by fright.

NUX VOMICA, for choleric persons, and if attended with derangement of the stomach, nausea, or constipation.

ARSENICUM, PULSATILLA, and SEPIA, are often useful.

DOSE.—Administer the above remedies, usually in water, one drop of the dilution, or six globules, in ten spoonfuls of water, give a spoonful every half hour for four hours; afterwards, every night and morning a dose, for one week. If the fits continue to recur, select some other remedy.

Toothache

Is a very common affection, and can generally be relieved by medicine. If Chamomilla, Mercurius, Nux vomica, or Pulsatilla, do not relieve, consult a physician, or see the article Toothache, page 162. It is not always best to extract hollow or decayed teeth. Fill the cavity with raw cotton, crowding it closely in with some suitable instrument; remove it every hour, and supply its place with another dossil. After the irritation subsides, fill the cavity again with soft white wax, and give the appropriate remedies. Permanent relief will often be obtained.

The cavities of hollow teeth, should always be kept perfectly clean, and all the decayed portions should frequently be scraped off with some suitable instrument; the mouth, teeth, and gums, should be well washed in the morning and at night, in cold water, also, after meals; the finger or a piece of cotton cloth forms a sufficient tooth-brush.

Pains in the Back and Side during Pregnancy.

This is also a common affection; more frequently in the right side, under the ribs, or in the small of the back, or near the hips; an indescribable, aching pain, or a dull heavy pressure, as if caused by a dead weight resting on the part. These pains are sometimes very severe; they may be sharp and cutting, or burning,—generally worse from the fifth to the eighth month. For the pains in the back, Kali carbonicum will generally be found efficacious; if insufficient, give Bryonia; if worse on movement, Rhus toxicodendron; if aggravated by rest, Belladonna, or Pulsatilla; to feeble, scrofulous persons, Nux vomica, or

Sepia, or Sulphur, and if complicated with hæmorrhoids, or in case of constipation.

For pains in the side, Aconite, Chamomilla, Phosphorus, or Pulsatilla.

DOSE.—Of the selected remedy, give one drop, or six globules, in ten spoonfuls of water, a spoonful every four hours, two days; if no relief is obtained, select some other remedy.

Cramps,

In the legs, abdomen, hips, or back, are very frequent, and very annoying.

REMEDIES.—For cramps in the legs, Calcarea carbonica, Chamomilla, Colocynth., Graphites, Hyoscyamus, Nux vomica, or Sulphur. For those of the back, Ignatia, Opium, and Rhus toxicodendron; and Belladonna, Colocynthis, Hyoscyamus, Nux vomica, and Pulsatilla, for those of the abdomen.

DOSE and Administration.—The same as for pains in the back, &c.

Incontinence of Urine.

Frequent desire to pass water, or total inability to retain it, will generally be relieved by Pulsatilla. If not give Belladonna, or China, Silicea or Stramonium.

ADMINISTRATION.—Give four doses of the selected remedy, either dry or in solution, at intervals of four hours. If not better, select another remedy.

Hæmorrhoids or Piles,

May occur during pregnancy when the persons are not at other times liable to it, on account of some obstruction to the circulation. Nux vomica, will generally, in such cases, afford relief. If the pains extend high up, with itching and crawling in the parts, Ignatia should be given; also, if the bowels protrude greatly at each evacuation. If there be much bleeding, give

Aconite, Arnica, Belladonna, Hamamelis virg., and Sulphur, either in alternation or succession, or according to their respective symptoms, until the bleeding subsides. If the discharge be great, and the patient become very weak, give China.

ADMINISTRATION.—Give one drop of a dilution, or six globules, in ten spoonfuls of water, a spoonful every hour in extreme cases, in others every six hours, until relief is afforded.

Swelling of the Veins. Varicose Veins. Varicose Tumors.

This is an affection also to which many females are subject. It usually commences about the ankle, and extends upward towards the thigh. This swelling may involve all the veins of one or both limbs, or it may be confined to those below the knee, or it may appear in circumscribed tumors, generally of a bluish color, and all the veins implicated usually present an uneven knotted appearance. When the patient stands the swelling generally increases, and diminishes on lying down. The swelling may at length become very painful, the veins may burst, and large quantities of blood be discharged. After delivery the swelling subsides, and the veins often assume nearly their natural size and color.

Remedies which may be depended on in this affection are Arnica, Hamamelis virg., Nux vomica and Pulsatilla; also Apis mel., Arsenicum, Lachesis and Lycopodium.

ARNICA will almost always be useful at first, and also after the limbs or the veins feel sore, the circulation having been long impeded; *Hamamelis virg.* also the same as *Arnica*, in desperate cases where the bleeding is profuse.

NUX VOMICA, if there is enlargement of the abdomen,

hemorrhoids, constipation, and frequent bearing down pains.

PULSATILLA.—Veins much swollen, with swelling of the limb; and if the parts assume a bluish color, with pain and inflammation.

ARSENICUM and LACHESIS, after *Pulsatilla.* (See article on Varicose Veins.)

Much good will frequently result from bathing the parts frequently in a weak solution of Tincture of Arnica, or with an extract from the Ham. virg. and at times from the application of a bandage or laced stocking; the bandage should be applied when there is the least swelling, commencing at the foot and proceeding upward with a gentle and equal pressure. It is less useful after the swelling has been of long continuance than in more recent cases.

In severe cases the patient should remain in a recumbent posture, or should keep the limb in a horizontal position.

DOSE.—Of any of the indicated remedies, one drop, or six globules, dissolved in half a tumbler of water, give a spoonful every four hours for two days; if no relief is obtained, select another remedy.

Depression of Spirits.

This unhappy state of mind may frequently be alleviated by cheerful conversation, by exercise in the open air, attention to diet, &c.; but when these means fail, recourse must be had to medicines, for which consult the following remedies :

ACONITE, when fear of death and depression from fright are prominent symptoms.

AURUM, if there be desire to die, inclination to weep, anxiety of mind prompting the patient to suicide, despondency, mental weakness, shortness of memory, &c.

BELLADONNA.—Agitation and restlessness at night, with fear of ghosts, or fear with disposition to hide; involuntary laughter or singing, or passion and rage; frightful visions; not disposed to exertion.

PULSATILLA.—Against depression, with sadness and weeping; uneasiness at the pit of the stomach; sleeplessness; oppressed with a multitude of imaginary cares; dislike to conversation; heartburn and headache.

SULPHUR.—Lowness of spirits, with anxiety on religious subjects, and despair of salvation; forgetfulness of names and words, when about to speak them; disposition to anger.

DOSE and Administration.—Of either of the remedies one drop of the dilution, or six globules, in ten spoonfuls of water, give a spoonful every six hours, until amelioration or change.

Flooding. (*Menorrhagia.*)

Either during pregnancy or at delivery. Many of the remedies resorted to in this truly dangerous condition are almost equally dangerous, and even when they appear to give relief are of greater injury than benefit. Long continued applications of cold water produce congestions followed by inflammation, from the effects of which the patient frequently never recovers. Ether, as usually administered, induces to affections of the nervous system. Alum is productive of indurations, and introducing pieces of linen to close up the passage is seldom of benefit. Let the woman lie down quietly, and move as little as possible. Let her mind be kept free from care, and quietness be preserved in the room and in the house. Tie handkerchiefs immediately around the upper part of the thighs and arms, (silk handkerchiefs are to be preferred.) Give a few mouthfuls of cold water, and let the patient hold a mouthful for some little time in her mouth, spitting it carefully upon a hand. kerchief, that she may not be obliged to move even her head. If the face become pale a single drop of brandy or of wine may be administered at a dose until reaction is observed to take place, but not more than three or four doses. A few drops of vinegar applied to the nose, just sufficient that the patient may get the smell of it, may be of service.

REMEDIES.—Arnica, Bryonia, Belladonna, Chamomilla, China, Crocus, Ferrum, Hyoscyamus, Hamamelis virg., Ipecacuanha and Platina.

ARNICA is always indicated if the affection originates in mechanical injury, as a strain, blow, fall, misstep, &c., and may frequently be given with advantage in other cases, especially if there be nausea, shiverings, giddiness, agitation and trembling.

DOSE.—One drop of the dilution, or six globules, in ten spoonfuls of water, give a spoonful every half hour, in desperate cases every fifteen minutes, until relief is afforded. Lengthen the intervals as improvement becomes manifest, and if no improvement take place in from three to six hours, change the remedy. In chronic cases or in those not immediately urgent, the intervals should be from six to twelve hours, and the same remedy continued from two days to two weeks, according to the nature of the case, when if there be no improvement another remedy should be chosen.

BELLADONNA.—When there is pressure as if every thing would fall out from the private parts; pains in the small of the back, as if it would break; pale or flushed face; dulness, heat about the head, thirst, and palpitation of the heart.

BRYONIA.—Great quantities of dark red blood, with violent pressive pain in the small of the back, and headache, particularly in the temples, as if the head would burst; also if attended with constipation.

CHAMOMILLA, when the discharge is accompanied by pains similar to those of labor, or after *Ipecacuanha*, when that remedy has produced little or no improvement.

CHINA, in the most dangerous cases attended with heaviness of the head, or giddiness; loss of consciousness, or drowsiness; sudden weakness; faintness; coldness of the extremities; paleness of the face; convulsions or contortions of the mouth and eyes; or if the face and hands turn blue; or jerks pass through the body; also if the blood escape by starts, with spasms or pains like those of labor passing to the anus, the discharge taking place afresh at every pain; or if accompanied by colic, frequent urging to pass water, and sore tension of the abdomen. It is also serviceable after other remedies for the debility remaining after the flooding has ceased.

FERRUM MET.—Blood alternately black and clotted, or liquid, with pains like those of labor, and red face.

HYOSCYAMUS.—Pains resembling those of labor; with drawings in the thighs, and small of the back, or in the limbs; puffiness of the veins of the hands or face; heats over the whole body, with quick, full pulse; trembling; numbness of the limbs; twitchings and jerkings, alternating with stiffness; loss of consciousness; delirium; darkness or confusion of sight; great uneasiness, or excessive liveliness,

IPECACUANHA is frequently a most valuable remedy, especially if the flooding is very copious, and long continued, with cutting pains around the navel; pressive and bearing down pains; chills, and coldness of the body, or feeling of heat rising into the head; great weakness with inclination to lie down; especially if the above symptoms occur during pregnancy, or after delivery.

HAMAMELIS VIRG. may follow *Arnica* when that has failed, or it may be administered at first, when the flooding is copious, or it may be found useful in most cases, even when other remedies have failed.

PLATINA.—Discharge dark and thick, but not clotted; pain in the back, drawing towards the groin, and a sensation of inward pressure towards the private parts, which are extremely sensitive; and when the flooding has been produced by violent mental emotions.

For long continued menorrhagia, for females of advanced age, who are not pregnant, it is better to avoid all warm drinks, to drink milk which is quite cold, several times a day; cold, sour milk, or buttermilk, if agreeable, and to avoid all stimulating articles of diet, &c.

A drop of tincture of cinnamon, in half a tumbler of water, giving a teaspoonful every fifteen minutes for one or two hours, may often be of use; or a piece of cinnamon may be chewed for a few minutes, if the tincture is not at hand, after which take a piece of loaf-sugar, in the mouth, till the burning caused by the cinnamon subsides, then give *Arnica* or *Hamamelis virg.*, as above directed.

DOSE and Administration.—Of any of the above remedies, the same as above given for *Arnica*.

Miscarriage. Abortion.

Although miscarriage may occur at any period of pregnancy; it is much more common about the third or fourth month. At this period it is not very dangerous, although frequent miscarriages weaken the constitution, and may engender some chronic affection. Miscarriages at a later period are much more serious, and frequently dangerous, and those who have miscar-

58*

ried two or three times are exceedingly liable to do so again.

This event may take place from mechanical injuries, as a blow, fall, &c.; from the use, or rather the abuse of drugs; often from purgative medicines; from excessive exertions; from the too free use of stimulating food or drinks; from exposures to cold, late hours, confined heated air, or want of exercise. The early symptoms are chilliness, followed by fever and bearing down pains; cutting pains in the loins and abdomen, resembling the pains of labor; discharge of mucus and of blood, at times of a red color; at times dark and purple, or clotted, followed by emission of a serous fluid; with this serous discharge the miscarriage usually takes place, and if not checked by appropriate remedies, it may continue for hours and endanger the patient's life. If miscarriage is threatened, the patient should at once be placed in a horizontal position, where she should remain until all the danger has manifestly passed over; and if it has already occurred, she should still retain the same position for several days, until the parts have time to recover somewhat of their natural condition, and all danger from hemorrhage has ceased.

TREATMENT.—The remedies, treatment, &c., are very similar to those for menorrhagia, the indications for which may often be consulted with advantage.

Arnica, Belladonna, Bryonia, Chamomilla, China, Crocus, Ferrum metallicum, Hyoscyamus, Ipecacuanha, Nux vomica, Platina, Sabina and Secale.

ARNICA, in cases of mechanical injury, as a fall, blow, strain, over-lifting, great physical exertion, &c. (See the article Menorrhagia.)

BELLADONNA.—Violent severe bearing down pains

throughout the entire abdomen, as if all its contents would be forced out, and very profuse discharge.

BRYONIA.—For persons of dark complexion, subject to affections of the liver or spleen, and to frequent constipation.

CHAMOMILLA.—If there are periodical pains, like labor pains, each pain being followed by a discharge of dark coagulated blood, or of blood mixed with mucus; also if there are violent pains in the whole abdomen, extending to the sides, with a sensation as if about to evacuate the bowels or the bladder, and especially for irritable persons.

CHINA.—When the patient is weak and exhausted, with giddiness and fainting, or with drowsiness, coldness of the extremities, and loss of consciousness; and after the discharge has been checked by other remedies, it is a valuable aid in restoring the wasted energies of the patient, and promoting a speedy recovery. It is thought to be indicated by discharges which take place at intervals, or by starts with spasmodic bearing down pains.

CROCUS.—Discharge of dark and clotted blood, increased by the least exertion, with a fluttering sensation around the navel; also in protracted cases after other remedies have failed.

FERRUM METALLICUM.—If there be fever, pains like labor pains, with discharge of blood.

HYOSCYAMUS.—Spasms and convulsions of the whole body, with loss of consciousness, discharge of light red blood, mostly worse at night.

IPECACUANHA.—Spasms without loss of consciousness; discharge of bright red blood, profuse and continuous, with pressure downwards; cuttings around the navel; nausea and vomiting; chills and heat, with disposition to faintness.

NUX VOMICA. — For persons of sanguine, irritable temperament, subject to dyspeptic, hepatic and gastric diseases, with constipation and hemorrhoids.

PLATINA.—If attended with drawings in the groins. (See Flooding, page 676.)

SABINA.—If the pains are forcing and dragging, extending to the back and loins; profuse discharge of bright red blood; faint, sinking feeling in the abdomen; diarrhœa, or frequent desire to go to stool; nausea and vomiting, or fever with chilliness and heat.

SECALE CORN.—After miscarriage for feeble, debilitated persons, the discharge consisting of dark liquid blood, and the pains being slight.

DOSE.—Of the selected remedy, one drop, or six globules, in ten spoonfuls of water, give a teaspoonful, every fifteen or twenty minutes in severe cases, in milder ones every two hours, and in the early stages when no danger is apprehended, every six or twelve hours. In milder cases, if relief be not obtained, change the medicines not oftener than once in four or six days, in severer ones every six hours.

Regimen and attendance nearly the same as for Flooding, which see, page 676.

Care of the Breast and Nipples before Confinement.

A proper attention to the breast and nipples before confinement, will often prevent much trouble and suffering afterwards. Whilst the breasts are gradually increasing in size to fit them for their future function, whilst the nipples are gradually enlarging and becoming more prominent, there is also frequently more or less pain and soreness. If at this time they receive no attention, the foundation may be laid for abscesses, tumefactions, excoriations, cracks, inflammations and eruptions, which may require long and careful attention on the part of the physician, as well as much patient endurance on the part of the woman.

For several weeks previous to confinement, the entire breast and chest should receive daily ablutions in water, cold water, if the patient can bear it, if not the chill should be removed and the water applied on retiring at night, and on rising in the morning.

If there be tenderness, soreness, or slight excoriations, bathe also after the ablution in a weak tincture of Arnica, made by dropping ten drops of the tincture in a dessert-spoonful of water, or wet a piece of muslin in water, and after squeezing it until it will not drip, drop on a few drops of Tincture of Arnica, and apply it to the exco-riated surfaces, covering the breasts warmly, on retiring at night, and relief will generally be obtained. For acute pain shooting into the mammæ, Aconite, Belladonna, Bryonia, Chamomilla and Rhus tox. are the principal remedies.

ADMINISTRATION.—One drop of the dilution, or six globules, in ten spoonfuls of water, a spoonful every four hours, until the pains sub-side. See also Abscess of the Breasts.

For swelling, burning, itching, cracks, eruptions, &c., Bryonia, Graphites, Lycopodium, Mercurius, Hepar sulph., Rhus tox. and Sulphur will generally be found sufficient. For their symptomatic indications, see the article Sore Nipples, page 694.

DOSE, and Administration.—The same as above.

False Pains.

Frequently precede the setting in of labor, and are often much more severe and unendurable than true labor pains. In healthy females they precede labor but a few hours, in others they may come on weeks before delivery. They may be distinguished from the true pains of labor by the irregularity of their recurrence, often by their location, whilst they do not regularly increase in intensity like true labor pains, and under the action of appropriate remedies, they will frequently entirely subside. To distinguish between true and false pains may at times be difficult, but it is altogether unnecessary, for the proper administration of the appropriate remedy, whilst it will relieve the false, will also by harmonizing the action of nature's laws, give strength and power to the true and natural pains of labor. The exciting causes of these pains are too numerous to mention in this place.

The remedies are Aconite, Bryonia, Belladonna, Dulcamara, Nux vomica and Pulsatilla.

ACONITE, for young, full, strong, plethoric persons, with full pulse, congestion to the head, flushed face, &c.

BELLADONNA, after *Aconite*, for similar symptoms, and when the pains are spasmodic, and the abdomen very sensitive to the touch.

BRYONIA, especially after a fit of passion, and when the pains in the abdomen are followed or accompanied by dragging pains in the back and loins; constipation; for persons of dark complexion, black hair, and subject to biliary affections; pains aggravated by motion.

DULCAMARA, pains arising from the effects of cold, a chill, or from getting wet,—acute and violent, seated in the small of the back, coming on or aggravated at night.

NUX VOMICA, pains similar to those of *Bryonia*, for persons of a more sanguine character, passionate and lively; pains as from a bruise in the lower part of the abdomen, occurring chiefly at night, and for those who indulge in stimulants, highly seasoned food, wine, coffee, porter, and ardent spirits.

PULSATILLA, pains in the abdomen and loins, as if from continued stooping, with a feeling of stiffness and dragging in the thighs; constipation and diarrhœa; for persons of a mild disposition, and after eating fat indigestible foods.

DOSE and Administration.—One drop of the dilution, or six globules, in half a tumbler of water; give a teaspoonful every half hour, in severe cases, in others every four hours, until a change is effected or another remedy selected. After the above remedies always give *Sulphur*, one dose in the morning.

Childbirth. Labor. Parturition.

Natural labor usually takes place, at the end of the ninth month after conception. True labor-pains usually occur at regular intervals, gradually increasing in intensity, and perhaps in frequency, and delivery is completed in from four to six hours. Variations from this, are however, very common; in some cases, the whole time occupied, being less than half an hour, whilst in others, it has required several days; in a few rare instances, two or three pains have completed the process.

The time from conception to delivery, is about two hundred and eighty days, or forty weeks, reckoning from the last menstrual period. Morning sickness usually first occurs about six weeks, and quickening about twenty weeks after conception; during the eighth month the child sinks lower down in the abdomen, and the woman gradually becomes smaller around the waist; this sinking is often so sudden, as to be specially observable in one or two days; labor may then be expected, in from three to four weeks.

Agitation, trembling, lowness of spirits, and disposition to weep, are frequently premonitory symptoms of the approach of labor; flying pains, with frequent inclination to pass water, or involuntary urination sometimes occur; diarrhœa, or looseness of the bowels, for a day or two, if it occur, should not be interfered with. A slight discharge of reddish mucus, called the show, is the most certain indication.

Most of the sufferings attendant upon child-bearing, arise from ill health, or from those habits of life, which reason would teach any woman, must be injurious. Healthy women of regular habits, who pay proper attention to the cultivation of their physical powers, always suffer much less than others; some athletic, muscular women, accustomed to the open air, suffer but little.

Protracted Labors.

It is not easy to draw any exact line of demarcation, between what should be termed a natural and a protracted labor. In general, if the labor continue more than twelve hours, and if it be attended with much suffering, by which the patient becomes exhausted, and especially if in this exhausted condition, the force of the true labor pains comes to be partially diminished, or if by some obstruction delivery is delayed, it may be properly called a protracted labor. Such labors are more likely to occur in a first confinement, and in persons of slender form, and delicate, sensitive habits.

The remedies adapted to this condition, are Aconite, Belladonna, Chamomilla, Coffea, Nux vomica, Opium, Pulsatilla, and Secale.

ACONITE, if the person be of sanguineous temperament, the pains extremely violent but ineffectual; also, in rapid succession, with restlessness.

BELLADONNA, if there be a rigid, unyielding condition of the parts; or spasms, especially in the neck of the uterus; or if the pains diminish or cease entirely, after having been for some time violent.

CHAMOMILLA, often after *Aconite*, when there is great

sensibility to pain, anguish and discouragement, or mental excitement.

COFFEA, for symptoms similar to *Aconite* or *Chamomilla*, and if there is great agitation, restlessness and tossing about.

NUX VOMICA, if the pains are irregular and insufficient, and if there is constant disposition to pass water, or desire for stool.

OPIUM, if the pains cease suddenly with congestion to the head, redness of the face, stupor, and snoring.

PULSATILLA, if the pains are feeble, occurring at long intervals, or diminishing in strength and frequency; or if attended with vomiting, or with spasms in the stomach; acute pain in the back and loins, or painful drawings in the thighs.

SECALE, for symptoms similar to *Pulsatilla*, and when that remedy has failed.

DOSE and Administration.—One drop, or six globules, of the properly selected remedy, in ten spoonfuls of water, give a spoonful every half hour. If no relief follow the third or fourth dose, it will generally be expedient to select another remedy.

All drugs, stimulants, perfumery, spirituous liquors, &c., should be carefully excluded from the chamber of the patient, as they always increase the dangers, and diminish the prospects of life and health; also all cataplasms, and all similar appliances. Protracted labors should always be expected to terminate favorably.

Cramps. Convulsions. Spasmodic Pains.

These not only occasion suffering, but they frequently materially retard delivery. They will generally yield, however, to the application of medicines.

REMEDIES.—Belladonna, Chamomilla, Cocculus, Hyoscyamus, Ignatia, Ipecacuanha, and Stramonium.

BELLADONNA,—Excessive bearing down pains, with convulsive movements; great agitation and tossing, with congestions to the head, and even with frantic rage and delirium; throbbings; distension of the blood vessels; face red and bloated; with profuse sweat.

CHAMOMILLA.—Pains, mostly of a cutting character, extending from the loins to the lower part of the abdomen; spasmodic convulsions; redness of one cheek, or of the whole face; sensitiveness; excitement, especially of the nerves.

COCCULUS.—Cramps and convulsions in the lower part of the abdomen, in the limbs, or in the whole body; with heat and redness, and puffiness of the face.

HYOSCYAMUS.—Convulsions; loss of consciousness; cries; anguish; and oppression of the chest.

IGNATIA.—Confused feeling in the head, with sensation of suffocation; convulsions; spasmodic and compressive pains.

IPECACUANHA.—Nausea or vomiting; with paleness or bloatedness of the face; spasmodic convulsions.

STRAMONIUM.—Tremblings of the limbs, and convulsions, without loss of consciousness.

DOSE and Administration.—Any of the above remedies may be administered in water, a dose every fifteen minutes in extreme cases, or a few globules of the selected remedy may be placed upon the tongue during the paroxysm, and the remedies frequently changed if relief be not obtained.

Treatment after Delivery.

After delivery, the patient should be perfectly quiet. All noise, strong light, odors, and even conversation, should be carefully avoided. After an hour or two of rest, if no unpleasant symptoms exist to prevent, she may be changed and placed in bed. If the bandage has not been applied previously, it should be immediately after delivery, taking care to disturb the patient as little as possible. It is safe, in order to anticipate and prevent soreness as much as possible, to administer a little Arnica internally; for this purpose, a single drop of the dilution of Arnica may be infused in ten spoonfuls of water, and a spoonful be given every half hour for four hours. Benefit may also be derived from the external use of a lotion, made by mixing ten to twenty drops of Arnica in two tablespoonfuls of water, and applying it to the sore parts by saturating a small cloth with this solution. If the patient is prevented from sleep by nervous excitement, a dose or two of Coffea will commonly afford relief. Should there be any symptoms of fever, give Aconite. For other irregularities, consult the following articles.

Flooding after Delivery.

REMEDIES.—Belladonna, Chamomilla, China, Cinnamon tincture, Crocus, Hamamelis virg., Platina, and Sabina. For the particular indications of which, see the article Flooding, page 676.

After Pains.

These pains rarely occur with first children; afterwards, with some females they become more and more distressing with each successive labor, whilst others suffer but little inconvenience from them even after having borne several children. Some one of the following remedies will usually afford relief.

Arnica, Belladonna, Chamomilla, Coffea, Nux vomica, Pulsatilla and Secale.

ARNICA.—For violent pains, with a feeling of soreness; retention of urine, with pressure.

BELLADONNA.—If with much bearing down there be fulness about the head; disposition to sleep; abdomen very sensitive to the touch, with fulness.

CHAMOMILLA.—If *Arnica* prove insufficient, and the patient is irritable or excitable, restless and tossing about.

COFFEA.—If there is much nervous excitement, and the pains are very violent, or followed by convulsions, with coldness and rigidity.

NUX VOMICA.—After *Chamomilla*, or alternately with it, especially when the pains are like the pains of colic, and occur in persons of a positive or sanguine disposition; *Chamomilla* may be given in the forenoon, *Nux vomica* in the afternoon.

PULSATILLA.—For pains recurring at long intervals; protracted; continuing several days; for persons of mild disposition.

SECALE.—For the most violent cases in women who have bore many children.

DOSE and Administration.—One drop, or six globules, of the selected remedy, may be given in ten spoonfuls of water; a spoonful every half hour in severe cases, in others every four or six hours, until relief be obtained or a new remedy be chosen.

Remarks.

During the first week it is generally safest for the mother to keep her bed; after that, if her condition is favorable, she may sit up awhile at first whilst the bed is making, afterwards longer, spending most of her time in bed, or at least half reclining for at least two weeks. She may now be permitted to walk about her room occasionally, and if she feels strong and well to engage in conversation, reading, and perhaps very light employment, but should on no account be permitted to go up and down stairs, take long walks or laborious exercise for five or six weeks; some cases may even require a much longer period.

During the first week the diet should consist of such

articles as gruel, farina, panada, toast, toast-water, &c. Every thing stimulating, and all strong odors, flowers, and aromatic substances should be positively prohibited from her chamber. During the second week if there be no fever, and her appetite is good, she may be allowed chicken or beef broths, a light mutton chop or broth, but no spices, summer savory, nutmeg, cinnamon, or other articles having flavor, must on any account be mixed with her food or drink. The third week her diet may be more substantial; and on the fourth, in very favorable cases, she may return to her accustomed food, provided all stimulating and savory articles are carefully avoided.

Of the Lochia.

The Lochia is a healthy discharge which takes place after confinement, and is in color and appearance at first similar to the menstrual secretion, but gradually becomes lighter colored, yellowish, and before its final cessation, whitish in appearance. It also varies considerably in different females. It is at times thin and scanty, and ceases in a few days. At other times it continues several weeks, and is so profuse as almost to amount to hemorrhage.

If it continue too long, is too profuse, or if it be suddenly suppressed, medical aid is requisite.

REMEDIES. — Aconite, Belladonna, Bryonia, Crocus, Carbo animalis, Calcarea carb., Dulcamara, Opium, Platina and Pulsatilla.

ACONITE, if the discharge is too profuse, and of a bright red color, will often be sufficient, and in from one to three days the discharge may assume a healthy state.

59*

BELLADONNA, when it continues too long and becomes thin, fetid and offensive, and also if it excoriates the parts.

BRYONIA, for suppressed lochia, with headache, fulness and heaviness, or with pressure in the temples and forehead, throbbing in the head, aching in the small of the back, and scanty urination. Also useful when the lochia is too profuse, if the color be deep red, with burning pains in the region of the womb, or deep and low down in the abdomen.

CROCUS, if the discharge be too profuse, too long continued, and too dark colored, or nearly black, also if it be viscid.

CALCAREA CARB., after *Aconite*, and especially when there are itchings felt deep in the stomach.

CARBO ANIMALIS, after *Belladonna*, and for similar symptoms.

DULCAMARA, for suppression from exposure to cold or damp, and before or after *Pulsatilla*.

OPIUM, for suppression arising from fright, with congestion to the head, and dulness.

PLATINA, suppression from mental emotions, with dryness and uncommon sensitiveness of the sexual organs.

PULSATILLA, sudden suppression from mental emotions, dampness, or from any incidental cause, particularly if followed by febrile symptoms, headache, chiefly on one side of the head, coldness of the feet, frequent desire to pass water; worse towards evening, and better in the morning. Also if the discharge be scanty, without being entirely suppressed.

SECALE, for symptoms similar to *Pulsatilla*.

DOSE.—Dissolve a powder, or one drop of the dilution, in ten spoonfuls of water, give a spoonful every hour until relief is afforded ; in milder cases every four hours.

Coming of the Milk.—Milk Fever.

The coming of the milk is frequently attended by sufferings which require medical attention. It usually takes place about the third day after delivery, though it may appear even before delivery, or not until a much later period than the third day.

For the sufferings usually attendant, the following remedies are adapted: Aconite, Arnica, Bryonia, Belladonna, Chamomilla, Pulsatilla, Rhus toxicodendron.

ACONITE, if there be fever, with hot dry skin; breasts hard or in cakes; restlessness or anxiety.

ARNICA, given internally, and applied to the breasts externally as a lotion, ten drops of *Tincture of Arnica*, in ten teaspoonfuls of water, will be found useful, if there is much distension, hardness, and soreness.

BRYONIA, when the symptoms have been partially removed by *Aconite*, and if there be oppression, headache, constipation, &c.

BELLADONNA, after or in alternation with *Bryonia*, and for similar symptoms, especially if there be great sensitiveness to every movement or to noise.

CHAMOMILLA, much nervous excitement, restlessness, tenderness of the breasts, inflammation of the nipples.

PULSATILLA, for the most severe cases, and when fever is threatening; swelling of the breasts, soreness, and rheumatic pains.

RHUS TOXICODENDRON, when *Pulsatilla* or *Bryonia* is indicated; breasts swollen and hard, headache, stiffness of the joints, and general disturbance of the system.

DOSE and Administration.—One drop of the dilution, or six globules, of the selected remedy, in ten spoonfuls of water, give a spoonful every two hours, in severe cases; in other cases, every four hours until relief is obtained; afterwards, gradually cease medication.

Suppression of the Milk.

This secretion may be suddenly suppressed, either from exposure to cold, powerful emotions of the mind, or from any causes inciting the system to fever; as determination of the blood to other parts, local congestions, &c.

These symptoms usually indicate the approach of child-bed fever, for which, the immediate administration of Pulsatilla, is almost a specific remedy.

DOSE.—One drop of the dilution, or six globules, in ten spoonfuls of water, give a spoonful every two to four hours, for twelve hours. If the symptoms become favorable, diminish the frequency of the doses for twenty-four or forty-eight hours longer. If any unpleasant symptoms remain, give *Calcarea carbonica,* or *Zincum metallicum,* four doses, at intervals of twelve hours, each dose.

If, notwithstanding, feverish symptoms should appear, give Aconite, every hour, for six hours; afterwards, every two or four hours, according to the severity of the symptoms.

DOSE.—The same as *Pulsatilla.* If there be great restlessness, give *Coffea.*

Excessive secretion of Milk, or Involuntary Emissions.

When the secretion of milk is too abundant, and the breasts are painfully swollen, the milk constantly escaping of its own accord, Calcarea carb. or Phosphorus will generally afford relief. If there be much fever, Aconite or Rhus tox. may be given.

DOSE and Administration.—One drop of the dilution, or six globules, in ten spoonfuls of water, give of *Calcarea carb.* a teaspoonful every twelve hours, of *Zincum* or *Rhus tox.,* every six hours, a dose, of *Aconite* every two hours, four doses of the remedy chosen, then wait the result. If not relieved, select another remedy.

For involuntary emission of milk, not accompanied by the above symptoms, either one of the foregoing remedies may be given as above, a dose every twelve hours, or for debilitated persons from loss of fluids, *China*, and for females of mild, easy disposition, *Pulsa- tilla* may be administered in the same manner.

Diarrhœa.

Too frequent motion or too great looseness of the bowels during the lying-in period, is to be regarded as a highly dangerous condition, and means should be taken to prevent it as speedily as possible.

REMEDIES.—Antimonium crud., Dulcamara, Hyoscya- mus, Phosphorus, Phosphoric acid, Nux vomica Rheum, and Hepar sulph.

ANTIMONIUM CRUD., is useful against thin, watery, offensive discharges, after which give *Rhus*.

DULCAMARA, if preceded by exposure to cold or damp- ness.

HYOSCYAMUS, for painful, involuntary evacuations.

PHOSPHORUS or PHOSPHORIC ACID, in very obstinate cases, the evacuations being watery, painless and almost involuntary. For diarrhœa with whitish, curdled, sour smelling and musty discharges, frequently attendant upon nursing, with sore mouth, Pulte recommends Nux vomica and Hepar sulph. in alternation, every three hours, until relieved, or until six doses of each are taken, the patient being kept perfectly at rest, and in a recum- bent posture.

DOSE.—Give a drop, or six globules, of the selected remedy, in six spoonfuls of water, a spoonful every two hours, or after every discharge from the bowels, until relief be obtained.

Constipation.

The bowels should remain unmoved for a few days after delivery. This is a natural condition, and should never be disturbed, as it serves to promote the patient's strength. If the patient has no evacuation for five or six days, and complains of pain in the bowels or fulness in the head, one or two doses of Bryonia will generally afford relief. Should this prove insufficient, give a dose of Nux vomica at three o'clock in the afternoon, and a dose of Sulphur at six o'clock the following morning. Continue this treatment until evacuations occur. In a very obstinate case, attended with severe sufferings, and when other medicines had failed, immediate relief was afforded by the administration of Podophyllum peltatum.

Retention of Urine, or Painful Urination.

If after delivery, there be retention or painful emission of urine, Arnica, Belladonna, Nux vomica, or Pulsatilla, will generally afford relief. See Retention or Painful Emission of Urine.

DOSE.—Of a solution of the selected remedy, a teaspoonful every three hours.

Setting over a chamber which contains warm water, will sometimes be sufficient.

Sore Nipples.

In the majority of cases, if the preparatory treatment recommended on page 680, be adopted, sore nipples will be prevented. If there is a tendency to excoriation and soreness notwithstanding, give Arnica, every twelve hours a dose, and bathe the nipples and the breast around, with a solution of Arnica in water, ten drops to ten teaspoonfuls of water, always after nursing having previously washed them in clean water. Should this prove insufficient, administer some one of the following remedies; Calcarea carb., Graphites, Lycopodium, Mercurius, Nux vomica, Sepia, Silicea, and Sulphur.

The symptomatic indications of many of the above

remedies are very similar. If the nipples are very sore and chapped with deep fissures around the base, bleeding and burning, give Sulphur, every twelve hours a dose, four doses; if not relieved, give Calcarea in the same manner, or Graphites for similar symptoms in persons of general defective circulation, and unhealthiness of the skin, to whom Calcarea seems not to be adapted; Nux vomica, if there be painful excoriation, or rawness of the adjacent parts. Lycopodium, Mercurius, Sepia, or Silicea, in very obstinate cases.

DOSE and Administration.—One drop, or six globules, of the selected remedy, infused in ten spoonfuls of water; give a teaspoonful every six hours for twenty-four hours; if the pains are alleviated, continue the remedy twenty-four or forty-eight hours longer; if not, change the medicine.

Gathered Breasts.—Abscess in the Breasts.

This may arise at any time during the nursing period, or even previously. The exciting causes are numerous, —colds, passion or anger, and fright, a bruise, putting the child to the breast too late, or taking it from the breast too suddenly in weaning, or the death of the child, &c.

When any irritation arises, the breasts should be kept properly drawn. For this purpose, a breast-pipe may be used, or still better, the lips of the nurse.

The most valuable remedies are, Bryonia, Belladonna, Hepar sulphur, Mercurius, Phosphorus, and Sulphur.

BRYONIA, when the breasts become hard, swollen, and heavy, with shooting pains, dry skin, thirst, and oppression of the chest.

BELLADONNA after *Bryonia*, or when the swelling assumes an erysipelatous hue with shootings.

HEPAR SULPHUR after suppuration commences; known by throbbing pains, frequently preceded by a chill.

PHOSPHORUS after *Hepar sulphur*, if the discharge be very profuse.

SILICEA, if the discharge be thin and watery, with several fistulous openings, not disposed to heal.

SULPHUR, in inveterate cases, the discharge being profuse; with emaciation and hectic fever.

DOSE.—One drop of the dilution, or six globules, of the selected remedy, may be infused in ten spoonfuls of water, and a spoonful given every four hours, until amelioration or change.

Falling off of the Hair,

Which sometimes occurs while nursing, generally arises from some delicacy of the constitution.

The remedies are Calcarea, Lycopodium, Sepia, Silicea, and Sulphur.

ADMINISTRATION.—Give a dose each morning, four mornings in succession, then wait four days, and if not better, give another remedy.

CHAPTER XV.

DISEASES OF NEW-BORN INFANTS AND YOUNG CHILDREN.

Introductory Remarks.

SINCE it has been so well established, that the infant organism is susceptible to the influence of both morbific and medicinal agents, it seems requisite that a plain, judicious mode of treatment should be pointed out, which will serve not only as curative means to be employed for incidental ailments, but which will also have a tendency to correct in some measure, congenital difficulties.

It would seem plausible that any constitutional taint might be more readily destroyed in the germ, by well selected, specific remedies, than afterwards when it becomes more fully developed, and consequently of more powerful influence in the system.

The advantage which homœopathy possesses over all other modes of treatment in infantile cases, is well worthy of remark. For the minuteness, and yet sufficiency of the dose, effectually does away with all necessity for violent measures, so often productive of hurtful consequences, either from overdosing or by mistaking the remedy intended to be employed. It also, from its tasteless nature, does not produce that disgust, which the nauseous medicines, in the old mode of practice, so frequently creates.

Treatment of the Child immediately after Birth.

The child, as soon as born, should be wrapped in a soft linen covering, and enveloped in fine flannel; both of which should be previously warmed, so as to avoid any chilling effects upon the delicate skin of the new born babe. This seems the more requisite that the infant may become accustomed to the surrounding atmosphere by degrees; after which the skin should be gently washed with luke warm water, softened with bran, applied with fine soft sponge. The first washing should be without soap of any kind, so as to cleanse the surface without producing irritation. The room should be quiet, free from noise, brilliant light, and strongly scented substances. The body should be dried immediately after washing, by gentle wiping with soft linen, or a down brush and pearl powder, and after the first washing the child should be bathed twice a day, to keep up the healthy action of the skin. The temperature of the water may be somewhat lessened as the child advances in age.

The morning is the most suitable time for bathing children, when first taken from the bed; and also on returning to the bed for the night. The best mode of bathing is to immerse the whole body in water, taking suitable care to protect the eyes, nose, and mouth; for to immerse only one-half of the body at a time when bathing, leaving the other half exposed, is much more likely to produce the disagreeable consequences usually resulting from a chill on account of exposure to rapid evaporation in the surrounding atmosphere.

Very young children should only have what clothing the wants of their bodies require. It is hurtful to load them with unnecessary flannels and bandages. Improper clothing is the fruitful source of deformity of the limbs, and weakness in after life.

Apparent Death of New-Born Infants. (*Asphyxia.*)

It sometimes happens that a new-born infant does not breathe, its blood does not seem to circulate, and there is no apparent motion. This may be termed the first danger to which the infant is subject, on its entrance into the world; a suspension of vitality.

CAUSES.—Difficult and severe labor; injury from the forceps; pressure of the umbilical cord around the neck; natural debilty; accumulation of mucus or other matters in the throat; too sudden an alteration of temperature, the respiratory action of the lungs not having com- menced.

If the child does not breathe for several minutes after delivery, and is apparently dead, the body and limbs should immediately be wrapped in warm cloths, and the hands and chest rubbed gently with soft flannel, or per. haps more properly with the naked hand. Should slight pulsation manifest itself in the cord after this process, and the beating of the heart become apparent, breathing will soon follow, and nothing further will be required; but should these efforts prove a failure after five minutes, cut the cord, and immerse the child in a warm bath; rub and press the chest, working it like a bellows; also rub the limbs gently. These are generally the best manual operations.

TARTER EMETIC will be found useful when the child shows no signs of life, or there is but feeble pulsation of the cord, relaxed limbs, or pale face; or on the other hand, if the face is purple and swollen; also if the air passages seem to be obstructed with phlegm.

DOSE.—Place one globule on the tongue of the infant, or dissolve one drop, or six globules, in a tablespoonful of water, and moisten the tongue with a drop or two of the solution.

OPIUM.—Should no favorable change take place, and if the face is livid and bluish.

DOSE·—Dissolve a drop, or six globules, in a tablespoonful of water, and drop two or three drops into the mouth every ten or fifteen minutes, until a change of some kind is observed.

NOTE.—At times breathing may be induced by inflating the lungs of the child, or by placing the mouth over the mouth of the child, and thus forcing air into the lungs, which being suffered to escape, and if two or three times repeated, incites the action of the heart and lungs, and restores the child to consciousness; also pouring a small stream of cold water on the child's breast, will often succeed in promoting the action of the lungs, and the establishment of respiration

CHINA is indicated if the face be *pale* during the sus pension of animation, and also when the infant shows signs of life and respiration commences, if a similar pale- ness presents itself.

DOSE.—The same as *Opium*.

ACONITE is of service when the child is reviving and beginning to breathe, provided the face has been previously flushed or of a bluish tint.

DOSE.—One drop, or six globules, in a spoonful of water; drop a few drops of the solution upon the tongue, and repeat if necessary at longer or shorter intervals, in accordance with the effects produced.

Swelling of the Head, with Echymosis. *Blood Spots.*

The head of the infant after birth appears more or less swollen, but in most cases it proves a trifling and ephemeral affection requiring no treatment.

ARNICA internally, when the affection disappears tardily, will materially hasten its disappearance.

DOSE.—Dissolve one drop, or six globules, in a spoonful of water, and drop a few drops into the mouth.

RHUS TOX. is of service when there is considerable swelling of the anterior, or *fontanel.*

DOSE.—The same as for *Arnica.*

Benefit will also result when necessary from rubbing the tumefied portion of the scalp with the naked hand, or with a weak solution of *Arnica,* ten drops in a spoonful of water, by which means not only the swelling, but the naturally attendant soreness and pain will be greatly diminished. The same treatment will be effectual for all cases of echymosis, or spots of blood created by pressure during delivery, either from the smallness or irregularity of the pelvis, or from the use of instruments or other incidental causes.

Of the Meconium.

The first discharge from the bowels of the infant is called the meconium. It is of a dark or bottle green color, and usually occurs eight or twelve hours after birth, or within a few hours after first receiving its mother's milk. Should a temporary delay occur, it affords no cause of alarm, nor should any violent means be resorted to for hastening its expulsion.

If an unusually long period elapse, say twenty-four or forty-eight hours after birth, and the child appear restless and uneasy, give a dose of Nux vomica in the afternoon, both to the mother and child, and a dose of Sulphur on the following morning. This will generally afford sufficient relief. In obstinate cases, where the mother has long been of a costive habit, Bryonia, Lycopodium, Opium and Silicea may be found useful.

DOSE and Administration.—In ordinary cases it will be found sufficient to place a few globules of the selected remedy on the tongue once or twice in the twenty-four hours. In more obstinate cases it may be administered in water, six globules, or one drop of the dilution, in ten spoonfuls of water, and give a spoonful to the mother, and a few drops, say half a teaspoonful, to the child, every four hours, until relief is afforded.

Of Nursing.

That every healthy and well organized woman should support her child from the natural secretion from her own bosom, is the dictate both of nature and reason.

It is difficult to estimate the evils which may result from depriving the infant of this its natural nourishment, as no artificial food, however carefully prepared, can fully supply its place.

And again, the constitution of the mother rarely suffers from nursing her child, whilst the health of many women is materially benefited by it, and a very large portion of those women who think they suffer from this cause, really suffer only from the stimulants and other poisons they take to support their strength, as they call it, or to create an unnatural flow of milk, and not at all, as they imagine, from the effects of nursing alone.

60*

The child should usually be put to the breast within twelve (*often about six*) hours after birth. Instinct will then direct it what to do, and the advantages of its incipient labors are many and important. If there be no nilk in the breasts, the act of sucking will expedite the ecretion, and the mother be saved much of the pain onnected with their distension, whilst the child will aave commenced an action it will not easily forget, and it will not be likely afterwards to refuse the breast when its instinctive efforts shall be rewarded with a full supply of the wholesome beverage; but if the child be not put to the breast until the breast is distended with milk, the nipple itself will at times almost entirely disappear, the child has in a measure lost its instinctive capacity for nursing; it makes perhaps a few almost ineffectual efforts to lay hold of the half concealed nipple, the mother cringes under the excessive pain it occasions, and if it finally succeeds, another source of suffering called sore nipples, almost invariably follows.

Obstacles to Nursing.

These may sometimes exist on the part either of the mother or the child. If the mother is of consumptive tendencies, or of a strumous habit, the child ought, for its own sake, to derive its nourishment from other sources.

Also if the weakness of the mother be so great that she cannot endure the loss of fluids consequent thereupon without too great prostration of the vital force. But many of the obstacles to nursing a little perseverance will enable the mother effectually to overcome. There may also be obstacles on the part of the child. If the child refuse the breast, give Cina, and afterwards Mercurius, if necessary, one or two doses of each, both to the mother and child. It will generally be found effica_ cious in the course of a few hours. Aethusa cynapium is adapted when the child takes the breast readily, but throws up immediately afterwards; also Silicea. If these remedies fail, and the child does not thrive, other nourishment must be provided, and the child weaned.

DOSE, and Administration.—Of the selected remedy, one drop or six globules, in four spoonfuls of water, give a spoonful every six hours If relief does not follow in twenty-four hours, select another remedy.

Mental Emotions affecting the Milk.

Numerous examples attest the well established fact that mental emotions may change the milk of the mother from a source of nourishment into a most injurious substance to the infant. Mothers ought never to suckle their children when suffering from fright or passion; and after such suffering a portion of the milk should, if possible, be drawn from the breast before it is again given to the child. Homœopathy presents prompt and efficacious remedies for evils of this nature, which should be immediately administered to the mother according to the cause and symptoms, for the particular indications of which see Mental Emotions, page 660.

Deficiency or Suppression of the Secretion of Milk.

If this arise from inflammation of the breasts, see that article on page 692, but if it arise from want of energy and power, either functional or general, suitable remedies will generally produce a healthful flow. Pulsatilla is one of the most useful medicaments. It should be administered in water, one drop, or six globules, in ten spoonfuls of water, a teaspoonful to be given every four hours. After Pulsatilla, Silicea should be given in the same manner. Should the above medicines fail to re-establish the flow, give Asafœtida, Iodium or Sulphur, each four doses as above, and if no improvement take place, employ a regular homœopathic physician.

Deterioration of the Quality of the Milk.

If the milk become poor and watery, and distasteful to the child, give Cina and Mercurius alternately every twelve or twenty-four hours, for three or four days. If not better, give Sulphur, and afterwards Calcarea carb., or Silicea, especially if the infant vomit immediately after taking the breast.

RHEUM, if the milk become thick and yellow, and render the child restless and fretful.

DOSE.—One drop of the dilution, of the selected remedy, or six globules, in a spoonful of water, every twelve hours, two days, wait one day, if no change, select another remedy.

Treatment of Mothers who do not nurse their Children.

If a mother from any cause find herself under the disagreeable necessity of not suckling her child, the slightest regard to her own health should admonish her to be careful of her diet, until after the flow of milk into the breasts has completely ceased. The internal administration of Pulsatilla will often be sufficient with a spare diet to check any unpleasant consequences which might otherwise arise. If inflammation ensue, Bryonia, Belladonna and Phosphorus are appropriate remedies; also Rhus tox.

DOSE.—One drop, or six globules, of the selected remedy, in six spoonfuls of water, give a spoonful every three hours, and see *Inflammation of the Breasts*.

CALCAREA, if the breasts are much distended with milk. See also *Weaning*, page 709.

DOSE·—Of *Calcarea*, as above, one drop, or six globules, in four spoon. fuls of water, a spoonful every six hours, four doses, if not better give some other remedy.

Laurie recommends dry cupping at the outer surface of the arm, a little below the shoulder, or at the feet, in obstinate cases, to hasten the suppression; and Williamson, if the breasts become distended and painful, the application of hot lard enveloped in raw cotton. It may well be doubted whether either of these applications are homœopathic. Others practice the application of spirits of camphor externally to the breasts and about the arms, which often affords prompt relief. If such remedies are used at all, it should be with great caution, and all their effects carefully noted.

In cases where the objections to nursing on the part of the mother are insuperable, or when the death or disability of the mother appear to render it necessary, the following directions may not be found unimportant for

The Choice of a Nurse.

Let the nurse from whose breast the child is to derive its nourishment, be a healthy woman, free from any discoverable tendency to chronic diseases, about the same age or younger than the mother, and delivered at least within a few months of the same time. Let her complexion be clear, skin smooth and healthy, eyes and eyelids free from any redness or swelling. She should be of an amiable disposition, not irritable, nor prone to anger or passion, of regular habits, not indulging in any of the forms of dissipation, naturally kind and fond of children.

Diet during Nursing.

The mother or nurse, should always exercise proper discretion in regard to the nature and quality of her food. This should always be nutritious and healthful, and should never be partaken of, simply for the sake of increasing the natural flow of milk, but only according to the reasonable demands of the appetite. This is sometimes done by ignorant mothers and nurses, and can never fail to produce injurious effects upon the delicate organism of the young infant. The diet should be simple and nourishing, not too rich, nor too stimulating, and should be taken at regular intervals. Meats should generally be used sparingly; bread, fruits, and vegetables freely; and the homœopathic regimen should be strictly observed. All porter, ale, brandies, and all stimulating liquors and drinks, sarsaparilla, mead, beers, &c., should be positively prohibited. No idea can be more erroneous, than that women, during the nursing period, stand in need of stimulants to support their strength, under which impression, wine, malt liquors, and especially porter, are frequently resorted to. These are not only injurious from their stimulating properties, but the latter especially, from the nature of the drugs of which it is composed, can scarcely fail to engender obstinate and formidable chronic diseases, both of the mother and child. The relief afforded by such stimulants, if indeed it can be called relief, is of very short duration; it is invariably followed by a greater degree of weakness and depression, demanding a repetition of the same, or of more powerful stimulants, which destroy the tone of the stomach, deteriorate the quality of the milk, rendering it altogether unsuited to the delicate organism of the tender infant.

Supplementary Diet of Infants.

If the mother possess sufficient milk for the nourish. ment of her child, its stomach should never be loaded with other condiments, or with food of any kind, until it is at least five or six months old; but if the mother have an insufficient supply of milk, and if the child do not thrive, but become lean and emaciated, and is apparently hungry, it becomes necessary to give it some additional nutriment; also, at times, in case of mothers who, from the nature of their avocations, are separated from their children a considerable portion of the twenty-four hours.

In this case, the selected food should resemble as nearly as possible, the milk of a healthy nurse. The milk of a good cow, diluted with one third water, and a little sugar being added, is probably the best substitute. If there is any doubt of the purity or freshness of the milk, if it has stood many hours, or been transported a considerable distance, it should be boiled, and afterwards diluted. Its temperature is also important; it may be tried with the finger, to which it should neither feel hot nor cold, but very gently warm, or about the tempera-ture of the warmer parts of the body. Arrow-root, rusk, water from well toasted bread, sweetened with loaf sugar, may occassionally furnish a substitute for milk, but generally, the milk is to be preferred, and few changes of diet should be permitted. No portion of the prepared food, should be retained for the subsequent meal, and the milk should be renewed or rescalded, at least twice in the twenty-four hours. This is easily done by placing it in a covered vessel, and setting the vessel in a basin of boiling water.

After the fifth or sixth month, the food may become gradually of a more solid or substantial character, giving such articles only as are found by experience not to disagree. Sago, arrow-root, panada, a piece of well made stale bread, milk and cream, will generally afford a sufficient variety. Roasted apples, stewed or boiled fruits, may at times be permitted. If any article of food is found not to agree, it should be immediately withheld. But little variety should be introduced, and generally one kind of food only, or at most, two kinds, should be allowed at a meal. Milk should never be given with meats, nor before nor after acid fruits. The utmost regularity should be observed with regard to the hours of feeding, as well as the quantity of food. A child should never be fed because it cries, but always at regular intervals, and in a given quantity. Potatoes and other wholesome vegetables may be cautiously given after the second, and meats after the third year; but the quantity of meat should always be limited, and should only be allowed once each day, until the seventh year, when more freedom in diet may be permitted.

Very young infants should be allowed the breast every three hours. At the age of seven months the time may be extended to six hours, which should generally be continued during the nursing period. The child should be continued at the breast about thirty minutes, during which, no avocations should divert the attention of the mother from her offspring. It should then be removed, and no cries, entreaties, or persuasions, on the part of the child, should induce the mother again to give it the breast, until another time for nursing shall arrive.

Children managed in this way will seldom be subject to diarrhœas, dysenteries, or other morbid conditions of the bowels. The dreaded second summer will be to.

them as the first. They will be plump, healthful, and happy, and with comparatively little care will pass through the trying periods of childhood.

Weaning, or Period of Suckling.

Infants should usually be continued at the breast until they arive at the age of from fifteen to twenty months. The teeth then are generally sufficiently developed to enable them to masticate their food; their digestive organs if not previously overloaded, have become harmoniously developed, and the milk of the mother often becomes less adapted, at about this period, to the wants of her offspring. If, however, the menses reappear, and the milk diminish in quantity, or the mother again becomes pregnant, the child may be weaned at an earlier period.

On the other hand, however, the child should not be weaned while it is suffering from teething, or any other acute disease, unless the health of the mother or other circumstances, appear to render it indispensable. After the child is seven months old, it may gradually be accustomed to a small, but regular supply of other food, which should be of the most simple, but nourishing character, as bread, milk, sago, arrow-root, or farina, oatmeal or barley; meats should not be allowed until the child is three or four years old.

When once taken from the breast, the child should not on any account be permitted again to taste it. Perfect regularity should at once be adopted in regard to the hours of feeding. The stomach should not be overloaded, and for a few days the child may very properly receive a little extra attention and care. In from two days to a week, the weaning process will be completed.

61

Sleep.

The most important business of the young infant appears to be to eat and sleep, and if the child is in health, if it appear cheerful and lively on waking, its sleep should not be interfered with, but should be left to nature. Forcing children to sleep by excessive feeding, and long continued rocking, is only robbing yourself of a present pleasure, the innocent prattle of a young child, for the sake of bringing upon yourself and child future pain and suffering. Drugging it with opiates, stimulants, &c., is still worse, and a few such administrations will generally be sufficient to procure a fretful, impatient, restlessness for weeks afterwards. Carminatives, and all patent or quack medicines, sanctioned though they be by medical names of high repute, are fraught with mischiefs the more pernicious, because the composition of the article being a secret, the nature of the poisons administered cannot be understood, nor the proper anti-dotes administered to their death-producing influences. .

Children should early be accustomed to regular hours of sleep as far as practicable, and for sleep in the day-time, the forenoon is the most suitable, say from eleven to one o'clock, rather than the afternoon. They should be taught in infancy the habit of early rising in the morning, and until at least two years of age, should be allowed to sleep in the middle of the day. The hours of rest should not be so long continued as to interfere with the sleep at night.

During the first six weeks, especially in winter, the infant may be allowed to sleep by the side of its mother or nurse, from which it should early be removed to a suitable bed or cradle, where it can easily receive proper care and nourishment. It should never be burdened with too large a supply of clothing, nor have its face and head covered with the bed-clothes, exposing it to a vitiated atmosphere, if not to suffocation. Both mother and child will enjoy better health by sleeping apart, as it is gene. rally acknowledged that it is detrimental to the health of the young to sleep with old people.

Children should never be rocked long for the sake of causing them to sleep, neither should they be rocked when asleep. If, notwithstanding an attendance to the foregoing, the child is restless, sleepless and uneasy, or fretful, (see the articles Sleeplessness, Cries of Infants, &c., in subsequent portions of this chapter.)

Exercise.

As the infants' powers are developed, and its strength increases, it gradually manifests a disposition to raise itself to an upright position, which we may safely indulge, taking care not to overtask its strength by allowing it to exert itself too long at a time. It soon learns to stretch itself, to spring upon its feet, and to delight in jumping, or being dangled, springing up and down in the arms of its mother or nurse, all of which exercises are healthful, if indulged with moderation, but may become highly injurious if too long continued, or too violent, and without proper caution. The bony system is at this age soft and spongy, and will easily yield to external force, whilst a wrench or bruise upon any of these structures may lay the foundation for permanent derangement in after life.

When it is four or six weeks old, it may be carried out in pleasant weather, if it be healthful; at first a few minutes at a time, until it has become accustomed to the air, after which the time may be lengthened. Many children suffer from the foolish idea of making them hardy by exposure. They should be cautiously guarded against sudden changes of temperature, against exposure to cold, night air, and dampness.

In learning to walk, children should not be incited to too great exertions, nor to a premature exercise of their powers, from which, curvature of the limbs, or diseases of the spinal column, might perhaps result; but by giving nature time to act, the faculties of the child will be more gradually, but at the same time, more fully developed; it will walk with more firmness and independence, and with greater confidence.

Children should early be taught to walk in an upright position, so as to give full play and expansion to the chest and lungs.

In very early life, they should also be trained to healthful sports of an active character, calculated to expand the chest, as well as to give activity and agility to the body; running, walking, marching, jumping, &c., will give power to the lower limbs; reaching, stretching, pulling, climbing, &c., to the arms; drawing in and expiring large draughts of air, holding in the breath for a long time, and then suddenly forcing it out from the chest, talking or reading as long as possible at a single breath, singing, halloing, &c., will give strength to the lungs and chest. These sports will be an hundred fold more useful, as well as more pleasing to the child, if participated in, and guided by, the mother, the father, the nurse, or some older person, and the child will often be found afterwards, practising them voluntarily, or of its own accord. Parents should frequently unite with their children in sportive exercises.

Industrious avocations are also in the highest degree

useful as exercise, and the child cannot be put at such employments too young, nor employed in them with too much regularity and order; but children should not be put to work alone; they should always be taught avoca- tions in which they can participate with their parents or guardians, and should be encouraged with the idea of making themselves useful, much more frequently than they are chidden for awkwardness and inattention.

Neither exercise nor labor, should be too long con- tinued, till the powers of nature become exhausted. There is a difference however, between fatigue and exhaustion, and children of five or six years old, may properly be compelled to labor, even after they begin to feel fatigue. Their employments, as well as their sports and exercises, should be frequently changed, and health- ful rest from labor may often be best obtained from healthful exercises.

The mind, as well as the body, should be trained by exercise, and the nursery should be made a school of knowledge, as well as a scene for sports, hilarity and pastime. Parents should never rely too much upon the schools, for the mental training of their children, for although our schools are a glory to our land, yet much more useful and salutary instruction, should be given at home, and in almost all the departments of knowledge. The acquisition of knowledge, will thus be made delight- ful. Wisdom will be eagerly sought for by the child, and the schools become only an adjuvant to parental influences, in enlarging and expanding the opening minds of the young.

61*

Maternal Marks. (*Neavi.*)

Marks or spots on different parts of the body of the child at birth, indicating a failure on the part of some of the secretory organs of the skin to perform their functions, may frequently be removed by the administration of remedies. The most appropriate are Calcarea carb., Silicea and Sulphur, and the earlier they are given, the greater is the probability of success.

CALCAREA CARB. is the most important, and should be first administered, unless some important indication point to another remedy.

DOSE and Administration.—One drop of the dilution, or six globules, in four spoonfuls of water, may be administered every six hours, two days, a teaspoonful, (*or even a few drops placed in the mouth, or two globules placed upon the tongue, will be found sufficient;*) afterwards a dose every morning, one week; after which, give *Sulphur.* If no improvement take place, give four doses of *Silicea,* one dose every morning, and consult diseases of the skin.

Deformities. Monstrosities, &c.

In all cases administer first Sulphur, four doses, a dose every morning, then wait four days without medicine, and afterwards give Calcarea carb. in the same manner; many deformities may by this means be corrected, and after a few weeks will begin to disappear, the healthy action of the vital forces creating a resolution of the deformities.

The medicines may be repeated, one dose every alternate four days, for some weeks, unless some manifest change be observable. If so, discontinue the medicine, and await its action. If no change, give Silicea, especially if the osseous or bony system be involved; or consult some skilful and experienced homœopathic surgeon. After the case has been treated for some weeks, medicines, if continued at all, should be given at much longer intervals.

Cyanosis. (*Blue Skin. Blue Disease.*)

A passage between the right and left sides of the heart, is always open before birth, called the foramen ovale. After birth the circulation changes, and this passage usually becomes closed. When from any cause this closure does not take place, the venous and arterial blood become, to some extent, commingled, giving rise to a disease called cyanosis, the characteristic of which is an unnatural blueness of the whole surface of the body.

REMEDIES.—First, give Sulphur, one dose, a drop, or six globules, in a teaspoonful of water every morning, four days, and afterwards give Calcarea carb. in the same manner, then wait four or eight days, and if necessary return again to Sulphur. Or give Digitalis after Sulphur, or in alternation with Calcarea carb., and in the same manner. These remedies by exciting a healthy action, will generally promote a closure of the foramen, when the disease ceases.

Rupture. (*Hernia.*)

Of this there are three kinds, umbilical, inguinal and scrotal. The first consists in an unnatural protrusion at or about the navel, *umbilicus*. The second may be on several other parts of the abdomen, usually in the groin. The third is in the scrotum, into which the intestines frequently protrude in considerable quantity, producing a very much enlarged, puffy or bladder-like appearance to that organ. In either case, long-continued crying very much increases the protrusion. The intestines may be sometimes returned with the hand, and supported for a few days with a bandage, or a small piece of pasteboard wrapped in soft muslin may be bound over the part. It may generally be cured in a few weeks by medicines. First give Sulphur one dose each day, four days, in the morning, afterwards give Nux vomica in the same manner at three o'clock in the afternoon. In eight days more if there is not very manifest improvement, repeat the remedies. If there is also diarrhœa, Chamomilla will prove successful; if caused by external violence, Arnica or Rhus tox. may be given.

DOSE.—One drop, or six globules, in a teaspoonful of water, to be given every four alternate days, in case of *Nux vomica* or *Sulphur*. For *Chamomilla, Arnica* or *Rhus tox,* a solution of one drop, or six globules, in four spoonfuls of water, give a teaspoonful every four hours, until a change is effected, or some other remedy chosen.

Sore Eyes. Ophthalmia. (*Ophthalmia neonatorum.*)

The first symptoms are usually a slight weakness of the eye, with agglutination of the lids, frequently occurring the second or third day after birth. It at times becomes very troublesome and obstinate, producing opacity of the cornea, loss of vision, and even ulceration of the cornea; from which the contents of the globe of the eye have escaped, followed by a shrinking of the eye-ball and permanent blindness and deformity.

TREATMENT.—See the article Opthalmia.

Crying.

The crying of children is, it is true, almost the only means which nature has given them when very young, of making known their wants; and when it is only occasional and not protracted, it is not to be regarded as a symptom of disease. If, however, it becomes excessive; if the child is always peevish and irritable, and prone to cry without apparent cause; if it scream out suddenly, or cry incessantly, or have frequent paroxysms of loud and continuous crying, it is a sufficient indication that something should be done, and it is the duty of the nurse, the mother and the physician, to endeavor to discover the cause and afford relief. Having paid every proper attention to its dress, and carefully examined its little person to discover if there is any external or visible cause; having considered the condition of all the secretions and evacuations, if nothing abnormal can be discovered, but if every thing has the appearance of health and comfort, it becomes our duty under such circumstances to consider crying as a symptom, and to prescribe for it with the same care and wise attention to remote and concealed causes that we would prescribe for a cough, for diarrhœa, or for any other symptom by which a diseased condition is made manifest.

It would require a treatise too long for this work, to consider the remedies which might prove useful in this condition, and the various reasons which might influence the selection. If either of the parents are affected with any chronic disease, such affection might greatly influence the diagnosis, and modify the treatment; as for instance, if they were subject to glandular swellings, sore throats, and tumefactions, Belladonna and Mercurius might be the remedies which would afford the child relief; if to hepatic complaints, with pains in the side, or epigastrium, Bryonia, Nux vomica, or Pulsatilla; if to psoric eruptions, Sulphur; or if to erysipelatous conditions, Rhus tox. might be the remedy. If no cause can be discovered, it would be safe to give first Chamomilla, four doses of three globules, one every four hours, to be followed the next morning, by one dose of four globules of Mercurius; if relief be not obtained within two days, give Belladonna in the same manner, and afterwards again give Mercurius or Sulphur. If these remedies fail, give Coffea or Aconite as above, and if not yet relieved, and a renewed examination leads to no new view of the condition, give Arsenicum. Some of the above remedies will almost always alleviate or cure.

Sleeplessness.

Like crying, sleeplessness is to be regarded as a symptom, and treated always upon similar principles. It will generally be relieved by one of the above remedies, if not, give *Stramonium*, *Hyoscyamus*, or if a stupid, half wakeful state prevail, give *Opium*.

DOSE and Administration.—The medicine may be given in water, one drop, or six globules in four spoonfuls of water, a spoonful every four hours; if no relief is afforded, select another remedy. Or it may be given dry by placing a powder containing two or three globules of the selected remedy upon the tongue of the child every four hours, until four powders have been given.

It may be remarked, that crying and sleeplessness are at times occasioned by the condition of the mother's milk, or its want of adaptation to the condition of the child, when the difficulty is to be remedied by medicines given to the mother; or, if they prove ineffectual, by weaning the child.

Regurgitation of Milk.

Infants, at times overload their stomachs, and afterwards throw up a portion of the milk they have taken; for which, medical assistance is not always requisite. But if this change into vomiting, and nearly all the nourishment appears to be thrown up, or if followed by vomiting of mucus or bile, this condition should receive attention, and be relieved by the appropriate remedies. The first remedy in importance, is Ipecacuanha, which will generally afford relief. It is also useful if there be diarrhœa or flatulence, or distension of the abdomen. After Ipecacuanha, give Pulsatilla, or Antimonium crud. if only partial relief is afforded.

CHAMOMILLA will often be useful when there are rest-lessness, convulsions, diarrhœa with greenish stools, and pains in the stomach or abdomen.

BRYONIA or NUX VOMICA, if the affection be also attended with constipation, uneasiness, and where the condition of either of the parents is such as to lead one to suppose these remedies might be indicated. Also *Rhus tox.*

Calcarea carb., Carbo veg., Lachesis, Phosphorus, and Sulphur, are also appropriate remedies.

DOSE and Administration.—The remedy selected may be given either dry or in water, four doses in twenty-four hours, or as directed for sleeplessness, then wait twenty-four hours; if relief be not obtained select another remedy.

Obstruction of the Nose. Coryza. Cold in the Head.

This is often a distressing affection, as it prevents the child from nursing, often causing it to let go the nipple in order to breathe, and rendering the child irritable and peevish, sometimes excoriation of the nipple follows, causing the nurse also to suffer. If the case be pro-tracted, the child sometimes ceases to thrive, its breathing is labored, and its sleep prevented. This malady is frequently obstinate, and requires remedies adapted to the different groups of symptoms which may be ob-served, as well as to the different circumstances by which those symptoms may be modified and understood.

In general, *Nux vomica* is a most reliable remedy, especially if the obstruction be attended with dryness, or obstruction at night, and slight discharge by day, and if the child be fretful, peevish and irritable, worse in the morning.

SAMBUCUS, after *Nux vomica*, if it fail to relieve, or if a thick and viscid mucus accumulate in the nostril.

TARTAR EMETIC, after *Sambucus*, if a suffocating cough or wheezing, or quick and laborious breathing, still remain. For a watery discharge, with redness of one cheek, soreness of the nostrils, and fever, give *Chamomilla;* if the discharge be greenish or yellowish, give *Pulsatilla;* or if attended with frequent sneezing, *Calcarea carb., Carbo veg., Mercurius* and *Sulphur,* are sometimes adapted.

DOSE and Administration.—One drop, or six globules, of the selected remedy, in ten spoonfuls of water, give a spoonful every four hours for two days, and await the action of the remedy one day, if there be no relief, select some other remedy.

Inflammation of the Eyes. (*Ophthalmia Neonatorum.*)

The causes of this affection are various: it may arise from cold, or it may be epidemic; it may originate in some constitutional condition of one or both parents, from long continued leucorrhœa on the part of the mother, or from a syphilitic taint on the part of the father or mother. There is usually at first an inflammatory redness of the inner surface of the lid, which speedily extends to the ball of the eye, and is soon followed by profuse secretions; the eyes are generally very sensitive to light.

· REMEDIES.—ACONITE should usually be the first remedy administered, and will often be found efficacious; after which, if the disease continue to increase, give Sulphur; or Calcarea and Sulphur may be given in alternation after Aconite, especially when Sulphur does not prove alone sufficient, and also in scrofulous or syphilitic subjects.

CHAMOMILLA may at times be called for when the intolerance to light is very great, and if the eyelids are red, swollen and inflamed. If there be erysipelatous inflammation, *Rhus tox.;* if there be excessive secretion, *Argentum nit.;* and in inveterate cases, *Lycopodium* may be found useful.

DOSE and Administration.—The same as for Obstructions of the Nose, which see.

Aphthæ, or Thrush.

Commences with an eruption of small round whitish vesicles, which soon become confluent and form a thin white crust, which lines the mouth at times throughout its whole extent, and also the throat, frequently extending to the stomach, and even the whole length of the alimentary canal; at times portions of the mucus coat appear to slough off, forming ulcers. It generally communicates itself also to the nipples of the mother, where it produces excoriations and soreness. It may arise from want of cleanliness, from improper food, or from any of the causes enumerated in the preceding article. (See Inflammation of the Eyes, page 720.)

One of the remedies homœopathic to this affection is *Borax*, with a weak solution of which, when practicable, the mouth may be frequently washed, when no other internal administration will be essential, as the child will generally swallow sufficient to perfect the cure. If this be not sufficient, give Mercurius, especially if there be profuse salivation or a manifest tendency to ulceration. If the symptoms do not improve, give Sulphur, and afterwards Sulphuric acid. In very bad cases, especially if the ulcerations assume a livid redness, give Arsenicum; and if the mouth and throat become covered with ulcerations which do not yield to Arsenicum, give Nitric acid.

CHAMOMILLA, BRYONIA, or RHUS TOX. will often prove sufficient, or they may be followed by *Sulphur* or *Caclarea; Nux vomica* and *Pulsatilla* are also useful in many cases.

DOSE.—One drop of the dilution of the selected remedy, in six spoonfuls of water, give a spoonful every four hours ; continue the medicine as directed for Obstruction of the Nose, page 719, which see.

Excoriations. Intertrigo.

These may generally be avoided, by cleanliness and care. When, however, they do occur, give Chamomilla, or if either the mother or child have been dosed with chamomile tea, give Pulsatilla, or Ignatia.

MERCURIUS, if *Chamomilla* be insufficient, especially if the skin of the child be of a yellowish tinge.

SULPHUR, in obstinate cases, not relieved by the above, or after any of the other remedies.

CARBO VEG., LYCOPODIUM, SEPIA, SILICEA, will often be useful.

Bathe the parts frequently and very thoroughly, after which, wash with a weak solution of *Arnica*, say ten drops to ten spoonfuls of water. Where the excoriated surfaces overlap each other, they should be kept apart by some soft substance, or covered with flour or powdered chalk, which must be frequently and carefully removed by washing.

DOSE and Administration.—One drop of the dilution, or six globules, in four spoonfuls of water, give a spoonful every six hours ; then wait its action twenty-four hours ; if not better give some other remedy.

The Gum.

This is also a disease of infancy, usually resulting from inattention to cleanliness, keeping the child too warm and too close, or giving it herb-teas, and other poisons, It consists of an eruption of red pimples, generally occupying the face, neck and arms, but may extend to the whole body.

ACONITE will be requisite, if the eruption be extensive, and if there be fever. If not, give *Rhus toxicodendron*, four doses, and afterwards *Sulphur*.

DOSE and Administration.—The same as for Excoriations which see.

Heat Spots. Prickly Heat,

Consists of small vesicles or eruptions, generally about the size of a small millet seed, filled with a watery fluid, and situated upon a red, inflamed base. These may break, form thin scabs, and not unfrequently ulcerate. This disease, often very annoying, being attended with severe itchings and burnings, and may be accompanied with fever. Its development is favored by heat, warm rooms, or excess of clothing, and especially by confined and unwholesome air, and bad food. Frequent bathing and proper care, may prevent or remove it; if not, Aconite or Chamomilla, will generally afford relief, or Rhus tox., and Sulphur, may be given, as directed in the last article, page 722, which see. If the eruption still continue, give Arsenicum, and if it frequently return, give Sulphur.

DOSE and Administration.—Give four doses of the selected remedy in water, as above, a dose of three globules every six hours; then wait twenty-four hours. If better, wait twenty-four hours longer, after which give *Sulphur,* one or two doses, of three globules, to complete the cure. If not better, select another remedy.

Scurf on the Head.

This is a dark, dirty looking incrustation, usually appearing at first, on the top of the head, and extending over most of its surface. On removing any portion, the skin beneath, will be found red and inflamed. It occasions itchings, irritation, and uneasiness, and frequently emits an offensive smell. Removing it forcibly, as by combing, usually makes it worse. The disease which occasions it, should first be cured. Its causes are the same as have already been alluded to, under the article prickly heat, and it may often, though not always, be prevented, by attention and care. .

The principal remedy is Sulphur, night and morning, four days. If not sufficient, give Rhus tox., and afterwards again give Sulphur.

DOSE and Administration.—The same as in the last article.

Soreness Behind the Ears.

This is, generally, another form of excoriation, which see, and pursue the treatment therein delineated.

If the complaint prove obstinate, give Graphites, and if relief do not follow, give Arsenicum; or if the child be of scrofulous tendencies, give Calcarea carb. or Baryta carb.

DOSE and Administration.—The same as for Excoriations.

Milk Crust.

This affection is distinguished by an eruption of numerous small white pustules upon a red ground, appearing in clusters, first on the face, especially on the cheeks and forehead, and at times spreading over the entire body. These pustules at length assume a yellow hue, or become dark-colored, burst and form thin yellow crusts. There is often redness and swelling and distressing itchings. The child rubs off the scabs, which form anew, but with increased thickness and aggravations, until perhaps the face becomes nearly covered with a thick scab or incrustation. Occasionally the eyes and eyelids, the parotid and mesentary glands, become inflamed, and dangerous marasmus may follow. Aconite, Arsenicum, Hepar sulph., Rhus tox. and Sulphur, are the principal remedies. Also, Belladonna, Euphrasia, Graphites, Lycopodium, Staphysagria, Sambucus, and Viola tricolor.

ACONITE.—Redness of the skin, with inflammation,

restlessness, excitability. After *Aconite* give *Rhus tox.* or *Viola tricolor.*

ARSENICUM, after *Rhus tox.*, in some obstinate and complicated cases.

HEPAR SULPH. may follow *Aconite* or *Rhus tox.*, if there is slight discharge and tendency to suppurate, in which case *Lycopodium* may. also be useful.

RHUS TOX. may follow *Aconite* when that proves insufficient, or if the incrustations also involve portions of the hairy scalp.

SULPHUR, after *Rhus tox.* in ordinary cases, and where necessary to complete the cure.

VIOLA TRICOLOR may generally follow *Aconite*, and is one of the most reliable remedies after *Rhus tox.*

DOSE and Administration.—One drop of the dilution, or six globules, in ten spoonfuls of water, a spoonful to be given every six hours, two days, afterwards, night and morning. Omit medication one or two days. If no improvement follow in four or six days from the commencement of the treatment, another remedy should be chosen.

Erysipelas. *(Induration of the skin.)*

Commences with red spots usually at first on the nates or the extremities, afterwards on the abdomen and private parts. The skin becomes indurated, and the muscles of the mouth affected, so that the child cries with difficulty. There is fever, and the skin at times becomes nearly as dry and stiff as parchment; or instead of the fever there may be an extraordinary degree of coldness. It usually occurs during the first two or three months after birth; its duration is from four to fourteen days, and if not promptly relieved it generally proves fatal.

REMEDIES.—Aconite, Arsenicum, Belladonna, Hepar sulph., Lachesis, Nux vomica, Rhus tox., Silicea and Sulphur.

62*

ACONITE, at the commencement always, if there is fever, *Belladonna* or *Rhus tox.* may follow *Aconite*, or *Aconite* and *Belladonna* may be alternated at the commencement of the treatment, giving a dose of each every four hours, for twenty-four hours, and afterwards followed by *Rhus tox.*, which may be sufficient to complete the cure.

ARSENICUM, after *Rhus tox.*, if that prove ineffectual; also if the stomach reject food, if the evacuations are green, watery, acrid and offensive, or a tendency to gangrene, with lividity, vesications, &c., and when it especially affects the scrotum.

HEPAR SULPH.—If there be also glandular enlargements and tumefactions, or if there be symptoms of an abscess.

LACHESIS may be useful after *Belladonna* and *Aconite*, especially if there be much swelling, and symptoms generally worse after sleeping. If instead of the fever there is coldness, either general or partial, *Arsenicum* or *Lachesis* should be exhibited.

NUX VOMICA is indicated when it effects mostly the joints, especially the knee and ankle joints, or if the bowels are costive.

RHUS TOX., in almost all cases, for the administration of which see *Belladonna*.

SULPHUR, always after treatment, and if there be torpidity of the bowels or any psoric or constitutional taint, in which cases, as also when there are indurations, *Silicea* may be found useful.

The skin and the whole surface of the body should be kept as dry as possible, and dry lint may be applied to the affected portions; the nourishment should be of the simplest kind and only a little at a time.

DOSE and Administration.—Prepare the selected remedy by carefully infusing one drop of the dilution, or six globules, in ten spoonfuls of water. *Aconite* or *Belladonna* may be given, a spoonful of each in alternation, every two hours, for twenty-four hours, after which give *Rhus tox.* a spoonful prepared in the same manner, every four hours. *Aconite, Belladonna* and *Lachesis* may be given at frequent intervals every two hours, or even every hour. *Arsenicum, Hepar sulph., Nux vomica* and *Rhus tox.*, at intervals of four hours, and *Silicea* and *Sulphur* at intervals of twelve or twenty-four hours, continuing each remedy one or two days. This is generally correct in all acute skin diseases.

Running from the Ears. Abscess in the Ear. (*Ottorrhœa.*)

Children are sometimes attacked with violent pain in the ear, causing them to scream, to roll and toss the head, to start suddenly from sleep, and frequently to put the hand to the head. The cause of these attacks, at times remains undiscovered, until after some days, a purulent discharge from the ear makes known the source of the malady, which is only in fact, an abscess or gathering in the head, so situated as to discharge itself through the ear. The matter is generally white, at times greenish, or dark colored, and often very offensive.

The remedies are Belladonna, Chamomilla, Calcarea carbonica., Mercurius, Pulsatilla, Rhus toxicodendron, and Sulphur.

If the complaint arise from a cold, give Belladonna, Chamomilla, Mercurius, or Rhus tox.

If it follow some exanthematous disease, Belladonna, Pulsatilla, Rhus tox., or Sulphur, may be indicated.

If the discharge be offensive, give Carbo veg.

For further indications, see Ottorrhæa.

Rupture of the Navel. Umbilical Hernia

An unnatural protrusion of the navel, unattended with fever or pain, but much more manifest if the child cry, scream, or hold its breath, from any cause, is generally characteristic of this affection.

TREATMENT.—A piece of pasteboard, sheet lead, or other hard substance, may be covered with silk or velvet, and placed over the navel. Over this, place several folds of muslin, or other soft substance, and secure the whole properly with a bandage. Give a dose of Nux vomica, every other day, at three o'clock, P. M., until four doses are taken. Afterwards, give Aurum in the same manner. Continue this treatment for a few weeks, or until a cure is effected.

Soreness of the Navel.

Sometimes, from the neglect of the nurse, or other cause, the navel becomes sore and takes on inflammation, with purulent or other discharge. This is generally a simple excoriation, and should be treated as such. See Excoriations, page 722.

Swelling of the Breasts,

In young infants, may exist at birth, or occur after-wards. It may be created by external pressure, and is frequently caused by ignorant nurses, who are in the habit of squeezing the breasts, for the purpose of pressing something out of them. By this means, the breasts of some females have been destroyed forever. If the breasts are swollen, a linen rag may be wet with sweet oil, and applied to them, which will often be sufficient to effect a cure in a few days, or in addition give a few doses of Belladonna, or Chamomilla, and if suppuration ensue, give Hepar sulphur, and after two or three days give Silicea or Sulphur. Rhus tox., if there be erysipe-latous inflammation, followed by Sulphur or Hepar sulphur, will be found efficient.

DOSE and Administration.—Of the selected remedy, dissolve one drop, or six globules, in ten spoonfuls of water, give a spoonful every four hours, until four doses are taken; then wait twenty-four or forty-eight hours, and if not better, select another remedy.

White Discharge from the Private Parts. (*Leucorrhœa.*)

A discharge of whitish mucus, in female infants, resembling the leucorrhœa of adults. It is generally of constitutional origin, though it may at times, be induced by want of care and attention to cleanliness.

Bathe the parts frequently, in water slightly warm, and give Calcarea carb., every morning, for four days. After waiting four days without medicine, if not better, give Pulsatilla, in the same manner, at night, four days; afterwards wait one or two weeks, and repeat the remedies, or give Sulphur.

Inflammation of the Privates. Inflammation of the Labia

Young girls are not unfrequently, subject to an inflammatory swelling of the private parts, attended with dryness, heat, and burning or shooting pains.

One of the most valuable and efficient remedies is Rhus tox. Give a teaspoonful every four hours of the solution, one drop in ten spoonfuls of water, one day, after which, if more medicine be necessary, give Mercurius in the same manner. Belladonna, or Nux vomica, may at times be useful; also, Sulphur. See Inflammation of the Labia.

Itchings and Burnings in the Private Parts. Pruritus.

This affection may be unattended with swelling, and be very distressing, causing the child to cry with pain, whilst it rubs itself with the greatest violence and force, or it may be less severe, and the child, if young, may often be observed to be at work with its hand, about the privates. Rhus tox., and afterwards Sulphur, given, as directed for Rhus tox., and Mercurius, in the last article, will generally afford relief, if the affection be acute and the sufferings great, in a few days; if chronic, in a few weeks. See also, Pruritus.

Inflammation of the Foreskin. Swelling of the Prepuce. Phimosis.

This is a similar affection in boys to the inflammation of the labia in girls, and will be cured by the same remedies. (See Inflammation of the Labia, page 729.)

At times a portion, or perhaps the whole of the extremity of the prepuce takes on a puffy, bladder-like appearance. Rhus tox, given as directed above will effect a cure; afterwards give Sulphur.

Retention of Urine. Scanty and Painful Urination.

For this affection Aconite is often sufficient, if not Pulsatilla will be found useful, or Cantharis, and afterwards Sulphur. (See Retention of Urine.

Profuse Urination.

For profuse urination, give Apis mel.; if insufficient, give Rhus tox., and afterwards Sulphur, Argentum met. Baryta carb., Iodium, and Squilla may also be found useful.

DOSE.—One drop, or six globules, in ten teaspoonfuls of water, give a teaspoonful every three hours, until amelioration or change.

Wetting the Bed. Nocturnal Urination.

If this result from inattention and indifference, the parent is referred to Solomon for advice, Prov. xxix., 15. But if the result of a constitutional weakness or disease, as is often the case, it may generally be alleviated by medicine. First give Pulsatilla, every night, a dose of three globules, four nights; afterwards Silicea every morning, four mornings; alternate these remedies a few weeks. If improvement follow, wait a few weeks, if no improvement, give Rhus tox. and Sulphur, or Cina and Causticum in the same 'manner. Also Carbo veg., Iodium, Calcarea carb., and Natrum mur., may be adapted to different cases of this complaint.

Discharges of Blood from the Anus or Rectum.

This is perhaps not a very common affection. When it occurs give first Rhus tox., and afterwards Arsenicum; or Hamamelis virg. and Ferrum, Kali carb. and Graphites, or Pulsatilla and Sulphur, may be found useful.

DOSE and Administration.—For any of the above affections, one drop, or six globules, of the selected remedy, in ten spoonfuls of water, give a spoonful every four hours, in acute cases, and when not otherwise directed, until amelioration or change. In chronic cases, every twelve or twenty-four hours.

Jaundice.

In this disease the white of the eye is at first noticed to have a yellowish tinge, also the urine, and at length the entire skin becomes yellow or sallow, and pale; the bowels may be costive, or loose, and the stools are generally light or clay colored.

The remedies are Chamomilla, China, Mercurius, Nux vomica and Sulphur.

CHAMOMILLA, always at first, if the bowels are loose, the stomach distended, the child nervous or irritable, to be followed after twenty-four hours by *Mercurius;* if relief be not obtained, or if after waiting two days the relief be but partial, and there be need of further medication.

CHINA, after any other remedies for remaining symptoms, especially if the child be weak, if there be distention of the hypochondria, and if the accompanying fever is intermittent.

MERCURIUS, after *Chamomilla*, when that proves insufficient, and especially for scrofulous children, and generally for obstinate cases.

NUX VOMICA may be given at the outset, if the child is costive, irritable and passionate, and afterwards *China* or *Sulphur*.

DOSE.—One drop of the dilution, or six globules, in ten spoonfuls of water, a spoonful to be given every four hours, two days, then wait two days, or select some other remedy.

Constipation.

Is frequently caused by improper diet, either given to the child or to the mother, or where mothers do not nurse their own children, to the nurse, when a change in this respect is the proper remedy. If, however, the bowels are not moved daily, give Bryonia, and if it prove insufficient give Nux vomica or Opium, and if costiveness still continue, give Sulphur In very obstinate cases, Lycopodium, Alumina or Natrum mur. may be found useful.

ADMINISTRATION.—Give a dose of three globules of the selected remedy, daily, for four days. If no favorable change takes place, select some other remedy. Injections of lukewarm water may sometimes be administered with benefit.

Diarrhœa.

A healthy infant may have from three to six evacuations in twenty-four hours. If the discharges become more frequent, so as to appear exhausting, or are changed in character, becoming green, yellow, white, brown, frothy, watery, mucus or bloody; or if the child appear to suffer, becoming haggard, irritable, or exhibit any symptoms of a diseased condition, it is time to interfere, and one of the following remedies will usually be found appropriate.

REMEDIES.—Aconite, Belladonna, Chamomilla, Ipeca. cuanha, Mercurius and Rheum.

ACONITE, especially if there be fever, with hot skin and rapid pulse, will frequently be sufficient to control the disease.

BELLADONNA, after *Aconite*, if the child scream out with pain, start suddenly from sleep, and is very rest- less.

CHAMOMILLA.—If there be acidity of the stomach; constant crying, and restlessness; drawing up of the legs; frequent evacuations, bilious, watery, slimy or frothy, and whitish, yellowish or greenish, with sour, offensive smell, or like rotten eggs; hardness, tension and fulness of the abdomen. Also if excited by improper food, or occurring during teething. Often preferable to *Belladonna* and after *Aconite*.

IPECACUANHA.—Especially when arising from change of food, as at the period of weaning, or if there be frequent vomiting, with bilious, slimy or dark colored discharges, or mixed with blood, or evacuations like fermented matter mixed with flocks or flakes, and fol- lowed by straining.

MERCURIUS.—After *Chamomilla*, when that remedy proves insufficient, or if there be severe colic, with tenesmus and protrusion of the bowels, and especially if it has arisen from giving cathartic medicines.

RHEUM. —- Especially if there is acidity, with indi- gestion, and flatulent distension of the bowels; colic, crying and tenesmus, before and after evacuation; and when a sour smell is constantly emitted from the child; also when magnesia and similar poisons have been pre-

63

viously administered. Against poisonous doses of *Rheum* give *Chamomilla* or *Mercurius*. For further indications see article *Diarrhœa*, page 732.

DOSE and Administration.—Of the selected remedy, one drop, or six globules, in ten spoonfuls of water, give a spoonful every two hours, until amelioration or change; afterwards every four or six hours, until recovery, or some other remedy be chosen.

Summer Complaint. *Cholera Infantum.*

Sickness at the stomach, gagging, and fruitless efforts to vomit, or vomiting, first of food, afterwards of mucus; and evacuations very frequent, greenish, or yellowish, or white, slimy, and perhaps mixed with blood, or very thin and watery; or evacuations of undigested food, with very offensive smell, are common characteristics of this complaint. The thirst for cold water is usually very great, but all drinks are often ejected as soon as taken. The head is hot, the feet and hands cold, the abdomen generally hot and distended. If the disease continue the child loses flesh, the skin hangs about it in folds, and emaciation, hectic fever, usually worse towards evening, with sunken eyes, half closed during sleep, proclaim the dangerous nature of the complaint. The usual exciting causes, are want of proper food or clothing, or of fresh air, changes of temperature, stimulating drugs, taken as food or medicine, and teething. Children are most subject to it during their second summer. At this period every attention should be given to diet, exercise, clothing, &c., if the child still nurse, both for the mother or nurse, and for the child. All stimulants should be carefully avoided, the clothing should be adapted to the changes of the weather, and the child frequently taken into the open air.

REMEDIES.—Antimonium crud, Arsenicum, Bryonia,

Carbo veg., Dulcamara, Ipecacuanha, Mercurius, Nux vomica, Veratrum. and sulphur.

ANTIMONIUM CRUD.—White or yellow coated tongue; mouth dry and thirsty; nausea and vomiting; distension of the abdomen, and flatulence, with offensive stools; and frequent passages of urine.

ARSENICUM.—Cold extremities; loss of appetite; intense thirst, drinking little at a time; discharges yellow and watery, or white or brownish, worse after midnight, or after eating; and especially if the child has become weak, pale, and emaciated.

BRYONIA. — Diarrhœas in hot weather, with much thirst, or diarrhœa with colic; the stools having a putrid smell, and being whitish or brownish, and lumpy.

CARBO VEG., if *Bryonia* do not afford relief, and if the discharges are very thin, and offensive, with burning pains.

DULCAMARA, if the complaint recur on every change to cold, or arise from drinking cold water, worse at night.

IPECACUANHA.—Nausea and vomiting; vomiting of food and drink, or of mucus and bile, with diarrhœa; stools are fermented with white flocks, tinged with blood; coated tongue; dislike to all food; raging thirst. After *Ipecacuanha* give *Arsenicum*.

MERCURIUS.—Discharges worse before midnight, with colic; straining when at stool; perspiration scanty; greenish, sour evacuations, and nausea.

NUX VOMICA, after *Ipecacuanha*, when that remedy fails, and especially if the discharges are very frequent, small, and with straining.

VERATRUM.—Nausea and vomiting, with faintness and weakness; great exhaustion, with vomiting after swallowing the least liquid, or making the slightest movement; thirst for cold water; sensitiveness at the pit of the stomach; colic with burning pains; loose, watery stools, and at times unnoticed.

SULPHUR, for lingering cases; evacuations frequent, thin, watery, slimy, or greenish or whitish.

DOSE and Administration.—One drop of the dilution, or six globules, in ten spoonfuls of water, give a spoonful every half hour, until a change is effected; after the acute symptoms subside, give the remedies less frequently.

During the treatment the greatest care should be taken not to overload the stomach with food or drink; the patient should be kept quiet as possible, and all exposures carefully avoided.

Colic.

Extremely violent attacks of pain in the bowels, manifested by crying, writhing, drawing up the limbs, coldness of the feet, and generally distension of the abdomen. It may be attended by costiveness or diarrhœa.

REMEDIES.—Chamomilla, China, Ipecacuanha, Nux vomica and Pulsatilla.

CHAMOMILLA may be given in most cases, especially if there be writhing and twisting, irritability, &c.

CHINA.—When the abdomen is very hard and distended, and the attacks are intermittent.

IPECACUANHA.—Colic, with nausea and diarrhœa.

NUX VOMICA.—Colic, with constipation.

PULSATILLA. — Flatulent colic, rumbling of wind, shiverings, paleness, tenderness of the abdomen to the touch.

ADMINISTRATION.—Give the medicines in water as directed above, a teaspoonful every fifteen minutes, in violent cases, or give a dry powder every hour, until relief is afforded.

Infantile Remittent Fever.

The usual symptoms are languor, irritability, want of appetite, nausea, thirst, heat of the skin, and very rest. less nights. At length these symptoms become aggra- vated; there is hurried and oppressed breathing; rapid pulse; occasionally flushed face; vomiting; distension of the stomach; obstinate constipation, or diarrhœa, or frequent but ineffectual desire for stool; discharges dis- colored or fetid, or mucus, or mixed with blood; hands and feet cold, whilst other parts of the body are hot, dry and parched; head hot and heavy, and often symp- toms resembling hydrocephalus, such as coma; tongue moist, loaded, and often red along the margins, or becoming dry at the point; fever, with remissions and exacerbations; if worse at night, usually attended with violent twitchings or jerking, if by day, with stupor and drowsiness; sometimes a cough, with wheezing, &c.

The patient at times may appear to be steadily reco- vering, and may afterwards, without apparent cause, take a relapse, and these changes may alternate for con- siderable time, until if the disease be not checked, the glandular system becomes affected, or dropsical effusion take place, or the brain takes on active inflammation, the child becomes emaciated, the vital powers give way, and death closes the scene.

ACONITE, if there be fever with thirst, skin dry and hot, and if the bowels are regular and healthy.

DOSE.—One drop of the dilution, or six globules, in ten spoonfuls of water; a spoonful to be given every two hours, until amelioration or change.

BELLADONNA, if there be flushed face, dry heat, espe- cially of the head, coma or sleeplessness; tongue coated white or yellow in the centre, red at the edges; pulse

63*

very quick and full; great heat of the abdomen, with tenderness on the slightest pressure.

DOSE.—A teaspoonful of a solution, of one drop, or six globules, in water, as above every four hours.

BRYONIA, after *Aconite;* febrile heat, with chills, worse at night; head hot, heavy and painful; thirst; dry tongue; hiccough; retching; vomiting; colic; and constipation.

DOSE.—The same as for *Belladonna.*

CHAMOMILLA, often if there is diarrhœa or vomiting; after *Ipecacuanha,* or *Nux vomica;* or if the tongue is red and cracked, or coated yellow; lethargic or restless sleep, with starts and jerks; or if the head is hot and heavy, the face flushed, and the skin dry and parched; sensibility to pain; irritability; shortness of breath.

DOSE.—The same as for *Belladonna.*

CHINA is useful, after *Chamomilla* or *Ipecacuanha;* when the discharges have been exhausting; the bowels are tympanitic; and the fever is attended with manifest remissions and exacerbations.

DOSE.—The same as for *Bryonia.*

IPECACUANHA, often at the commencement, if there is loss of appetite, nausea, or vomiting; with headache; yellow coated tongue; restlessness; heat in the palms of the hands; night sweats; oppression for breath; languor and apathy.

DOSE.—One drop of the dilution, or six globules, in ten spoonfuls of water; give a spoonful every four hours, one or two days; afterwards, give *Pulsatilla,* if required.

LACHESIS, after *Belladonna;* if there be deep, prolonged sleep; grinding of the teeth; sleeplessness, alternated with sopor; distension and tenderness of the abdomen, especially in spots, or in a single spot; worse at night, and after sleep.

DOSE.—The same as *Belladonna*.

MERCURIUS, after *Belladonna*, if the heaviness and heat of the head continue; and if there is foul tongue; loss of appetite; nausea or vomiting; with tenderness of the abdomen; thirst; constipation; or diarrhœa, with tenesmus.

DOSE.—One drop, or six globules, in ten spoonfuls of water, give a spoonful every four hours, one day; afterwards, every six or twelve houis, according to the condition.

NUX VOMICA.—Bowels costive, with frequent inclination for an evacuation; scanty, watery stools, after much straining; abdomen swollen and painful; child peevish, obstinate, wilful; loss of appetite, or disgust at food; fever towards morning or evening.

DOSE.—The same as for *Mercurius*, or it may often be sufficient to give a single powder daily, at three o'clock in the afternoon,'continuing also, the indicated remedy, according to directions.

PULSATILLA, after *Ipecacuanha*, when that remedy has proved inefficient, or when there is a relaxed condition of the bowels; with whitish, bilious, or fetid discharge, or of variable color, and accompanied with gripings.

DOSE.—The same as *Mercurius*.

Spasms or Convulsions.

Children are more subject to these affections in infancy than at any other period of life. The exciting causes are numerous, among which may be mentioned bad air, unwholesome gases and vapors, unwholesome or irritating food or drinks, such as coffee, spices, sweatmeats, candies, &c., worms, glandular affections, repelled eruptions, mechanical injuries, and teething.

The remedies are Belladonna, Chamomilla, Coffea,

Cina, Hyoscyamus, Ignatia, Ipecacuanha, Mercurius, Opium, Stramonium, and Sulphur.

BELLADONNA, if the pupils are dilated, the body rigid, the forehead and hands dry and hot; at times, clenching of the hands, involuntary urination, the slightest touch often exciting an attack; and especially if the child starts frequently, and stares about.

DOSE.—Three globules, dry on the tongue, or in a teaspoonful of water, every half hour.

CHAMOMILLA, convulsive jerkings and twitchings; motion of the head from side to side; drowsiness; eyes half closed; loss of consciousness; restlessness; fretfulness; especially during dentition, and for children of a peevish, fretful disposition.

DOSE.—The same as *Belladonna*.

COFFEA, for weak, nervous children, and when the cause cannot be discovered, may be given after *Belladonna*, or *Chamomilla*.

CINA, if the child is subject to worms, to wetting the bed, itchings at the nose, or at the anus, spasms with rigidity of the whole body.

DOSE.—The same as for *Belladonna*.

HYOSCYAMUS, for convulsions caused by fright, or with loss of consciousness, thumbs clenched upon the palms.

DOSE.—The same as for *Belladonna*.

IGNATIA.—Sudden and violent starts from sleep, with loud screams; trembling; convulsions of single limbs, or of single muscles; fits returning every day, at the same hour, or every other day, at about the same time, followed by fever; for children of pale delicate appearance; alternations of laughter and sadness, crying and laughing almost in the same breath; during dentition, and when other remedies fail.

DOSE.—Three globules every half houi, until relieved or change.

IPECACUANHA, if there is great difficulty of breathing, nausea, aversion to food, and disposition to lie down.

DOSE.—The same as for *Ignatia.*

MERCURIUS. — Convulsions caused by worms; with distension of the abdomen; eructations; flow of water from the mouth; and great weakness.

DOSE.—The same as for *Ignatia.*

OPIUM. — Convulsions from fright, with trembling, tossing of the limbs, and loud screams; or if the child lie unconscious, as if stunned; breathing with difficulty; abdomen distended; and all the evacuations suppressed.

DOSE.—Three globules every half hour, until amelioration or change.

STRAMONIUM.—Symptoms similar to *Opium* or *Hyoscyamus,* and if there are involuntary evacuations of fœces and urine.

DOSE.—The same as for *Opium.*

SULPHUR, at the close of the treatment, or if the convulsions are caused by repelled eruptions.

DOSE.—Three globules every twelve hours.

External applications are of doubtful utility. Cold applications to hot surfaces, or hot applications to cold surfaces, although sanctioned by usage, may often be productive of injury, whilst their usefulness is not confirmed by any well authenticated evidence. And they certainly appear unphilosophical. If the shock caused by a stream of cold water upon the head, has ever produced apparent improvement, it must have been done by producing some powerful revulsion of the whole system, and have been attended with danger to other important organs. It is generally safer to trust to the administra‑ tion of medicines, or in extreme cases, relying on the homœopathic principle, to apply hot applications to hot surfaces; cold applications to cold surfaces.

Frequent and constant rubbing downwards, from the head towards the extremities, will produce a much more favorable reaction than extremes of cold or heat.

Lock-jaw.

This affection, under the old school treatment, often proves fatal. The child at first is apparently unable to suck, or if it succeed, the milk escapes from the mouth. On examination the lower jaw can not be depressed, the muscles are rigid, the jaws gradually close, the whole body becomes rigid, and death ensues, usually in from two to four days.

TREATMENT.—If any local irritation can be discovered to have caused the attack, give Aconite, and at the same time bathe the injured part with a weak solution of the Tincture of Arnica.

If from the condition of the mother's milk, give Lachesis, and afterwards Belladonna. If no cause can be assigned or discovered give Belladonna.

After Belladonna, if the improvement be not satisfac‑ tory, give Mercurius.

If the affection appear to arise from a cold, give Chamo‑ milla; or if catarrhal symptoms are present, give Nux vomica. Hyoscyamus may also be useful after Nux vom. or Belladonna. (See Lockjaw, page 517.)

Spasms in the Chest. (*Spasmodic Asthma.*)

This differs from ordinary spasms or convulsions, inas. much as the chest and respiratory organs are principally affected; and from Millar's asthma, because this last named disease principally affects the upper portion of the windpipe.

In an attack of spasmodic asthma, the child wakes suddenly from sleep, with a shrill cry, and appears to be suffocating; the countenance is often livid, and the expression anxious. There is generally cough, dull, hollow and dry, and the breathing is rapid, laborious, and painfully distressing.

IPECACUANHA is the first remedy to be administered, and if relief follow, do not repeat it until the symptoms are again aggravated; but if there be no relief in thirty to forty minutes, give *Sambucus.* If there be aggravation after the administration of a medicine, wait a short time; if the aggravation be caused by the medicine, relief will soon follow; if not, repeat the remedy or select another.

ARSENICUM may in many cases follow *Ipecacuanha,* when partial relief only has been obtained, also *Lachesis.*

DOSE.—A drop of the selected remedy in four teaspoonfuls of water, give a teaspoonful or less every ten or fifteen minutes, until improvement is manifest; or a few globules may be placed upon the tongue of the child every ten minutes.

Asthma of Millar,

Differs from croup in the extreme suddenness of the attack, and in the cessation from suffering the patient enjoys during the intervals, whilst after croup is established the sufferings are continuous; croup also appears to consist in a stoppage of the throat, by what is called false membrane, whilst in this affection there seems to be a spasmodic contraction of the upper portion of the windwipe.

The attacks are distinguished by spasmodic inspirations, accompanied by a crowing noise much like croup, but with less rattling of mucus in the early stages; the face and extremities at length become purple, the thumbs are clenched, the toes drawn in, giving a distorted appearance to the foot; the attacks recur frequently at short intervals, until if relief be not obtained, the child dies in one of the paroxysms.

This disease has as yet received too little attention. The remedies which have been found efficacious are Aconite, Arsenicum, Ipecacuanha, Moschus, Pulsatilla and Sambucus.

ACONITE, if there be fever, with symptoms of congestion of blood to the head.

ARSENICUM, after *Ipecacuanha*, especially if there be anguish, cold perspiration, and prostration of strength; or if these indications are very prominent, it may be given at the commencement.

IPECACUANHA.—Anxious, short and sighing respiration; purple color of the face and rigidity of the frame; spasmodic symptoms, and suffocation.

MOSCHUS, appears to be adapted, and has been given with success for spasmodic constrictions of the larynx, with difficult and short breathing; also in many cases attended with spasms in the chest, inclination to cough, the spasms becoming exacerbated after the cough.

SAMBUCUS.—Livid hue of the face; dry heat of the body; twitchings and jerkings of the muscles; small irregular intermittent pulse; no thirst; ineffectual inclination to sleep; or lethargy, with oppression for breath; and wheezing; if *Sambucus* fail, give *Pulsatilla*.

DOSE and Administration.—Give any of the above remedies, dry or in water, by infusing one drop, or six globules, in ten spoonfuls of water, and placing a small quantity, from a few drops to a teaspoonful, on the tongue, every ten minutes, until relief is afforded. If given during the intervals between the paroxysms, give a teaspoonful every hour, or every two hours, according as they occur, more or less frequently.

For further indications, see Asthma, page 421.

Hiccough,

Is frequently troublesome to the child, and occasions anxiety to the mother. It may often be relieved by wrapping the child up more warmly, giving it the breast, &c. If it become troublesome, give a teaspoonful of sweetened water, or a little white sugar. If it frequently recur, its cause is to be sought and treated with remedies adapted to the condition of the patient. Nux vomica or Moschus, Ipecacuanha or Sambucus, administered at intervals of twenty-four or forty-eight hours, two globules at a dose, for four or eight days, will often afford relief. It is essentially spasmodic in its character, and is to be relieved by similar remedies. (See Spasms, page 740.)

DOSE.—The same as for Spasm in the Chest.

Loss of Flesh. Atrophy. Marasmus.

SULPHUR, followed by *Calcarea carb.* or *Arsenicum*, will generally afford relief. (See Atrophy.

Head-fall.

Some children with open fontanelles, and of weak or cachetic habits, whilst they appear gradually sinking away, manifest among other symptoms of exhaustion a peculiar depression between the bony structures of the head, as if the brain were too feeble to hold itself in position, and which has hence been denominated head-

64

fall. It more commonly occurs in very early life, and appears to consist in a lack of vital energy, or nerve power, and like most other diseases, may more properly be considered a symptom than a disease.

When this condition is manifested, the attention of the physician should be directed to such remedies as appear adapted to restore the vital force.

BELLADONNA, MOSCHUS, NUX VOMICA and PHOSPHO-RUS, are among the more active remedies. *Calcarea carb.*, *Mercurius*, *Silicea* and *Sulphur*, will also be found efficient.

DOSE and Administration.—Give a dose, two globules, of the selected remedy, once in four hours, two days; if improvement be observed in the general condition, continue the remedy once in twelve or twenty-four hours, for one or two weeks; if there be no improvement select another remedy

Dentition.

The commencement of teething is very variable as to time; some children cut their teeth very young, and in others the period of their appearance is long deferred. In general, at about the age of five to seven months they may be expected. The appearance of the teeth is usually preceded by restlessness; flushes of heat, or paleness; difficulty of sucking; gums swollen and hot; disposed to bite; drivelling at the mouth, and looseness of the bowels. During this period, if by cold or other cause, the secretions become suppressed, a tendency of blood to the head is usually manifest, which, if not speedily checked, may terminate in inflammation of the brain.

The teeth usually appear in the following order:— First, the two middle lower teeth; next, the two middle upper teeth, usually two or three weeks afterwards; third, the two lower teeth, one on each side the first two, and very soon the corresponding teeth above. About two months after this the jaw teeth begin to appear before the stomach and eye teeth, which are cut shortly after the four front jaw teeth, and at about the age of two and a half years, the four back jaw teeth complete the set.

With proper exercise and diet on the part of the mother and child, in healthy children, this period should pass over without much danger or suffering; but mothers who insist on feeding their children with various condiments from the table, or candies, sweetmeats, &c., from the shops, as well as those who dose them with the drugs of the apothecary, may be sure that this period will be full of suffering, dangers and anxieties, unless nature shall reverse her ordinary laws, and procure for them an exemption they have no reason to anticipate. The infant should take no other nourishment but the breast until after it cuts its stomach teeth, and the mother should abstain from all stimulating drinks, coffee, pepper, spices, &c.

If medicines are required, the following will be found useful:

Aconite, Belladonna, Chamomilla, Calcarea carbonica, Coffea, Cuprum, Mercurius, Nux vomica, Sulphur and Zincum.

ACONITE, if there be fever, restlessness, sleeplessness, with cryings and startings.

BELLADONNA, for convulsions followed by sound and long-continued sleep; or if the child start suddenly from sleep and look around as if terrified, pupils dilated, the child stares, the body becomes stiff, and the temples and palms of the hands are hot.

CHAMOMILLA.—Child restless at night, tosses about, drinks frequently; spasmodic twitchings and jerkings when asleep, starts from the slightest noise; agitation, groaning, breathing rapid and difficult, hacking cough;

diarrhœa, with green slimy or watery evacuations, and all the symptoms worse at night.

CALCAREA CARB.—Dentition slow and difficult for children of light complexion and inclined to flesh, or for those of scrofulous habit, with tendency to rachitis or to glandular diseases.

COFFEA.—If *Belladonna* or *Chamomilla* fail, and for children of excitable temperament; or if the child is sleepless, fretful and lively by turns, irritable and difficult to please.

CUPRUM, if there are cerebral symptoms, and the child clenches the cup almost spasmodically with its gums.

MERCURIUS, for copious drivelling, redness of the gums, and diarrhœa, with greenish evacuations after *Chamomilla*.

NUX VOM., also after *Chamomilla* or *Belladonna*, when there is costiveness or diarrhœa, with scanty evacuations and gripings.

SULPHUR may be given after almost any of the foregoing remedies, and especially for children of thin and meagre habit, and with tendency to eruptions.

ZINCUM, for apparently hopeless cases, with symptoms of incipient paralysis of the brain; sopor; eyes half closed, or motionless; coldness of the whole body; bluish color of the skin; respiration obstructed, and pulse nearly extinct; in grain doses every two hours, until the temperature of the body begins to return, when the intervals may be lengthened or some other remedy be alternated with it, as *Belladonna* for instance, for the remaining symptoms.

DOSE.—Of any of the above remedies, give one drop of the dilution, or six globules, in ten spoonfuls of water; a spoonful every four hours, or oftener in extreme cases, until amelioration or change.

Weaning.

It is generally appropriate to the condition of both the mother and child to continue the period of nursing eigh. teen or twenty months; but if the mother be delicate, the supply of milk diminished, or its quality degenerated; if the menses have reappeared, or the mother complain of great prostration after nursing, the child may be weaned at an earlier period.

The child should not however be weaned whilst suffer. ing from teething, or from any other acute attack, unless the condition of the mother absolutely requires it. The spring and fall afford the most suitable season for wean. ing. The child should gradually become accustomed to the use of food after it is about a year old, that the diges. tive organs may be the more fully developed; but its diet should be simple, such as bread, milk, ripe fruit, farina, &c. Meat should not be given until the child is from three to five years old, and then very sparingly once each day. Ripe and wholesome fruits may be allowed at a much earlier period.

The mother, after the child is removed from the breast, should be careful of her diet, and avoid unusual or unne- cessary exposure.

If the breasts become distended and painful, they should be bathed in lard, or wrapped up in raw cotton; one or two applications of a camphorated spirit bath may also be useful. They should be drawn occasion- ally with a breast pipe, or by the lips of another child, or a nurse. Bryonia, Pulsatilla or Rhus tox., will also be useful, if internally administered.

. **DOSE.**—Give one drop, or six globules, in a spoonful of water, every night and morning; or if there be severe inflammation, every four hours, until the swelling and inflammation subside

64*

Vaccination.

That vaccination affords another illustration of the great homœopathic law, all homœopathists will no doubt readily admit. Of its influence to protect the child from the contagion of small-pox, we think there is abundant evidence.

All persons should be vaccinated twice, once in infancy, and again at about the age of eighteen years. The first vaccination should be performed when the child is from four to six months old, unless the prevalence of small-pox or some other circumstance renders an earlier or later period more desirable or convenient.

The vaccine matter should be obtained direct from the cow, or from a child perfectly free from eruptions or disease of any kind.

Successful vaccination manifests itself about the fourth or fifth day. A slight redness, and a small elevation or pimple is perceived, which begins to fill about the seventh or eighth day, soon after which it is surrounded by a red circle or areola, which increases until the tenth day, when it attains about the size of a dollar.

The fluid in the vesicle now begins to dry up, and by the twelfth day the scab appears, which gradually becomes dry and hard until the eighteenth day, when it can frequently be removed, or it falls off of itself.

The indisposition attendant upon genuine vaccination, commences on the sixth or seventh day, consisting generally of slight rigors; pain and soreness under the arm; lassitude; headache; occasionally nausea; loss of appetite; general fever and restlessness. These symptoms seldom continue more than two or three days, and should not be interfered with. They subside as the vesicle fills; Hahnemann recommends that a dose of Sulphur be given on the eighth day, to prevent the development of any eruptive disease, as erysipelas.

Spurious vaccination progresses from the time of the insertion of the matter. It runs its course in a shorter time than the genuine; the scab is of a lighter color; there is no hardened, depressed speck in the centre; it is more brittle and mealy; and the indisposition, if it appears at all, comes on at an earlier period.

To perform vaccination properly, it is only necessary to insert a small quantity of the true vaccine virus beneath the skin.

CHAPTER XVI.

RANGE OF USE OF THE MORE PROMINENT REMEDIES USED IN THIS WORK.

1.—Aconitum.

RANGE OF USE.—Acute inflammation; rush of blood to the head; evil effects of fright or anger, or from a chill produced by a dry cold air; inflammatory bilious and nervous fevers; derangement of the mind in expectation of death; dizziness; first stage of croup, and the first stage of hooping-cough; measles; small-pox; erysipelas, and all the eruptive diseases; darting pains, aggravated or renewed by wine or other stimulants; pains and restlessness at night; painful affections, with thirst and redness of the cheeks; irritable; considerable languor and disposition to lie down; red, hot, shining swellings; rash; burns, &c., when attended with violent fever; inability to sleep; constantly restless; tossing about, and anxiety; dry heat over the entire surface of the body; heat; thirst; short breathing; quick pulse; redness of the face and cheeks; disposition to uncover oneself; chilliness soon after going to bed, or in the evening; attacks of feverish redness of the cheeks; severe thirst; inflammatory fevers, attended with quick pulse and great irritability; anguish, with apprehensions of death; trembling state of mind; bitter wailing; great tendency to start; sensitive and irritable; merry at times; vertigo, with reeling; darkness of sight, or nausea; ful-

(753)

ness and sense of weight in the forehead, with sensation as though all the contents of the skull would issue through the forehead; sensation as if the senses were about to depart, with crampy sensation in the forehead, or above the root of the nose; great fulness of the head, with heat and redness of the face; dilated pupils; aversion to light; very painful inflammation of the eyes, with discharge of water; inflammation caused by foreign bodies penetrating into the eyes; red, hard swelling of the lids; intolerance of noise and humming in the ears; bleeding at the nose of plethoric persons; stoppage from cold; bloated red face; red cheeks; sweat on the forehead; pain in the teeth, caused by exposure to a sharp wind; throbbing on the painful side, with redness of the face; rheumatic pains in the face and teeth, and toothache after drinking some heating beverage; dryness of the mouth and tongue; tingling, burning and stinging on the tongue; spitting of blood; burning and stinging in the throat, with inflammation; bitter taste; loss of appetite; burning unquenchable thirst; inflammation of the stomach; pressure at the pit of the stomach as if from a weight; vomiting of blood; inflammation of the liver; sense of tightness; pressure and fulness of the bowels; pressure in the region of the liver; oppressed breathing; inflammation of the bowels; inflammation attendant on strangulated rupture, with vomiting of bitter bilious matter; watery diarrhœa, with flowing piles; urinary organs; inflammation of the neck of the bladder; difficult and scanty emission of urine; deep red hot urine, without sediment, or with a brickdust deposit in the vessel; pain in the testicles as if bruised; profuse menses, and fear of death during pregnancy; short dry cough, excited by titillation of the throat after midnight; bloody and slimy expectoration when coughing; influenza and sore-throat; short breath when sleeping; fetid breath; pleurisy; anxious, difficult and sobbing breathing; acute pains in the chest; inflammation of the lungs; intense anguish in the chest; palpitation of the heart, with intense anxiety; pain in the small of the back as if bruised and beaten; the arms feel lame as if beaten; pain in the hips as if beaten; inflammatory swelling of the legs.

2.—Arnica Montana.

RANGE OF USE.—Affections arising from mechanical injuries; bruises, sprains and wounds, principally inflicted by blunt instruments, bites, dislocations, sprains and fractures; stings of insects; corns, by an external use, when sensitive and painful; rheumatism, with tearing pains; tingling, burning pains, as if bruised; affections arising from a shock or fall, or bruise, or from lifting; rushes of blood to the head; heat in the head, and cold feet; pains aggravated by talking or gentle exercise, and apoplexy; wounds caused by bruises, bites or boils; hot, hard, shining swellings; drowsiness in day-time, and in the evening at an early hour; anxious and frightful dreams; chilliness in the evening, and fever; intermittent fevers, with a good deal of thirst, the fever preceded by pains in the limbs and bones as if bruised; puerperal fever; anxious and sad, hypochondriacal and inconsolable; vertigo when walking; pressing headache, especially in the forehead; jerking, tearing and stitching in the head; rush of blood to the head, with burning heat in the head, the body being cool or naturally warm; headache caused by a fall; external tingling of the scalp upon the top of the head; tingling around the eyes; inflammation of the eyes from injury; swollen lids; eyes

without lustre, and profuse discharge of burning tears;
pain in the ears as if bruised; long stitches in and behind
the ears; roaring in the ears, and deafness after injuries;
sensation as if the nose were bruised; swelling and bleeding of the nose; countenance pale and sunken; redness
of one cheek only; beating or tingling of the cheeks;
swelling of the cheeks; cracked borders of the lips;
pain in teeth, with swelling of the cheeks; disagreeable
tingling of the gums; spitting of blood; dry or white
coated tongue; burning in the throat; putrid taste in the
mouth; bitter taste in the morning; aversion to meat;
bitter or putrid risings, or empty risings from the stomach;
gulping up of bitter mucus; inclination to vomit early in
the morning; empty retching and inclination to vomit;
vomiting of coagulated food; and vomiting of milk and
blood after drinking; fulness in the stomach; stitches in
the pit of the stomach, with pressure extending to the
back, and tightness of the chest; stitches in the left side
when walking, arresting the breath and painful; colic
after lifting; pain in the sides of the abdomen as if
bruised; watery diarrhœa, and involuntary at night;
thin stools after several ineffectual attempts; unable to
urinate, with pressure in the bladder; brown urine, with
brick-dust sediment; blood mixed with the urine; blue
red swelling of the penis and scrotum; swelling of the
testicles, and dropsy of the testicles; *and in females*, premature courses, and after-pains in women who have been
confined, very severe and of long duration; dry cough,
after crying of children; hooping-cough; expectoration
of blood, with oppressed breathing; shooting stitches and
pains in the head when coughing; oppressed breathing;
anxious panting or short breathing; fetid breath; stitches
in the chest that interrupts the breath; rheumatic pains

MORE PROMINENT REMEDIES USED.   757

in the side as if sore and bruised; soreness of the nipples;
pain as if beaten in the small of the back; tingling along
the spine; pain in the arm as if bruised, with tingling in
the arm and sprains of the wrist; bruised, painful feeling
in the hands; bruised feeling in the legs and feet; drawing and weariness in the thighs; tearing pains in the
knee, and a feeling as if the tendons were too short,
aggravated when walking; tingling in the feet; swelling
and erysipelas of the feet; toes hot, red and swollen,

3.—Arsenicum Album.

RANGE OF USE.—Burning, chiefly in the stomach or
in the other interior parts affected; sharp drawing pains;
night pains, almost unbearable, creating despair; aggravation of suffering in the evening in bed, or lying on the
part affected, or when asleep; mitigation by heat applied
externally and by moving about; loss of strength, great
weakness, the energies entirely prostrated; skin dry as
parchment, or cold and bluish, ulcers with raised and
hard edges; fetid smell; irritating suppuration; bleeding,
putridity and bluish or greenish color of the ulcers; dry
burning; blue and cold skin; blood-blisters, and itch-like
pimples; spots upon the skin; black pustules, as if near
mortification; festering itch, with burning pain; burning
ulcers, with acrid discharges; ulcers that have been so
much inflamed as to present a black appearance, extremely
painful, with stinging and burning; sleepless and restlessness at night; starting and twitching of the limbs, or of
the whole body during sleep, or on the point of falling
asleep; restlessness and anguish about the heart every
night; anxious dreams; general coldness; sinking of the
pulse, and clammy perspiration; very chilly; without
thirst; generally after drinking, with paroxysms of pain,

or followed with other symptoms; vertigo, with fever
following, and humming in the ears; intermittent fevers,
where each paroxysm commences with chilliness and heat
at the same time; great restlessness and thirst; typhus
fevers; very restless in mind, and anxious about every
thing, causing one to walk to and fro in the daytime;
in bed and out at night, especially after first going to
bed; irritable, especially after taking brandy too freely;
disposition to be troubled about other people's faults;
feels confused and heavy; vertigo, and throbbing in the
head; beating pain in the forehead; swelling of the head,
and scald head; inflammation, with burning in the eyes
and inner surface of the eyelids; disposition to shed tears,
and the lids become stuck together during sleep every
night; specks upon the eye near the sight; humming in
the ears as if the ears were stopped; burning in the nose;
excessive discharge of burning, acrid, thin mucus; bluish
face; sunken eyes; cadaverous look; bloated below the
eyelids; cancer on the face; the lips blackish, cracked
and dry; swelling of the glands of the under jaw; pain
in the teeth at night, aggravated by lying in bed on the
affected side, mitigated by sitting near a warm stove;
grating of the teeth; sore mouth; inflammation of the
little follicles, with burning and fetor; cracked tongue;
dry streak in the middle of the tongue; sore throat when
swallowing, as from an internal swelling; ineffectual
attempts to swallow; burning in the throat, and some
pain; bitter taste after eating; constant desire for drinks;
desire for sour things, or brandy; hiccough and empty
risings; nausea and weak feeling, compelling one to lie
down; habitual vomiting of the food from the stomach;
green vomitings; black vomitings; violent vomiting of
burning acrid bile; pressure at the pit of the stomach,

very painful to the touch, with anguish; cancer of the stomach; swollen and distended; excessive pain in the bowels; anguish and hardness of the bowels; colic pains like cutting sensation, with internal heat and external coldness; violent burning pains in the whole abdomen; urgent desire for stool; watery stool; greenish, yellowish, fetid, putrid and very offensive stools; burning stools, with violent colic; burning humor around the anus, extending up the rectum; stoppage of the urine in consequence of paralysis of the bladder; at other times burning urine, with slimy sediment; burning eruptions upon the scrotum; profuse flow during the *courses;* sore throat, with dry, burning sensation in the throat, unable to raise anything from coughing; very dry cough after drinking; tightness of the chest; spasmodic asthma; suffocating asthma in the bed at night, sensation as if the chest were contracted; burning in the chest; palpitation of the heart, with great anguish, especially at night; cancer of the heart; violent burning in the back; tearing or drawing pain in the back, running up under the shoulder blades, obliging one to lie down; swelling of the arms, covered with black pocks; burning ulcers at the top of the fingers; severe pains in the hip-joint, accompanied with much heat and burning; old ulcers upon the legs; neuralgia pains in knee-joints; burning and swelling of the feet.

4.—Belladonna.

RANGE OF USE.—Ailments caused by cold; rheumatic pains in the limbs; bilious derangement of the stomach, and severe pain in the head; inflammations of any of the internal organs, inviting the blood to any part; tendency to rush of blood to head; or quinsy, or epilepsy, or fits;

excited senses; noises unbearable; lock-jaw; convulsions of children; spasms from teething; inflammation of the throat, and inflammation of the brain; scarlet red eruptions upon the skin, with dryness, heat, burning, bloated appearance of the surface; smooth genuine scarlet fever, and erysipelas of the skin; scarlet rash over the whole body, and hot swellings, boils, and highly inflamed pocks; restless at night; ineffectual effort to sleep; starting as if from fright; disturbed by anxious dreams; alternate chilliness and heat; chilliness that runs down the back; rush of blood to the head, and pressure in the forehead; continuous burning heat and restlessness; throbbing of the blood-vessels; inflammatory fevers affecting the nose, lungs and head, with violent delirium; typhoid fever; melancholy and lowness of spirits, crying as if from rage, anguish and restlessness; trembling, diffidence and despondency; mania; headstrong; loss of consciousness and stupid; mania and ludicrous gesticulations; illusions of fancy; feeling about the head as if intoxicated, and reeling; vertigo, with anguish and falling; headache after dinner, and after taking cold in the head; stupefying headache, with loss of consciousness; periodical nervous headache, and pressure from within; outward rush of blood to the head; inflammation of the brain; dropsy of the brain; disposition and effort to bury the head in the pillow; pains in the eyes and in the balls; violent aching through the eyes; inflammation of the eyes; dilated pupils; strabismus or cross-eyed; dread of light; swelling of the parotid glands; hardness of hearing resulting from a cold in the head; inflammatory swelling of the nose, internally and externally; dry nose, one nostril stopped up; bleeding from the nose and mouth; redness of the face, somewhat bluish and bloated; distorted fea-

tures, expressive of anguish; violent cutting aching of the
face; swelling of the face from erysipelas; dark red lips;
eruptions at the corners of the mouth; swelling of the
glands of the under-jaw; pain in the teeth from cold; neuralgia of the teeth; mouth dry, without thirst; considerable quantity of tough mucus in the mouth; swelling and
redness of the tongue and palate; sore-throat and spasms
of the fauces or back portion of the mouth, preventing the
act of swallowing: swelling of the uvula and tonsils;
absence of taste; slimy, insipid taste; thirst, but unable
to drink; aversion to food; nausea and loathing of food;
empty gagging; vomiting of mucus; pressure at the pit
of the stomach, and bleeding after eating; painful distension of the abdomen, and painful as if raw and sore;
flatulent colic; constipation; mucus stools; involuntary
stools; stoppage of the urine, but constant sensation as
if urged to urinate; urine dark, torbid or flaming red;
urging to urinate in the afternoon, with pale yellow
urine; involuntary emission of urine; nocturnal emissions and weakness of the male genital organs; bearing
down pains; falling of the womb; flow of blood from
the womb; hemorrhage of bright red blood from the
womb; short, hurried and anxious respiration; danger
of suffocation when swallowing; the throat excessively
painful, as if filling up; rough, hoarse voice; short cough
and night cough; hooping-cough, and cough after midnight; oppression of the chest and short breath; stitches
throught the chest; uneasiness and beating in the chest;
rush of blood to the chest; inflammation of the lungs;
milk fever, or copious discharges of milk from the breasts;
stiffness of the neck; painful swelling of the neck and
nape of the neck; painful swelling of the glands of the
neck and those under the arms; paralysis of the arms;

65*

scarlet redness of the arms and hands; violent pain, with pressure in the shoulder; pain in the hip-joint, worse at night; violent pains in the knees; heaviness and lameness of the legs and feet.

5.—Bryonia.

RANGE OF USE.—Rheumatic fevers; typhoid fevers; bilious, intermittent and typhus fevers; shining swelling of individual parts; ailments arising from having a chill; a chill caused by anguish; general coldness of the body; hysteric spasms; pain on moving about, and drawing through the whole body; erysipelas and rash; itching, smarting and burning pimples on the skin; spots as in malignant fever; ulcers, with feeling of coldness; disposed to be drowsy, and yawn in the daytime; unable to sleep before midnight; thirst so intense during sleep as to awaken; vexatious dreams; delirium at night; talking and walking in the sleep; chilliness and coldness of the body when in bed; shaking chill, with heat in the head; red face and thirst before; vertigo and headache and stretching; general dry heat, internally and externally; intermittent fevers, with coldness prevailing; inflammatory, bilious, typhoid, milk and childbed fevers; profuse sweats; morning and evening perspiration, with a sour smell; restlessness of mind, and dread of future; a good deal of crying; irritable, vexed, vehement; delirious talk about business; head dull, confused; great fulness and heaviness of the head, with digging pressure in the direction of the forehead; pressing in the brain, either from within outwards, or from without inwards; inflammation of the brain, headache worse when in motion; pressure in the eyes in the evening; burning of the eyes; inflammation of the eyes and lids, and particularly of new born infants; itching tetter upon the lids; painful and red swelling of the lids; stick together after sleeping; dread of light; intolerance of noise and humming in the ears; inflammation up within the nostrils, and bleeding at the nose from suppression of the courses; chronic dry discharge from nose; red and burning; swelling of the face; lips cracked; pain in the teeth at night in bed; drawing, jerking, sensation as if the teeth were loose and elongated; dryness of the mouth and throat; stinging pains in the throat; flat, insipid and foul taste in the mouth; everything tastes bitter, either at the time or after taking it in the mouth; between meals or early in the morning; violent thirst after drinking beer; longing for wine and sour drinks and coffee; enormous appetite, or loss of appetite after eating a mouthful; bitter and sour risings from the stomach; gulping up the food; inclination to vomit, especially after eating food well liked; empty efforts to vomit; vomiting undigested food from the stomach, and glary liquid, bitter vomiting of blood: pressure in the stomach as from a stone, after eating; heartburn; stitching pains at the pit of the stomach when treading or making a wrong step, or when lying on the side; burning in the stomach during motion; pain in the right side; painful sensation when being touched, or coughing or drawing a breath; inflammation of the liver; abdominal spasms and cramps; inflammation of the bowels; loud rumbling in the abdomen; constipation; costiveness of long standing; diarrhœa; violent colic attending the discharge of undigested food; small quantity of urine, red or brown, and hot; an irresistible desire to urinate; suppression of the courses, and at other times too early, and profuse bleeding from the uterus; puerperal fever; hoarseness; cough; titillation of the throat; spasmodic and suffocating cough, with vomiting food from the stomach; cough with stitches in the sides of the chest, with aching pains in the head as if it would fly to pieces; yellowish expectoration, with pure blood or blood-streaked mucus, with little lumps of blood; difficult breathing; paroxysms of asthma; pressure at the chest as from a load; stitches in the chest and sides of the chest when coughing, or when drawing a long breath, or lying on the back, or in motion; palpitation of the heart; milk fever; pain in the small of the back, like a painful stiffness; stitching in the back and small of the back; rheumatic stiffness and tightness in the nape of the neck; tearing in the shoulder joints and upper arms, with tightness and stiching and swelling of the parts; swelling of the arm at the elbow-joint; pain in the wrist-joint as if sprained, when moving it; swelling of the hands; drawing pains in the thighs; stitches in the thighs from the seat to the ankles, with intolerance of contact or motion; perspiration; stiffness and swelling of the knees; tensive stitching and tearing in the calves of the legs down to the ankles; swelling of the legs down to the feet, pain as if sprained; swelling of the feet, with redness, heat, and stitching pain; sensation of parts being stretched during motion.

6.—Calcarea Carbonica.

RANGE OF USE.—Tearing in the limbs and joints; numbness of single parts liable to straining by lifting; ailments from teething; swelling and curvature of the bones; pains excited or aggravated by washing in cold water; subject to being easily impressed from cold air; chronic eruptions; scald head; nettle-rash; humid and scurfy eruptions or tetters; hard spots on the skin; warts or corns, with burning pain; itching of the skin; drowsy in the daytime, and early in the evening; lascivious dreams or fancies, and wanderings of the mind, with anxiety; difficult breathing at night, and thirst; Chilli- ness internally, with frequent flushes of heat and anguish; profuse perspiration in the daytime, from moderate exer- tion of the body; night or morning sweat; weeping; anxiety and anguish, and horrible disagreeable feelings on waking; despairing of success, and dread of sickness, wretchedness and accidents; sensitive and out of humor; chronic dulness of the head; dizziness before breakfast, with trembling; vertigo when ascending an eminence; pain in the head after lifting; pain in one side of the head, with belching of wind and inclination to vomit; stupefying or throbbing headache from mental efforts; icy coldness in and about the head; fulness and rush of blood to the head; falling out of the hair, and evening sweat about the head; pressure in the eyes; smarting in the eyes when reading by candle-light; sore eyes from mechanical injuries or cold; dilated pupils; dimness of sight, as if caused by a fog; discharge of pus from the ears; hardness of hearing; ulcerated scurfy nostrils yellow complexion, and humid scurfy eruptions on the lips and cheeks; toothache caused by the extremes of heat and cold; dry tongue, and very red; spasmodic con- struction of the throat; very sour taste in the mouth, and very thirsty all the time, and complete loss of appetite; belching of wind and heartburn after eating any kind of food; nausea in the morning; sour vomiting of young children; vomiting of the contents of the stomach; pain in the stomach, with cramp and vomiting of food, espe- cially after eating; swelled at the pit and region of the stomach; pains in the liver, and a tension in both the right and left side, unable to bear tight clothing at all; fulness of the bowels, as if distended with wind; bowels swollen hard, with colic and spasms; the bowels are sometimes constipated, at others loose, amounting to a diarrhœa; excessive, pungent, burning and fetid urine; weakness of the sexual power; leucorrhœa before the menses; frequent hoarseness and accumulation of mucus in the chest, and also cough without expectoration, as if some dust were in the throat; cough, with yellow fetid expectoration; suppuration of the lungs and bloody cough; stitching in the chest, and in the sides of the chest during motion; sore pain in the chest when drawing breath; palpitation of the heart after eating; pain in the small of the back and nape of the neck, after straining the parts by lifting, or pains as if sprained; curvature of the spine; swelling of the glands of the neck; rheumatic pains and weakness in the arms, hands or fingers; the legs are disposed to bend in children; they feel heavy and crampy; the knees swell, the feet feel numb in the evening, sometimes ulcers on the legs.

7.—Carbo Vegetabilis.

RANGE OF USE.—Rheumatic pains in the limbs and bones, with burning and prostration; lameness in the morning; burning of the skin here and there; dry itch; fetid ulcers; sleepless the fore part of the night, but falls asleep late; chilliness and coldness of the body; intermittent, with thirst during the cold stage; night-sweats; anguish and restless in the evening, and dread of ghosts; whirling of the head; pain in the head from heat; heaviness and oppression of the head; tearing in the outer parts of the forehead and back part of the head; nightly sticking of the lids; burning pressure of the eyes, and bleeding from them; want of ear wax; fetid discharge from the ear; itching of the nose, and frequent bleeding, with pale face; cracked lips; toothache; chronic loose. ness of the teeth, and bleeding of the gums; humor upon the tongue; dryness or flow of water in the mouth; scraping and burning in the throat and palate; bitter taste; chronic aversion to meat; acidity in the mouth after eating; sweat when eating; nausea in the morning; water-brash and vomiting of blood; burning and aching heartburn; pain in both sides, below the ribs and disten- sion of the bowels, and sometimes colic; bowels costive and difficult to move, with burning at the anus; thin, pale-colored slimy stool; wetting the bed; copious flow of urine; premature menses, and too profuse; con- tinual hoarseness, sore-throat, dry cough, and cough in the evening; short breathing, with tightness and oppres- sion of the chest; burning in the chest and dropsy; rheu- matic drawing pains in the back and nape of the neck; drawing and tearing in the arms and wrists and fingers; lameness of the wrist-joints; laming, drawing pains in the lower limbs; crampy feeling in the legs and soles of the feet; sweaty feet, and redness and swelling of the toes.

8.—Chamomilla.

RANGE OF USE.—Bilious derangements; various ail- ments of females; pregnant and lying-in women; teeth- ing children and new-born infants; irritable, restless and sensitive conditions of the nervous system; bad effects of disappointment or chagrin; rash in young children; soreness of children; sleep with open eyes, or half open; restlessness at night, with paroxysms of anxiety; crying, screaming and starting and tossing about during sleep; shuddering of single parts, and shuddering with internal heat; burning heat and sour sweat; bilious fevers; lung fevers; fevers in children when teething; anxious moaning and tossing about; vexed and whining mood, with crying; crying of new-born infants; confused state of the head, unable to comprehend; whirling early in the morning, and attacks of vertigo, as if one would faint; headache in the morning; heaviness; pains drawing and tearing on one side of the head; rush of blood to the head, with beating in the brain; inflammation of the eyes and margins of the lids; hemorrhage from the eyes; spasmodic closing of the lids; twitching of the eyes and lids; distortion of the eyes; pains in the ears; inflammatory swelling of the parotid glands; very sensitive smell, nose sore and ulcerated; frequent change of color, red face, one cheek red; erysipelas of the face, bloated, with hardness and throbbing of the cheek; convulsions of the face; twitchings of the lips; toothache after eating and drinking; after coffee and warm drinks; difficult dentition, producing spasms in children; toothache at night, with swelling of the cheeks; frothing at the mouth, as in spasms of teething children; convulsive movement of the tongue; tightness of the throat, with soreness, caused by a cold; little inclination to take food; bitter taste in the mouth; inclination to·vomit early in the morning, or with suffocating fits after drinking coffee; bilious vomiting; heartburn; colic, pain at the pit of the stomach, as if from a stone, after a meal; cutting pains and colic, above the navel; spasms of the bowels; rupture in either groin; watery, greenish diarrhœa, or like the yolks of eggs; undigested stools; excoriations around the arms in children; hot and burning and excoriating in children; yellow urine, with floculent sediment; profuse discharge of blood from the womb; thirst during the cold and hot

stage, and during the sweating stage; fevers commencing
with other ailments; bilious and typhoid fevers; fevers
that occur in the morning, with small feeble pulse; sweating during exercise and sleep; anguish; loss of courage;
excessively nervous, with low spirits, and intolerance of
noise, despising everything, and everything seems flat;
ideas and plans crowd upon the mind, with slow development of ideas when thinking; dulness of the head as of a
cold, and loss of sleep; whirling of the head when raising
it; headache from cold, and as if the head would split;
headache, with sleeplessness at night; rush of blood to
the head, with heat and fulness; the scalp and even the
hair are sensitive to contact; sore eyes and incipient
blindness; dread of light; humming and ringing in the
ears; frequent bleeding from the nose and mouth; nose
hot and red; pále or livid or dark yellow; sunken with
hollow eyes; dry parched lips, with a black streak; jerking, tearing toothache, when in contact with the open air;
distressing dull pain in hollow teeth; slimy, flat-watery
taste; spitting blood; yellow coated tongue; stinging sore
throat; everything in the form of food and drink has a
bitter taste; feeling as if satisfied and averse to taking
food and drink, much thirst, unable to decide upon dain-
ties, but craves them; fulness of the bowels after eating,
which causes oppression and drowsiness; sense of pressure after eating; belchings of a bitter taste; heartburn;
vomiting of blood; enlargement of the liver; pain in the
left side under the ribs; the bowels feel pressed and full
after a meal; dropsy and swelling of the bowels; flatulent
colic; fetid flatulence; scanty, slow and difficult stools;
watery yellow or mucus diarrhœa; undigested diarrhœa
stools, sometimes involuntary; disposition to urinate when
asleep; sexual desires excited with lascivious ideas; pro-

fuse menstruation; inflammation of the ovaria; painful hardness of the neck of the womb; leucorrhœa, watery or bloody; hoarseness, husky voice, deep when singing; suffocating cough at night, with pains in the chest; expectoration streaked with blood; bleeding from the lungs; matter formed in the lungs; suffocation from mucus in the air tubes; wheezing when breathing; pressure at the the chest; stitches at the chest and sides; inflammation of the lungs, with typhoid symptoms; violent rush of blood to the chest and palpitation of the heart; dull pains in the small of the back at night: great weakness of the arms, hands and fingers, with jerking of the muscles and bones: weakness and unsteadiness in the hip, knee and ankle-joint: swelling of the joints, and painful to the touch; red, hard swelling of the feet.

9.—Cina.

RANGE OF USE.—Pains in the extremities of a drawing, laming, cramping character; convulsions and worm affections; sleepless at night and tossing about; frequent shuddering, even near a warm stove; intermittent fever, with vomiting of food and canine hunger; disposition to cry and be restless, cannot bear to be touched; delirium during fever; pressure upon the head, and headache from reading; dimness of sight when reading, passes off by rubbing the eyes; crampy twitching in the outer ear; disposition to bore in the nose; fluent discharge; sickly and pale appearance around the eyes, bloated, bluish; toothache caused by air and cold drinks; inability to swallow; canine hunger, bitter taste, voracious; vomiting of worms and pinching pain in the stomach; soft stools, but not watery; wetting the bed; courses too early and excessive; dry spasmodic cough, with anxiety; stitching and boring in the chest; oppressed respiration; pain as if bruised in the small of the back; crampy tearing in the arms and hands; spasmodic stretching or tearing of the lower limbs.

10.—Coffea Cruda.

RANGE OF USE.—Excessive irritability of the body and mind, especially of lying-in women; ailments and pains after taking cold; aversion to the open air; convulsions; affections arising from excessive emotions; ill effects from intoxication; irritability of the skin of a nervous character; sleepless and wakeful; sleepless infants, with crying; chilliness, with feverish temperature of the body; whining mood, with cries, tossing about, anguish about the heart; pain in one side of the head; toothache, with restlessness; jerking in the teeth; heartburn and flatulent colic of infants; colic, with acute sensitiveness, driving one to despair; diarrhœa during teething; excessive labor-pains, and violent after-pains; short, hacking, dry cough; suffocating catarrh; trembling of the hands and feet; crampy affections in both the upper and lower extremities; tearing pains in the teeth and gums; tearing pains in the back part of the mouth; flow of watery saliva; the tongue feels heavy, stiff and insensible; inflammation of the tonsils and throat; mucus in the mouth and throat; fainting nausea from the smell of eggs and fat meat; vomiting of food; stomach sensitive to touch, and burning feeling in the stomach, and a feeling of coldness; pressing pains in the bowels from within outwards; dropsy of the abdomen; indolent stools; dysenteric diarrhœa; tearing in the anus; diminished secretion of dark urine, straining and burning; painful emission of a little hot urine, and burning in the urinary passages;

oppression of the chest, with difficult breathing; spasm of the chest; violent palpitation of the heart; pain in the small of the back when touching it, as if sore; tearing in the arms, hands and fingers; lame feeling in the arms; tingling in the fingers; tearing in the legs, feet and toes; hot swelling of the legs, and tingling in the toes.

11.—Colocynthis.

RANGE OF USE.—Painful crampy contraction of the bowels, with drawing up of the extremities; troublesome itching, with great restlessness; lowness of spirits, anguish and restlessness; pressing in the fore part of the head; aching of one half of the head, with nausea and vomiting; burning and cutting in the eyes; pain at the pit of the stomach; distension of the bowels; crampy pain and constriction in the bowels; violent colic after chagrin; dysenteric diarrhœa, with colic; diminished in quantity; impotence in the male; suppression of the discharges after childbirth, brought on by excitement; dry, hacking cough; acute and chronic pains in the hip and region of the kidneys, extending down the thighs; voluntary limping; stiffness of the knees, not allowing one to squat down.

12.—Drosera rotundifolia.

RANGE OF USE.—Emaciation, pains in the bones and joints gnawing and stinging, all the limbs feel bruised and outwardly painful; throat consumption; frequent starting during sleep; snoring when lying on the back; intermittent fever; constant chilliness when at rest; anxiety, especially when alone, with fever; dread of ghosts; pain in the forehead; sore scalp; bitter taste; thirst; aversion to fat food; vomiting of bile, or mucus, after a fit of coughing; rough scraping; feeling of dryness and inclination to cough; hoarseness; chronic inflammation of the larynx and windpipe, with much phlegm; cough and hoarseness after measles; night cough; hooping cough; spasmodic cough, with effort to vomit; tightness of the chest and contraction when talking; pain in the back as if lamed and bruised; the joints of the arms and wrist-joints feel as if lamed and bruised, and in the ankle-joints as if dislocated.

13.—Dulcamara.

RANGE OF USE.—Ailments arising from a cold; swelling and induration of the glands; dropsical swelling of the whole body, occurring rapidly after acute diseases; nettle-rash; suppurating humid tetters; dry scaby tetter; very drowsy in the daytime, wakes very early; dry heat and burning in the skin; mucus fever after a cold; internal uneasiness; impatience; delirium at night; gradual failing of the sight from weakness of the optic nerve; bleeding at the nose; milk-crust upon the face; profuse flow of saliva, preceded by dry tongue; paralysis of the tongue; thickness of the speech and swelling of the tongue; violent thirst for cold liquids, generally with dry tongue; colic from cold; vomiting tenacious mucus; diarrhœa after a cold, with colic; green slimy diarrhœa; scanty fetid urine, with slimy sediment; hooping-cough after a cold; mucus expectoration; humid cough; violent tightness of the chest; dropsy of the chest; dull stitches in the chest on both sides; violent pain in the loins above the hips during rest; lameness of the arm; herpetic eruption and warts on the hands; sweaty palms of the hands.

66*

14.—Helleborus Niger.

RANGE OF USE.—General dropsy after scarlatina; convulsive movements of the muscles; typhus fever, with
softening of the muscles; silent melancholy; excessive
anguish as if one would die; hypochondria; dullness and
a bruised pain in the head; dropsy of the head; painful
feeling of the scalp on the back part of the head; boring
of the head into the pillows; heaviness in the eyes pressing from above downwards; dread of light, mouth, &c.;
profuse flow of saliva; rigid and swollen tongue; nausea,
with great desire to eat and aversion to food; distension
of the stomach and bowels; distress at the pit of the
stomach; heavy breathing; dropsy of the chest; sense of
constriction of the chest; boring and stinging in the
wrists and hands; in the knees and joints of the feet.

15.—Hepar sulphuris calcis.

RANGE OF USE.—Ulceration of the glands; suppuration of inflamed parts; pains aggravated at night; scrofulous complaints; erysipelas of external parts; burning
and itching over the body; blotches; ulcers that bleed
readily; cracks in the skin; very drowsy early in the
morning and evening, with convulsive yawning; starting
at night as if for want of air; dry heat at night, or night
sweat; anguish in the evening; weak memory; vertigo;
stitches when stooping, and boring headache; blotches
on the head, sore to the touch; stinging in the eyes;
inflammation of the eyes and lids, also erysipelatious and
scrofulous inflammation; spasmodic closing of the lids;
dread of light; discharge of fetid pus; humming in the
ears; inflammation of the nose, sore to the touch, and
fetid discharge of mucus; bright red hot face; erysipelas

and swelling of the face, sore when touched; drawing, jerking toothache; feverish flow of saliva; hawking up mucus; sore throat as from a plug; stinging in the throat; bitter taste; dyspepsia; belching of wind; pressure at the stomach; distention in the pit of the stomach; inflammation of the kidneys; contractive pain in the bowels; stool hard and dry; sour, whitish diarrhœa in children; dysenteric stools; dark red, hot urine; nightly wetting the bed; bloody urine; soreness and dampness between the thighs and scrotum; discharge of a thin milky matter after a hard stool; soreness of the female parts; rush of blood to the womb; dry evening cough; paroxysms of dry hoarse cough, with anguish and retching; cancer of the heart; drawing in the back; ulceration of the auxiliary glands; pain in the arms above the elbows as if lamed and bruised; swelling of the finger joints; pain in the hips and thighs; swelling of the knees.

16.—Hyoscyamus niger.

RANGE OF USE.—Inflammation of internal organs, with typhoid symptoms; spasms also caused by worms, or in the case of women in childbed; epileptic fits; ill effects of unfortunate love, with jealousy; morbid sleep, as in contagious typhus fevers; inclined to laugh at every thing; jealous imbecility; mania lasciviousness; inflammation and stupor of the head; dropsy of the brain; the head shakes to and fro; eyes red, squinting; spasmodic closing of the lids; far-sighted; objects seem larger; bloated red face; lockjaw; throbbing toothache after a cold; pain in the gums; frothing at the mouth; red tongue, parched and dry; constriction of the throat, with inability to swallow liquids; canine hunger; aversion to drinks; vomiting of bloody mucus and dark red blood;

colicky spasms in the bowels; watery diarrhœa; involun
tary stools and discharge of urine; frequent urging to
urinate; hysteric spasms previous to the menses; sterility;
dry spasmodic cough, or catarrh upon the lungs; dry
cough at night, or cough without irritation; spasms of
the chest, and typhoid inflammation of the lungs; painful
spasms of the thighs and calves.

17.—Ignatia amara.

RANGE OF USE.—Bad effects of chagrin, grief or fright,
or unhappy love; ailments from abuse of coffee; hysteric
debility and fainting fits; itching which disappears by
scratching; nettle-rash; deep stupifying sleep; spasmodic
yawning; restless sleep; chilliness, heat all over except
the feet, no thirst either during heat or sweat; silent
grief; inclines to start; delicacy of feeling and conscience; alternate mirth and sad weeping mood; vertigo;
aching above the nose, lessened by bending the head
forwards; pressing in the head from within outwards;
headache as if from a nail in the brain; the head inclines
backwards; pressure in the eyes as from sand; scrofulous
sore eyes; convulsive movement of the eyes and lids;
dread of light; swelling of the parotid gland; sore nostrils; redness and burning heat of one cheek; alternate
redness and paleness; lips dry and chapped; convulsive
twitchings of the corners of the mouth; difficult dentition;
mouth and throat inflamed and red; sore-throat as from
a plug; stinging sore-throat and soreness of the throat,
only when swallowing; empty and weak feeling in the
pit of the stomach; fulness and distension of the bowels
at the sides, and spasms of the bowels; hard fæces, whitish
yellow; diarrhœa consisting of mucus blood; falling out
of the rectum; itching and creeping in the rectum; fre.

quent discharge of watery urine; spasms of the womb, brought on by grief, &c.; cough from constriction of the throat-pit; dry cough; asthmatic breathing; spasmodic constriction of the chest; convulsive twitchings of the arms and lower limbs.

18.—Ipecacuanha.

RANGE OF USE.—Attacks of illness, with loathing of food and great prostration; bleeding from various organs; ill effects of arsenic and quinine; lockjaw; convulsions; moaning in the sleep and frightful dreams; coldness, especially of the hands and feet; thirst only during the chilliness; intermittent fevers, and also after the abuse of peruvian bark; peevish and contemptuous and impatient; pain in one side of the head; nausea and vomiting; stitching headache, with heaviness of the head; pressure of the head; twitching of the eyelids; bleeding from the nose; pale face; convulsive twitchings of the muscles of the face; convulsive twitching of the lips; aversion to every kind of food; nausea; vomiting of thin bile or jelly-like mucus; vomiting, with diarrhœa; violent distress in the stomach and pit of the stomach; sensation as if a hand with fingers spread out were pressing on the abdomen, and the anterior joints were boring into the bowels, aggravated by motion; diarrhœa; fermented stools; bloody bilious, mucus diarrhœa; bleeding from the womb; miscarriage; stoppage of the nose, or inveterate acrid discharge; dry cough; racking spasmodic cough, with arrest of breathing; expectoration of blood with the cough; anxious hurried breathing; spasmodic tightness of the chest, with constriction of the throat, and panting, sobbing breathings; asthma and palpitation of the heart; convulsive twitchings of the legs and feet.

19.—Lycopodium.

RANGE OF USE.—Tearing of the limbs at night and during rest; stinging pains; numbness and insensibility of the limbs; dropsical swelling of single parts and organs; internal weakness; weakness of the limbs, especially during rest; itching when getting heated; dry skin; livid spots; humid tetter; boils; sore skin; frequent yawning; drowsy in the daytime; restless; weary on waking; flushes of heat; typhoid fever; night sweat, sometimes fetid and clammy; anxiety when people come too near; irritable, sensitive and obstinate; impeded activity of the mind; pain as if from a nail in the head; tearing headache; rush of blood to the head; eruptions on the head suppurating profusely with fetid smell; pressure in the eyes and smarting at candle-light; inflammation of the eyes and lids; agglutinations or sticking of the lids at night, with flow of tears in the daytime; discharge from the ears; excessive sensitiveness of the hearing; roaring in the ears; hardness of hearing; excessive sensitiveness of smell; pale face; sallow face, with deep wrinkles; circumscribed redness of the cheeks; frequent flushes of heat in the face and itching eruption; swelling of the glands on the under jaw; dull toothache; dry mouth; tetter of the mouth; dry throat; sores in the upper part of the throat and mouth; eating ulcers upon the tonsils; no appetite; food tastes sour, or canine hunger and fulness of the stomach and chest after eating; sour belchings; heartburn; paroxysms of violent hiccough; water-brash; pressure at the stomach after every meal; swelling at the pit of the stomach, with painfulness of contact; pinching in the abdomen and inguinal hernia; rumbling: chronic constipation: itching and tension of the anus; passing urine drop by drop, sometimes bloody; chronic dryness of the vagina; excessive or deficient sexual desire; hoarseness, with soreness of the chest when talking; nightly cough, affecting the head, stomach and diaphragm; titillating cough, excited by long breath, with salt, yellowish-grey expectoration; purulent expectoration; bloody cough; shortness of breath; oppression; constant pressure in the chest; stitches in the chest, especially the left; palpitation of the heart; drawing pains; swelling of the cervical and axiliary glands; drawing pain in the arms; the arms and fingers are liable to go to sleep; dry skin on the hands, and twitch-ing of the fingers; tearing in the thighs and knees during the night; stiffness of the knee; swelling of the knee; inveterate ulcers on the legs; swelling of the feet; corns, with stinging pain.

20.—Mercurius vivus.

RANGE OF USE.—Rheumatic arthritic drawing at night; shining red swelling of the joints; jaundice and bilious complaints; lymphatic affections; rickets; pains rendered intolerable by warmth in the bed; fall dysentery, &c.; itch-ing aggravated by the warmth of the bed; eating ulcers, bleeding freely; eruptions; malignant sores; uneasy superficial sleep, and anxiety at night; fever; chills; night fevers; mucus fever; inflammatory fevers, with disposition to perspire; profuse night-sweats; anguish; obstinate; impatient; full of disputation; vertigo, with nausea in the evening; headache as if the head would fly to pieces; tearing headache on one side, stinging down to the teeth and muscles of the neck; stitching in the hairy scalp and forehead, the hair falls off; pain under the lids as if from some cutting body; burning in the eyes; chronic sore·eyes; intolerance of the glare of fire; swollen eyes; scurfs around the eyes; incipient blindness; stitching pain in the ears; purulent discharge from the ears; hardness of hearing; rushing in the ears; red shining swelling of the nose, with itching; profuse excoriating watery discharge; pale complexion; livid cheeks; dingy yellow crust in the face; continued itching day and night, and bleeding after scratching; malignant milk-crust; cracks in the lips; ulcerated corners of the mouth; pimples on the chin; toothache, aggravated by cold or warm things, or at night in bed, becoming intolerable; swollen receding gums; tetter of the mouth; inflammatory swelling of the inner mouth; pimples in the mouth; little white blisters upon the tongue; fetid saliva flowing in profusion; sore-throat; burning in the throat as if a hot vapor were rising from the bowels; loss of voice; inflammation of the tonsils; ulcers in the throat; sweet taste in the mouth; violent burning thirst for cold drinks; canine hunger; aversion to food, especially to warm and solid food; very weak digestion; nausea; inclination to vomit, with sweetish taste in the mouth and throat; bitter bilious vomiting; pressure in the stomach, with sensation as if dragged down, also after the lightest kind of food; inflammation of the liver; dropsy of the abdomen; ineffectual urging, with tenesmus, especially at night; hard lumpy stool; sour smelling, green slimy or bloody stool; diarrhœa; dysenteric stools; discharge of bright red blood at stool; sudden urging to urinate; excessive disposition to make water, but can pass but a few drops at a time; involuntary emission of urine; dark red fetid urine, which soon becomes turbid; prolapsion of the rectum; rush of blood to the uterus; falling of the passage to the womb; purulent corrosive leucorrhœa; swelling of the veins of the penis; sores on the gland of the penis; white slime constantly collecting underneath the skin of the penis; hoarse husky voice; loss of voice; catarrh, with cough and sore-throat; bloody expectoration from the chest; ulceration of the lungs; spasms of the chest; palpitation of the heart; swelling and ulceration of the nipples; shingles; small blisters forming a belt and extending entirely around the whole abdomen; gouty, red, hot swelling of the fore-arm; itch-like eruption on the hands; tearing and stitching in the lower limbs, at night and during motion, with sensation of coldness in the affected parts; shining, transparent, dropsical swelling of the thighs and legs; painful swelling of the bones.

21.—Nux vomica.

RANGE OF USE.—Rheumatism and stiffness of the limbs; convulsions; bilious difficulties; jaundice; congestions; paralysis; sedentary habits, such as onanism, effects of inebriation from spirits, coffee, tobacco, and taking cold; nervous irritation; great prostration and heaviness; blue spots; boils; chilblains, with burning, itching, &c.; very drowsy in the daytime; inability to sleep on the account of ideas pressing upon the mind; anxious horrid dreams; chilliness, evening or night, after drinking or any emotion; chilliness, with heat in the head or redness of the cheeks; chilliness, with or without external coldness; blue skin and blue nails; the chill is attended with pain in the small of the back; fever, attended with yawning, stretching; gastric symptoms and headache; intermittent fever; hectic, puerperal or typhoid fevers; anguish and restlessness, and inclination to suicide; irresolute, excessive sensitiveness to

67

external impressions; tendency to start; irritable; very
lazy, with dread of work; cloudiness of the head, as if
from drunkenness; the head feels weary, as if from mental
labor; vertigo of various descriptions, the head turning
round as if intoxicated; headache increased by motion or
reflection; headache, with nausea; heaviness of the head;
pain in one side of the head, and sour vomiting; pressure
of the head from within outwards; rush of blood to the
head, with humming in the ears, worse in stormy weather;
burning and smarting in the eyes; sore eyes from scrofula,
or in gouty persons; spots on the pupils; bleeding from
the eyes; painful short stitches in the ears; ringing in the
ears; inflammation of the inner nose, with discharge of
fetid pus; bleeding of the nose early in the morning;
sickly, pale, sallow complexion; yellowish tint around
the nose and mouth; glowing redness of the face, with
heat; pain in the cheek-bones; painful peeling off of the
lips; lockjaw; toothache caused by a cold; dull aching
of the teeth; excited cold drink; stinging in decayed
teeth; loose teeth; putrid bleeding and swelling of the
gums; small blisters upon the tongue; sore mouth; sensation as if a plug were in the throat, especially between
swallowing; sour taste after eating or drinking; foul
taste; thirst; aversion to food; depressed after eating,
and drowsy; bitter, foul, sour eructations; frequent violent hiccough when eating; nausea and inclination to
vomit, especially early in the morning and after eating;
empty retching, especially in the case of drunkards;
periodical attacks of vomiting; vomiting and nausea of
pregnant females; vomiting of the contents of the stomach; bleeding from the stomach; distension and pressure in the stomach and at the pit, as if from a stone,
after eating; painful feeling as if from contraction at the

cardiac orifice; contractive griping, tearing heartburn; the clothes press upon the sides; beating in the region of the liver; acute inflammation of the liver; affections of the kidneys; distension of the bowels; spasmodic colic; hernia; strangulated hernia; wind colic; constipation of a chronic character; watery diarrhœa; dysenteric stools; frequent small mucus stools, with straining; piles; strangury, urging to urinate, ending in discharge of blood; inflammation and swelling of the testicles, with spasmodic constrictive strangulation; sexual desire easily excited; congestion of blood to the womb, and weight and heat; inflammation of the female organs; falling of the womb; too early menses; excessive labor pains; catarrhal hoarseness; constrictive spasm of the larynx; cough, which is excited or aggravated by excessive reading and thinking; cough, with titillation, most violent early in the morning; racking cough as if the head would split; continual cough, dry in the afternoon and at night, with expectoration; oppressed breathing; anxious oppression of the chest; spasmodic asthma of adults; palpitation of the heart; pains in the small of the back as if bruised; burning, tearing in the back; lameness of the arm; numbness and want of power to move the arms; pain in the hips; drawing and stinging in the lower limbs; unsteadiness of the lower limbs, and giving away of the knees and trembling weakness; cramp in the calves at night.

22.—Opium.

RANGE OF USE.—General torpor of the nerves; diseases of drunkards; affections incident to old age; convulsions and spasms, also epileptic fits; spasms of lockjaw; ill effects of fright; dropsical swellings of the whole body; bluish skin, with blue spots; constant itching of

the skin; stupor; sleep with half consciousness; sleeplessness; disturbed sleep, with lascivious dreams; the skin
feels cold; burning heat of the body, with redness of the
face, pulse generally slow, full, intermittent or quick and
hard; typhus, with delirium; absence of all care; bold-
ness during courage; tendency to start; fearfulness; loss
of consciousness; illusions of fancy; delirium; delirium
tremens; delirious talk, rage, imbecility, as if idiotic,
after scarlatina; dulness of the head, as after intoxication; stupifaction, as if intoxicated; rush of blood to the
head; heaviness of the head; congestion, with violent
throbbing; red inflamed eyes; half opened, distorted,
staring eyes, dilated pupils, obscuration of sight; pale
and sallow countenance; dark red, hot, burning face;
the muscles of the face hang down relaxed; convulsive
motion of the muscles of the face; twitchings at the
corners of the mouth; lockjaw; profuse flow of saliva;
paralysis of the tongue, inability to swallow; violent
thirst; seasons of intense hunger, with no inclination to.
eat; vomiting, with violent pains at the stomach and
convulsions; vomiting of fæces and urine; heaviness in
the stomach; the stomach distended like a drum head;
colic, strangulated rupture; constipation chronic with
children; black fetid stools; retention of urine, as if the
bladder were closed; increased sexual desire, with erections and emissions; suppressed labor pains; chest and
respiration; heaviness; cough when swallowing or drawing a breath; cough, with frothy expectoration; interruption of the breast, with great anguish; paroxysms of suffocation and construction of the chest; convulsive motion
of the arms and trembling of the hands; convulsive
motion of the lower limbs.

23.—Phosphorus.

RANGE OF USE.—Trembling of the limbs; rushes of blood; congestions; bleeding from different organs; heaviness of the limbs; lazy feeling; intolerance of the open air, especially when cool; pains settling in when the weather changes; boils; profuse bleeding of small scratches or cuts; chilblains; corns; sleepless the fore-part of the night; falls asleep late; uneasiness and anxiety on waking; unrefreshing sleep; anxious, heavy and fret-ful dreams, somnambula-like; anxious or flying heat; heat at night; night and morning sweat; anxious and uneasy when alone, or during a thunder storm; melan-choly; out of temper; dread of labor; dizzy; vertigo, with nausea; morning headache; stupifying headache, with pressure from within outwards; rush of blood to the head; shooting pains on one side of the temples; the hair falls out; burning in the corners of the eyes next to the nose; sore eyes; nightly sticking together of the lids; see better by night than by day; black spots before the eyes; beating, throbbing and stitching in the ears; hard of hearing; the nose is red and swollen; bad smell; bleeding from the nose, or blood blown from the nose; sunken pale face; blue streaks around the eyes; bloated face; sores at the corners of the mouth; pains in the face bones; stitching toothache in the open air, or in the evening or at night; ulceration, swelling or bleeding of the gums; soreness of the inner mouth and spitting of blood; dry throat, with burning and hawking of mucus in the morning; sour taste after eating; want of appetite; empty belching from the stomach; sour risings of food after being taken into the stomach; vomiting, with pains in the stomach; fulness of the stomach and pressure;

67*

burning in the stomach and pit of the stomach; inflammation of the stomach; distension after dinner; tearing in the abdomen; alternate sensation of heat and cold in the bowels; wind colic, attended with mucus diarrhœa; chronic looseness of the bowels; bloody diarrhœa; bleeding cracks of the arms; increase of watery urine; bloody urine; burning in the urethra; tearing and stitching from the passage to the womb and the womb itself; sterility; menses·too early and too profuse; constant desire for embrace; hoarse rough cough; loss of voice; croup; cough, with stinging in the throat; dry racking cough, or with saltish purulent expectoration, or with bloody mucus; chronic bronchitis, or mucus consumption; heaviness, fulness and tightness of the chest; inflammation of the lungs; abscesses on the breasts; pains in the small of the back and back as if broken; burning of the arms and hands; trembling of the arms and hands; chilblains; drawing and tearing in the knee; swelling of the feet; pain in the soles of the feet; chilblains.

24.—Pulsatilla.

RANGE OF USE.—Rheumatic pains in damp weather that shift about; ill effects of suppressed measles; diseases of the mucus membrane; itching of the skin; chicken pox; rash from eating bacon; feverish, heavy sleep; sleepless at night; frightful dreams; chilliness, without thirst; paroxysms of anxious heat; dread of company; diffidence; low spirits; loss of consciousness; severe effects of mental labor; vertigo from intoxication; vertigo, with inclination to vomit; pain in one side of the head; rush of blood to the head; painful inflammation of the glands of the lids; dryness of the lids; inflammation of the outer ear; purulent discharge from the ears;

ulcerated humid discharge from the nose; bleeding at the nose; complexion pale or yellowish; drawing, jerking toothache; stitches in the gums; toothach abates in the open air; flow of saliva; tongue coated yellow, and covered with tough mucus; stinging sore throat, and tough mucus in the throat; taste flat, bitter or putrid; hunger, with no choice of food; belchings and vomiting of food after being received into the stomach, especially in the evening and at night; spasms of the bowels; violent colic; painful rumbling; bilious diarrhœa; frequent urging to stool; watery discharges from the bowels at night; stoppage of the urine; frequent urging to urinate; ineffectual effort to urinate; wetting the bed; inflammation of the testicles; dropsy of the testicles; suppression of the menses; delay of the menses in young girls; false spasmodic labor pains; dry cough with gagging and vomiting; stoppage of breath; paroxysms of suffocation at night; palpitation of the heart; typhoid inflammation of the lungs; vanishing of the milk; pain in the small of the back and parts; spinal difficulties; pains in the shoulders, arms and joints; inflammatory swelling of the knee; weariness of the legs; swelling of the feet.

25.—Rhus Toxicodendron.

RANGE OF USE.—Rheumatic and gouty affections; paralysis; red shining swellings; burning pain as if the flesh had been detached from the bones by blows; inflammatory typhoid diseases; erysipelas; shingles; burning itching; nettle-rash; frequent spasmodic yawning; sleepless before midnight; digging, pinching colic and vomiting; chilliness and coldness; shaking chill in the open air, with violent thirst; double tertian fever;

pains in the limbs during chilliness; headache; typhus and typhoid fevers; night and morning sweats; sadness and anxiety; delirium; swimming of the head; fulness and heaviness of the head; stinging headache day and night; swelling of the head; dry tetter on the hairy scalp; violent itching at night; inflammation of the eyes and lids with redness and sticking together at night; swelling of the whole eye and the surrounding parts; inflammatory swelling of the parotid glands; inflammation and bleeding of the nose; erysipelas and swelling of the face; dry mouth and thirst; inclination to vomit; pressure in the stomach; watery diarrhœa; bearing down and straining when at stool; inability to urinate, though frequent urgings; swelling of the penis; morning cough after waking; cough caused by tickling in the air-passages, generally short and dry; anxious oppresssion of the chest; tremulous feeling about the heart; burning pain in the small of the back; rheumatic stiffness of the nape of the neck; burning and lameness in the shoulder and arm; coldness and immobility of the arm; cracks on the back of the hand; heaviness of the lower limbs, and spraining pain in the ankles; swelling of the feet.

26.—Sepia Succus.

RANGE OF USE.—Bad effects of chagrin; stiffness of the joints; hysteric spasms and other ailments; affections of pregnant females, restlessness in all the limbs; throbbing and rush of blood at night; want of strength when waking; sensitive to cold air and liable to take cold; sticking and soreness in the joints; boils; painful ulcers; sleepiness in the day time; frequent waking without any apparent cause; restless sleep with rush of blood; deficient animal heat; chilliness; flushes of heat; intermit.

tent fevers with thirst during the chill; profuse sweat during the least exercise; night sweat; morning sweat also with sour smell; sad, depressed in spirits; anxious, with flushes of heat in the evening, and for one's health indifference; weak memory; dulness of the head; vertigo; pain in one side of the head; morning head-ache; weight in the head; sick headache; rush of blood to the head; itching of the scalp; paralysis of the eyes; pressure in the eyeballs; sore eyes with stinging; inflammation, redness and swelling of the lids; profuse tears nightly; sticking of the lids (or agglutination); far sighted; stitching and roaring in the ears; swelling of the nose; ulcerated nostrils; bleeding at the nose; pale face; yellow saddle across the cheeks and nose; milk crust; drawing pains in the face; yellowness or tetter around the mouth; toothache of pregnant females; fetor from the mouth; sore throat and sensation as if a plug were in the throat; hawking up phlegm; putrid taste; voracious appetite, or else loathing of food; distention of the bowels; sour belchings; nausea before breakfast; vomiting of food and bile; pressure as if from a stone; heartburn; pains in the region of the liver, and in both sides under the ribs; colic of pregnant females; abdominal spasms; pressure and weight in the lower bowels; ineffectual urging of discharge of mere wind and mucus; chronic constipation, or else soft stool or weakening diarrhœa; prolapsion of the anus; frequent urging, but unable to urinate; pressure in the bladder; smarting in the urinary passage; gleet; frequent nocturnal emissions; soreness of the female parts between the thighs; falling of the womb; suppressed menses, or disposition to miscarry; hoarseness with catarrh; dry cough as if from the stomach; pulmonary consumption;

oppression of the chest, owing either to frequent or stagnant perspiration; stitches in the chest and at the sides when coughing or drawing a breath; rushes of blood to the chest and palpitation of the heart; soreness of the nipples; burning tearing pains in the small of the back; stiffness of the neck; pain in the arms and wrists; stiffness of the elbow joints; itching scurfs at the elbow and on the hands; gouty pains in the finger joints; cold legs and feet; jerking stitches in the thighs; boils in the bends of the knees; burning of the feet; ulcers on the heels.

27.—Silicea.

RANGE OF USE.—Epilepsy; worm affections of scrofulous persons; pains worse at the full of the moon; restlessness of the whole body after sitting; nervous debility; sensitiveness of the skin; itching of the whole body; fetid ulcers; stinging sores; sleeplessness and heat in the head; anxious dreams; starting of the body when asleep as if from fright; chilliness; intermittent fever with violent heat; worm fever in scrofulous children; profuse night sweats and with sour smell; anxious, restless, and want of cheerfulness; gloominess of the head, and wearied by mental labor; vertigo; headache ascending from the nape of the neck to the vertex; heaviness of the head and pressure as if the head would fly to pieces; throbbing headache with rush of blood; enlarged head with open fontanelles; itching humid scald-head; swelling of the tear passages; fungus cancer of the eyes; paralysis of the optic nerve, and blindness; black spots before the eyes and dread of light; discharge from the ears and stoppage when blowing and opening again with a report; gnawing pains high up in the nose; ulcers of the nose; scurfy eruptions on the face and chin; swelling of the glands of the under jaw; dry mouth; coated tongue of a brown color; loss of taste; bitter mouth in the morning; large quantity of phlegm in the throat with soreness; violent thirst; aversion of food; loathing of meat; acidity in the mouth after eating; pressure at the stomach, water-brash and vomiting; nausea and vomiting; the pit of the stomach is painful to the touch; griping at the pit of the stomach; distended bowels; colic with constipation or with diarrhœa; constipation and hard stool; itching at the anus; pressing and straining from the bladder; dropsy of the testicles; itching humid spots on the scrotum; chronic suppression of the menses; itching of the female parts; miscarriage; leucorrhœa; acrid excoriating leucorrhœa; stoppage of the nose, or fluent discharge of hot liquid secretion from the nose; cough with purulent expectoration; pulmonary consumption; stoppage of breath when lying on the back; shortness of breath during slight labor; oppression of the chest; pain in the small of the back; curvature of the spine; heaviness of the arms and legs; felons upon the fingers; whitlow upon the fingers and toes; coldness and swelling of the feet.

28.—Spongia tosta.

RANGE OF USE.—In diseases of the windpipe; pain in the larynx when touching it or when turning the neck; membraneous croup; hollow barking cough; throat consumption; cough day and night; wheezing respiration; burning in the chest from below upwards; rush of blood to the chest; painful tension and stiffness of the muscles of the neck; goitre or swelling of the neck.

29.—Sulphur.

RANGE OF USE.—Gouty swelling of all the joints; inflammation, swelling and suppuration, and hardness of the glands; decayed bones or teeth; hysteria and hypochondria; paralysis; fainting fits; pains felt at night, or worse when standing; emaciation of children; pains when the weather changes; dread of being washed; itching of the skin; eruptions after cow-pox; itch; nettle-rash; liver-colored spots; tetter; chilblains; corns; irresistible drowsiness; one sleeps too long; unrefreshing sleep; jerking and starting of the extremities during sleep; chilliness very much increased at night; profuse sweat in the day-time during work; melancholy; tendency to start; irritable; weak memory; philosophical and weak fancies; vertigo, especially when sitting or early in the morning with nose-bleed; headache with nausea; nightly headache; feeling of fulness and weight in the head; drawing and tearing in the head; stitching headache; throbbing headache, with heat in the head, caused by rush of blood to the head; coldness of the scalp; scald-head; pain in the eyes as if from sand; pressure in the eyelids; itching, smarting or burning in the eyes, lids and corners (canthi); inflammation of the eyes and lids; ulceration of the lids; dryness of the eyes, or else profuse tears; twitching of the lids; gauze before the eyes; incipient blindness; dread of light; short-sighted; purulent discharge from the ears; dull hearing, roaring and humming in the ears; inflamed and swollen nose; bleeding of the nose, especially on blowing of the nose; pale, sickly complexion; heat of the face; erysipelas in the face; chronic eruption of the face; crusta lactea; swelling of the lips; cancer of the lips; swelling of the glands of the under jaw; toothache; stitches, tearing, drawing, burning and boring in the teeth; toothache in the evening and at night; swelling of the gums with throbbing pain; salivation from the use of mercury; bad smell from the mouth after eating; blisters in the mouth; white coated tongue; sore throat as from a plug; painful feeling of contraction; dryness of the throat; sweetish foul taste or sour taste in the mouth; too much appetite; canine hunger; aversion to meat, sweet and sour things; oppression across the chest after eating; empty belch- ings; sour risings of the food after eating; nausea; water-brash; vomiting of partly digested food from the stomach; pressure at the stomach; contractive heart- burn immediately after eating; stinging in the region of the liver; colic immediately after eating or drinking; weight in the abdomen as from a lump; violent pressure in the abdomen; stitching colic when walking; dropsy of the abdomen; wind lodged in the stomach or intes- tines; loud rumbling; constipation; frequent urging and hard lumpy insufficient stool; itching, stinging and burning in the anus and rectum; frequent urging to urinate; wetting the bed; bleeding from the urinary passage with stinging and burning soreness between the thighs; discharge of purulent matter from the urinary passage; matter around the head of the penis; swelling of the prepuce ; suppressed menses, or else too soon, preceded by headache; sterility; miscarriage; excoria- ting leucorrhœa; dryness of the nose; discharge of burning water; hoarseness and roughness in the throat; tingling in the larynx, exciting a cough; suffocating catarrh of children; cough with strangling and vomiting; dry cough, or with bloody expectoration; frequent stop- page of breath; oppression and suffocation at night;

68

weakness of the chest; palpitation of the heart, which is frequently visible and attended with anxiety; cracks in the nipples; stitches in the back and small of the back; stiffness of the neck; rickety curvatures of the spine; fetid sweats under the arms; swelling and suppuration of the glands in the arm-pits; drawing, tearing and stitching in the shoulders, arms, hands and fingers; swelling of the arms; trembling of the hands; cracked skin on the hands; deadness of the fingers; heaviness of the lower limbs; large shining swelling of the knee; cramp in the calves and soles; cold feet; cold and sweaty feet; ulcers on the back of the foot; shining swelling of the toes.

30.—Tartarus emeticus.

RANGE OF USE.—Gastric or bilious affections; prostration; languor; fainting spells; pustules resembling small-pox; very drowsy; irresistible somnolence with deep stupid sleep; light sleep with fantastic dreams; jerks and shocks during sleep; chilliness and coldness prevail; violent heat of the whole body; intermittent fever and cold sweats; oppressive constrictive headache as if the brain were formed into a ball; chronic trembling of the head; pressure on the eyes; incipient stage of blindness; dimness of sight with flickering before the eyes; the face pale and sunken; good appetite; great desire for acids and fresh fruits; loathing of food, or inappetency, especially for milk; empty rising and tasting of bad eggs; nausea also, continually, with inclination to vomit; violent vomiting, attended with great straining; vomiting of mucus; stomachache as if the stomach were overloaded; pressure in the stomach and pit of the stomach; colic with great bodily and mental nneasiness; fulness and pressure in the abdomen as from stones, especially when sitting bent; colic as if the bowels would be cut to pieces; thinnish stools; mucus diarrhœa; bloody stools; violent and painful urging to urinate; scanty emission of urine; inflamed and red urine, or of a dark brown color; profuse discharge of acrid matter from the nose; a quantity of rattling mucus in the chest; paroxysms of cough with suffocation; arrest of breathing; cough with vomiting of food; rattling hollow cough, and with expectoration of mucus; paralysis of the lungs; rattling, breating palpitation of the heart; pain in the back and small of the back when sitting; trembling of the hands; cramps in the legs.

31.—Veratrum album.

RANGE OF USE.—Pain in the limbs which do not bear the warmth of the bed, which cease on rising and walking about; trembling of the limbs; convulsive movements; sporadic and Asiatic cholera; general prostration; excessive debility; fainting turns; general emaciation; dry itch-like eruptions upon the skin, or coma vigil nightly; sleeplessness with great anguish; coldness all over, with cold clammy sweat; intermittent fevers with coldness only on the outside; chilliness with thirst, followed by heat and constant thirst; slow pulse, small and scarcely perceptible; excessive anguish and oppression, with forebodings and anxiety of conscience; tendency to start with fearful mood, moving about to and fro as if very busy; very much out of humor or disposed to be silent; deficiency of ideas; mental alienation; delirium; vertigo; pain in one side of the head with nausea and vomiting; oppressive headache in the top of the head; sensitivness of the hairs; cold sweat on the forehead; painful sore eyes; the lids very dry; profuse flow of tears; paralysis of the lids; contracted pupils, or else dilated; sight of one eye obscured; deafness, as if the ears were stopped; face pale, cold, sunken, with pointed nose; burning heat and sweat of the face; lips dry, blackish and cracked; locking of the jaws; grating of the teeth; profuse flow of saliva; froth at the mouth; cold feeling or burning in the mouth and on the tongue; red, swollen or dry blackish cracked tongue; speechless; burning in the tonsils and gullet; putrid taste in the mouth, also cooling and smarting taste as if from peppermint; great thirst for cold drinks; canine hunger and voracious appetite; constant and intense desire for sour or cooling things; vomiting and diarrhœa; violent empty belchings, sometimes sour or bitter; violent nausea with desire to vomit; violent vomiting with constant nausea; prostration; vomiting of the ingesta or food from the stomach; vomiting of black bile and blood; constant vomiting with diarrhœa; pressure in the pit of the stomach; and burning colic in the region of the navel; soreness of the bowels to the touch; colicky abdominal spasms; cutting in the abdomen; inguinal hernia; flatulent colic; constipation caused by torpor of the rectum; violent diarrhœa; also painful unperceived discharge of thin stool during the emission of flatulence; excessive languor during stool; involuntary emission of urine, and burning during the time; menses too soon and too profuse, or else suppressed; cough in the evening; hot dry cough; deep hollow cough; paroxysms of hooping cough; stoppage of breath; oppression; a good deal of oppression on the chest; painful spasmodic constriction of the chest; paroxysms of excessive anguish about the heart; laming weakness of the muscles of the back of the neck; laming and bruising pains of the lower limbs; cramps in the calves; stitching in the big toes.

INDEX.

A.

68*   (797)

E.

O.

P.

810 INDEX.

R.

S.

W.

Y.

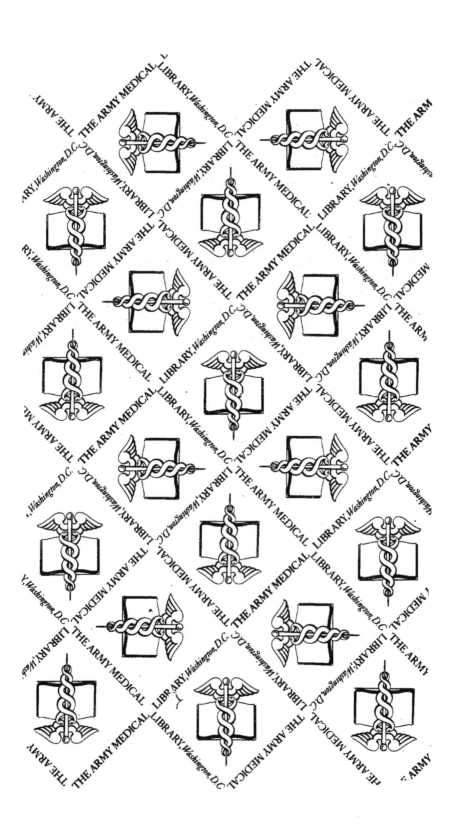

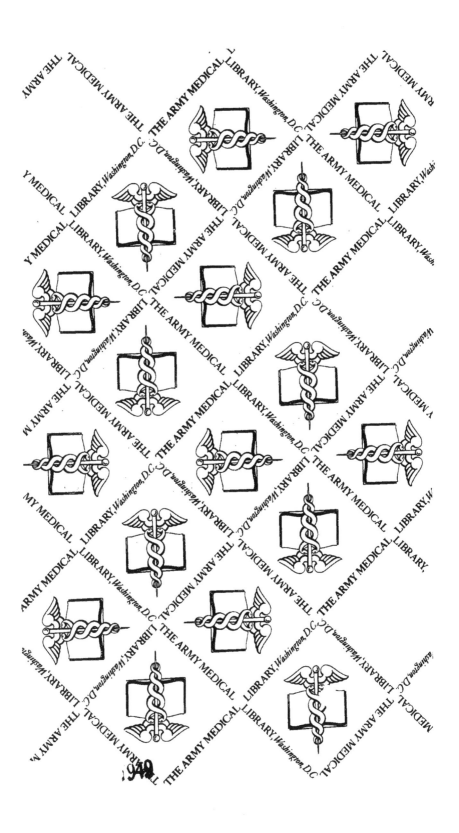